DEDICATION

To the contributors to this and future editions, who took time
to share their knowledge, insight, and humor for the benefit of students.

and

To our families, friends, and loved ones, who supported us
in the task of assembling this guide.

Contents

CONTRIBUTING AUTHORS

Keli L. Beck
Wake Forest School of Medicine
Class of 2011

Shalini Bumb
Wake Forest School of Medicine
Class of 2011

Po-Hao "Howard" Chen
Harvard Medical School
Class of 2012

Michael S. Clemens
Wake Forest School of Medicine
Class of 2012

Michael Coulter
Harvard Medical School
Class of 2014

Annie Dude
Pritzker School of Medicine
University of Chicago
Class of 2011

Daniel J. Durand, MD
Instructor and Fellow
Radiology and Radiological Sciences
Johns Hopkins University School of Medicine

Shantanu K. Gaur
Harvard Medical School
Class of 2012

Thomas Hickey
Harvard Medical School
Class of 2011

Katie Lee Hwang, MSc
Harvard/MIT MD-PhD Program
Harvard Medical School

Vamsi K. Kancherla
Perelman School of Medicine
University of Pennsylvania
Class of 2011

Robert M. Koffie, PhD
Harvard Medical School
Class of 2013

Wendy W. Liu
Harvard/MIT MD-PhD Program
Harvard Medical School

Justin H. Lo
Harvard/MIT MD-PhD Program
Harvard Medical School

Behrouz Namdari, MD
Duke Psychiatry Residency
Class of 2014

Jason B. O'Neal
Wake Forest School of Medicine
Class of 2011

Jason M. Paluzzi
Wake Forest School of Medicine
Class of 2012

Derek T. Peters
Harvard/MIT MD-PhD Program
Harvard Medical School

Matthew J. Sagransky
Wake Forest School of Medicine
Class of 2012

Walter F. Wiggins
MD-PhD Program
Wake Forest School of Medicine

FACULTY REVIEWERS

Mebea Aklilu, MD
Assistant Professor
Hematology and Oncology
Comprehensive Cancer Center
Wake Forest Baptist Health Center

Robert L. Barbieri, MD
Chairman, Obstetrics and Gynecology and Reproductive
  Biology
Kate Macy Ladd Professor of Obstetrics, Gynecology and
  Reproductive Biology
Department of Obstetrics and Gynecology and Reproductive
  Biology
Brigham and Women's Hospital
Harvard Medical School

Bryann Bromley, MD
Associate Clinical Professor of Obstetrics, Gynecology and
  Reproductive Biology
Department of Obstetrics, Gynecology, and Reproductive Biology
Massachusetts General Hospital
Harvard Medical School

David Lopes Cardozo, PhD
Assistant Professor, Neurobiology
Department of Neurobiology
Associate Dean for Graduate Studies
Department of Basic Sciences and Graduate Studies
Course Director, Human Nervous System and Behavior
Harvard Medical School

Kenneth Christopher, MD
Instructor in Medicine
Department of Medicine
Brigham and Women's Hospital
Harvard Medical School

Michael S. Glock, MD
Associate Professor, Pediatrics
Wake Forest Baptist Medical Center
Wake Forest School of Medicine

John R. Hoyle, MD
Associate Professor
Department of Cardiology
Wake Forest Baptist Medical Center
Wake Forest School of Medicine

Kaarkuzhali Babu Krishnamurthy, MD
Director, Human Subjects Protection Office
Director, Women's Health in Epilepsy
Assistant Professor of Neurology
Department of Neurology
Beth Israel Deaconess Medical Center
Harvard Medical School

Stephen H. Loring, MD
Associate Professor of Anesthesia
Department of Anesthesia, Critical Care and Pain Medicine
Beth Israel Deaconess Medical Center
Harvard Medical School

Shannon A. Novosad, MD
Hospitalist
Duke Hospital Medicine Program
Medical Instructor
Duke University School of Medicine

Kenneth S. O'Rourke, MD
Associate Professor, Rheumatology and Immunology
Wake Forest Baptist Medical Center
Wake Forest Medical School

Steve Sazinsky, PhD
Postdoctoral Fellow
Boston University

Adam Schaffer, MD
Instructor in Medicine
Department of Medicine
Brigham and Women's Hospital
Harvard Medical School

Steven Schlozman, MD
Assistant Professor of Psychiatry
Department of Psychiatry
Co-Director of Medical Student Education in Psychiatry
Associate Director of Training, Child and Adolescent Psychiatry
Massachusetts General Hospital
Harvard Medical School

Vivek Unni, MD, PhD
Instructor in Neurology
Department of Neurology
Massachusetts General Hospital
Harvard Medical School

Preface

With this second edition of *First Aid for the Basic Sciences: Organ Systems,* we continue our commitment to providing students with the most useful and up-to-date preparation guides for the USMLE Step 1. For the past year, a team of authors and editors have worked to update and further improve this second edition. This edition represents a major revision in many ways, including the following:

- Every page has been carefully reviewed and updated
- New high-yield figures, images, tables, and mnemonics have been added
- Hundreds of user comments and suggestions have been incorporated
- Increased emphasis on integration and linkage of concepts

These books would not have been possible without the help of the hundreds of students and faculty members who contributed their feedback and suggestions. We invite students and faculty to please share their thoughts and ideas to help us improve *First Aid for the Basic Sciences: Organ Systems.* (See How to Contribute, p. xv.)

Tao Le
Louisville

Kendall Krause
Denver

How to Use This Book

Both this text and its companion, *First Aid for the Basic Sciences: General Principles*, are designed to fill the need for a high-quality, in-depth, conceptually-driven study guide for the USMLE Step 1. They can be used either alone, or in conjunction with the original *First Aid for the USMLE Step 1*, *First Aid Cases for the USMLE Step 1*, or *First Aid Q&A for the USMLE Step 1*. In this way, students can tailor their own studying experience, calling on either series, according to their mastery of each subject.

Medical students who have used the previous edition of this guide have given us feedback on how best to make use of the book.

- **It is recommended that you begin using this book as early as possible** when learning the basic medical sciences.
- As you study each discipline, **use the corresponding section in *First Aid for the Basic Sciences: Organ Systems*** to consolidate the material, deepen your understanding, or clarify concepts.
- As you approach the test, use *First Aid for the Basic Sciences: Organ Systems* and *First Aid for the Basic Sciences: General Principles* to review challenging concepts.
- Use the margin elements (ie, Flash Forward, Flash Back, Key Fact, Clinical Correlation, Mnemonic) to test yourself throughout your studies.

To **broaden** your learning strategy, you can **integrate** your *First Aid for the Basic Sciences: Organ Systems* study with *First Aid for the USMLE Step 1*, *First Aid Cases for the USMLE Step 1*, and *First Aid Q&A for the USMLE Step 1* on a chapter-by-chapter basis.

Acknowledgments

This has been a collaborative project from the start. We gratefully acknowledge the thoughtful comments and advice of the residents, international medical graduates, and faculty who have supported the editors and authors in the development of *First Aid for the Basic Sciences: Organ Systems.*

We wish to extend sincere and heartfelt thanks to our managing editor, Isabel Nogueira, who, once again, was truly the backbone of this project. Without her enthusiasm and commitment, the extensive update of this project would not have been possible. For support and encouragement throughout the process, we are grateful to Thao Pham and Louise Petersen.

Furthermore, we wish to give credit to our amazing editors and authors, who worked tirelessly on the manuscript. We never cease to be astounded by their dedication, thoughtfulness, and creativity.

Thanks to Catherine Johnson and our publisher, McGraw-Hill, for their assistance and guidance. For outstanding editorial work, we thank Linda Davoli. A special thanks to Rainbow Graphics for remarkable production work.

We also thank the faculty at Uniformed Services University of the Health Sciences (USUHS) for use of their images.

Tao Le
Louisville

Kendall Krause
Denver

How to Contribute

To continue to produce a high-yield review source for the USMLE Step 1, you are invited to submit any suggestions or corrections. We also offer paid internships in medical education and publishing ranging from three months to one year (see below for details). Please send us your suggestions for:

- New facts, mnemonics, diagrams, and illustrations
- High-yield topics that may reappear on future Step 1 examinations
- Corrections and other suggestions

For each entry incorporated into the next edition, you will receive a $10 gift certificate, as well as personal acknowledgment in the next edition. Diagrams, tables, partial entries, updates, corrections, and study hints are also appreciated, and significant contributions will be compensated at the discretion of the authors. Also let us know about material in this edition that you feel is low yield and should be deleted.

The preferred way to submit entries, suggestions, or corrections is via our blog:

www.firstaidteam.com.

Otherwise, please send entries, neatly written or typed, or on disk (Microsoft Word), to:

**First Aid Team
914 N. Dixie Avenue, Suite 100
Elizabethtown, KY 42701
Attention: First Aid General Principles**

NOTE TO CONTRIBUTORS

All entries become property of the authors and are subject to editing and reviewing. Please verify all data and spellings carefully. In the event that similar or duplicate entries are received, only the first entry received will be used. Include a reference to a standard textbook to facilitate verification of the fact. Please follow the style, punctuation, and format of this edition, if possible.

AUTHOR OPPORTUNITIES

The author team is pleased to offer opportunities in medical education and publishing to motivated medical students and physicians. Projects may range from three months (eg, a summer) up to a full year. Participants will have an opportunity to author, edit, and earn academic credit on a wide variety of projects, including the popular *First Aid* series. English writing/editing experience, familiarity with Microsoft Word, and Internet access are required. Go to our blog **www.firstaidteam.com** to apply for an internship. A sample of your work or a proposal of a specific project is helpful.

Alistair Mackenzie Library
Wishaw General Hospital
50 Netherton Street
Wishaw
ML2 0DP

Cardiovascular

Embryology

DEVELOPMENT OF THE HEART

Embryonic Heart Structures and Adult Derivatives

The primitive heart tube is formed by the lateral folding and fusion of the endocardial heart tubes. It forms dilatations that eventually become the structures of the adult heart (Table 1-1).

Formation of Septa

ATRIAL SEPTUM

The atrial septum is responsible for the initial division of the primitive atrium into the left and right atria. The steps of development are as follows (Figure 1-1):

1. The **septum primum** begins to grow toward the atrioventricular (AV) cushions. The space between the leading edge of the septum primum and the AV cushions is termed the **ostium primum.** The ostium primum is obliterated when the septum primum reaches the AV septum.
2. The **ostium secundum** is formed as tissue degenerates in the superior septum primum.
3. The **septum secundum** forms alongside the right edge of the septum primum.
4. The septum secundum contains the **foramen ovale,** which allows blood to be shunted from the right atrium (RA) to the left atrium (LA) during fetal life. After birth, the increase in pressure in the LA closes the foramen ovale.

An **atrial septal defect (ASD)** is an opening in the atrial septum, allowing blood to flow between the atria (Figure 1-2). The most common form is the **ostium secundum** type due to excessive resorption of the septum primum or inadequate formation of the septum secundum. Patients are typically asymptomatic until adulthood, but the clinical course depends on the size of the defect.

TABLE 1-1. Embryonic Heart Structures and Adult Derivatives

EMBRYONIC STRUCTURE	ADULT STRUCTURE
Truncus arteriosus	Ascending aorta and pulmonary trunk
Bulbus cordis	Smooth parts of left and right ventricle
Primitive ventricle	Trabeculated parts of left and right ventricle
Primitive atrium	Trabeculated parts of left and right atria
Left horn of sinus venosus (SV)	Coronary sinus
Right horn of SV	Smooth part of right atrium
Right common cardinal vein and right anterior cardinal vein	Superior vena cava

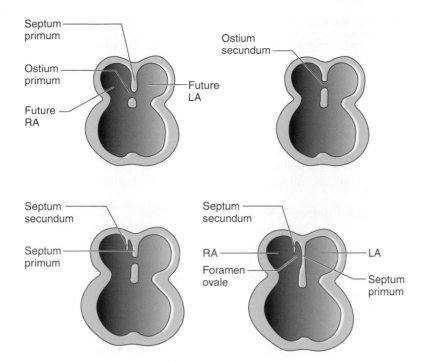

FIGURE 1-1. Embryologic development of the septum.

Classic signs of ASD include the following:

- Wide, fixed splitting of S_2
- Systolic ejection murmur heard best in the second intercostal space along the left sternal border

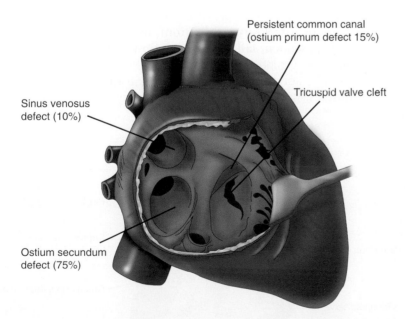

FIGURE 1-2. Various forms of atrial septal defects viewed through the lateral wall of the right atrium.

INTERVENTRICULAR SEPTUM

The interventricular septum consists of two parts: the **muscular** portion and the **membranous** portion.

- The **muscular** interventricular **septum** forms as an upward expansion of the base of the primitive ventricle. It extends toward the AV septum but does not reach it; the resulting gap is the interventricular foramen.
- The **membranous** interventricular **septum** is created by the fusion of the aorticopulmonary septum with the muscular intraventricular septum. It grows downward from the AV cushions and fuses with the muscular interventricular septum, obliterating the interventricular foramen.

Ventricular septal defect (VSD), an abnormal opening in the interventricular septum, is the most common congenital heart malformation (Figure 1-3). The most common location is in the membranous interventricular septum, resulting from incomplete fusion of the AV cushions in the conotruncal region. Clinical manifestations of a VSD vary depending on the size of the defect. Most are small and resolve spontaneously. Larger VSDs result in left-to-right shunting of blood.

- A classic symptom is **easy fatigability.**
- Cardiac auscultation reveals a **harsh holosystolic murmur** heard best at the left lower sternal border.

AORTICOPULMONARY SEPTUM

The **aorticopulmonary (AP) septum** is derived from **neural crest cells** that migrate into the conotruncal ridges. It is responsible for **separating the truncus arteriosus** into the aorta and pulmonary trunk. As the septum descends, it **spirals** so that the aorta becomes the left ventricular outflow tract and the pulmonary trunk becomes the right ventricular outflow tract. Failure of spiraling leads to congenital malformations.

- **Persistent truncus arteriosus** results from abnormal migration of neural crest cells and subsequent **failure of formation of the AP septum.** Therefore, separation of the left ventricular and right ventricular outflow tracts never occurs. The aorta and pulmonary trunk form a common tract leaving the ventricles, which allows mixing of oxygenated and deoxygenated

KEY FACT

Neural crest cells are also important in craniofacial development. Therefore, many newborns with abnormal migration of neural crest cells will have concurrent facial and cardiac defects.

MNEMONIC

The 5 T's of early cyanosis (right-to-left shunts):
Tetralogy of Fallot
Transposition of the great vessels
Truncus arteriosus
Tricuspid atresia
TAPVR (Total Anomalous Pulmonary Venous Return)

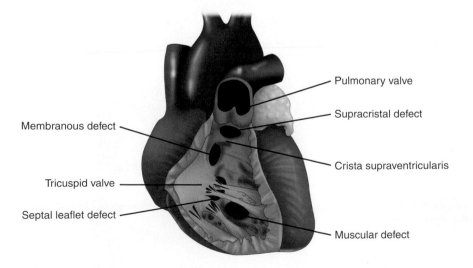

FIGURE 1-3. **Ventricular septal defects.** Notice the inferiorly located muscular defect and the more superior membranous defect.

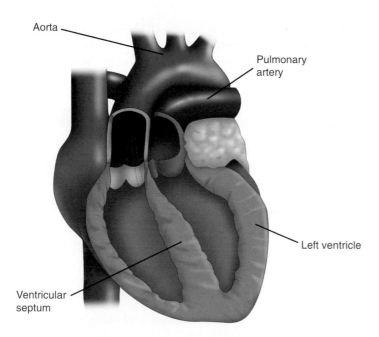

FIGURE 1-4.   Transposition of the great vessels.

blood. This congenital malformation leads to **right-to-left shunting** of blood and **early cyanosis** in the newborn period.

■ **Transposition of the great vessels** occurs with **failure of spiral development of the AP septum.** The left ventricle (LV) is connected to the pulmonary trunk, and the right ventricle (RV) is connected to the aorta (Figure 1-4). This condition results in a complete **right-to-left shunt** and **early cyanosis.**

■ **Tetralogy of Fallot** is caused by anterior displacement of the AP septum.

■ The four abnormalities are overriding aorta, pulmonic stenosis, RV hypertrophy, and VSD (Figure 1-5).

■ The primary defect is termed an **"overriding aorta,"** because the misplaced aorta partially obstructs the right ventricular outflow tract, leading to **right ventricular outflow obstruction (pulmonic stenosis).** Pulmonic

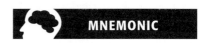

MNEMONIC

Tetralogy of Fallot—

PROVe
Pulmonic stenosis
RV hypertrophy
Overriding aorta
VSD

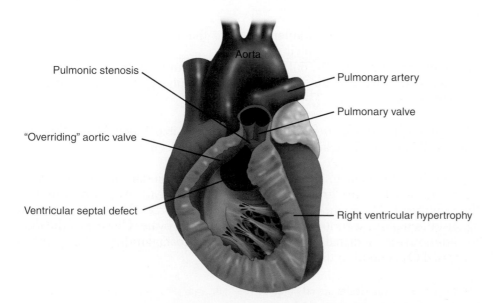

FIGURE 1-5.   Tetralogy of Fallot viewed through the right ventricle.

stenosis leads to increased pressures in the RV and subsequent **right ventricular hypertrophy.** The **membranous VSD** results from a failure of fusion between the AP septum and the muscular portion of the intraventricular septum (IVS). **Right-to-left shunting** results in **early cyanosis.**

FETAL ERYTHROPOIESIS

Organ Involvement

Fetal erythrocytes are produced in different locations throughout the life of the fetus.

- Yolk sac (3–8 weeks) during organogenesis
- Liver (6–30 weeks)
- Spleen (9–28 weeks)
- Bone marrow (28 weeks–adult)

Hemoglobin

Fetal hemoglobin consists of two alpha subunits and two gamma subunits (α_2 and γ_2). Because it has a lower affinity for 2,3-bisphosphoglycerate (2,3-BPG) than does adult hemoglobin, and thus a higher affinity for oxygen, the transfer of oxygen across the placenta from maternal to fetal circulation is ensured.

FETAL CIRCULATION

Deoxygenated blood leaves the fetus via the **umbilical arteries.** The umbilical arteries travel through the umbilical cord toward the placenta. **Oxygenated blood** (approximately 80% saturated with O_2) returns from the placenta toward the fetus via the **umbilical vein** (Figure 1-6). Blood from the umbilical vein **bypasses the liver** by flowing through the **ductus venosus** and empties into the inferior vena cava (IVC). The IVC brings blood into the right atrium. Since this blood is already oxygenated, the pulmonary circulation is unnecessary and can be bypassed. In the fetus, pressures in the right heart are greater than those in the left heart due to high resistance in the pulmonary circulation. The pressure gradient drives right-to-left shunts, allowing the bypass of the pulmonary circulation. Blood in the RA has **two methods** of bypassing the pulmonary circulation:

1. **Flowing through the foramen ovale** to the LA, continuing to the LV, aorta, and eventually supplying the head.
2. Continuing into the RV, out the pulmonary trunk, and then **through the ductus arteriosus** to the aorta, primarily supplying the trunk and lower extremities.

The aorta sends blood to fetal tissues. Deoxygenated blood leaves the iliac arteries via the umbilical arteries to return to the placenta.

After birth, as the neonate begins to breathe, the pulmonary arterial resistance decreases. For the first time, pressures in the left heart exceed pressures in the right heart. The increase in left atrial pressure forces the septum primum against the septum secundum, closing the foramen ovale. Closure of the ductus arteriosus is mediated by **falling levels of prostaglandins** subsequent to increased O_2 content in the circulation.

MNEMONIC

Young **L**iver **S**ynthesizes **B**lood.

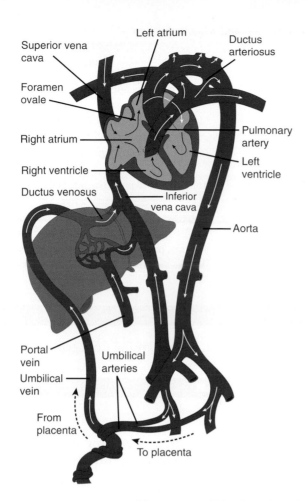

FIGURE 1-6. **Fetal circulation.** Most of the oxygenated blood reaching the heart via the umbilical vein and inferior vena cava is diverted through the foramen ovale and pumped out the aorta to the head, while the deoxygenated blood returned via the superior vena cava is mostly pumped through the pulmonary artery and ductus arteriosus to the feet and the umbilical arteries. (Modified with permission from Barrett KE, Barman SM, Boitano S, Brooks H: *Ganong's Review of Medical Physiology*, 23rd ed. New York: McGraw-Hill, 2010, Fig. 34-18: 628.)

FETAL-POSTNATAL DERIVATIVES

Some important fetal structures and their postnatal counterparts follow:

- Umbilical vein → ligamentum teres hepatis
- UmbiLical arteries → **mediaL** umbilical ligaments
- Ductus venosus → ligamentum venosum
- Ductus arteriosus → ligamentum arteriosus
- AllaNtois → urachus—**mediaN** umbilical ligament
- Foramen ovale → fossa ovalis
- Notochord → nucleus pulposus of intervertebral disk

TABLE 1-2.   Aortic Arches and Adult Derivatives

AORTIC ARCH	ADULT STRUCTURE
First	Part of maxillary artery
Second	Stapedial artery and hyoid artery
Third	Common carotid and proximal internal carotid artery
Fourth	Aortic arch and proximal part of the right subclavian artery
Fifth	Regresses in humans
Sixth	Proximal pulmonary arteries and ductus arteriosus

AORTIC ARCH DERIVATIVES

Table 1-2 describes the adult structures arising from each of the aortic arches.

DEFECTS IN THE ARTERIAL SYSTEM

Coarctation of the Aorta

This abnormal narrowing of the aorta in the area surrounding the ductus arteriosus manifests in two types: **preductal** and **postductal.**

- **Preductal coarctation** is constriction of the aorta proximal to the ductus arteriosus. In this type, the ductus arteriosus typically remains patent, resulting in a right-to-left shunt with sufficient blood supply to the lower extremities.
- **Postductal coarctation** is constriction of the aorta distal to the ductus arteriosus (Figure 1-7). It is characterized by elevated blood pressure (BP) in the arms, decreased BP in the legs, and weak or absent femoral pulses. Collateral circulation develops to route blood to the lower extremities. Blood flows from the proximal aorta to the legs via the subclavian artery to the internal thoracic artery, then the intercostal artery, the superior epigastric artery, the inferior epigastric artery, and the external iliac artery. The increased blood flow to the intercostal arteries causes them to dilate and eventually erode into the ribs. This process results in the characteristic **"rib notching"** associated with coarctation of the aorta.

Patent Ductus Arteriosus

Patent ductus arteriosus (PDA) is the failure of the ductus arteriosus to close. A connection persists between the left pulmonary artery and the aortic arch. Since the left heart has higher pressures than the right heart, a **left-to-right shunt** develops, with blood flowing from the aorta into the pulmonary artery. It is most common in premature infants and does not result in early cyanosis. Administration of prostaglandin inhibitors (eg, indomethacin, NSAIDs) enhances closure of the PDA.

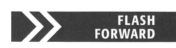

FLASH FORWARD

Indomethacin, a nonsteroidal anti-inflammatory drug (NSAID), is used to close a patent ductus arteriosus (PDA). Exogenous administration of prostaglandins is used to keep a PDA open.

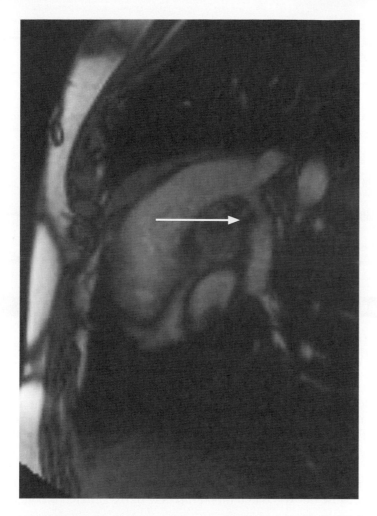

FIGURE 1-7.   Postductal coarctation of the aorta. Sagittal bright blood MRI demonstrates narrowing of the aorta immediately distal to the take-off of the left subclavian artery (*arrow*). (Reproduced with permission from USMLERx.com.)

RIGHT-TO-LEFT SHUNTS: EARLY CYANOSIS

The 5 T's:

1. Tetralogy of Fallot (most common cause of early cyanosis)
2. Transposition of the great vessels
3. Truncus arteriosus
4. Total anomalous pulmonary venous return
5. Tricuspid atresia

These cardiac malformations each result in **shunting of deoxygenated blood** from the pulmonary circulation (or right heart) **into oxygenated blood** in the systemic circulation (or left heart). The addition of deoxygenated blood to oxygenated blood decreases the partial pressure of O_2 in the systemic circulation and causes **early cyanosis.**

Squatting increases systemic vascular resistance (or left-sided pressure) by compression of the femoral arteries; this decreases the pressure gradient and thus may alleviate symptoms of right-to-left shunts.

TABLE 1-3. Disorders and Associated Cardiac Defects

DISORDER	CARDIAC DEFECT
22q11 Deletions	Truncus arteriosus, tetralogy of Fallot
Down syndrome	VSD, ASD, AV septal defect (endocardial cushion defect)
Turner syndrome	Coarctation of the aorta
Offspring of a diabetic mother	Transposition of the great vessels
Congenital rubella	Septal defects, PDA, pulmonary artery stenosis
Marfan syndrome	Aortic insufficiency (late complication)

LEFT-TO-RIGHT SHUNTS: LATE CYANOSIS

- VSD (most common congenital cardiac anomaly)
- ASD (loud S_1; wide, fixed split S_2)
- PDA

If these defects do not close and high flow continues through the pulmonary circulation, the pulmonary arterial system becomes hypertrophic and even fibrotic. **Pulmonary hypertension** and subsequent RV hypertrophy result. When the right heart pressures become higher than the left heart pressures, the shunt reverses and becomes right to left. This shunt reversal is termed **Eisenmenger syndrome** and causes **late cyanosis.** Right-to-left shunts cause cyanosis because deoxygenated blood mixes with oxygenated blood.

CONGENITAL CARDIAC DEFECT ASSOCIATIONS

Certain disorders are associated with particular congenital cardiac malformations (Table 1-3).

Anatomy

SURFACES AND BORDERS OF THE HEART

- The **anterior (sternal) surface** is formed by the RV (Figure 1-8).
- The **posterior surface** is formed by the LA and is in close proximity to the esophagus.
- The **right border** is formed by the right atrium.
- The **left border** is formed by the LA and LV.
- The **apex** is formed by the LV.

KEY FACT

Enlargement of the LA, a characteristic finding in mitral valve (MV) insufficiency, may cause dysphagia.

KEY FACT

In cardiomegaly the apex is shifted laterally, therefore the point of maximal impulse (PMI) is palpated more lateral than the midclavicular line.

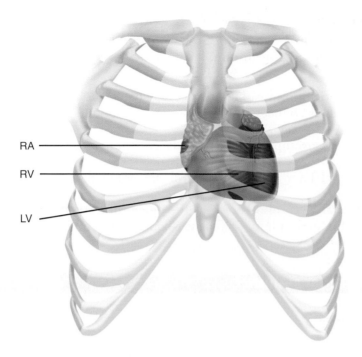

FIGURE 1-8. **Anatomic relationships of the heart.** LA, left atrium; RA, right atrium; RV, right ventricle.

RELATIONSHIPS OF THE HEART AND GREAT VESSELS

- The **right border** is located between the third and sixth ribs along the right sternal border.
- The **left border** is located between the third and sixth ribs between the midclavicular line and left sternal border.
- The apex is located at the fifth intercostal space, midclavicular line. The point of maximal impulse (PMI) is normally palpated here.
- The **aortic arch** is located at the level of the sternal notch, corresponding to vertebral level T2.
- The **superior vena cava (SVC)** enters the RA at the level of the third rib.

LAYERS OF THE HEART

The heart is composed of three layers: **endocardium, myocardium,** and **pericardium.**

Endocardium

The endocardium is the innermost layer and contacts the blood in the heart chambers. It is composed of simple squamous epithelium (endothelium) and underlying connective tissue.

Myocardium

The myocardium is the middle layer composed of myocytes, the contractile cells responsible for pumping blood through the heart.

CLINICAL CORRELATION

Q: A 30-year-old magician swallows an open safety pin as part of his show. Which chamber of the heart is most likely to be punctured?
A: The left atrium.

CLINICAL CORRELATION

Q: An 18-year-old male is stabbed with a knife just to the right of the sternum between the fourth and fifth ribs. Which cardiac structure is penetrated by the knife?
A: The right atrium.

CLINICAL CORRELATION

Cardiac tamponade is the compression of the heart by fluid (ie, blood) in the pericardial sac, leading to decreased cardiac output (CO). Classic signs include decreased mean arterial pressure (MAP), distended neck veins due to inability of the SVC to drain, pulsus paradoxus, and an ECG showing electrical alternans. Treatment is pericardiocentesis.

? CLINICAL CORRELATION

Pericarditis is inflammation of the pericardium; causes of which vary and include systemic lupus erythematosus (SLE), rheumatoid arthritis, myocardial infarction (MI), tuberculosis, and malignancy. Findings include chest pain and friction rub on auscultation, and the ECG shows diffuse ST elevations in all leads.

? CLINICAL CORRELATION

Subendocardial infarctions result from repeated episodes of temporary occlusion of a coronary artery (eg, unstable angina) or from severe anemia or hypotension. ECG findings show ST-segment depression. Histologic findings include fibrosis and vacuolization of the subendocardial area.

Pericardium

The pericardium is composed of two layers: the outer **fibrous pericardium** and the inner **serous pericardium.** It covers the heart and proximal portion of the great vessels.

- **Fibrous pericardium** is the tough connective tissue that tethers the heart in place via its connections to the sternum anteriorly and the central tendon of the diaphragm inferiorly.
- **Serous pericardium** comprises two layers: the parietal layer and the visceral layer.
- The parietal layer is continuous with the internal aspect of the fibrous pericardium.
- The visceral layer, also known as the **epicardium,** is the thin innermost layer of the pericardium. This layer contains the major branches of the coronary arteries.

CORONARY ARTERY ANATOMY

Major Branches

The coronary arteries arise from the proximal portion of the aorta (the aorta's first branches) as the **right coronary artery (RCA)** and the **left coronary artery (LCA)** (Figure 1-9). These vessels lie just deep to the epicardium on the surface of the heart.

The heart receives a dual blood supply: The **epicardium** and **myocardium** are supplied by the **coronary arteries** and their branches, whereas the **endocardium** receives O_2 and nutrients from direct contact with blood inside the heart chambers.

When flow through a coronary artery is compromised, the subendocardial tissue is most vulnerable to ischemic injury because it lies in the zone farthest from either blood supply.

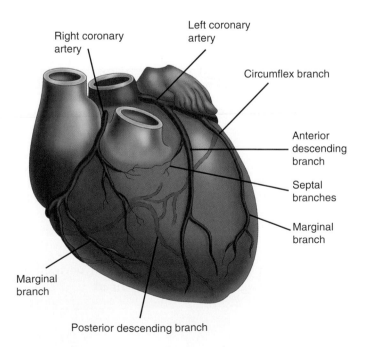

FIGURE 1-9.   Coronary artery circulation.

TABLE 1-4.   **Arterial Supply of the Heart in Right-Dominant Coronary Circulation**

LAD	LEFT CIRCUMFLEX	RCA
Apex	Lateral wall of LV	Lateral wall of RV
Anterior wall of LV	Posterior wall of LV (20%)	Posterior wall of LV (80%)
Anterior two thirds of IVS	Posterior one third of IVS (20%)	Posterior one third of IVS (80%)
		SA node
		AV node

AV = atrioventricular; IVS = interventricular septum; LAD = left anterior descending; LV = left ventricle; RCA = right coronary artery; RV = right ventricle; SA = sinoatrial.

Flow through the coronary arteries occurs mainly during diastole. The contraction of the myocardium during systole increases external pressure on the vessels and inhibits blood flow through them.

Major branches of the LCA are the left anterior descending artery (LAD) and left circumflex artery.

Major branches of the RCA are the **marginal artery** and the **posterior descending artery.**

Dominant Circulation

Table 1-4 summarizes the arterial supply of the heart. This **right-dominant coronary circulation** occurs in 80% of the population.

Myocardial Infarctions

The coronary artery **most commonly occluded** (40–50%) is the **LAD,** resulting in infarction of the anterior portion of the ventricles, the cardiac apex, and/or the IVS. The RCA is the second most commonly occluded, followed by the left circumflex. Infarction results in characteristic ECG changes demonstrated in Figure 1-10 and Table 1-5.

KEY FACT

Tachycardia shortens diastole so the heart receives less blood supply.

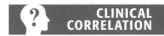

CLINICAL CORRELATION

Acute MI of the inferior portion of the heart (RV) is associated with characteristic ECG findings of ST-segment elevation in leads II, III, and aVF.

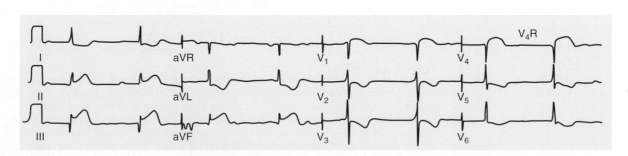

FIGURE 1-10.   ECG findings in acute myocardial infarction of the right ventricle. (Modified with permission from Fuster V, et al. *Hurst's The Heart,* 11th ed. New York: McGraw-Hill, 2006: 300.)

TABLE 1-5.   **ECG Findings With Myocardial Infarction**

Area of Infarct	Coronary Artery Involved	Leads With ST Elevation
Inferior wall (RV)	RCA	II, III, aVF
Septum	LAD	V_2, V_3
Lateral wall (LV)	Left circumflex	I, aVL, V_5, V_6

aVF = augmented voltage foot; aVL = augmented voltage left arm; LAD = left anterior descending; LV = left ventricle; RCA = right coronary artery; RV = right ventricle.

CONDUCTION SYSTEM

The cardiac conduction system is responsible for distributing electrical impulses throughout the heart so that the atria and ventricles function in concert as an effective pump (Figure 1-11).

Sinoatrial Node

- The SA node contains specialized myocytes that depolarize rhythmically and serve to initiate the spread of electrical impulses throughout the heart.
- It is located at the junction of the RA and SVC just beneath the pericardium and is supplied by the **SA nodal artery**, typically a branch of the RCA.

KEY FACT

The SA node receives input from both the sympathetic nervous system (accelerating its rate of depolarization) and the parasympathetic nervous system via the vagus nerve (slowing its rate).

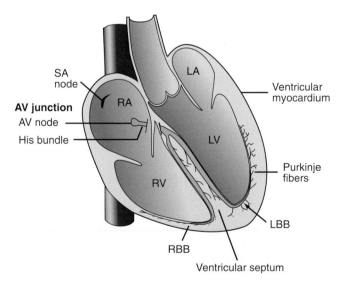

FIGURE 1-11.   **Anatomy of the conduction system in the heart.** To initiate a contraction, the sinoatrial (SA) node fires at an intrinsic rate of 100–120 beats/min. The impulse travels through the atrial myocardium and arrives at the atrioventricular (AV) node, located at the base of the right atrium. The impulse stalls at the AV node, then propagates through the His bundle along the interventricular septum, into bifurcating paths called the right bundle branch (RBB) and left bundle branch (LBB). These bundles subdivide into Purkinje fibers that relay the impulse to the ventricular myocardium. The Purkinje fibers conduct the most quickly, to enable a rapid and synchronized ventricular contraction. LA, left atrium; LV, left ventricle; RA, right atrium; RV, right ventricle. (Modified with permission from Kasper DL, Braunwald E, Fauci AS, et al. *Harrison's Principles of Internal Medicine*, 16th ed. New York: McGraw-Hill, 2005: 1311.)

■ From the SA node, the impulses disperse across the atrial septum to the LA and toward the AV septum of the right heart. The impulse eventually reaches the **AV node**.

Atrioventricular Node

■ The **atrioventricular (AV) node** is located in the subendocardial connective tissue in the interatrial septum near the ostium of the coronary sinus.
■ It receives blood supply from the **AV nodal artery,** also a branch of the RCA.
■ The AV node is responsible for dispersing the electrical signal to both ventricles, which it accomplishes via the AV bundles (**bundles of His**).
■ Conduction through the AV node is relatively slow, which allows time for the atria to depolarize and fully empty their contents into the ventricles before ventricular contraction. This is key for efficient systolic pumping.
■ If the SA node is diseased or fails to fire, the AV node initiates cardiac contractions at a rate of 40–60 beats/min.

Bundles of His

The **bundles of His** travel parallel to the interventricular septum deep to the endocardium, eventually terminating as the **Purkinje fibers** in the walls of both ventricles.

HEART VALVES AND SITES OF AUSCULTATION

The four heart valves are the **aortic, pulmonic, mitral, and tricuspid valves** (Table 1-6). It is important to understand how valve movement relates to the cardiac cycle.

Many cardiac diseases and valvular lesions result in abnormal heart sounds. Heart sounds are due to blood flow; therefore, the site of auscultation (Figure 1-12) of a particular valve is downstream to the direction of flow through that valve.

TABLE 1-6. Characteristics of Heart Valves

Valve	Location	Structure	Site of Auscultation	Phase When Valve Is Open
Aortic	Between LV and aorta	Semilunar (3 cusps)	Right second intercostal space (IS) at the sternal border (SB)	Systole
Pulmonic	Between RV and pulmonary trunk	Semilunar (3 cusps)	Left second IS at the SB	Systole
Mitral	Between LA and LV	Bicuspid	Left fifth IS at the midclavicular line	Diastole
Tricuspid	Between RA and RV	Tricuspid	Left fifth IS at the SB	Diastole

CLINICAL CORRELATION

Damage to the AV node (most often caused by ischemia) may result in complete heart block. Impulses are unable to get from the RA to the RV; thus, ventricular rate is slowed and cardiac output is low. Treatment is usually insertion of a permanent pacemaker.

MNEMONIC

All Patients Take Meds
Aortic
Pulmonic
Tricuspid
Mitral

CLINICAL CORRELATION

Aortic stenosis (AS) causes a crescendo-decrescendo systolic ejection murmur. The murmur is best heard at the right second intercostal space and typically radiates toward the carotid arteries and/or the cardiac apex.

CLINICAL CORRELATION

Mitral regurgitation (MR) causes a holosystolic blowing murmur, heard best at the cardiac apex. It can sometimes be confused with tricuspid regurgitation; however, the murmur of tricuspid regurgitation becomes louder with inspiration.

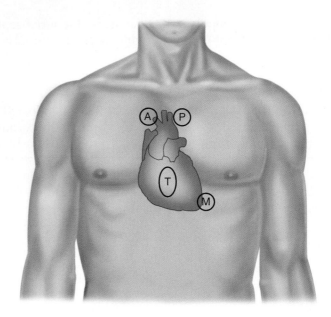

FIGURE 1-12. **Sites of cardiac auscultation.** A, aortic valve; P, pulmonic valve; T, tricuspid valve; M, mitral valve.

Physiology

The cardiovascular (CV) system, which can be modeled as a pump (heart) and a set of tubes (blood vessels), distributes O_2, nutrients, and other substances to the tissues while removing metabolic by-products from the tissues.

CARDIAC ELECTROPHYSIOLOGY

Cardiac nodal cells and myocytes are excitable cells that generate characteristic action potentials. Nodal cells share similar qualities with excitable cells such as neurons in that both rely on cationic Na^+ inflow to reach the threshold membrane potential to fire action potentials. However, cardiac nodal cells have a more negative action potential threshold and therefore can be stimulated to depolarize by a relatively smaller influx of Na^+. The membrane potential can spontaneously depolarize as Na^+ enters the cell, accounting for the automaticity of the SA and AV nodes. Cardiac myocytes resemble the skeletal myocyte in that both rely on Ca^{2+} inflow for contraction, but key differences include the action potential's shape (plateau in atrial and ventricular myocytes due to inward Ca^{2+} current) and electrical coupling via gap junctions.

Resting Membrane Potential

The membrane potential (V_m) in all cells is based on:

- The relative permeability of the cell membrane for certain ions (eg, K^+, Na^+, Ca^{2+}). This determines which ion's equilibrium potential predominates. The membrane potential at any point in the action potential is determined by the relative contribution of different ion conductances.
- The relative intracellular and extracellular concentrations of these ions.

The resting membrane potential is determined primarily by the potassium (K^+) conductance, $[K^+]_{intracellular}$ ($[K^+]_i$), and $[K^+]_{extracellular}$ ($[K^+]_e$). Since $[K^+]_i \gg [K^+]_e$, K^+ diffuses out of the cell and down its concentration gradi-

KEY FACT

Inward current → positive charge (eg, K^+, Na^+) enters cell → depolarizes V_m (makes less negative).

Outward current → positive charge leaves cell → hyperpolarizes V_m (makes more negative).

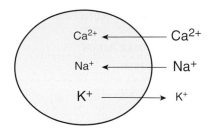

FIGURE 1-13. **Relative intracellular and extracellular concentrations of Ca²⁺, Na⁺, and K⁺.**

ent, causing the V_m to become more negative (losing positive charge to the outside). At a certain membrane potential, the net force driving K⁺ along its electrochemical gradient equals the net concentration gradient driving ions across the membrane. This potential at which there is no net movement of ions across the membrane is the **equilibrium (or Nernst) potential** and can be calculated:

$$V_m = 61.5\log \frac{[K^+]_e}{[K^+]_i} \text{ mV}$$

In contrast, since the [Na⁺] is higher in the extracellular space, Na⁺ tends to enter the cell and make the membrane potential more positive. The Na⁺-K⁺-ATPase pump maintains the ionic gradient across the cell membrane by pumping 3 Na⁺ out for every 2 K⁺ pumped in. This sets up an Na⁺ gradient such that [Na⁺]_e is greater than [Na⁺]_i (Figure 1-13).

Cardiac Action Potentials

The heart has two populations of excitable cells: one produces a fast-response action potential, and the other produces a slow-response action potential (Figure 1-14). These action potentials (AP) differ in their shape and conduction velocity (Table 1-7).

KEY FACT

The most important difference between fast- and slow-response cardiac action potentials is the ion responsible for the phase 0 upstroke:
Fast-response action potential = fast inward Na⁺ current
Slow-response action potential = slow inward Ca²⁺ current

FLASH FORWARD

The four classes of antiarrhythmia drugs target specific channels/receptors:
Class I: Na⁺ channel blockers
Class II: β-Blockers
Class III: K⁺ channel blockers
Class IV: Ca²⁺ channel blockers

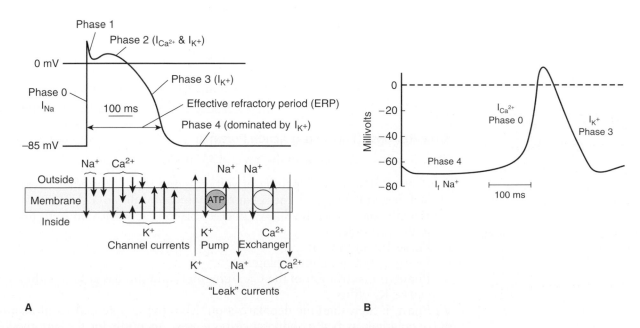

FIGURE 1-14. **Fast response (A) and slow response (B) cardiac action potentials.** I, inflow of the specified ion through the ion channel. (Modified with permission from Ganong WF. *Review of Medical Physiology*, 22nd ed. New York: McGraw-Hill, 2005.)

TABLE 1-7. **Comparison of Slow and Fast Action Potentials**

	SLOW PACEMAKER ACTION POTENTIAL	FAST ACTION POTENTIAL
Length of AP	150 ms (SA, atria), 250–300 ms (AV, ventricular)	100 ms
Conduction velocity	0.3–3.0 m/sec	0.01–0.10 m/sec
Tissues involved	SA and AV nodes	Atria, ventricles, bundle of His, Purkinje fibers
Phases	0 $G_{Ca^{2+}}$	0. Increased G_{Na^+}
	III I_{K^+}	I. Decreased G_{Na^+}
	IV I_f	II. Increased $G_{Ca^{2+}}$
		III. Increased I_{K^+}, decreased $I_{Ca^{2+}}$
Targeting antiarrhythmics	Class II β-blockers (phase IV), class IV Ca channel blockers (phase 0)	Class Ia, Ib, Ic (phase 0), class III (phase III)

AV = atrioventricular; SA = sinoatrial.

FAST-RESPONSE (VENTRICULAR) ACTION POTENTIAL

Fast-response action potentials occur in the atrial and ventricular myocytes, the bundle of His, and Purkinje fibers.

- Phase 0: Rapid upstroke. Voltage-gated Na^+ channels open.
- Phase 1: Initial repolarization. Inactivation of voltage-gated Na^+ channels. Voltage-gated K^+ channels begin to open.
- Phase 2: Plateau. Ca^{2+} influx through voltage-gated Ca^{2+} channels balances K^+ efflux. Ca^{2+} influx triggers Ca^{2+} release of intracellular Ca^{2+} from sarcoplasmic reticulum and myocyte contraction.
- Phase 3: Repolarization. Massive K^+ efflux due to opening of voltage-gated slow K^+ channels and closure of voltage-gated Ca^{2+} channels.
- Phase 4: Resting potential. High K^+ permeability through K^+ channels.

SLOW-RESPONSE (PACEMAKER) ACTION POTENTIAL

Slow-response APs occur in the SA and AV nodes.

- Phase 0: Upstroke. Opening of voltage-gated Ca^{2+} channels. These cells lack fast voltage-gated Na^+ channels, which results in a slow conduction velocity that is used by the AV node to prolong transmission from the atria to the ventricles.
- Phase 1: Not present.
- Phase 2: Not present (no plateau).
- Phase 3: Inactivation of the Ca^{2+} channels and increased K^+ conductance causes K^+ efflux.
- Phase 4: Slow diastolic depolarization. Membrane potential spontaneously depolarizes as Na^+ conductance increases. Accounts for the automaticity of the SA and AV nodes.

CARDIAC PACEMAKERS

Due to its slow-response AP, the SA node is the intrinsic pacemaker of the heart with the highest intrinsic rate of firing, determined by the slope of phase 4 depolarization. The slope of phase 4 in the SA node determines the heart rate (HR). Acetylcholine (Ach) decreases the rate of diastolic depolarization and decreases HR, whereas catecholamines increase depolarization and increase HR.

In contrast, the AV node and His-Purkinje systems are latent pacemakers; they take over as pacemaker cells if the SA node is suppressed. The primary, secondary, and tertiary pacemaker cells are related to their rates of phase 4 depolarization: SA node > AV node > His-Purkinje.

CONDUCTION VELOCITY

Depends on the size of the inward current during the AP upstroke (ie, phase 0); a larger inward current corresponds to a faster conduction velocity. It is fastest in the Purkinje system and slowest in the AV node. A slower conduction velocity in the AV node means that the excitation of the ventricles is delayed. The AV nodal delay enables the atria to empty fully into the ventricles prior to depolarization of the ventricles, thus improving ventricular filling and increasing cardiac output in a given beat.

REFRACTORY PERIOD

The period of the AP in which cardiac cells cannot be excited; it can be defined in three ways (Figure 1-15):

- **Absolute:** Begins at phase 0 and ends after phase 2 (plateau); reflects time in which no AP can be generated, regardless of the amount of inward current delivered.
- **Effective:** Period in which a **conducted** AP cannot be generated; slightly longer than the absolute refractory period.
- **Relative:** Period in which an AP can be generated with a larger-than-usual amount of inward current.

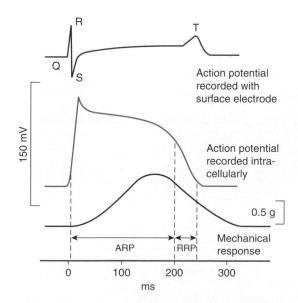

FIGURE 1-15. **Absolute (ARP), effective (ERP), and relative (RRP) refractory periods in the ventricle.** The refractory period sets the rate of firing, and consequently, the heart rate. Longer refractory periods lead to slower heart rates. (Modified with permission from Ganong WF. *Review of Medical Physiology*, 22nd ed. New York: McGraw-Hill, 2005: 80.)

> **KEY FACT**

Overdrive suppression: Because the SA node fires the fastest, at a rate of 100–120/min, by default it sets the heart rate (HR) unless diseased (ie, RCA infarct). In that situation, the AV node fires at 40–60/min, and the Purkinje system comes in last at 30–40/min.

CARDIAC MUSCLE AND CONTRACTION

Contraction of the cardiac muscle cell is initiated by the AP signal acting on intracellular organelles to evoke the generation of tension and shortening of the cell. These APs are profoundly different from those of skeletal muscle cells. For example, they can be self-generating, can propagate directly from cell to cell, and have longer durations.

Excitation-Contraction Coupling

Coupling depends on several structures in the myocardial cell that coordinate the contraction response to the cardiac AP.

- **Sarcomere:** Contractile unit of myocardial cell that runs from Z line to Z line (Figure 1-16). Composed of thick filaments (myosin) and thin filaments (actin, troponin, tropomyosin).
- **T tubules:** Parts of the cell membrane that invaginate at the Z lines. They carry APs into the cell interior.
- **Sarcoplasmic reticulum:** Intracellular site of storage and release of Ca^{2+}, which is used in excitation-contraction coupling.
- **Intercalated disks:** Located at the ends of cells. Mediate adhesion between cells.
- **Gap junctions:** Occur at the intercalated disks. Provide a path of low resistance for APs to rapidly spread between cells.

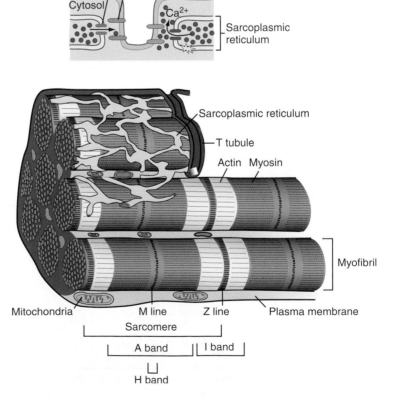

FIGURE 1-16. **Schematic of cardiac myocyte.**

MYOCARDIAL CONTRACTION AND RELAXATION

The cardiac myocyte translates the electrical signal (AP) into a physical response (contraction) through the following steps: Extracellular Ca^{2+} enters myocardial cell $\rightarrow$ Ca^{2+} induces intracellular Ca^{2+} release $\rightarrow$ myocardial contraction, and finally myocardial relaxation.

- **Influx of extracellular Ca^{2+} into myocardial cells:** Action potential spreads from cell membrane into the T tubules. During the plateau (phase 2) of the AP, extracellular Ca^{2+} enters the cell through voltage-gated Ca^{2+} (L-type Ca^{2+}) channels.
- **Ca^{2+}-induced Ca^{2+} release:** The influx of extracellular Ca^{2+} is not sufficient to induce muscle contraction. Therefore, extracellular Ca^{2+} binds to ryanodine receptors on the sarcoplasmic reticulum (SR), inducing a conformational change that releases Ca^{2+} from the SR (calcium-induced calcium release).
- Amount of Ca^{2+} released from the SR depends on:
    - Size of inward current during plateau of the AP
    - Amount of Ca^{2+} stored in SR
- **Myocardial contraction:** Ca^{2+} release from the SR increases intracellular $[Ca^{2+}]$. Ca^{2+} binds to troponin C, which causes a conformational change and moves tropomyosin out of the myosin-binding groove on the actin filament. Myosin binds the newly exposed actin. The bound myosin head then releases its bound ADP and undergoes a change in shape that moves the thin filament (power stroke) and shortens the sarcomere. Contraction results in HIZ shrinkage—aka H, I, and Z band contraction (Figure 1-17), but the A band remains the same length.
- **Myocardial relaxation:** Occurs when Ca^{2+} is pumped back into the SR via Ca^{2+}-ATPase. This reduces intracellular $[Ca^{2+}]$ and removes Ca^{2+} from troponin.

KEY FACT

The contractility (inotropy) that can be generated by cardiac muscle is related to intracellular $[Ca^{2+}]$.

KEY FACT

During contraction, the H, I, and Z bands shorten. Only the A band stays constant throughout the cycle.

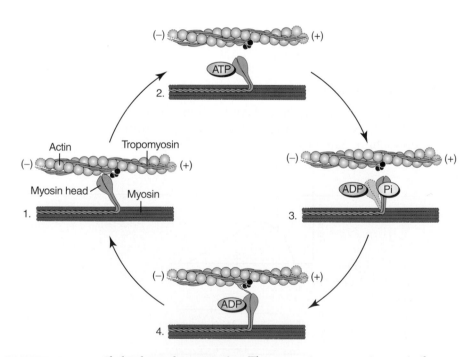

FIGURE 1-17. Skeletal muscle contraction. The process in myocytes is very similar.

Cardiac and skeletal muscles differ physiologically. In contrast to skeletal muscle:

- Cardiac muscle AP has a plateau, due to Ca^{2+} influx.
- Cardiac nodal cells spontaneously depolarize, resulting in automaticity.
- Cardiac myocytes are electrically coupled to each other by gap junctions.
- Cardiac muscle cells have more mitochondria.
- Cardiac muscle increases contractile force through changes in fiber contractility (compared with increasing the number of skeletal muscle fibers activated).

Contractility

Contractility is the amount of force cardiac muscle can generate at a given muscle length and is related to intracellular $[Ca^{2+}]$. It can be estimated by the ejection fraction (EF, normal > 55%). It increases with increased HR, sympathetic stimulation, and cardiac glycosides.

$$EF = \frac{\text{stroke volume}}{\text{end-diastolic volume}} \text{ (normal = 55\%)}$$

Contractility and, by proxy, stroke volume (SV) are increased with:

- **Increased HR.** As HR increases, Ca^{2+} clearance is less efficient during relaxation after contraction, and intracellular Ca^{2+} builds up.
- **Sympathetic stimulation.** Stimulation leads to increased Ca^{2+} influx and also increases the activity of the SR Ca^{2+}-ATPase.
- Cardiac glycosides (digoxin).

Conversely, contractility and SV are decreased in the setting of:

- β-Blockade, calcium channel blockers
- Heart failure
- Parasympathetic nervous system stimulation
- Acidosis, hypoxia, hypercapnia

Length-Tension Relationship in Ventricles

Sarcomere length affects the force of contraction (Figure 1-18). At the optimal length, there is maximal actin-myosin overlap, which results in the maximum systolic contraction. Sarcomere length is related to **preload.**

FLASH FORWARD

Cardiac glycosides such as digitalis increase the force of contraction by inhibiting Na^+-K^+-ATPase in the myocardial cell membrane. This results in increased intracellular $[Na^+]$ and decreased $[Na^+]$ gradient across the cell membrane. Since Ca^{2+} extrusion relies on the $[Na^+]$ gradient (Na^+–Ca^{2+} exchange), less Ca^{2+} is removed, and intracellular $[Ca^{2+}]$ is increased.

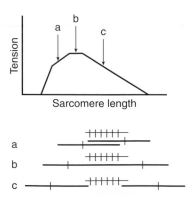

FIGURE 1-18. **Effect of sarcomere length on the force of contraction.** There is an ideal length that maximizes the overlap between actin and myosin (b) and maximizes contraction. If the sarcomere is too short (a) or too long (c), the myosin and actin do not interact as well.

PRELOAD

The volume of blood within the left ventricle while the heart is in its relaxed state. It represents the stretch on the filled ventricle during diastole, before contraction takes place. Related to left ventricular end-diastolic volume (LVEDV) and left ventricular end-diastolic pressure (LVEDP). An acute increase in preload in diastole stretches the myocytes and causes optimized overlapping of actin-myosin complexes, leading to increased force of contraction in systole.

AFTERLOAD

Load against which the myocytes must contract to generate cardiac output. Represents the force that must be generated to push blood from LV into the aorta. Related to peak LV pressure. An acute increase in afterload reduces the volume of blood that is ejected during systole.

FRANK-STARLING RELATIONSHIP

The greater the venous return, the greater the cardiac output. It can be thought of as the length-tension relationship applied to the whole heart: The force of systolic contraction is proportional to the initial length of cardiac muscle in diastole (preload).

- **Molecular/cellular level:** Sarcomere length is proportional to the force of contraction that it can generate: The longer it is, the more cross-bridges that form, and the greater the tension that can develop. The increased stretch that the myocytes see when the ventricle is filled translates into optimized overlapping of the actin-myosin filaments, which generate increasing force of contraction when the cross-bridges recycle. Up to a certain point, the increased stretch/preload leads to greater contractility.
- **Organ level:** Increased venous return or end-diastolic volume (preload) leads to increased ventricular fiber length and increasing tension, which increases stroke volume and cardiac output. The Frank-Starling curve can be shifted up or down when the heart is in a state of increased or decreased contractility, respectively (Figure 1-19).
- **Caveat:** This rule holds up to a certain threshold preload. The heart at its strongest and contracting most vigorously can handle only so much venous return before it becomes overstretched. At a preload beyond this threshold value, actin-myosin overlap is no longer optimal, as the cross-bridges

KEY FACT

Preload increases with exercise (slightly), increasing blood volume (overtransfusion), and excitement (sympathetics).

KEY FACT

In the LV, afterload is equivalent to aortic pressure and MAP/systolic pressure.
In the RV, afterload is equivalent to pulmonary artery pressure and LVEDV.

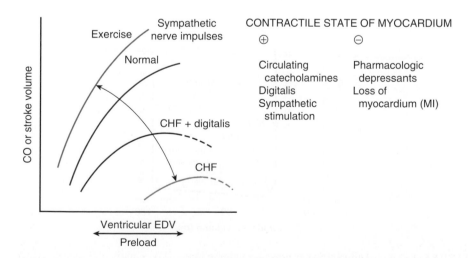

FIGURE 1-19. Frank-Starling curve and the effect of positive and negative inotropic agents. CO, cardiac output; CHF, congestive heart failure; EDV, end-diastolic volume; MI, myocardial infarction.

KEY FACT

Increased venous return →
increased cardiac output.

cannot form. As a result, contractility decreases as the preload continues to increase. This accounts for the descending limb of the length-tension curve at excessively high preloads.

PRESSURE-VOLUME LOOPS

Pressure-volume (PV) loops describe the relationship between LV volume and pressure during the five phases of the cardiac cycle (Figure 1-20). The bottom curve, which is the compliance curve, defines how the pressure in the LV changes as it is filled in diastole (LVEDV). The five phases and how they relate to systole and diastole are as described in the following sections.

Diastole

Mitral valve (MV) opens, and the ventricle rapidly fills until the pressure of the LV is greater than that of the LA and the **MV closes.** Corresponds to P and PR intervals on ECG.

Isovolumetric contraction is the period between MV closure and aortic valve (AoV) opening. Since the MV and AoV are closed, the LV is a closed chamber and contracts under a constant volume. Eventually, LV pressure is greater than that in the aorta and the AoV opens. Corresponds to the QRS on ECG and is the period of highest O_2 consumption.

Systole

AoV has opened:

- **Systolic ejection:** Period between AoV opening and closing. Volume ejected from the LV in this phase is the **SV** (width of pressure-volume loop). LV pressure decreases and the **AoV closes.** Corresponds to ST on ECG.
- **Isovolumetric relaxation:** Period between AoV closing and MV opening. LV is a closed chamber with both the MV and AoV closed. LV relaxes until pressure in the LV drops to that of the LA, the **MV opens,** and blood moves from the LA to the LV. Corresponds to T wave on the ECG.

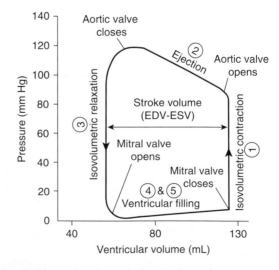

FIGURE 1-20. **Left ventricular pressure-volume loop.** EDV, end-diastolic volume; ESV, end-systolic volume. (Modified with permission from Ganong WF. *Review of Medical Physiology,* 22nd ed. New York: McGraw-Hill, 2005.)

TABLE 1-8.   Variables That Affect Stroke Volume in the Pressure–Volume Loop

VARIABLE	EFFECT ON STROKE VOLUME
Increased preload and venous return (eg, aortic insufficiency)	↑
Increased afterload (eg, hypertension, aortic stenosis)	↓
Increased contractility (eg, exercise)	↑

- **Rapid filling:** Period just after MV opening.
- **Slow filling:** Period just before MV closure.

SV can be altered with changes in preload, afterload, or contractility (Table 1-8 and Figure 1-21).

CARDIAC AND VASCULAR FUNCTION CURVES

The cardiac function and vascular function curves plot how cardiac output (CO) and venous return change with respect to right atrial pressure or end-diastolic volume (Figure 1-22). The factors affecting these functions include:

- **Cardiac function curve (Frank-Starling length-tension relationship):** Increased preload/venous return leads to increased CO, and decreased preload leads to decreased CO.
- **Vascular function curve:** Increased right atrial or systemic pressure and/or decreased blood volume decreases venous return to the heart (decreased preload), and vice versa.
  - **Decreased blood volume** (hemorrhage, shock) shifts the vascular function curve left and downward, leading to decreased potential venous return and increased mean systemic pressure through sympathetic stimulation.
  - **Exercise** shifts the vascular function curve upward and to the right, in addition to increasing systemic pressure through sympathetic stimulation.

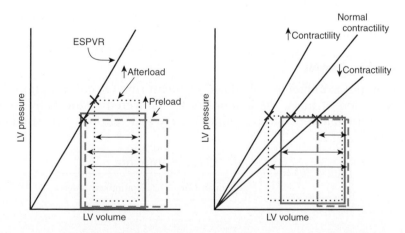

FIGURE 1-21.   Effect of changes in preload, afterload, and contractility on stroke volume (width of pressure-volume loop). ESPVR, end-systolic pressure-volume relationship; LV, left ventricular. (Modified with permission from Kasper DL, Braunwald E, Fauci AS, et al. *Harrison's Principles of Internal Medicine*, 16th ed. New York: McGraw-Hill, 2005: 1363.)

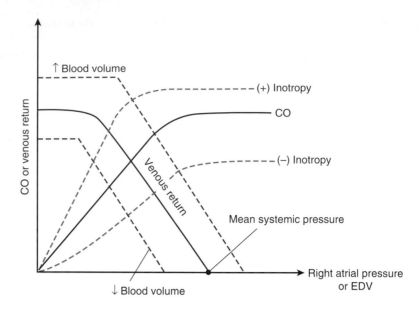

FIGURE 1-22. **Cardiac and vascular function curves and dependence on inotropy and blood volume, respectively.** Changes in inotropy affect the cardiac function curve. Changes in blood volume affect the venous return curve. Changes in total peripheral resistance (TPR) affect both curves. Increased TPR causes a counterclockwise rotation of the venous return curve and a clockwise rotation of the cardiac output curve. CO, cardiac output; EDV, end-diastolic volume.

- **X-intercept of the vascular function curve yields mean systemic pressure:** Pressure in the RA when there is no blood flow through the CV system (heart has stopped); pressure is equal throughout the CV system (ie, there is no pressure gradient).
- **Intersection of cardiac and vascular function curve yields the equilibrium point:** Occurs when CO = venous return. Provides the resting CO.

CARDIAC OUTPUT

KEY FACT

Mean systemic pressure is increased by:
- Increased blood volume
- Decreased venous compliance (blood shifted from veins to arteries)
- Exercise (sympathetic stimulation)

The volume of blood pumped per minute from either ventricle, which should be equal in the absence of pathology, is known as **cardiac output (CO)**. Normal resting CO is 4–8 L/min and can increase five- to sixfold during exercise. CO can be calculated using SV and HR (CO = SV × HR) or measured using Fick's O_2 method.

Fick's Cardiac Output

Cardiac output is indirectly calculated by measuring O_2 consumption. Based on conservation of mass, the amount of O_2 delivered to the body (product of CO and the difference in pulmonary artery and vein $[O_2]$) must equal O_2 consumed.

$$\text{Fick's CO} = \frac{O_2 \text{ consumption}}{([O_2]_{\text{pulmonary vein}} - [O_2]_{\text{pulmonary artery}})}$$

TABLE 1-9. **Factors Affecting Contractility and Stroke Volume**

CONTRACTILITY AND SV ↑ WITH	CONTRACTILITY AND SV ↓ WITH
■ Catecholamines (↑ activity of the Ca^{2+} pump in sarcoplasmic reticulum)	■ β_1-Blockade ■ Heart failure
■ ↑ Intracellular Ca^{2+}	■ Acidosis
■ ↓ Extracellular Na^+	■ Hypoxia/hypercapnia
■ Digitalis (↑ intracellular Na^+, causing ↑ intracellular Ca^{2+})	

SV = stroke volume.

Stroke Volume

Stroke volume is the difference between end-diastolic volume and end-systolic volume, or the volume of blood ejected by the LV during a heartbeat. It varies directly as a function of contractility and preload and varies inversely with afterload. SV increases with increased preload, decreased afterload, or increased contractility. Other variables that affect SV and contractility are summarized in Table 1-9.

Ejection Fraction

The ejection fraction (EF) is the fraction of blood received by the LV (end diastolic volume) that is ejected (SV) and directly reflects the state of contractility of the heart. A larger percentage of LV blood volume ejected (larger EF) reflects an increased contractile state.

$$EF = \frac{\text{stroke volume}}{\text{end-diastolic volume}} \ (\text{normal} = 55\text{–}80\%)$$

$$SV = \frac{CO}{HR} = EDV - ESV$$

$$EF = \frac{SV}{EDV} \times 100\%$$

KEY FACT

Factors that increase O_2 consumption:
- Increased afterload
- Increased contractility
- Increased HR
- Increased size of heart (increases radius → increases tension via LaPlace's law)

MNEMONIC

SV CAP
Stroke **V**olume affected by:
Contractility
Afterload
Preload

THE CARDIAC CYCLE

PV loops divide the cycle into five phases: (1) isovolumetric contraction, (2) systolic ejection, (3) isovolumetric relaxation, (4) rapid filling of the LV, and (5) slow filling of the LV (see Figure 1-20). The heart cycle can be traced from systole through diastole with PV loops, pressure tracings in the heart, and heart sounds.

Pressure Tracings During the Cardiac Cycle

PRESSURE CHANGES IN DIASTOLE AND SYSTOLE

Ventricular diastole begins with AoV closure (S_2) and lasts through the MV closure (S_1), whereas **ventricular systole** is defined as the part of the cardiac cycle from MV closure (S_1) to AoV closure (S_2) (Figure 1-23).

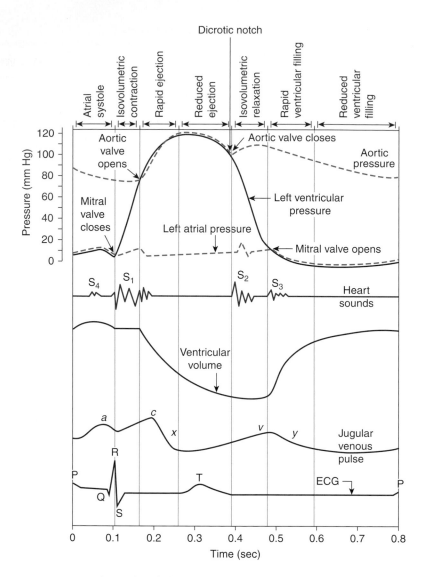

FIGURE 1-23. **Mechanical and electrical events of a single cardiac cycle.** The seven phases are separated by vertical lines. (Adapted with permission from Ganong WF. *Review of Medical Physiology*, 22nd ed. New York: McGraw-Hill, 2005.)

PRESSURE CHANGES IN JUGULAR VENOUS PULSES, LV, AND AORTA

- **Jugular venous pulses:** Provides another complementary pressure tracing to follow mechanical (as opposed to valvular) events of systole and diastole; consists of *a*, *c*, and *v* waves, and *y* descent (see Figure 1-23).

    a wave: **A**trial contraction

    c wave: RV **c**ontraction (tricuspid valve bulging into the RA)

    v wave: Increased RA pressure due to filling against closed tricuspid valve

    y descent: Corresponds to rate of atrial emptying as the tricuspid valve opens

- **LV pressure:** In diastole, during LV filling, P_{LV} equals P_{LA} until the MV closes. During isovolumetric contraction, P_{LV} rises dramatically until it exceeds aortic pressure (P_{Ao}), and then the AoV opens to initiate systole. As blood rushes out of the LV, the P_{LV} drops, continuing to decrease as the AoV closes, and continues to drop more as the LV relaxes, until it equals the P_{LA}. The MV opens once more, and diastole begins again.

KEY FACT

Jugular venous distention is seen in right heart failure (RHF).

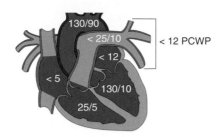

FIGURE 1-24. **Normal pressures in the heart in millimeters of mercury (mm Hg).** Superior vena cava, 5; right atrium, 5–10; right ventricle, 25/5; left atrium, 25/10; left ventricle, 130/10; aorta, 130/90. PCWP, pulmonary capillary wedge pressure.

- **Aortic pressure:** In diastole, P_{Ao} is greater than P_{LV}, and the AoV remains closed. When P_{LV} is equal to or greater than P_{Ao}, the AoV opens and P_{Ao} increases as blood (SV) is moved into the aorta. P_{Ao} begins to decrease as the ejection rate slows down, P_{LV} drops, and the AoV closes to begin diastole.

Pressures in the various heart chambers are measured with a Swan-Ganz catheter (Figure 1-24). The pulmonary capillary wedge pressure (PCWP) is a good approximation of LA pressure.

Heart Sounds

The state of valve closure, ventricular filling, or pathology can be extrapolated from four heart sounds (Table 1-10).

S₁ and S₂, Splitting

S_1 and S_2 are due to valve closures. S_1 is due to closure of the mitral and tricuspid valves; S_2 is due to closure of the aortic and pulmonic valves. S_1 is usually auscultated as a single sound. S_2, which is really composed of two sounds closely linked in time (AoV closure and pulmonic valve closure), exhibits a splitting.

> **KEY FACT**
>
> The slope of the *y* descent decreases in tamponade (ie, the RA empties slower) and increases in constrictive pericarditis.

TABLE 1-10. **Heart Sounds and Significance**

Sound	Significance
S_1	MV and tricuspid valve closure; the MV closes before the tricuspid, so S_1 may be split.
S_2	Aortic and pulmonary valve closure; the AoV closes before the pulmonic valve; inspiration causes increased splitting of S_2.
S_3	During rapid ventricular filling (early diastole); normal in children; in adults, associated with dilated ventricles (ie, dilated CHF) and increased filling pressures.
S_4	Late diastole; not audible in normal adults; its presence suggests high atrial pressure or a stiff ventricle (ie, ventricular hypertrophy). The left atrium must push against a stiff LV wall ("atrial kick").

CHF = congestive heart failure.

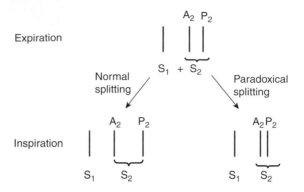

FIGURE 1-25. **S₂ splitting: Normal and pathologic states.** During inspiration, the pulmonic valve closes even later, augmenting the split between A_2 (aortic valve closure) and P_2 (pulmonic valve closure). However, in paradoxical splitting—which is associated with aortic stenosis—P_2 and A_2 come closer during inspiration.

- **Normal splitting:** S_2 splits during inspiration for two reasons:
  - Inspiration decreases intrathoracic pressure, which increases venous return to the heart and delays pulmonic valve closure (P_2 delayed).
  - Inspiration has the opposite effect on A_2 since blood wants to stay in the lung (lower intrathoracic pressure). This transiently decreases venous return to the LA and LV, reduces LV filling, shortens LV emptying, and results in earlier AoV closure (A_2) (Figure 1-25).
- **Wide splitting:** Seen with any condition in which RV emptying is delayed (pulmonic stenosis, right bundle branch block). The delay in RV emptying causes a delayed pulmonic sound (P_2), independent of breathing.
- **Fixed splitting:** Associated with ASD. The left-to-right shunt of ASD causes increased flow through the pulmonic valve such that pulmonic valve closure is significantly delayed. Fixed splitting is independent of breathing.
- **Paradoxical splitting:** Seen with any condition in which LV emptying is delayed (aortic stenosis, left bundle branch block). Due to delayed aortic valve closure, the P_2 sound is heard before the delayed A_2 sound. Inspiration causes the delayed A_2 and earlier P_2 sounds to move closer, effectively eliminating the split.

REGULATION OF ARTERIAL PRESSURE

Arterial pressure varies in a pulsatile pattern during the cardiac cycle. It is assessed by measuring systolic pressure and diastolic pressure; both values are used to calculate pulse pressure and MAP (Figure 1-26).

- **Systolic pressure:** Highest arterial pressure of the cardiac cycle. Measured after the heart contracts and blood has been ejected into the arterial system. In older patients, it is increased due to age-related stiffening of large arteries. In younger patients, it is increased due to increased SV. Decreases with dehydration, β-blockers, diuretics, and blood loss.
- **Diastolic pressure:** Lowest arterial pressure of the cardiac cycle. Corresponds to the time when the heart is relaxed and blood is returning to the heart via the venous system. Decreases with aortic stiffening (decreased compliance), which results in less blood volume in the aorta at the onset of diastole.
- **Pulse pressure:** Difference between systolic and diastolic pressure; depends mainly on SV. Decreased vessel capacitance secondary to aging

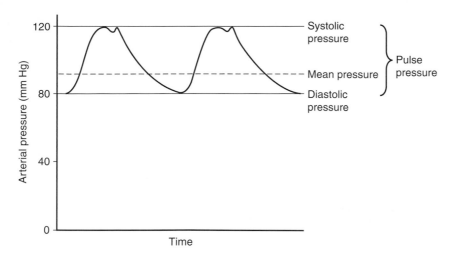

FIGURE 1-26. **Arterial pressure during the cardiac cycle.**

(think stiffer pipes) increases the pulse pressure since systolic pressure increases as diastolic pressure decreases.

$$\text{Pulse pressure} = \text{systolic pressure} - \text{diastolic pressure}$$
$$\textbf{MAP} = \text{diastolic pressure} + \tfrac{1}{3} \times (\text{pulse pressure})$$

Regulation of Mean Arterial Pressure

Changes in MAP are detected by either baroreceptors or the kidney as decreased extracellular circulating volume (ECV) (Figure 1-27). Decreased baroreceptor firing is centrally processed and relayed to the autonomic nervous system (ANS), whereas decreased ECV activates the renin-angiotensin-aldosterone system (RAAS). The baroreceptor reflex is neurally controlled and

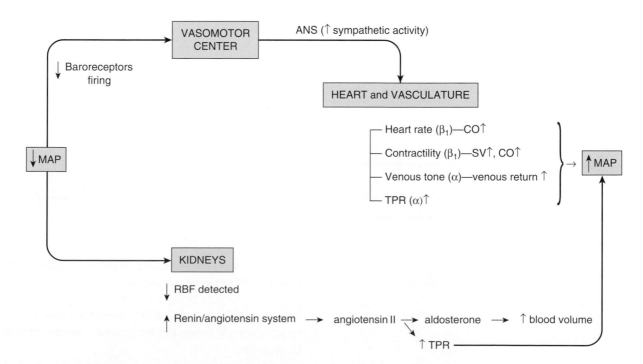

FIGURE 1-27. **Control of Mean Arterial Pressure (MAP).** ANS, autonomic nervous system; CO, cardiac output; RBF, renal blood flow; SV, stroke volume; TPR, total peripheral resistance.

Mechanisms to regulate BP:
- Baroreceptor reflex (short term): Baroreceptors in the sinus are always active, and increased activity indicates ↑ in BP
- RAAS (long term)
- Cerebral ischemia leading to hypercapnia
- Hypoxia with P_{O_2} < 60 mm Hg
- Severe volume depletion leading to ADH secretion
- Atrial stretch mediated by atrial natriuretic peptide (ANP)
- Autoregulation

has a fast (minute-to-minute) response, whereas the RAAS is hormonally controlled with a slower regulation response.

Mechanisms other than the fast baroreceptor reflex and slower RAAS to regulate arterial pressure are based on P_{CO_2}, P_{O_2}, blood volume, and atrial pressure (Table 1-11).

Baroreceptor Reflex: Short-Term Regulation of Blood Pressure

Stretch receptors located within the walls of the carotid sinus and aortic arch respond to both MAP and pulse pressure. Carotid sinus baroreceptors are tonically active, so increased activity indicates an increase in BP, and decreased firing indicates decreased arterial pressure. Changes in firing rate at the carotid sinus (transmitted by CN IX) and at the aortic arch (transmitted by CN X) are relayed to the vasomotor center of the brain stem and elicit an ANS response.

For example, decreased firing secondary to perceived drop in BP leads to decreased parasympathetic and increased sympathetic outflow to the heart, leading to increased HR, contractility, SV, and vasoconstriction of arterioles and veins (Figure 1-28).

Maneuvers that affect baroreceptor reflex:

- Increased sympathetic nervous system (SNS) output, decreased parasympathetic nervous system (PNS) output: leads to increase in blood pressure.
- Carotid occlusion, cutting afferents, orthostasis/lying to standing, and fluid loss.
- Increased PNS output, decreased SNS output: leads to a dramatic decrease in blood pressure).
- Carotid massage, volume loading, and weightlessness.

AUTONOMIC NERVOUS SYSTEM

The sympathetic and parasympathetic nervous systems of the ANS affect HR via the SA and AV nodes, conduction velocity, and blood vessel tone through

TABLE 1-11. **Other Mechanisms That Regulate Arterial Pressure**

TRIGGER	RESPONSE
↑ P_{CO_2} in brain tissue (cerebral ischemia)	↑ Sympathetic outflow to heart and blood vessels.
↓ P_{O_2} detected by chemoreceptors in carotid and aortic bodies	Vasoconstriction to increase total peripheral resistance (TPR) and arterial pressure.
↓ Blood volume (eg, hemorrhage)	Release of vasopressin (ADH) leads to vasoconstriction, which increases TPR and water reabsorption.
↑ Atrial pressure	Release of atrial natriuretic peptide (ANP) to relax vascular smooth muscle to reduce TPR and increase natriuresis to reduce blood volume.

ADH = antidiuretic hormone.

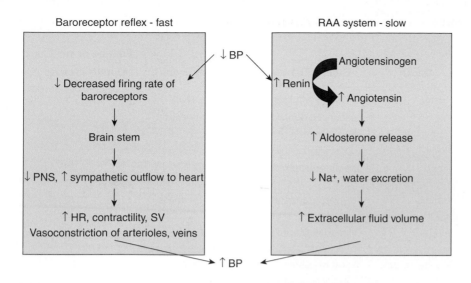

FIGURE 1-28. Effect of decreased blood pressure (BP) on baroreceptors and the renin-angiotensin-aldosterone (RAA) system. HR, heart rate; PNS, parasympathetic nervous system; SV, stroke volume.

action on β_1- and muscarinic acetylcholine receptors (mAChR), respectively (Table 1-12).

Renin-Angiotensin-Aldosterone System: Long-Term Regulation of Blood Pressure

Decreased BP activates the RAAS. Renin is secreted by the kidneys and increases conversion of angiotensinogen to angiotensin, which causes increased release of aldosterone from the adrenal cortex, decreased Na^+ and water excretion, resulting in increased extracellular fluid volume and BP (see Figure 1-28).

Autoregulation

Each organ has a different mechanism to maintain constant blood flow over a wide range of perfusion pressures (Table 1-13). Except for the pulmonary vasculature, in which hypoxia induces vasoconstriction, hypoxia causes vasodilation in all other organs, thus increasing delivery of blood and O_2 to starved tissues.

KEY FACT

Conduction velocity through the AV node is controlled by:
- SNS: ↑ conduction of APs from atria to ventricles, which may compromise ventricular filling time
- PNS: ↓ conduction leads to ↑ PR interval

CLINICAL CORRELATION

Angiotensin-converting enzyme (ACE) inhibitors impede the RAAS pathway and thus are commonly used in the management of hypertension.

KEY FACT

Circulation through organs:
Liver: Largest share of systemic cardiac output
Kidney: Highest blood flow per gram of tissue
Heart: Largest arteriovenous O_2 difference; ↑ O_2 demand met by ↑ coronary blood flow.

TABLE 1-12. Autonomic Effects on the Heart and Blood Vessels

	SYMPATHETIC	PARASYMPATHETIC
Heart rate	↑ via β_1-receptor	↓ via mAChR (contractility
Conduction velocity at AV node		decreased in atria only)
Contractility		
Vascular smooth muscle	Constriction via α_1-receptor	
	Relaxation via β_2-receptor	

AV = atrioventricular; mAChR = muscarinic aceytlcholine receptor.

TABLE 1-13. **Autoregulation in Various Organs**

ORGAN	FACTORS DETERMINING AUTOREGULATION	PORTION OF THE CARDIAC OUTPUT RECEIVED (%)
Heart	Local metabolites: O_2, adenosine, NO; enhanced during mechanical compression in systole	5
Brain	Local metabolites: CO_2 (pH)	15
Kidneys	Myogenic and tubuloglomerular feedback	20
Lungs	Hypoxia-induced vasoconstriction	100
Skeletal muscle	Local metabolites: lactate, adenosine, K^+ (also bundle of His, bradykinin)	20
Skin	Sympathetic stimulation	5

HEMODYNAMICS AND PERIPHERAL VASCULAR CIRCULATION

Physical factors such as blood flow, velocity, resistance, and capacitance govern blood flow within the circulatory system. The components of blood and the circulatory system (ie, types of vasculature) are reviewed briefly.

Blood

Normal adult blood composition is illustrated in Figure 1-29. Note that serum = plasma – clotting factors (eg, fibrinogen).

Components of the Vasculature

The vasculature includes arteries, arterioles, capillaries, venules, and veins, each of which has different composition and function (Table 1-14).

KEY FACT

Arterioles: Site of highest resistance in the CV system
Capillaries: Largest total cross-sectional and surface area (remember, this facilitates gas exchange!)
Veins: Highest proportion of blood in the CV system

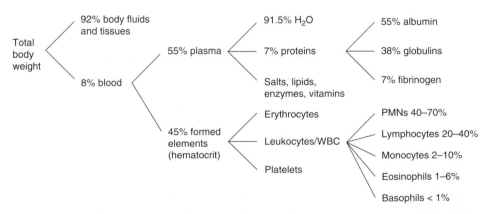

FIGURE 1-29. **Normal adult blood composition.** PMNs, polymorphonuclear neutrophils; WBC, white blood cells.

TABLE 1-14. **Function and Composition of the Vasculature**

	COMPOSITION	PRESSURE	FUNCTION
Artery	Thick-walled with elastic tissue, smooth muscle	High	Deliver oxygenated blood to tissues
Arteriole	Smooth muscle with innervation from autonomic nerve fibers	High	Smallest branches of arteries
Capillary	Single layer of endothelial cells, thin-walled	Low	Exchanges nutrients, water, and gases with surrounding tissues
Venule	Thin-walled	Low	Formed from merging capillaries
Vein	Thin-walled	Low	The largest vein, the vena cava, returns blood to the heart

Hemodynamic Parameters

VELOCITY OF BLOOD FLOW

$$v = Q/A$$

where

v is velocity (cm/sec)
Q is blood flow (mL/min)
A is cross-sectional area (cm^2)

Velocity is directly proportional to blood flow ($\uparrow$ blood flow $\rightarrow$ $\uparrow$ velocity), and inversely proportional to area (ie, blood flow velocity is > in the aorta [smaller cross-sectional area] than in the capillaries [larger total cross-sectional area]).

BLOOD FLOW

$$Q = \Delta P/R$$

Relationship is analogous to Ohm's law ($I = V/R$), where

Q (blood flow or cardiac output, mL/min)	$\leftrightarrow$	I (current)
ΔP (pressure gradient, mm Hg)	$\leftrightarrow$	V (voltage)
R (resistance, mm Hg/mL/min)	$\leftrightarrow$	R

- Blood flow is inversely proportional to blood vessel resistance and can be hormonally controlled. **Histamine** and **bradykinin** mediate arteriolar dilation and venous constriction, promoting blood flow to the site of their secretion, whereas serotonin causes arteriolar constriction. **Prostaglandins** have different effects—prostacyclin is a vasodilator in several vascular beds, but thromboxane A$_2$ acts as a vasoconstrictor.
- **Coronary blood flow:** During systole, coronary arteries are compressed $\rightarrow$ increased coronary vascular resistance $\rightarrow$ decreased coronary blood flow. The largest proportion of coronary blood flow occurs during diastole.

RESISTANCE (R)

$$\text{Resistance} = \frac{\text{driving pressure } (\Delta P)}{\text{flow } (Q)} = \frac{8\eta(\text{viscosity}) \times \text{length}}{\pi r^4} \text{ (Poiseuille's law)}$$

Resistance is inversely proportional to the fourth power of the blood vessel radius, so increasing the radius by 2 times decreases the resistance by a factor of $2^4 = 16$! Resistances in parallel or series can be calculated with the following equations:

- In **parallel** (eg, systemic circulation in which each organ is supplied by an artery that branches off the aorta)

$$1/R_{total} = 1/R_a + 1/R_b + \cdots + 1/R_n$$

- In **series** (eg, the arrangement of blood vessels in a given organ; the incoming large artery becomes arterioles, capillaries, and veins that are arranged in series)

$$R_{total} = R_{artery} + R_{capillaries} + R_{veins}$$

- The same volume of blood flows through each set of vessels (ie, blood flow through the largest artery is the same as through all the capillaries).

Arterioles have the largest proportion of resistance, and they are responsible for the largest drop in perfusion pressure.

CAPACITANCE (COMPLIANCE)

$$C = V/P$$

where

C is capacitance (mL/mm Hg)
V is volume (mL)
P is pressure (mm Hg)

Capacitance describes how distensible a blood vessel is and is inversely related to elastance. Since veins are more compliant than arteries, more blood is stored in veins than in arteries. With aging, vessels stiffen and become less compliant.

Laminar Versus Turbulent Flow

Laminar flow is streamlined (ie, travels in a straight line). Turbulent flow is not and causes audible vibrations (bruits). Turbulence is increased by:

- Decreased blood viscosity (eg, anemia)
- Increased blood velocity (eg, narrower vessel, increased CO)

Capillary Fluid Exchange

Fluid movement is determined by osmotic and hydrostatic pressures in the capillary and interstitial space, which are known as Starling forces (Figure 1-30). These include:

- P_c = Capillary pressure: Tends to push fluid out of the capillary
- P_i = Interstitial fluid pressure: Tends to push fluid into the capillary
- π_c = Plasma colloid osmotic pressure: Tends to pull fluid into the capillary
- π_i = Interstitial fluid colloid osmotic pressure: Tends to pull fluid out of the capillary

KEY FACT

Velocity $v = Q/A$
Blood flow $Q = \Delta P/R$
Resistance

$$R = \frac{\text{driving pressure } (\Delta P)}{\text{flow } (Q)} =$$

$$\frac{8\eta(\text{viscosity}) \times \text{length}}{\pi r^4}$$

(Poiseuille's law)

Capacitance $C = V/P$

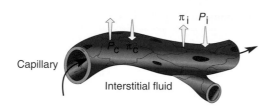

FIGURE 1-30. Capillary fluid exchange. P_c = capillary pressure; P_i = interstitial fluid pressure; π_c = plasma colloid osmotic pressure; π_i = interstitial fluid colloid osmotic pressure.

NET FILTRATION PRESSURE

The net filtration pressure (P_{net}) is the sum of the Starling forces. Note that the force is positive if entering the capillary (arteriolar end) and negative if leaving the capillary (venular end).

$$P_{net} = [(P_c - P_i) - (\pi_c - \pi_i)]$$

NET FLUID FLOW

The new fluid flow (J_v, mL/min) is determined by P_{net} and K_f, the filtration constant (capillary permeability). This relationship is known as the **Starling equation.** A positive J_v means net fluid movement out of the capillary (filtration).

$$J_v = K_f \times P_{net} = K_f[(P_c - P_i) - (\pi_c - \pi_i)]$$

LYMPHATICS

Lymph from the right side of the upper body empties into the right lymphatic duct. All other lymph from the rest of the body empties via the **thoracic duct** into the venous system. Lymph has the same composition as the surrounding interstitial fluid.

EDEMA

Occurs when volume of interstitial fluid > capacity of lymphatics and filtration; caused by increased K_f, increased P_c, and/or decreased π_c (these all increase J_v) (Tables 1-15 and 1-16).

TABLE 1-15. Causes and Examples of Edema

CAUSE	EXAMPLES
↑ P_c	↑ Venous pressure
	Standing, which causes edema in the dependent limbs
↓ π_c	↓ Plasma protein concentration secondary to:
	▪ ↓ Synthesis (liver disease)
	▪ ↓ Intake (protein malnutrition)
	▪ ↑ Excretion (nephrotic syndrome)
↑ K_f	Burns
	Inflammation

TABLE 1-16. Types of Edema

	TRANSUDATE	EXUDATE
Mechanism	↑ Capillary pressure (P_c) or ↓ oncotic pressure (π_c).	More permeable vessels (↑ K_f). Due to lymphatic obstruction, inflammation, etc.
	Fluid from the vessel is either pushed out or leaves based on differences in osmotic pressure.	The vessel becomes leakier; therefore both protein and fluid leave.
Composition of fluid	Protein-poor. Hypocellular. Specific gravity < 1.012.	Protein-rich. Cellular. Specific gravity > 1.020.

ELECTROCARDIOGRAPHY

Electrocardiograms (ECGs) are recordings of electrical impulses flowing through the heart. They provide information about cardiac structure and function. These impulses follow a distinct pathway, known as the cardiac conduction system:

- An electrical impulse begins at the **SA node.**
- The impulse traverses the atria to the **AV node.**
- The AV node conducts the impulse slowly, which allows atrial contraction to be completed before ventricular depolarization and contraction occur.
- Conduction continues through the **bundle of His** and into **right and left bundle branches.**
- Bundle branches divide into **Purkinje fibers,** which stimulate myocardial cell contraction.

KEY FACT

Locations and corresponding leads:
Inferior = II, III, aVF
Septal (anterior) = V_1, V_2
Anterior = V_3, V_4
Lateral = I, V_5, V_6, aVL

Electrocardiogram Lead System

Twelve leads record along set axes—six leads on the **frontal** plane (I, II, III, aVR, aVL, and aVF) and six on the **transverse/horizontal** (V_1–V_6) plane of the body, also known as the chest, or precordial, leads (Figure 1-31). ECG is recorded on 1-mm graph paper at a speed of 25 mm of recording paper per

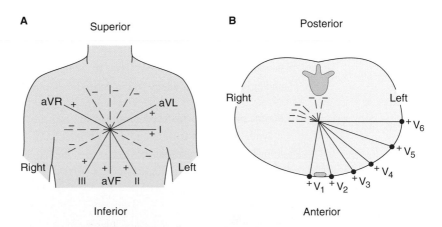

FIGURE 1-31.   (A) Frontal and (B) precordial leads. (Modified with permission from Kasper DL, Braunwald E, Fauci AS, et al. *Harrison's Principles of Internal Medicine,* 16th ed. New York: McGraw-Hill, 2005: 1312.)

TABLE 1-17. Electrocardiographic Intervals

INTERVAL	NORMAL RANGE
PR	0.12–0.20 sec (3–5 small boxes)
QRS	≤ 0.10 sec (≤ 2.5 small boxes)
QT	Corrected QT* ≤ 0.44 sec

*Corrected QT = QT/√(R-R), R-R = distance between two QRS complexes.

second. Each millimeter (small box) corresponds to 0.04 second, and 5-mm grid lines indicate 0.2 second.

Electrocardiographic Features

- **P wave:** Atrial depolarization.
- **PR interval:** Measured from onset of P wave to onset of QRS. Corresponds to the time it takes the electrical impulse to travel from the SA node, through the AV node, to the start of ventricular depolarization. Depends on both conduction velocity through the AV node and HR.
- **QRS interval:** Measured from beginning to end of QRS complex. Corresponds to ventricular depolarization.
- **QT interval:** Measured from beginning of QRS to end of T wave. Corresponds to mechanical contraction of the ventricles.
- **T wave:** Ventricular repolarization.
- **ST segment:** Isoelectric, ventricles depolarized.
- **U wave:** Seen in states of hypokalemia, bradycardia.

Normal interval lengths are listed in Table 1-17.

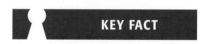

KEY FACT

↑ HR leads to ↓ PR interval.

ARRHYTHMIAS

Arrhythmias are abnormalities of electrical rhythm that result from alterations of **impulse conduction, impulse formation,** or both.

Wolff-Parkinson-White Syndrome

If an accessory pathway from the atrium to the ventricle is present (bundle of Kent), electrical impulses bypass the AV node, allowing the ventricle to partially depolarize earlier. This condition, known as Wolff-Parkinson-White syndrome, has a characteristic delta wave on ECG (Figure 1-32) and may result in a reentry current, leading to supraventricular tachycardia.

Disturbances of Impulse Conduction

Disturbances can be due to a delay or failure of conduction and can occur in any part of the cardiac conduction system; they are most common in the AV node (**AV block**) and bundle branches (**bundle-branch block**).

ATRIOVENTRICULAR BLOCK

- **First-degree AV block:** Conduction between atria and ventricles is delayed due to an abnormal AV node. Prolonged PR interval (≥ 0.20 sec), with each P wave followed by a QRS complex (Figure 1-33). Asymptomatic.

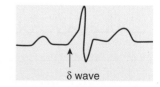

FIGURE 1-32. Characteristic delta wave seen in Wolff-Parkinson-White syndrome.

δ wave

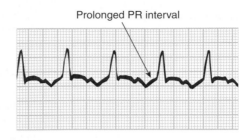

FIGURE 1-33. First-degree atrioventricular block.

Due to a wide variety of causes, including vagal stimulation, β-receptor antagonists, and infiltrative or degenerative conditions (eg, amyloidosis, sarcoidosis).

■ **Second-degree AV block:** Two types of second-degree AV block have been described (Figure 1-34).

■ **Mobitz type I (Wenckebach):** Intermittent failure of AV conduction. Progressive lengthening of the PR interval until a beat is "dropped" (P wave not followed by a QRS complex). Usually asymptomatic and rarely progressive to third-degree AV block.

■ **Mobitz type II (Hay):** Sudden, unpredictable loss of AV conduction. Dropped beats (QRS intervals) not proceeded by a change in the length of PR intervals (as seen with type I). It is often described as the ratio of P waves to QRS complexes, with 2:1 block most commonly seen. Often progresses to third-degree AV block and may require prophylactic pacing.

■ **Third-degree (complete) AV block:** Failure of any impulses to be conducted from atria to ventricles. Atria and ventricles beat independently of each other **(AV dissociation),** in which ventricles are depolarized by AV nodal or ventricular escape rhythm. As a result, both P waves and QRS complexes are present, but there is **no relationship** between P waves and QRS complexes (Figure 1-35). Atrial rate is faster than ventricular rate. Usually treated with a pacemaker.

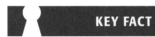

KEY FACT

In Mobitz type I second-degree AV block, PR intervals progressively lengthen before the dropped beat. In Mobitz type II, PR intervals are constant.

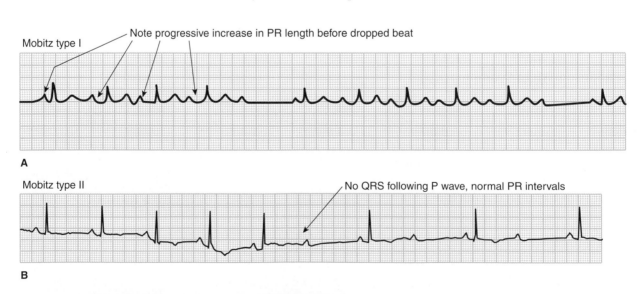

FIGURE 1-34. ECG tracings of second-degree atrioventricular block. (A) Mobitz type I, and (B) Mobitz type II.

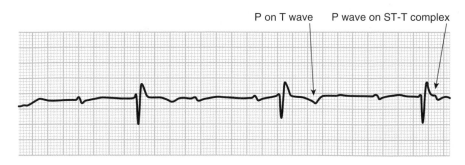

P on T wave   P wave on ST-T complex

FIGURE 1-35. ECG tracing of third-degree (complete) atrioventricular block.

BUNDLE-BRANCH BLOCK

Failure of impulse conduction through one of the bundle branches. Affected ventricle depolarizes much more slowly. For example, in left bundle-branch block (LBBB), the RV depolarizes before the LV.

Disturbances of Impulse Formation

Disturbances of impulse formation are due to an ectopic impulse originating from outside the SA node, which depolarizes the heart and causes an ectopic beat. These may originate from latent pacemaker cells (in the AV nodal area or His-Purkinje system) outside the SA node (**escape beats**), from the atria (**supraventricular arrhythmia**), or from the ventricles (**ventricular arrhythmia**).

ESCAPE BEATS AND RHYTHMS

Normally, pacemaker cells outside of the SA node (ie, AV node and His-Purkinje system) remain latent since their rate of depolarization is slower than that of the SA node; they are depolarized by the SA nodal impulse before they reach threshold and depolarize spontaneously.

However, if the SA nodal impulse fails to depolarize these pacemaker cells, they may reach threshold and produce an escape beat. Two types—junctional and ventricular escape beats—may occur, depending on their point of origin.

- **Nodal, or junctional, escape beats:** Originate from the AV nodal area and are conducted through the His-Purkinje system to the ventricles, producing a normal QRS complex. Junctional escape rhythms can be seen in third-degree (complete) AV block. Typical rate: 45–60/min.
- **Ventricular escape beats:** Originate from an ectopic ventricular focus (often Purkinje fibers). Abnormal QRS complex. Ventricular escape rhythm can be seen in third-degree (complete) AV block. Typical rate: 35–40/min.

SUPRAVENTRICULAR ARRHYTHMIAS

These originate above the ventricles and usually have normal QRS complexes.

- **Paroxysmal supraventricular tachycardia (PSVT):** Regular, rapid (150–250/min) arrhythmia that originates in atria or AV node. Often due to reentrant pathway in the AV node.
- **Atrial flutter:** Regular, rapid (250–350/min) arrhythmia originating from the atria. ECG shows a rapid succession of identical, back-to-back atrial depolarization waves, giving a **"sawtooth"** appearance (Figure 1-36).

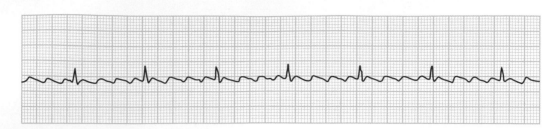

FIGURE 1-36. ECG tracing of atrial flutter.

KEY FACT

A mural thrombus adheres to a wall of the heart or major artery. Mitral stenosis is a risk factor for LA mural thrombus.

KEY FACT

Impulses that travel through the His-Purkinje system are associated with normal QRS complexes. Impulses that originate in the ventricles are conducted slowly through ventricular myocardium and produce an abnormal QRS complex.

Caused by reentry over a large anatomically fixed circuit. Not all atrial impulses are transmitted to ventricles because the AV node is in refractory period (physiologic AV block)—2:1 or 4:1 conduction. Attempt to convert to sinus rhythm; use class IA, IC, or III antiarrhythmics.

- **Atrial fibrillation:** Irregularly irregular, rapid (350–600/min) impulses from multiple atrial foci depolarize the atria. Chaotic and erratic baseline (**irregularly irregular**) with **no discrete P waves** and irregularly spaced QRS complexes (Figure 1-37). Associated with right or left atria enlargement. Atrial contraction is ineffective, causing decreased cardiac output and atrial stasis, and therefore predisposes for emboli formation and subsequent stroke. Treat with warfarin.

VENTRICULAR ARRHYTHMIAS

Arrhythmias that originate in ventricles and therefore have abnormal QRS complexes.

- **Premature ventricular contraction (PVC):** Ectopic ventricular pacemaker produces an ectopic beat before the next sinus beat occurs.
- **Ventricular tachycardia (VT):** Ectopic impulses originate in ventricles at a regular, rapid rate (100–250/min). Most frequently caused by reentry mechanism. Can deteriorate into ventricular fibrillation. **Torsades de pointes** is a form of VT in which QRS amplitude and axis change cyclically. Occurs most often in patients with prolonged QT interval.
- **Ventricular fibrillation:** Rapid, irregular ventricular depolarization due to impulses that originate from multiple ectopic ventricular foci. Completely erratic rhythm with no identifiable waves (Figure 1-38). Fatal arrhythmia without immediate defibrillation.

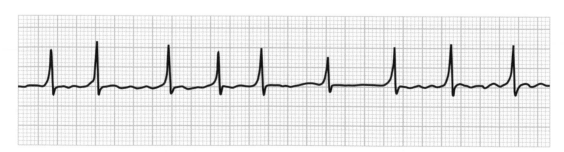

FIGURE 1-37. ECG tracing of atrial fibrillation.

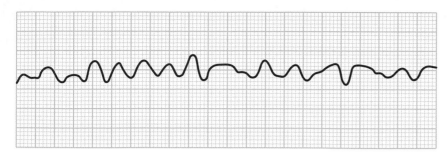

FIGURE 1-38. **ECG tracing of ventricular fibrillation.**

Pathology

HYPERTENSION

Hypertension affects more than 20% of the population and is a major risk factor for many CV diseases. It is defined as a sustained systolic pressure > 140 mm Hg and/or a diastolic pressure > 90 mm Hg. Risk factors include race (**African American** > Caucasian > Asian), obesity, **diabetes,** advanced age, **oral contraceptive use,** family history, excessive alcohol consumption, and **cigarette** smoking. Hypertension has several stages (Table 1-18).

Primary (Essential) Hypertension

Primary hypertension is the most **common** type of hypertension, comprising 95% of cases. Although there is no single identifiable cause, genetics, excessive salt intake, and increased **adrenergic tone** have all been implicated in primary hypertension.

Complications include atherosclerosis, **stroke, chronic kidney disease,** LV hypertrophy, **heart failure,** retinopathy, aortic dissection, and ischemic heart disease (IHD).

DIAGNOSIS

BP of > 140/90 mm Hg, confirmed on at least **three** separate occasions, or a single reading of > 170/110 mm Hg. Since it is a diagnosis of exclusion, secondary hypertension must be ruled out.

KEY FACT

The most common cause of atrial fibrillation in the United States is hypertension.

CLINICAL CORRELATION

For each 20-mm Hg ↑ in systolic or 10-mm Hg ↑ in diastolic pressure above 115/75 mm Hg, the CV disease risk doubles.

KEY FACT

Thiazide diuretics are usually the initial drug of choice for treatment of primary hypertension.

TABLE 1-18. **Stages of Hypertension**

	SYSTOLIC (MM HG)	DIASTOLIC (MM HG)
Normal	< 120	*and* < 80
Prehypertension	120–139	*or* 80–89
Stage 1	140–159	*or* 90–99
Stage 2	≥ 160	*or* ≥ 100

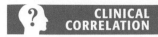

CLINICAL CORRELATION

ACE inhibitors have been proven to lower mortality and morbidity in diabetic hypertensives. They decrease renal hypertension by decreasing vasoconstriction of the efferent arteriole. This lowers intraglomerular pressure and helps prevent proteinuria.

TREATMENT

Initial treatment includes weight loss, decreased alcohol intake, increased exercise, reduced Na intake, and smoking cessation, collectively known as therapeutic lifestyle modifications.

Medical therapy involves the use of diuretics, β-adrenergic antagonists, angiotensin-converting enzyme (ACE) inhibitors, angiotensin receptor blockers (ARBs), calcium channel blockers, or α-adrenergic antagonists.

Secondary Hypertension

Secondary hypertension is increased systemic arterial pressure as a result of other identifiable conditions. Features of secondary hypertension may include onset of hypertension at **ages** < 20 or > 50 years old, BP > 180/110 mm Hg, abdominal bruits, and/or a **family history** of renal disease or **uncontrolled hypertension** despite maximal doses of three antihypertensive agents. Causes include:

- **Renal artery stenosis:** Causes include atherosclerosis (older patients, usually bilateral) and **fibrous dysplasia,** a "beaded appearance" on arteriogram (young women).
- **Renal parenchymal disease:** Treat with ACE inhibitors, which slow progression.
- Use of oral contraceptive pills, glucocorticoids, phenylephrine, and/or nonsteroidal anti-inflammatory drugs (NSAIDs) (preferentially constrict the afferent arteriole).
- **Pheochromocytoma:** Adrenal tumor secreting catecholamines. Manifests with **triad** of **hypertension, diaphoresis,** and **tachycardia.**
- **Primary aldosteronism (Conn syndrome):** Aldosterone-producing tumor causes **triad** of **hypertension, hypokalemia,** and **metabolic alkalosis** (increased aldosterone, decreased renin).
- Hyperthyroidism.
- Cushing syndrome.
- **Coarctation of the aorta:** Constriction of the aortic segment usually distal to the left subclavian artery. Leads to high BP in upper extremities, low BP in lower extremities, and differential cyanosis.
- **Fibromuscular dysplasia:** A disease resulting in narrowing of small and medium-sized arteries (primarily renal arteries), leading to hypertension. Often diagnosed in young women who present with headaches and uncontrollable hypertension.

PRESENTATION

Patients are usually asymptomatic but can present with signs and symptoms of end-organ damage, such as chest pain, peripheral edema, vision changes, and claudication. Additionally, the following may be found on physical exam and routine lab work:

- **Cardiac:** An S_4 heart sound due to increased resistance to ventricular filling and peripheral edema.
- **Renal:** Microalbuminuria, proteinuria.
- **Vascular:** Carotid bruits, hyaline arteriosclerosis, abdominal bruits.
- **Ophthalmologic:** Loss of venous pulsations, arteriovenous nicking, hemorrhages, and papilledema.

DIAGNOSIS

A thorough history and physical exam are necessary to detect clinical features of secondary hypertension. Specific diagnostic tests can also be very helpful.

- **Pheochromocytoma:** Symptoms of sweating and palpitations; increased urinary catecholamines, metanephrines, and **vanillylmandelic acid (VMA).**
- **Renal artery stenosis:** Auscultation of abdominal bruits on physical exam; increased plasma renin levels.
- **Hyperthyroidism:** Symptoms of **heat intolerance,** weight loss, weakness, and fatigue; decreased thyroid-stimulating hormone (TSH).
- **Coarctation of the aorta:** Absent or decreased femoral pulses on physical exam.

TREATMENT

Treatment varies depending on the underlying cause. Nonpharmacologic treatment includes weight loss, sodium restriction, smoking cessation, exercise, and reduction in alcohol intake. Antihypertensive medications include ACE inhibitors, ARBs, diuretics, vasodilators, calcium channel blockers, and α- and β-blockers.

Malignant Hypertension

Malignant hypertension is a severe, **rapid increase** in BP, usually > 240/120 mm Hg, associated with **organ damage** ("flea-bitten kidneys"). It is most often seen in young African American males. Clinically it is characterized by LV hypertrophy, papilledema, and retinal hemorrhages, as well as chest pain, dyspnea, angina, or headache. End-organ damage can manifest as pulmonary edema, azotemia, retinal hemorrhages, encephalopathy, seizures, and coma.

ARTERIOSCLEROSIS

Arteriosclerosis comprises a group of diseases that involve arterial wall thickening and loss of elasticity. They are divided into three categories (Table 1-19).

Mönckeberg Arteriosclerosis

A benign **medial** calcification of medium-sized (muscular) arteries that usually affects radial, ulnar, tibial, uterine, or femoral arteries in the elderly. It is normally asymptomatic and **benign** (unless associated with atherosclerosis).

Arteriolosclerosis

Affects the **intima** of small arterioles and arteries and is most often seen in the elderly and in those with diabetes, metabolic syndrome, or hypertension.

Microscopically there are two types of arteriolosclerosis:

- **Hyaline arteriolosclerosis: Protein** deposits seen in **essential hypertension** are visualized as pink arterial wall thickening with luminal narrowing.

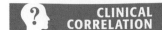

CLINICAL CORRELATION

Hypertensive urgency: BP > 180/120 mm Hg with no end-organ damage

Hypertensive emergency: BP > 180/120 mm Hg with end-organ damage

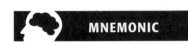

MNEMONIC

Mönckeberg is **M**edial calcification of the **M**edium-sized arteries.

TABLE 1-19. Features of Arteriosclerosis

	MÖNCKEBERG	**ARTERIOLOSCLEROSIS**	**ATHEROSCLEROSIS**
Artery size	Medium	Small	Medium to large
Affected layer	Media	Intima	Intima
Distinguishing feature	Calcification	Onion skinning	Foam cells

FLASH BACK

Metabolic syndrome is a group of risk factors in a single individual that increases risk for CV disease. These include insulin resistance, hypertension, abdominal obesity, dyslipidemia, and prothrombotic states.

FLASH FORWARD

In the kidney, hyaline arteriosclerosis is termed *benign* nephrosclerosis, and hyperplastic arteriosclerosis is termed *malignant* nephrosclerosis.

KEY FACT

Hyperlipidemia is defined as an excess of fat in the blood. These lipids can be triglycerides, cholesterol, cholesterol esters (compounds), or phospholipids.

KEY FACT

C-reactive protein (CRP) is a marker of inflammation, as seen in unstable plaques.

In diabetics, it is due to advanced glycosylation end products being deposited in the vessel's basement membrane. In patients with essential hypertension, it results from an increased pressure in the arteries that forces proteins into the wall, causing hardening of the artery.

- **Hyperplastic arteriolosclerosis:** Seen in **malignant hypertension,** it is visualized as an increase in smooth muscle proliferation and basement membrane duplication, leading to **"onion skinning"** (concentric wall thickening). Effects are especially prevalent in the renal arterioles (Figure 1-39).

Atherosclerosis

Usually affects **medium** and **large** arteries such as the aorta and the coronary, carotid, cerebral, and popliteal arteries. Lipid deposition, fatty streaks, and fibrous plaques form in the **intima** of medium to large arteries. Risk factors are divided into major and minor categories.

- **Major:** Hyperlipidemia, hypertension, smoking, diabetes, and obesity.
- **Minor:** Male gender, oral contraceptives, increased age, sedentary lifestyle, stress, elevated homocysteine level, family history, and infections (*Chlamydia pneumoniae*).

PATHOGENESIS

Endothelial cell injury → macrophages/platelets adhere to damaged endothelium and release cytokines → smooth muscle hyperplasia/migration of cells to the tunica intima → macrophages form **foam cells** within smooth muscle → fibrous cap develops → fibrous cap (plaque) calcifies dystrophically and ulcerates → platelets adhere to the ulcer, causing vessel thrombosis (Figure 1-40).

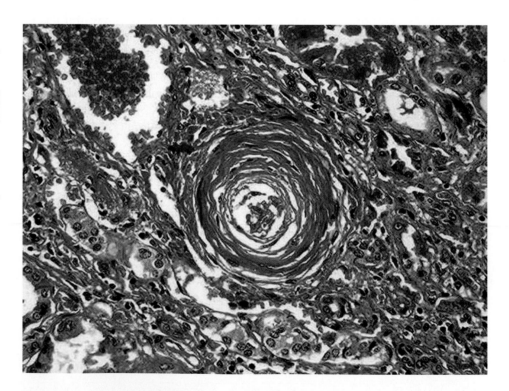

FIGURE 1-39. Hyperplastic arteriosclerosis. The basement membrane duplication and smooth muscle proliferation resemble the layers of an onion. (Reproduced with permission from USMLERx.com.)

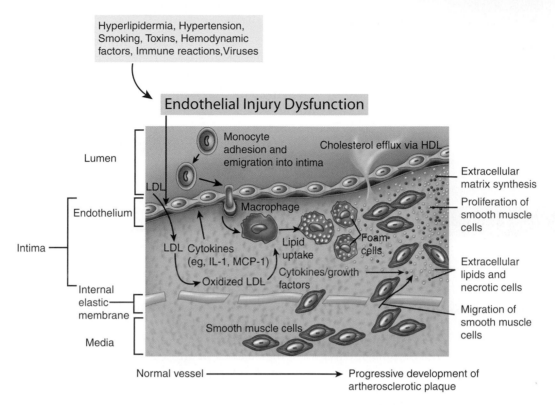

FIGURE 1-40. **Pathogenesis of atherosclerosis.** HDL, high-density lipoprotein; IL-1, interleukin-1; LDL, low-density lipoprotein; MCP-1, monocyte chemotactic protein-1.

HISTOPATHOLOGY

- Fatty streaks are flat and yellow and contain **foam cells, which can be visualized by microscopy** (lipid-laden macrophages).
- Fibrous plaques are elevated white plaques that contain a necrotic core of cholesterol, lipids, foam cells, and debris surrounded by a fibrous cap of collagen, smooth muscle, and lymphocytes (Figure 1-41).

KEY FACT

Aneurysm formation is often found below the level of the renal arteries since there are fewer vasa vasorum in the media of these vessels, leading to ↑ effect from ischemia.

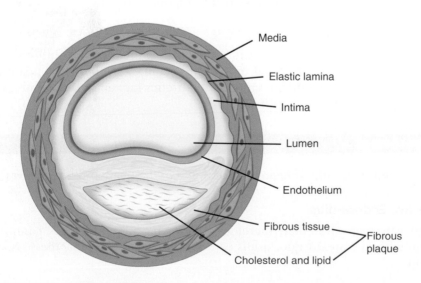

FIGURE 1-41. **Fibrous plaque.**

COMPLICATIONS

Plaque rupture, unstable angina, **myocardial infarction (MI)**, death, **stroke**, aneurysm formation due to artery wall degeneration, transient ischemic attacks, renal artery ischemia, peripheral vascular occlusive disease, impotence, **claudication**, proximal renal thrombosis → renin-angiotensin-aldosterone system (RAAS) activation and hypertension.

MYOCARDITIS

Myocarditis is inflammation of the heart muscle due to various causes, including infections, toxins, autoimmune diseases, and drug reactions. The most common cause of myocarditis in developed countries is a **viral infection** caused by coxsackie B virus, rubella virus, and cytomegalovirus; however, the most common cause worldwide is Chagas disease (caused by *Trypanosoma cruzi*).

Bacteria such as *Staphylococcus aureus*, *Corynebacterium diphtheriae*, and *Haemophilus influenzae* can also cause myocarditis.

Myocarditis in those with HIV can be caused by toxoplasmosis or Kaposi sarcoma metastasis. Other causes of myocarditis include Lyme disease, acute renal failure, rheumatic fever, lupus, and drugs such as doxorubicin.

PRESENTATION

Patients may present with any of the following: Chest pain, edema, and dyspnea from congestive heart failure (CHF); palpitations from arrhythmias; fever, diarrhea, and fatigue due to viral illness; a muffled S_1, an S_3, and a mitral regurgitation (MR) murmur.

DIAGNOSIS

ECG shows **diffuse** T wave inversions and ST segment elevations, which can mimic an MI or pericarditis. Biopsy is the gold standard, demonstrating edematous myocardial interstitium with lymphocytic infiltrate. Creatine kinase–myocardial bound fraction (CK-MB) and troponin may also be elevated.

TREATMENT

Supportive therapy for acute heart failure with diuretics, ACE inhibitors, or nitrates is often necessary. Viral myocarditis requires symptomatic treatment, including NSAIDs for inflammation and diuretics for ventricular failure. Bacterial myocarditis requires antibiotics.

ENDOCARDITIS

Endocarditis is an inflammation of the lining of the heart and heart valves.

Infective Endocarditis

Heart valves are avascular; therefore, if bacteria adhere, WBCs cannot be recruited to the area. Endocarditis can be acute (days) or subacute (weeks to months).

Acute infective endocarditis usually affects **normal heart valves** and is most often caused by *S aureus* or IV drug abuse because of the ability of *S aureus* to colonize normal valves.

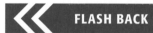

KEY FACT

Bacterial myocarditis is rare in patients who are immunocompetent.

FLASH BACK

Virulence factors of *S aureus* include **protein A** to inhibit phagocytic engulfment and **catalase** to enhance survival in phagocytes.

KEY FACT

Right-sided endocarditis suggests IV drug abuse. Since drugs are injected into the veins, the bacteria go to the right heart first.

Subacute infective endocarditis usually colonizes a **previously damaged valve** (in the setting of bacteremia from oral surgery or poor dentition). It is most often caused by viridans group of streptococci (Table 1-20).

PRESENTATION

Fever, chills, weight loss, systemic emboli, petechiae, **Janeway lesions** (painless peripheral hemorrhages on the palms and soles), **Osler nodes** (small, painful subcutaneous nodules on the fingers and toes), **splinter hemorrhages** (linear streaks under the fingernails and toenails), **Roth spots** (retinal seeding), and **valvular involvement** (mitral > aortic > tricuspid).

DIAGNOSIS

Duke criteria include positive serial blood cultures, prior endocardial involvement, IV drug use, fever, vascular or immune phenomena, and valvular lesions on echocardiography.

TREATMENT

Intravenous antibiotics targeted to the specific organism. For acute endocarditis, start antibiotics empirically—nafcillin and gentamicin provide good coverage. For subacute endocarditis, obtain blood cultures before starting antibiotics. Choices include ampicillin + gentamicin for native valves, and vancomycin, gentamicin, and rifampin for prosthetic valves.

Marantic Endocarditis

Nonbacterial endocarditis (nonbacterial thrombotic endocarditis [NBTE]) occurs when small, sterile fibrin vegetations deposit on the heart valves of people with debilitating disease. This is a paraneoplastic syndrome in which mucin-secreting tumors (usually of the colon or pancreas) cause mucin deposition on the heart valves, yielding a platelet-sticky nidus of infection. A major complication is a **sterile embolus,** which can lead to cerebral infarct. Marantic endocarditis has a poor prognosis.

FLASH FORWARD

Ring-enhancing brain lesions can be due to septic emboli from endocarditis; other causes include tumors, pyogenic abscesses, toxoplasmosis, and tuberculosis.

KEY FACT

Staphylococcus epidermidis mostly affects prosthetic valves within the first 6 months. After that, ***S aureus*** and the viridans group streptococci are the most likely culprits. In a patient with a prosthetic valve who develops a murmur, be sure to order both echocardiography and blood cultures.

TABLE 1-20. Bacterial Causes of Endocarditis

RISK FACTOR/PRESENTING FACTOR	BACTERIA TO CONSIDER
Prosthetic device	*Staphylococcus epidermidis*
Colon cancer	*Streptococcus bovis*
Dental procedure	Viridans group streptococci
GI surgery	*Enterococcus*
Total parenteral nutrition	Fungal
Alcoholics or the homeless	*Bartonella henselae*
Fastidious and culture negative	HACEK organisms

HACEK = *Haemophilus, Actinobacillus, Cardiobacterium, Eikenella,* and *Kingella.*

Libman-Sacks Endocarditis (LSE)

Libman-Sacks endocarditis is autoantibody damage to the heart valves from systemic lupus erythematosus (SLE). Sterile vegetations form on **both sides of the heart valves.** Often the patient is asymptomatic, but the condition can be picked up by the presence of a heart murmur.

Carcinoid Syndrome

Carcinoid tumors release an increased amount of serotonin, which leads to thickening, contraction, and decreased mobility of the **right-sided valves,** as well as blood vessel dilation. The left side of the heart is protected by serotonin inactivation in the lungs. The difference between **carcinoid syndrome** and **carcinoid tumors** is as follows:

- **Carcinoid syndrome** is a group of symptoms associated with carcinoid tumor. Its origin is most commonly in the terminal ileum, and the tumor is large enough to cause systemic effects such as abdominal pain, flushing, diarrhea, and wheezing.
- **Carcinoid tumor** is most commonly found in the appendix, but in general the tumor is too small to be symptomatic.

Diagnosis

Elevated levels of **5-hydroxindoleacetic acid (5-HIAA),** a serotonin metabolite, are detected in the urine. CT, MRI, and indium-111 pentetreotide scan (OctreoScan) can also be used in diagnosis.

Treatment

Surgery to remove the tumor is often first-line treatment. Octreotide (Sandostatin) injections can be used in those patients in whom surgery is not an option.

CARDIOMYOPATHIES

See Table 1-21.

TABLE 1-21.   Cardiomyopathies

	Dilated	**Hypertrophic**	**Restrictive**
Cause	Idiopathic, ethanol abuse, coxsackie B virus infection, cocaine abuse, Chagas disease, peripartum	Autosomal dominant	Senile/primary amyloidosis, sarcoidosis, Loeffler endomyocarditis
Clinical presentation	↓ EF and JVP, fatigue, cardiomegaly, dyspnea	Dyspnea, angina, S$_4$, syncope	Peripheral edema, dyspnea, ascites, JVD
Special notes	Most common form on chest film: balloon heart	Young athletes' chest film: banana-shaped LV	

EF = ejection fraction; JVD = jugular venous distension; JVP = jugular venous pressure; LV = left ventricle.

Dilated/Congestive Cardiomyopathy

The dilated variant represents approximately 90% of nonischemic cardiomyopathies. Echocardiography often reveals four-chamber enlargement.

Causes include: idiopathic (most common), alcohol abuse, thiamine deficiency, coxsackie B virus infection, Chagas disease, HIV, cocaine, doxorubicin, Lyme disease, sarcoidosis, hypothyroidism, Wegener granulomatosis, acromegaly, and peripartum cardiomyopathy.

PRESENTATION

Can manifest as right or left heart failure. Signs and symptoms can include decreased ejection fraction (EF), jugular venous distension (JVD), edema, orthopnea, hepatomegaly, or cardiomegaly.

DIAGNOSIS

Radiography shows an enlarged cardiac silhouette with pulmonary congestion. **Echocardiography** is the key diagnostic study and shows a dilated LV with a decreased EF.

TREATMENT

Similar to treatment of CHF: Digitalis, β-blockers, ACE inhibitors, ARBs, diuretics, vasodilators, or heart transplantation. Anticoagulation is used to prevent emboli.

Hypertrophic Cardiomyopathy (HCM)

This is usually an autosomal dominant disorder in which asymmetrical septal hypertrophy causes a decrease in LV compliance and diastolic dysfunction. Blood flows at an increased velocity over the hypertrophied septum, creating negative pressure, which draws the anterior mitral leaflet into the outflow tract, thereby causing subaortic obstruction to outflow via the Venturi effect. HCM can lead to sudden cardiac death seen in some **young athletes.**

PRESENTATION

Syncope, dyspnea, S_4 cardiac gallop due to an atrial kick into the noncompliant ventricle, cardiomegaly secondary to aberrant fibers in the myocardium, systolic murmur of mitral valve regurgitation (MR), and pain relieved by squatting and exacerbated by strenuous exercise.

DIAGNOSIS

The radiograph shows a dilated LA. **Echocardiography** is normally used for diagnosis and shows asymmetrical hypertrophy, MR, and diastolic dysfunction.

TREATMENT

The goal is to maintain ventricular filling in order to prevent obstruction. β-Blockers and calcium channel blockers are often used to slow the heart rate (HR) and increase diastolic filling time, as well as decrease myocardial O_2 consumption. Implantable cardioverter defibrillators (ICDs) are often implanted in high-risk patients to prevent sudden cardiac death.

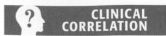

CLINICAL CORRELATION

Complications of dilated cardiomyopathy include cardiac arrhythmias, mural thrombi, CHF, bundle-branch blocks, and death.

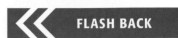

FLASH BACK

Vitamin **B₁** deficiency also leads to beriberi (see as **B**er1-**B**er1).

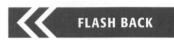

FLASH BACK

Chagas disease is caused by **T cruzi,** which is transmitted by the reduviid bug.

KEY FACT

Any maneuver that ↓ end-diastolic volume, such as Valsalva maneuver or exercise, ↑ the murmur's intensity in both mitral valve prolapse (MVP) and hypertrophic cardiomyopathy because the ↓ volume leads to a ↓ chamber size and ↑ obstruction.

KEY FACT

Primary amyloidosis is a disorder in which amyloid light-chain protein fibers are deposited in tissues and organs, impeding their function.

Restrictive Cardiomyopathy

The least common type of cardiomyopathy. It is caused by diseases that infiltrate the myocardium to impede diastolic filling of the heart. Common causes include **sarcoidosis, amyloidosis,** hemochromatosis, Loeffler endomyocarditis (most common worldwide), endocardial fibroelastosis (children), postradiation fibrosis, glycogen storage diseases (Pompe disease), inborn errors of metabolism (Fabry disease, Gaucher disease), and scleroderma.

PRESENTATION

Dyspnea, weakness, exercise intolerance, peripheral edema, ascites, JVD, S_4 gallop, pulsus paradoxus, CHF, and arrhythmias from conduction defects.

DIAGNOSIS

Radiography shows mild cardiomegaly. Echocardiography shows **thickening** of cardiac structures.

TREATMENT

There is no effective therapy except to treat the underlying disease. Heart transplantation is an option.

CONGESTIVE HEART FAILURE

KEY FACT

An S_3 heart sound is caused by vibration and turbulence as blood fills a ventricle that already has excess fluid due to systolic dysfunction.

CHF is defined as the inability of the heart to generate sufficient cardiac output to meet the metabolic demands of the body. It is a syndrome or diagnosis, not a specific disease. Heart failure can be the final manifestation of most cardiac disease, from hypertension to cardiomyopathy. The incidence in the United States is increasing due to the growing aging population and prolonged survival after cardiac insults. CHF is usually attributed to left heart failure; however, left and right heart failure often occur concurrently.

Left-Sided Heart Failure

There are two major causes of left-sided heart failure: (1) systolic dysfunction due to impaired contractility and/or increased afterload or (2) diastolic dysfunction due to impaired ventricular filling, relaxation, or compliance (Table 1-22).

TABLE 1-22. Etiology of Left-Sided Heart Failure

	SYSTOLIC DYSFUNCTION		DIASTOLIC DYSFUNCTION	
	IMPAIRED CONTRACTILITY	**INCREASED AFTERLOAD**	**VENTRICULAR RELAXATION**	**IMPAIRED VENTRICULAR FILLING**
Causes	Myocardial infarction	Hypertension	Ventricular hypertrophy	Mitral stenosis
	Myocardial disease	Aortic stenosis	Cardiomyopathy	Tamponade
	Myocardial ischemia Volume overload, mitral or aortic regurgitation	Hypertrophic cardiomyopathy	Myocardial ischemia	Pericardial constriction
Signs and symptoms	Dyspnea, orthopnea, fatigue, palpitations, ascites, S_3 gallop		Filling defect with increased or normal ejection fraction; S_4 gallop, edema, hepatomegaly	

PRESENTATION

Patients typically present with dyspnea on exertion, orthopnea, paroxysmal nocturnal dyspnea, pulmonary edema, reduced renal perfusion, and an S_3 heart sound. Most of these are due to failure of LV output and increased pulmonary venous pressure.

Microscopically, intra-alveolar hemosiderin-laden macrophages (heart failure cells), alveolar edema, and cardiac monocyte hypertrophy are seen. Complications include pulmonary congestion, cardiogenic shock, and hyperaldosteronism secondary to RAAS activation.

TREATMENT

Acute treatment involves relieving dyspnea and congestion with O_2, diuretics, nitrates, and morphine. Long-term management includes counteracting rise in hormone levels with β-blockers, ACE inhibitors, and ARBs.

Right-Sided Heart Failure

The most common cause of right-sided heart failure is left-sided heart failure. Other causes include cor pulmonale, which is right-sided heart failure **not** caused by left-sided heart failure, and pulmonary or tricuspid valve disease.

PRESENTATION

Patients usually present with splenomegaly, hepatomegaly/ascites ("nutmeg" liver), edema, and JVD. Renal hypoxia as well as right-sided pump failure leads to fluid retention clinically seen as pitting edema (first in the ankles), pleural effusions, and ascites (Figure 1-42).

Complications include cardiac cirrhosis due to long-standing congestion.

TREATMENT

Involves ACE inhibitors, which decrease afterload and prevent aldosterone-mediated salt and water retention. ACE inhibitors have been shown to

KEY FACT

ARBs are similar to ACE inhibitors in their effects; however, they do not increase bradykinin levels as do ACE inhibitors and thus do not have the side effect of dry cough.

KEY FACT

Cor pulmonale is an alteration of the structure and function of the right side of the heart secondary to chronic lung disorders, resulting in pulmonary arterial hypertension.

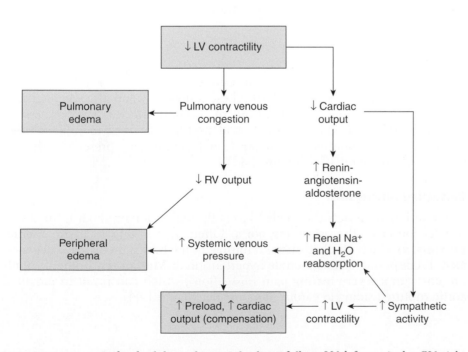

FIGURE 1-42. **Pathophysiology of congestive heart failure.** LV, left ventricular; RV, right ventricular.

MNEMONIC

To remember the treatments of acute decompensated CHF, think—

LMNOP
Lasix (furosemide)
Morphine
Nitrates
O$_2$
Position (better to sit up)

decrease mortality rates in CHF patients. Diuretics are also a mainstay in CHF treatment by preventing volume overloading. Digoxin is not used, as the EF in diastolic dysfunction is normal.

ANEURYSMS

Aneurysms are congenital or acquired **abnormal dilatations** of either an artery or vein due to weakness of the vessel wall. There are many types of aneurysms (discussed as follows). Complications of aneurysms include thrombus formation, erosion into nearby structures, and rupture leading to hypotension, shock, or death.

Abdominal Aortic Aneurysm (AAA)

Most common form of aneurysm. Typically affects men > 50 years old with **atherosclerosis** and occurs between the renal arteries and the aortic bifurcation. Classically manifests as a palpable pulsating abdominal mass. AAAs can become large, are filled with blood, and may result in **rupture** (with subsequent loss of massive amounts of blood into the peritoneal cavity), obstruction or compression of other structures, or **release of emboli** (resulting in stroke, MI). Abdominal ultrasound screening is recommended for past or active male smokers between 65 and 75 years old.

Atherosclerotic Aneurysms

Caused by atheroma formation leading to weakening of the media. Usually due to atherosclerotic disease or coronary artery disease (CAD) and associated with **hypertension.**

Syphilitic Aneurysms

Syphilis is a sexually transmitted disease (STD) that has primary, secondary, and tertiary stages. Seen in the tertiary stage, **syphilitic aortitis** is characterized by medial necrosis and **obliterative endarteritis** of the vasa vasorum, creating a functional deficit similar to atherosclerotic aneurysm. Usually involves the **ascending aorta** and aortic root. Involvement of the aortic valve (AoV) can lead to aortic insufficiency.

Berry Aneurysms

These are small, congenital, saccular lesions seen most often in the **circle of Willis.** Although not present at birth, these lesions develop at congenital sites of medial weakness at the **bifurcations of cerebral arteries.** They are associated with polycystic kidney disease, and rupture can lead to subarachnoid hemorrhage. A patient with a subarachnoid hemorrhage presents with "the worst headache of my life" (Figure 1-43).

Dissecting Aneurysms

Luminal blood dissects the medial layers through a longitudinal intimal tear usually found in the ascending aorta. Often, this is due to **cystic medial necrosis,** in which elastic tissue and muscle in the tunica media have degenerated. Predisposing factors include hypertension or **Marfan syndrome.** Patients present with a severe tearing pain (dissection), which can result in proximal aortic rupture leading to cardiac tamponade (Figure 1-44).

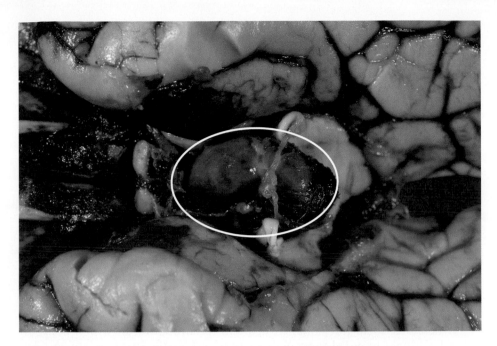

FIGURE 1-43. **Berry aneurysm.** Notice the grape-sized aneurysm (white oval) at the circle of Willis. (Reproduced with permission from USMLERx.com.)

Mycotic Aneurysms

Usually due to bacterial infection (most often salmonellosis) involving the abdominal aorta.

Microaneurysms

These are small aneurysms usually seen in diabetes and hypertension.

Arteriovenous Fistula

This is an abnormal communication between an artery and a vein, usually secondary to trauma. The diversion of blood can result in **ischemic changes,**

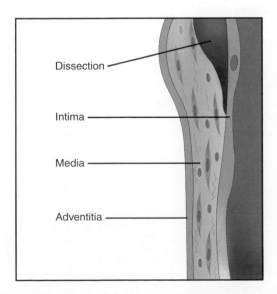

FIGURE 1-44. **Dissection.** A dissection occurs between the intima and media of a vessel.

KEY FACT

Sydenham chorea is an involuntary, purposeless contraction of the trunk muscles and extremities.

MNEMONIC

Group A STREP also causes rheumatic fever:
Sydenham chorea
Transient migratory arthritis
Rheumatic subcutaneous nodules
Erythema marginatum
Pancarditis

MNEMONIC

JONES PEACE

Major criteria:
Joints: migratory arthritis
Carditis: new-**O**nset murmur
Nodules, subcutaneous: extensor surfaces
Erythema marginatum
Sydenham chorea

Minor criteria:
PR interval, prolonged
ESR elevated
Arthralgias
CRP elevated
Elevated temperature (fever)

KEY FACT

Aschoff bodies contain both Aschoff cells and Anitschkow cells.

increased venous pressure causing **aneurysm** formation, and hypervolemia leading to **high-output cardiac failure.**

RHEUMATIC FEVER

Rheumatic fever is a multisystem inflammatory disease that may occur following pharyngeal infection with **group A β-hemolytic streptococci.** It usually affects children aged 5–10 years. It has been postulated that the streptococcal antigens elicit production of antibodies that cross-react with cardiac antigens.

PRESENTATION

Classically, patients complain of a pharyngeal infection 1–4 weeks prior and present with symptoms from the Jones criteria (Table 1-23 and Figure 1-45).

Acute Rheumatic Heart Disease

The most serious complication of rheumatic fever. It can be divided into:

- Fibrinous pericarditis.
- Myocarditis: focal interstitial myocardial inflammation in which collagen and fibrinoid material form nodules (**Aschoff bodies**) and are surrounded by macrophages (**Anitschkow cells**), lymphocytes, plasma cells, and multinucleated giant cells (**Aschoff cells**) (Figure 1-46).
- Endocarditis: The valve leaflets become red and swollen, and small verrucae (rubbery fibrin vegetations) form along the lines of closure. Eventually the valves become fibrotic, thickened, and calcified. Valvular disease can lead to either insufficiency or stenosis. Most often affected are the mitral and aortic valves since they see the greatest pressure gradient.

Chronic Rheumatic Heart Disease

Mitral and aortic valvular fibrosis causes valve thickening and calcifications, fusion of commissures, and short, thick chordae tendineae. The chronic form can lead to mitral stenosis (MS), MR, aortic regurgitation, and CHF. It can also predispose to infectious endocarditis.

TABLE 1-23. Jones Criteria

MAJOR CRITERIA	MINOR CRITERIA
Migratory polyarthritis	Arthralgia (most common)
Carditis	Fever
Subcutaneous nodules	High ESR/CRP
Erythema marginatum	Long PR interval
Sydenham chorea	ASO titer
	High WBC count
	Anemia

ASO = antistreptolysin O; CRP = C-reactive protein; ESR = erythrocyte sedimentation rate; WBC = white blood cell.

Two major criteria or one major and two minor criteria are needed for diagnosis.

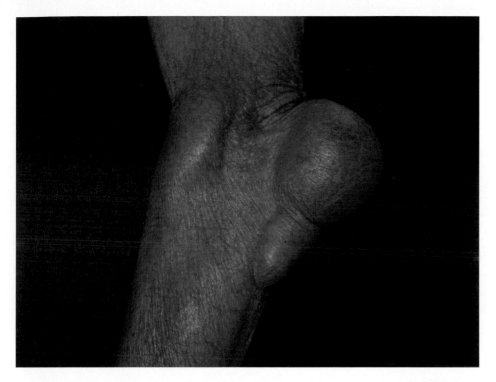

FIGURE 1-45. **Rheumatic subcutaneous nodule of the elbow.** (Reproduced with permission from USMLERx.com.)

DIAGNOSIS

Usually made through clinical suspicion and fulfilling the Jones criteria (see Table 1-23). A positive streptococcal antibody test can verify prior infection, and echocardiography can help in diagnosing CV problems.

TREATMENT

Symptomatic and involves:

- Treatment of group A streptococci with penicillin
- Use of steroids or salicylates for pain and inflammation
- Digitalis for heart failure
- Haloperidol for Sydenham chorea

 KEY FACT

Myocarditis leading to cardiac failure is a cause of death in acute rheumatic fever.

 KEY FACT

Erythema marginatum is seen as nonpruritic, serpiginous, erythematous rings on the patient's trunk and extremity, usually sparing the face.

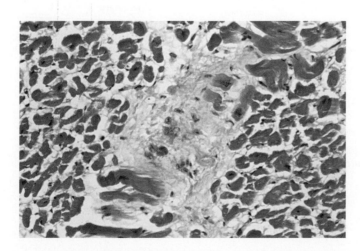

FIGURE 1-46. **Acute rheumatic heart disease.** Note the typical multinucleated Aschoff cells, which are modified histiocytes. (Image courtesy Dr. Ed Uthman.)

CLINICAL CORRELATION

The murmur of mitral valve prolapse (MVP), often seen in patients with Marfan syndrome and in young women, is exaggerated by the Valsalva maneuver.

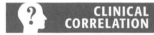

KEY FACT

An S_3 occurs in early diastole and implies volume overload in older adults. It can be normal in children and young adults.

CLINICAL CORRELATION

Tricuspid regurgitation is a blowing holosystolic murmur heard at the left lower sternal border that increases with inspiration due to the increase in venous return to the right side of the heart.

HEART MURMURS

Murmurs are normally generated by turbulent blood flow. If there are hemodynamic or structural changes in the heart, laminar flow may become turbulent, thus creating a heart sound. The most common hemodynamic or structural changes that occur to the heart are increased flow, decreased valvular area, regurgitation, dilated chambers, and shunting. Heart sounds are auscultated in four places on the anterior chest wall (Figure 1-47).

Murmurs can be divided into three groups (Table 1-24): Systolic (between S_1 and S_2), diastolic (between S_2 and S_1), and continuous (throughout the cycle or between S_1 and the next S_1).

Systolic Murmurs

MITRAL REGURGITATION (MR)

Insufficiency of the mitral valve allows for backflow of blood from the LV into the LA. Acute causes of MR include papillary muscle rupture, endocarditis, or ruptured chordae tendineae. Chronic causes include **rheumatic heart disease,** ischemic cardiomyopathy, dilated cardiomyopathy, hypertrophic cardiomyopathy, MVP, endocardial fibroelastosis, or endocarditis.

PRESENTATION

Clinically, patients can present with LV failure (dyspnea, orthopnea) and dilated LA due to increased volume. Chronic disease can lead to right-sided heart failure (peripheral edema or ascites).

On physical examination, an S_3 and a **holosystolic,** high-pitched, blowing murmur are heard best at the apex, radiating toward the left axilla. The murmur is holosystolic since LV pressure is always greater than LA pressure in systole. The increased flow in the LA can lead to increased LA pressure and **pulmonary edema** (Figure 1-48).

DIAGNOSIS

ECG changes include LV hypertrophy and LA enlargement. Echocardiography shows LA and LV enlargement.

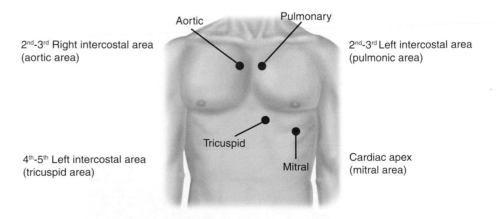

FIGURE 1-47. **Cardiac physical examination areas.**

TABLE 1-24. **Classification of Murmurs**

	SYSTOLIC			DIASTOLIC		CONTINUOUS
EJECTION	HOLOSYSTOLIC	LATE SYSTOLIC	EARLY	LATE	
Aortic stenosis	MR	MVP	Aortic regurgitation	Mitral stenosis	PDA
Pulmonic stenosis	Tricuspid regurgitation	HCM	Pulmonic regurgitation	Tricuspid stenosis	VSD

HCM = hypertrophic cardiomyopathy; MR = mitral regurgitation; MVP = mitral valve prolapse; PDA = patent ductus arteriosus; VSD = ventricular septal defect.

TREATMENT

The goal is to increase forward flow and decrease pulmonary venous hypertension. Medications include diuretics, ACE inhibitors, and digitalis. MV repair or replacement is usually required for symptomatic severe MR.

AORTIC STENOSIS (AS)

Usually due to thickening and calcification of the valves with age or rheumatic heart disease. More commonly seen with congenital bicuspid valves.

PRESENTATION

- Patients can have angina, syncope, or dyspnea from CHF.
- Crescendo-decrescendo systolic ejection murmur that begins shortly after the S_1 heart sound. Once the AoV opens, the murmur intensifies as the LV pressure increases (crescendo) and then subsides as the LV relaxes (decrescendo). The high-frequency murmur is best heard in the aortic area and usually radiates to the carotids (in the direction of turbulent blood flow) (Figure 1-49).
- Weak and delayed pulse at the carotid artery due to stenosis (pulsus parvus et tardus).

DIAGNOSIS

Echocardiography shows a thickened AoV with decreased systolic opening and LV hypertrophy.

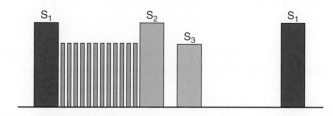

FIGURE 1-48. **Mitral regurgitation.** Note the holosystolic murmur followed by an S_3 heart sound.

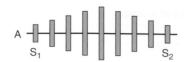

FIGURE 1-49. **Aortic stenosis.** Notice the crescendo-decrescendo pattern that is due to blood being forced through the narrowed aortic valve.

CLINICAL CORRELATION

Pulmonic stenosis is also a systolic ejection murmur that can radiate to the neck or shoulder and is loudest in the second and third left intercostal space.

FLASH BACK

A single ventricular chamber is divided into two chambers between the fourth and eighth weeks of gestation as muscle tissue forms from the apex to the cushion.

KEY FACT

Left-to-right shunting can lead to increased pulmonary and right atrial pressure; if these pressures eventually become greater than the left-sided pressures, the shunt will reverse and become right-to-left. This is called Eisenmenger syndrome.

TREATMENT

Surgical correction or balloon valvuloplasty.

VENTRICULAR SEPTAL DEFECT (VSD)

A developmental defect in the interventricular septum that allows the two ventricles to communicate. VSDs most often occur in the membranous ventricular septum.

PRESENTATION

A defect in this septum leads to left-to-right shunting of blood, which may result in increased pulmonary blood flow and pulmonary artery pressure. Infants with this congenital defect may present with a harsh systolic murmur, fatigue with feeding, poor growth, and respiratory infections.

DIAGNOSIS

The VSD murmur is a harsh, nonradiating holosystolic murmur best heard over the left sternal border at the third and fourth intercostal spaces. The smaller the VSD, the more turbulent the flow through it, resulting in a louder murmur over the entire precordium. Extremely large VSDs may be entirely silent (Figure 1-50).

TREATMENT

Surgery.

MITRAL VALVE PROLAPSE (MVP)

A common syndrome that affects up to 7% of women aged 14–30 years. Often called floppy valve disease, it occurs when the MV leaflets do not close properly and billow into the LA during ventricular systole. It can be an autosomal dominant disorder or acquired as part of a connective tissue disorder. The normal collagen and elastin are replaced by myxomatous connective tissue. Connective tissue disorders such as Marfan syndrome, SLE, the mucopolysaccharidoses, and Ehlers-Danlos syndrome can manifest with MVP.

PRESENTATION

Usually asymptomatic; however, it can cause chest pain, palpitations, labored breathing, or fatigue. The murmur heard in MVP is a late systolic murmur

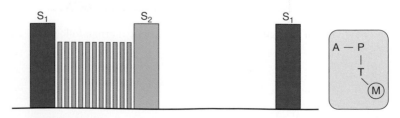

FIGURE 1-50. **Ventricular septal defect.** A, aortic valve; P, pulmonic valve; T, triscupid valve; M, mitral valve.

preceded by a midsystolic click that corresponds to the tensing of the mitral leaflet/chordae tendineae as they are forced into the LA. The murmur corresponds to the regurgitation of blood from the LV into the LA (Figure 1-51).

Valsalva maneuver decreases preload, and squatting increases preload. Any maneuver that decreases the volume of the LV, such as Valsalva or standing, allows the prolapse to occur sooner, causing an increase in the intensity of the murmur. Squatting, which increases venous return, increases ventricular volume, helping to maintain tension on the chordae tendineae and allowing the valve to stay shut longer, thus causing a decrease in the intensity of the murmur.

DIAGNOSIS

Doppler echocardiography can show systolic displacement of the mitral leaflets.

TREATMENT

β-Blockers for chest pain or arrhythmias. Surgical treatment is rare. Endocarditis prophylaxis is no longer indicated.

Diastolic Murmurs

AORTIC VALVE REGURGITATION (AR)

Allows backflow of blood from the aorta into the LV during diastole. It can be due to rheumatic heart disease, infectious endocarditis, aortic dissection, hypertension, syphilis, or Marfan syndrome. Regurgitation occurs during diastole, increasing the amount of blood the LV pumps out in the next cycle.

PRESENTATION

Patients typically present with:

- Dyspnea on exertion.
- Angina due to shorter diastole and decreased coronary artery filling.
- Fatigue.
- Wide pulse pressures.
- S_3 and an early diastolic decrescendo murmur heard best at the second right intercostal space (Figure 1-52).
- Austin Flint murmur, a mid-diastolic, low-pitched rumbling that occurs when the regurgitated blood hits the MV leaflet in diastole, preventing an opening snap (differentiating AR from MS).

AR → increased LV volume → increased LV diastolic pressure → increased LA and pulmonary pressure → pulmonary edema.

Midsystolic click

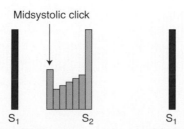

S_1 S_2 S_1

FIGURE 1-51. **Mitral valve prolapse.** Notice the midsystolic click that precedes the systolic murmur.

CLINICAL CORRELATION

MVP and hypertrophic cardiomyopathy are the only two murmurs with this paradoxic relationship. All other murmurs increase in intensity with increased preload (squatting) and decrease in intensity with decreased preload (Valsalva).

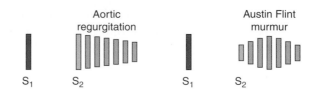

FIGURE 1-52. **Aortic regurgitation.** The murmur caused by aortic regurgitation has a decrescendo shape because there is a rapid diastolic relaxation of the left ventricle, and therefore a rapid pressure gradient is generated between the high-pressure aorta and the low-pressure ventricle. An Austin Flint murmur, however, has a crescendo-decrescendo pattern.

KEY FACT

Pulmonic regurgitation is usually due to pulmonary artery hypertension. It is also a decrescendo murmur and is heard best in the pulmonic area of the heart.

CLINICAL CORRELATION

Tricuspid stenosis is better heard at the lower sternum and ↑ with inspiration.

MNEMONIC

PASS and PAID
Pulmonary and **A**ortic **S**tenosis:
   Systolic murmurs
Pulmonary and **A**ortic **I**nsufficiency:
   Diastolic murmurs
Mitral and tricuspid murmurs are the
   opposite.

Chronic AR leads to LV dilatation. This dilatation allows the LV to accommodate more aortic regurgitation without further increases in diastolic pressure. The increase in LV systolic pressure without a concomitant increase in aortic diastolic pressure leads to a **widened pulse pressure.**

DIAGNOSIS

Echocardiography showing a dilated LV and aorta and aortic regurgitant flow. Regurgitation can cause a "pseudovalve" or "bird's-nest deformity" on the ventricular septum on pathologic examination.

TREATMENT

The goal is afterload reduction with ACE inhibitors and vasodilators. Diuretics and digitalis are also used. Valve replacement can help if EF decreases or symptoms develop.

MITRAL STENOSIS

Almost always due to rheumatic heart disease causing commissural fusion. Other causes, such as endocarditis with large vegetations and calcifications in the elderly, have also been noted as causes.

PRESENTATION

The stenotic obstruction in MS impedes LA emptying and leads to a pressure gradient between the LA and LV during diastole. Clinically, patients present with dyspnea, fatigue, and orthopnea. The characteristic murmur of MS is a high-pitched opening snap after S_2 followed by a decrescendo murmur or rumble that intensifies at the end of diastole and is best heard at the apex (Figures 1-53 and 1-54).

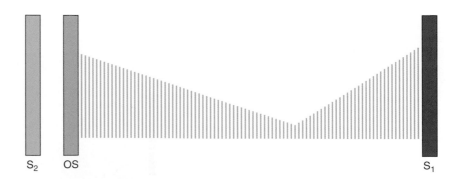

FIGURE 1-53. **Mitral stenosis.** The opening snap (OS) is due to the sudden tensing of the stenotic valve and chordae tendineae upon opening. The decrescendo murmur is caused by turbulent flow across the stenotic valve. The late diastolic intensification of the murmur is attributed to left atrium (LA) contraction at the end of diastole, which increases the pressure gradient between the LA and left ventricle.

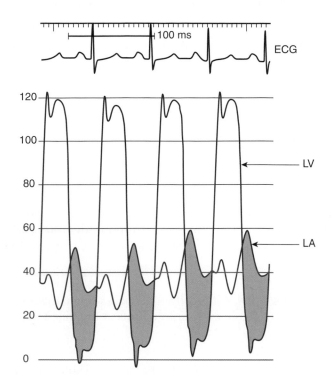

FIGURE 1-54. **Mitral stenosis pressure tracing.** This figure illustrates the difference in pressure between the left atrium (LA) and the left ventricle (LV). Also evident is the increase in pressure at the end of diastole, due to LA contraction. This is why there is a decrescendo-crescendo murmur associated with mitral stenosis.

DIAGNOSIS

Echocardiography shows thick MV leaflets and LA enlargement. ECG shows P mitrale (an **M**-shaped P wave) due to an enlarged atrium (Figure 1-55).

TREATMENT

Usually involves diuretics and a salt-restricted diet. Never use inotropes because MS is **not** equivalent to ventricular failure. Treatment also includes warfarin, β-blockers, and surgery/balloon valvotomy if needed.

Continuous Murmur

PATENT DUCTUS ARTERIOSUS (PDA)

Congenital disorder with persistent communication between the aorta and the pulmonary artery via a patent ductus arteriosus.

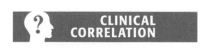

CLINICAL CORRELATION

In patients with a PDA, think about congenital rubella and prematurity. A common complication is endarteritis.

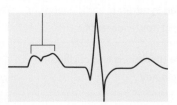

FIGURE 1-55. **P mitrale.** Note the **M**-shaped P wave (bracket) due to an enlarged atrium that is often seen in mitral stenosis.

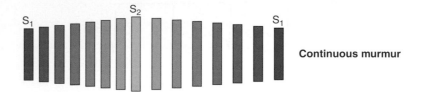

Continuous murmur

FIGURE 1-56. **Patent ductus arteriosus murmur.** Notice how the murmur spans both diastole and systole.

PRESENTATION

CHF and late cyanosis are often seen. Because the aortic pressure is always greater than pulmonary artery pressure in both diastole and systole, the machinery-like murmur is heard throughout the cardiac cycle (Figure 1-56).

DIAGNOSIS

Doppler echocardiography. Clinically, the well-known machinery-like murmur heard throughout systole and diastole hints at the diagnosis.

TREATMENT

Indomethacin is often used to close the PDA. See Table 1-25 for a summary of heart disease and associated murmurs.

MNEMONIC

Keep open with PGE; PGF closes.
E for the "**E**mpty" hand when open and **F** for the "**F**ist" that's closed.

TABLE 1-25. **Valvular Heart Disease**

VALVULAR DISEASE	ETIOLOGY	MURMUR
MR	**Rheumatic heart disease,** infective endocarditis, myxomatous degeneration, papillary muscle dysfunction, MVP, hypertrophic cardiomyopathy	Holosystolic blowing murmur radiating toward the apex
Mitral stenosis	**Rheumatic heart disease,** calcification, endocarditis	Late diastolic decrescendo rumble preceded by an **opening snap**
MVP	**Connective tissue disorder,** autosomal dominant	Late systolic murmur preceded by a **midsystolic click**
Aortic regurgitation	**Rheumatic heart disease, syphilis, Marfan syndrome,** aortic aneurysm, bicuspid AoV, endocarditis	Early blowing decrescendo diastolic murmur
Aortic stenosis	**Senile** (thickening and calcification), bicuspid AoV	Crescendo-decrescendo systolic ejection murmur

AoV = aortic valve; MR = mitral regurgitation; MVP = mitral valve prolapse.

CARDIAC TUMORS

Primary cardiac tumors are very rare (more rare than secondary tumors) and include myxomas and rhabdomyomas. Most cardiac tumors are metastatic from bronchogenic carcinoma, malignant melanoma, malignant lymphoma, and carcinoma of the pancreas and esophagus.

Cardiac Myxoma

The most common primary cardiac tumor in the **adult.** They are benign and found near the fossa ovalis in the **LA** in 90% of adults. They arise from endocardial mesenchymal cells, which proliferate and protrude into cardiac chambers. On microscopy, myxoma cells, endothelial cells, and smooth muscle cells are found in a mucopolysaccharide background. They may cause tumor emboli or **ball-valve** obstruction and syncopal episodes as they act on the MV (Figure 1-57).

Cardiac Rhabdomyoma

The most common primary cardiac tumor in **children.** They usually arise within the myocardium and are associated with **tuberous sclerosis.**

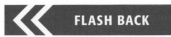

FLASH BACK

Tuberous sclerosis in an autosomal dominant disorder diagnosed in children that manifests with cortical tubers, hamartomas, hypopigmented "ash-leaf" skin lesions, renal angiomyolipomas, and cardiac rhabdomyomas.

VENOUS DISEASE

Varicose Veins

Varicose veins are tortuous, dilated, superficial vessels that normally involve the lower extremities. More common in women, they are thought to result from increased intraluminal pressure, intrinsic weakness of the vessel wall, or congenital defects of the valves that impair forward flow to the heart.

PRESENTATION

Patients have a history of pregnancy, prolonged standing, or obesity. Many people seek treatment for cosmetic reasons; however, symptoms can also include a dull aching pressure after long periods of standing, swelling and skin ulceration from valvular dysfunction, and thrombosis and hematoma from stasis of blood.

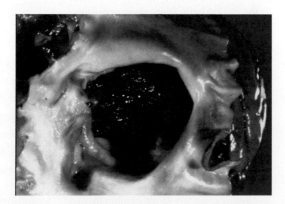

FIGURE 1-57. **Cardiac myxoma.** This image shows a cardiac myxoma attached by a small pedicle to the left atrial septum. They are normally single, pedunculated, and polypoid. (Courtesy of the Armed Forces Institute of Pathology [AFIP]).

TREATMENT

Treatment includes elevation of the legs, compression stockings to offset the increased venous hydrostatic pressure, and IV sclerosing agents. Surgical vein ligation and therapy is rare and only used in patients with symptomatic recurrent thrombosis or ulcers.

Deep Venous Thrombosis (DVT)

Blood clots most often occur in the calf veins, although they can also affect the popliteal, femoral, or iliac veins. Risk factors are summarized in **Virchow triad:** Stasis of blood flow, vascular damage, and hypercoagulability (Table 1-26).

PRESENTATION

Patients can be asymptomatic or present with calf or thigh discomfort, unilateral leg swelling, edema, erythema, and warmth or tenderness on palpation over the vein. Homans sign—dorsiflexion of the foot producing calf pain—is often used as a test but is unreliable.

DIAGNOSIS

Usually made through clinical judgment and laboratory testing. An increased D-dimer (fibrin degradation product) is sensitive but not specific. **Venous duplex ultrasonography** uses Doppler ultrasound to assess blood flow within the vein. This test is both sensitive and specific. The gold standard is angiography.

> **KEY FACT**
>
> The most common place for a DVT to develop is in the calves; however, it may also form in the deep veins of the thigh or even the upper extremities.

TABLE 1-26. Virchow Triad

SIGN OR SYMPTOM	EXAMPLES	PATHOGENESIS
Stasis/turbulence of blood flow	Immobilization (cast applied for bone fracture may cover damaged vessels as well); inactivity (postsurgery, long plane or car rides); hyperviscosity (polycythemia vera); turbulence (aneurysms) particularly common at the carotid bifurcation; deep sea diving (compression of legs and stasis).	Disruption of laminar flow increasing platelet-endothelium contact; there is a build-up of coagulation factors.
Vascular damage	Trauma, IV catheters, atherosclerosis.	Exposes collagen to increase von Willebrand factor binding and initiate the clotting cascade; endothelial damage also prevents antithrombotic secretions.
Hypercoagulable state	Clotting disorders (antithrombin III deficiency, antiphospholipid antibodies) high-estrogen states (pregnancy, oral contraceptives), smoking, neoplastic disease.	Malignancy involves necrotic tumor cells which secrete thrombogenic factors.

TREATMENT

The main objective is to prevent complications such as pulmonary embolism (PE) and postthrombotic syndrome. Elevation of the extremity helps reduce edema, and anticoagulation with heparin is started to prevent thrombus enlargement. For patients who cannot comply with anticoagulation or have medical conditions preventing anticoagulation, an intravascular filter is placed in the inferior vena cava (IVC) to prevent emboli from traveling from the extremity to the lungs.

Migratory Thrombophlebitis (Trousseau Syndrome)

Hypercoagulability secondary to malignancy resulting in venous thromboses appearing at one site, disappearing, and then reappearing in other veins. Occurs as a paraneoplastic syndrome (lung, pancreas, and colon).

Superior Vena Cava Syndrome

Symptoms include cyanosis, sensation of facial/head fullness, and dilation of head, neck, and arm veins. Caused by neoplasms (bronchogenic carcinoma and mediastinal lymphomas) compressing or invading the superior vena cava (SVC), leading to impaired drainage of the vessels above the level of the blockage. Often accompanied by respiratory distress (pulmonary venous compression).

Inferior Vena Cava Syndrome

Obstruction of the IVC manifests with edema in the legs, distention of the superficial veins of the lower abdomen, and, if renal veins are involved, massive proteinuria. Caused by neoplasms (liver and kidney cancers) or thrombi that compress or occlude the IVC.

EMBOLI

An embolus is a mass composed of tumor, air, blood clot, or vegetation, which travels in the bloodstream and is eventually trapped within the vasculature. Thromboembolism refers to the trapping of fragmented thrombi in various parts of human vasculature. Thrombi are the most common types of emboli; however, other forms such as fat emboli and gas emboli also occur.

Pulmonary Emboli

Pulmonary emboli usually arise from a DVT that has fragmented, with small portions traveling through the IVC and into branches of the pulmonary artery.

PRESENTATION

Often clinically silent, this diagnosis is frequently missed in the hospital setting. Patients can present with tachycardia, tachypnea, dyspnea, hemoptysis, cough, and/or chest pain.

DIAGNOSIS

Once clinically suspected, diagnostic tests include a $\dot{V}/\dot{Q}$ scan (which will reveal a ventilation-perfusion mismatch), spiral CT, pulmonary angiogram, or Doppler ultrasound.

KEY FACT

Red, or hemorrhagic, infarcts occur in tissues with collateral circulation, such as lung or intestine, or in tissues that are subsequently reperfused. Pale infarcts occur in solid tissue with a single blood supply, like the brain, kidney, or spleen.

FLASH BACK

Three congenital heart defects that do not cause cyanosis:
AS**D**
VS**D**
P**DA**

CLINICAL CORRELATION

Arterial embolism to an extremity → remember the 5 Ps
Pain
Pulselessness
Pallor
Paresthesias
Paralysis

TREATMENT

Options include anticoagulation therapy with heparin and warfarin or IVC filter placement to prevent future emboli. Thrombolytic therapy is also an option with substances such as tissue plasminogen activator or streptokinase; however, there is an increased risk of bleeding and stroke with thrombolytics.

PROGNOSIS

The majority of patients, if receiving the correct diagnosis, have no sequelae. Obstruction of the pulmonary artery can lead to a hemorrhagic pulmonary infarction in which the patient presents with shortness of breath, hemoptysis, and pleuritic chest pain. Sudden death occurs in cases of a saddle embolus, an embolus located at the bifurcation of the main pulmonary artery, and a minority of patients with multiple pulmonary emboli can have chronic pulmonary hypertension.

Arterial Emboli

An arterial embolus usually arises from a mural thrombus.

Arterial emboli often cause infarction involving the brain (branches of the carotid artery), kidney (branches of the renal artery), and the intestine (branches of the mesenteric artery). Other sites affected can include the spleen and lower extremities.

Paradoxical Emboli

Paradoxical emboli are venous emboli that cross over from the right side of the heart to the left side and access the systemic circulation. Most common coexisting defects are ASDs or a patent foramen ovale (PFO).

Fat Emboli

Bone marrow particles and fatty tissue travel to the lungs, brain, and kidney following severe long-bone fractures (occurs 24–48 hours post trauma). Patients present with petechiae, neurologic abnormalities, and pulmonary distress.

Gas Emboli

Caused by the introduction of air into the circulation. This is often seen in deep-sea divers who ascend from depth too rapidly. Nitrogen bubbles precipitate and block circulation, causing musculoskeletal pain also known as "the bends."

Amniotic Fluid Emboli

A complication of labor in which amniotic fluid leaks into the maternal circulation, most commonly after trauma or placenta abruptio. Complications include disseminated intravascular coagulation (80%) and death (20–90%).

SHOCK

Shock is a state of generalized hypoperfusion of tissues and cells in which O_2 delivery cannot meet O_2 demand. Initially the injury is reversible; however, as the hypoperfusion continues, the injuries become permanent and lead to multiple organ dysfunction syndrome (MODS). MODS can follow any type of shock and frequently involves the lung, kidney, heart, and liver (Tables 1-27 and 1-28).

TABLE 1-27. Types of Shock

TYPES OF SHOCK	PATHOPHYSIOLOGY	CLINICAL EXAMPLES	TREATMENT
Hypovolemic	Low circulating blood volume.	Hemorrhage, burns, vomiting, diarrhea, severe dehydration.	Fluid replacement and controlling fluid loss.
Cardiogenic	Pump failure, often due to the LV failure.	MI, arrhythmia, pulmonary embolism, cardiac tamponade.	IV inotropic agents to increase cardiac output, arterial vasodilators to reduce resistance.
Septic	Bacterial infection → endotoxin release → nitric oxide release, alternative complement pathway activation → polymorphonuclear leukocyte adherence to pulmonary capillaries → multiple organ dysfunction syndrome → tissue hypoxia.	Gram-negative septicemia, disseminated intravascular coagulation.	Fluid, vasopressors and antibiotics.
Neurogenic	Severe trauma → loss of sympathetic nervous system signals → peripheral vasodilatation.	Trauma involving spinal cord, brain stem, or cerebral injury.	Fluid and vasopressors.
Anaphylactic	Histamine release → increased venous capacitance.	Type I hypersensitivity reaction.	Epinephrine and securing the airway.

LV = left ventricle; MI = myocardial infarction.

PRESENTATION

Patients usually present with tachycardia, oliguria, hypotension, weak pulses, mental status changes, and cool extremities.

STAGES OF SHOCK

- **Compensation:** Reflex mechanisms maintain perfusion of vital organs. These mechanisms include increased HR, increased peripheral resistance, release of catecholamines, and activation of the RAAS.
- **Decompensation:** Reflex mechanisms can no longer compensate, leading to tissue hypoperfusion, reversible tissue injury, and metabolic imbalance (eg, metabolic acidosis and renal insufficiency).

TABLE 1-28. Hemodynamic Profile of Shock

TYPE OF SHOCK	CARDIAC OUTPUT	SVR	PCWP
Hypovolemic	↓	↑	↓
Cardiogenic	↓	↑	↑
Septic	↑	↓	↓
Anaphylactic	↑ or normal	↓	↓ or normal
Neurogenic	↓	↓	↓ or normal

PCWP = pulmonary capillary wedge pressure; SVR = systemic vascular resistance.

KEY FACT

Left anterior descending (LAD) infarction can cause left bundle-branch block (LBBB), anterior wall rupture, and mural thrombi. Right coronary artery (RCA) infarction can cause LV papillary rupture, posterior flail leaflet, and MR.

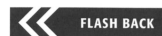

FLASH BACK

CO = HR × SV
SVR = (MAP − CVP) × 80 / CO

IRREVERSIBLE

Organ damage, organ failure, and irreversible tissue injury ultimately leading to death.

PATHOLOGY

- Kidney: Acute tubular necrosis, oliguria.
- Intestines: Mucosal ischemic necrosis and patchy hemorrhages, sepsis.
- Brain: Necrosis.
- Liver: Centrilobular necrosis ("shock liver").
- Adrenal: Waterhouse-Friderichsen syndrome with acute hemorrhagic infarction and adrenal insufficiency.

PERICARDIAL DISEASE

The pericardium is a double-layered sac that surrounds the heart, with the visceral pericardium lining the heart and the parietal pericardium on the outside. In between the two layers is pericardial fluid that helps to decrease friction.

Pericardial Effusion

Increased fluid accumulation sometimes occurs in the pericardial space. The volume of fluid, the rate of increase, and pericardial compliance all factor into the clinical symptoms of effusion. It can be acute or chronic (Table 1-29).

PRESENTATION

Usually asymptomatic, clinical features can include soft heart sounds, dullness over the posterior left lung and left-sided chest ache, or compressive symptoms such as dysphagia, hoarseness, or dyspnea.

DIAGNOSIS

Echocardiography can quantify the volume of fluid in the pericardial sac. ECG shows low voltages, and an increased cardiac silhouette is seen on chest radiograph.

TREATMENT

Involves treatment of the underlying disorder or pericardiocentesis.

TABLE 1-29. Acute Versus Chronic Pericardial Effusion

	ACUTE	CHRONIC
Cause	Pericarditis, cardiac surgery, uremia, and collagen vascular disease.	TB, cancer (lung, breast, or bone), SLE, HIV.
Presentation	Chest pain, pericardial friction rub, pericardiocentesis reveals small amounts of fluid.	With or without symptoms, large amounts of fluid on pericardiocentesis, symptom relief may or may not be seen after fluid is drained.

HIV = human immunodeficiency virus; SLE = systemic lupus erythematosus; TB = tuberculosis.

Cardiac Tamponade

A pericardial effusion with enough fluid and pressure to compress the heart chambers, leading to impaired cardiac filling. The most common causes include neoplasms; postviral uremia; CHF; and hemorrhage from trauma, ruptured LV following LAD MI, active tuberculosis, or dissecting aortic aneurysm.

PRESENTATION

Principal features include systemic venous congestion exhibited by JVD, peripheral edema and hepatomegaly, pulmonary venous congestion demonstrated by crackles (rales) on exam, and decreased cardiac output evidenced by hypotension and tachycardia. Other features include elevated diastolic intracardiac pressure, a quiet heart with decreased heart sounds, and pulsus paradoxus.

Normally with inspiration the intrathoracic pressure becomes more negative, leading to increased venous return and increased filling of the right heart. This leads to intraventricular septal bulging into the LV, causing decreased cardiac output and BP. Any disease that causes high negative intrathoracic pressures or impaired right ventricular filling or outflow will exaggerate this mechanism, causing a >10-mm Hg decline in systolic BP upon inspiration **(pulsus paradoxus)**.

DIAGNOSIS

Echocardiography can help evaluate for pericardial effusion. In tamponade, there is collapse of the RA and RV during diastole. Definitive diagnosis is by cardiac catheterization, which shows diastolic pressure equalization in all four chambers. ECG shows low voltage because the surrounding fluid blocks the signal and causes electrical alternans, which is an alternative beat variation due to alteration of the position of the heart in relation to the recording electrodes as a result of an enlarged pericardial sac.

TREATMENT

Removal of fluid through pericardiocentesis. The two locations for pericardiocentesis are in between the fifth or sixth intercostal space along the left sternal border or an infrasternal approach starting just inferior to the xiphoid process.

Acute Pericarditis

INFLAMMATION OF THE PERICARDIUM

There are four subtypes: serous, fibrinous, suppurative, and hemorrhagic. These may resolve or lead to scarring and chronic adhesive or chronic constrictive pericarditis (Table 1-30).

PRESENTATION

Patients present with retrosternal chest pain (worse on inspiration or coughing; relief while sitting or leaning forward), fever, hypotension, JVD, pericardial friction rub, and distant heart sounds.

DIAGNOSIS

Clinical suspicion with the presence of pleuritic and positional pain with a friction rub; ECG with diffuse ST segment elevation is often seen (Figure 1-58).

KEY FACT

The Beck triad of cardiac tamponade includes muffled heart sounds, elevated jugular venous pressure, and a fall in the systolic pressure.

FLASH BACK

Parasternal pericardiocentesis requires the needle to pass through the skin, superficial and deep fascia, pectoralis major muscle, external intercostal membrane, internal intercostal membrane, transversus thoracis muscle, fibrous pericardium, and the parietal layer of the serous pericardium.

MNEMONIC

Causes of pericarditis—

CARDIAC RIND
Collagen vascular disease
Aortic aneurysm
Radiation
Drugs (hydralazine)
Infections
Acute renal failure
Cardiac Infarction
Rheumatic fever
Injury
Neoplasms
Dressler syndrome

TABLE 1-30. Types of Pericarditis

DISEASE	EXUDATE	ASSOCIATIONS
Serous	Protein-rich, straw-colored, few inflammatory cells.	Associated with SLE, rheumatic fever, uremia, and viral infection (coxsackie B).
Fibrinous	Fibrin-rich with plasma proteins.	Associated with MI, uremia, or rheumatic fever; can lead to scar formation and diastolic filling defects.
Suppurative	Cloudy fluid with many inflammatory cells.	Caused by bacterial infection leading to erythematous serosal surfaces.
Hemorrhagic	Bloody and inflammatory fluid.	Due to tumor invasion or TB.

MI = myocardial infarction; SLE = systemic lupus erythematosus; TB = tuberculosis.

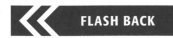

FLASH BACK

Dressler syndrome is a delayed pericarditis that develops 2–10 weeks after an MI.

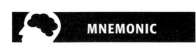

MNEMONIC

Konstrictive pericarditis presents with **K**ussmaul sign and a pericardial **K**nock.

TREATMENT

Treat the underlying cause, including NSAIDs for pain in viral pericarditis or Dressler syndrome.

Chronic Constrictive Pericarditis

Gradual resorption of acute pericarditis can lead to fusion of the pericardial layers and scar formation with possible calcifications leading to a stiff pericardium (see Table 1-29). This results in inhibition of diastolic filling, and signs similar to those of CHF may become evident. The most common cause worldwide is TB; however, it may also be secondary to pyogenic organisms or *Staphylococcus* spp. leading to obliteration of the pericardial cavity.

PRESENTATION

Patients present with fatigue, dyspnea on exertion, hypotension and tachycardia due to decreased cardiac output and JVD, and edema and ascites due to increased systemic venous pressure. Kussmaul sign is also seen, in which the jugular veins distend during inspiration. Heart sounds are distant, and a pericardial "knock" (early apical diastolic sound) is heard.

DIAGNOSIS

Chest radiograph may show an enlarged cardiac silhouette, and CT or MRI may show pericardial thickening. Confirmation is by cardiac catheterization showing increased diastolic pressures.

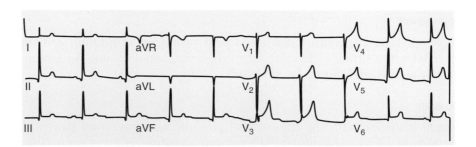

FIGURE 1-58. **ECG findings in acute pericarditis.** Notice the diffuse concave upward ST segment elevation.

TREATMENT

Effective treatment requires pericardial removal (pericardectomy).

PERIPHERAL VASCULAR DISEASE

Polyarteritis Nodosa (PAN)

A necrotizing immune complex inflammation and polymorphonuclear infiltration of the small to medium arteries that involves destruction of the media and internal elastic lamina. It most commonly affects middle-aged to older men, peaking at 50 years of age. It is common in patients with hepatitis B infection ($\leq$ 30% are infected).

PRESENTATION

Symptoms are either inflammatory in nature (eg, fever and musculoskeletal pain) or due to decreased organ blood flow (eg, headache, abdominal pain, and hypertension). Ischemia of vessels can lead to distal disruption including **ischemic heart disease, arthritis,** and **renal lesions.** There is **no lung involvement.**

DIAGNOSIS

Definitive diagnosis is by biopsy of the affected vessels. Antineutrophil cytoplasmic antibodies (ANCA) are highly suggestive of microscopic PAN.

TREATMENT

Immunosuppressants, prednisone.

Temporal Arteritis

Also known as giant-cell arteritis, temporal arteritis involves nodular inflammation, intimal fibrosis, and granulomas containing multinucleated giant cells in the medium to large arteries, most commonly of the carotid and aortic branches. Most often affects older women.

PRESENTATION

Often affects the temporal artery. Symptoms include headache and sudden-onset visual defects, absence of pulse, facial pain, and jaw claudication. Ophthalmic artery involvement can lead to blindness. Patients can also have polymyalgia rheumatica, characterized by severe stiffness and aches in the axial skeleton (neck, shoulder girdle, and pelvic girdle).

DIAGNOSIS

Definitive diagnosis is by biopsy of the affected vessel, usually the temporal artery, showing granulomatous inflammation. Elevated erythrocyte sedimentation rate (ESR) and CRP levels are also seen due to inflammation.

TREATMENT

First confirm elevated ESR, then immediately start high doses of systemic steroids to prevent loss of vision while awaiting biopsy results.

Takayasu Arteritis

Also known as pulseless disease, Takayasu arteritis is an inflammation of the aorta and its branches, usually affecting Asian women younger than 40 years old. It affects elastic arteries. (The most elastic arteries are the aorta and upper branching vessels.)

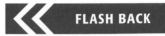

FLASH BACK

Cytoplasmic antineutrophil cytoplasmic antibody (c-ANCA) is often associated with Wegener granulomatosis.

Perinuclear antineutrophil cytoplasmic antibody (p-ANCA) is often seen in Churg-Strauss syndrome, microscopic polyangiitis, and primary sclerosing cholangitis.

KEY FACT

Raynaud phenomenon occurs when cold or stress exposure induces vasoconstriction of the digital arteries, causing the fingers/toes to turn white or blue. Primary Raynaud phenomenon (Raynaud disease) occurs in the absence of an underlying cause and is usually found in women, whereas secondary Raynaud phenomenon is usually found in men with a secondary systemic disorder.

MNEMONIC

Kawasaki Disease–

Remember CHILD
Conjunctivitis
Hyperthermia (fever) > 5 days
Idiopathic polymorphic rash
Lymphadenopathy (cervical)
Dryness and redness (lips, mouth, palms, and soles)

KEY FACT

The triad of Wegener is (1) focal necrotizing vasculitis, (2) necrotizing granulomas of the lungs and upper airway, and (3) necrotizing glomerulonephritis.

KEY FACT

Microscopic polyarteritis is a small-vessel vasculitis that is part of the Wegener granulomatosis spectrum. It presents with similar symptoms, ANCA, and histologic findings as Wegener, but without the respiratory findings.

PRESENTATION

Loss of the carotid, ulnar, and radial pulse leads to the distinctive "pulseless disease" designation. Inflammation of the affected vessels can lead to myocardial ischemia, hypertension, and visual defects. Systemic inflammatory effects such as fever, night sweats, arthralgia, and weight loss are also seen, most commonly in young Asian women.

DIAGNOSIS

Angiography.

TREATMENT

Steroids and cytotoxic drugs are used to reduce inflammation.

Thromboangiitis Obliterans

Also known as Buerger disease, thromboangiitis obliterans is a full-thickness inflammation of the distal extremity medium-sized arteries, veins, and nerves. It is strongly associated with **young men** who are **heavy smokers.**

PRESENTATION

Triad of distal arterial occlusion, Raynaud phenomenon, and migrating superficial vein thrombophlebitis. May be so severe that it progresses to gangrene.

DIAGNOSIS

Arteriography may show distal stenotic corkscrew vessels. Definitive diagnosis involves tissue biopsy.

TREATMENT

Smoking cessation.

Kawasaki Disease

A mucocutaneous disease characterized by acute necrotizing inflammation of the small, medium, and larger arteries. It is often found in children younger than 4 years. The most serious sequelae include coronary vessel involvement, leading to aneurysms.

PRESENTATION

Symptoms include fever present for at least 5 days, rash, fissured lips, cervical lymphadenopathy, edema, **desquamation of hands and feet,** bilateral conjunctivitis, oral erythema, and development of coronary artery aneurysms.

DIAGNOSIS

Diagnosis is made clinically; coronary angiogram is performed to diagnose coronary artery aneurysms.

TREATMENT

Aspirin and IV immunoglobin aid as anti-inflammatory agents. Long-term treatment in those with CAD includes aspirin and antiplatelet therapy. Anticoagulation is used in those with coronary aneurysms.

Wegener Granulomatosis

A necrotizing granulomatous lesion affecting the small vessels in the kidney, lung, and upper respiratory tract.

PRESENTATION

- Renal: Red blood cell casts in the urine, proteinuria
- Pulmonary: Cough, nasal septum ulcers/perforation, sinusitis, dyspnea, hemoptysis
- Skin: Purpura

DIAGNOSIS

Ninety percent of patients are c-ANCA-positive, and definitive diagnosis is made through biopsy showing necrosis and granuloma formation. Chest radiography shows nodular densities. Hematuria/red cell casts also aid in diagnosis.

TREATMENT

Prednisone, methotrexate, and cyclophosphamide.

Henoch-Schönlein Purpura (HSP)

A small-vessel IgA- and immune complex-mediated vasculitis that often follows upper respiratory infection in young children.

PRESENTATION

Symptoms include skin lesions that progress from blanching macules to petechiae to **palpable purpura,** often found on the **buttocks and legs** (nearly pathognomonic). Patients may also complain of edema, polyarthritis, colicky abdominal pain, hematuria, and hypertension.

DIAGNOSIS

The diagnosis is made clinically, since laboratory tests are often normal.

TREATMENT

Supportive therapy and the use of corticosteroids for GI symptoms.

Churg-Strauss Syndrome

A small- to medium-sized granulomatous vasculitis associated with antibodies to neutrophil cytoplasmic antigens (p-ANCA).

PRESENTATION

Patients present with asthma, cough, allergic rhinitis, arthralgias, and purpura. GI symptoms include bleeding, diarrhea, and colitis. Cardiac manifestations and peripheral neuropathy are also seen.

DIAGNOSIS

Criteria include asthma, peripheral eosinophilia, paranasal sinusitis, pulmonary infiltrates, histologic proof of vasculitis, and polyneuropathy. Often p-ANCA-positive (70%).

TREATMENT

Supportive therapy and glucocorticoids.

FLASH BACK

The main side effect of **C**yclophosphamide is **C**ystitis. Mesna is used to prevent cyclophosphamide-induced cystitis by binding to the metabolite acrolein in the bladder.

KEY FACT

Platelet counts are often normal or elevated in HSP, whereas they are decreased in idiopathic thrombocytopenic purpura (ITP).

KEY FACT

Cryoglobulinemic vasculitis is a small-vessel disease in which serum proteins precipitate out in the cold. Often due to hepatitis C infection, it is diagnosed with purpura, low complement, and immune deposits in vascular walls. Treatment involves plasmapheresis and hepatitis C treatment (interferon-alfa and ribavirin).

ISCHEMIC HEART DISEASE

IHD involves an interruption of arterial blood flow to the heart, leading to an inadequate supply of O_2; it is often due to atherosclerotic narrowing of the coronary arteries. Risk factors include hypertension, family history, smoking, hypercholesterolemia (LDL > 160 mg/dL or HDL < 35 mg/dL), diabetes mellitus, age (male > 45 years old or female > 55 years old/postmenopausal), and tobacco use. IHD can present as angina pectoris, chronic IHD, or MI.

Angina Pectoris

Episodic chest pain caused by a disparity between cardiac perfusion and cardiac demand, leading to transient hypoxia of the myocardium.

PRESENTATION

Typically manifests as retrosternal chest pain or pressure that can radiate to the neck, jaw, or left arm, and lasts anywhere from 15 seconds to 15 minutes. Patients are often diaphoretic and nauseated. Symptoms are very similar to patients with MI, but the ECG does not show any acute changes. Precipitating factors include cold, food, and stress, whereas relieving factors include rest and nitroglycerin. There are three types: stable angina, unstable angina, and Prinzmetal angina.

- **Stable angina:** The most common form in which pain is **induced by exertion** (usually the same amount of exertion causes pain); the pain is **relieved by rest** or nitroglycerin. Pain is thought to be due to **stenosis** of the atherosclerotic coronary arteries, which can no longer supply enough O_2 to meet the increased demands of the heart during exertion. If pain occurs with exertion, the coronaries are generally > 70% stenotic; if pain occurs at rest, the arteries are > 90% stenotic.
- **Unstable angina:** Pain at **rest** or with increasing frequency or duration during activity. Thought to be induced by a ruptured atherosclerotic plaque that leads to thrombosis and embolization. Unstable angina is more likely to lead to **MI** than is stable angina. Diagnosis is clinical with an angina-like presentation; however, no ST segment elevations are seen on ECG. Treatment involves aspirin, nitrates, β-blockers, and statins for lipid management. Heparin or glycoprotein IIb/IIIa inhibitors are also used. Patients are often sent for coronary angiography.
- **Prinzmetal angina:** Also called variant angina, it presents as **intermittent chest pain at rest** that is not related to activity, stress, or BP. Often occurs during the night. It is thought to be due to **coronary artery vasospasm.** Cardiac catheterization may not demonstrate atherosclerosis, and spasm can be precipitated with ergonovine. Definitive diagnosis involves exaggerated spasm of coronary arteries after injection with provocative agents, such as ergonovine, during coronary angiography. Treatment includes calcium channel blockers and nitrates.

DIAGNOSIS

Many diagnostic modalities are available. ECG may show prior MI or ischemia. Stress tests may reveal inducible ischemia, and coronary obstruction can be visualized on cardiac catheterization.

TREATMENT

Modification of risk factors is always helpful. Medical therapy for stable angina is shown in Table 1-31.

Surgical therapy includes coronary artery bypass graft and percutaneous transluminal coronary angioplasty.

TABLE 1-31.   **Drug Treatment for Stable Angina Pectoris**

DRUG	REASON FOR USE	SIDE EFFECTS
Nitrates	Venous dilation to ↓ preload, arteriolar dilatation to ↓ afterload, and coronary artery dilatation to ↑ O_2 supply.	Orthostatic hypotension, reflex tachycardia, blushing, headache.
β-Blockers	↓ Sympathetic drive will ↓ myocardial O_2 demand and improve survival.	Bronchoconstriction, insomnia.
Calcium channel blockers	↓ Preload and afterload.	Hypotension, reflex tachycardia, flushing, headache.

MYOCARDIAL INFARCTION

MI is due to myocardial necrosis secondary to inadequate cardiac tissue perfusion. This leads to microscopic changes in the heart and release of myocardial enzymes into the bloodstream. Risk factors include increasing age, hypercoagulable states, vasculitis, and those that predispose to atherosclerosis.

PRESENTATION

Patients describe prolonged (> 30–45 minutes) crushing chest pain similar to angina, but **not relieved by nitroglycerin,** as well as nausea, vomiting, sweating, shortness of breath, and weakness. There are two patterns of myocardial involvement: nontransmural and transmural (Table 1-32).

TABLE 1-32.   **Gross and Microscopic Changes to the Heart in Myocardial Infarction**

TIME	GROSS CHANGES	MICROSCOPIC CHANGES
0–6 h	None	Vascular congestion, wavy monocyte fibers, contraction bands.
12–24 h	Slight pallor, swelling, and softening	Start neutrophilic infiltration, **coagulation necrosis at 12 h.**
1–7 d	Yellow pallor	Neutrophilic infiltrate replaced by macrophages on day 4.
7–10 d	Yellow center softening surrounded by red border	Young fibroblastic growth and new vessel infiltration.
10–28 d	Red connective tissue replacing yellow necrotic tissue	Continued phagocytosis, collagen synthesis.
Months	Gray-white firm scar	Fibrous tissue replaces infarcted tissue that will not rupture because fibrosis adds to its strength.

FLASH BACK

Atherosclerosis risk factors include hypertension, hypercholesterolemia, age, cigarette smoking, and diabetes.

KEY FACT

Cocaine can cause MI by precipitation coronary vasospasm and thrombosis.

KEY FACT

Red infarcts occur in tissues with collateral circulation, such as the lungs or intestines.

Pale infarcts occur in solid tissues with a single blood source, such as brain, heart, and kidney.

- **Non-ST-elevation myocardial infarct (NSTEMI):** Also known as non–Q wave MI. This is a MI that is limited to the inner one-half to one-third of the LV wall. Coronary artery atherosclerosis results in decreased coronary blood flow and loss of perfusion to the wall. **ST-segment depression** is seen on ECG.
- **ST-elevation myocardial infarct (STEMI):** This occurs following atherosclerotic plaque rupture and thrombosis leading to complete vessel occlusion (no blood flow!). Necrosis of the entire myocardial wall is seen. ECG is characterized by Q waves and **ST-segment elevation** (Figure 1-59).

Coronary artery thrombosis affects LAD > RCA > left circumflex coronary artery.

DIAGNOSIS

ST segment elevation is seen in transmural infarcts. ECG changes include:

- Tall peaked T waves starting immediately and lasting up to 1 day
- ST segment elevation starting shortly after MI, due to injured myocytes
- Prolonged Q waves starting 1–4 days after MI, due to coagulative necrosis
- T wave inversion starting within 1 day, signifying ischemia at the periphery of the infarct

Echocardiogram can show ventricular wall hypokinesia or akinesia.

Cardiac enzymes are widely used for diagnosis (Figures 1-60 and 1-61).

- Troponin starts to elevate 4–6 hours after the pain starts and lasts 7–10 days. It is more specific than CK-MB.
- CK-MB is a specific enzyme for myocardial damage. Elevation starts 4–6 hours after the pain begins, peaks within 1 day, and lasts up to 3 days. It

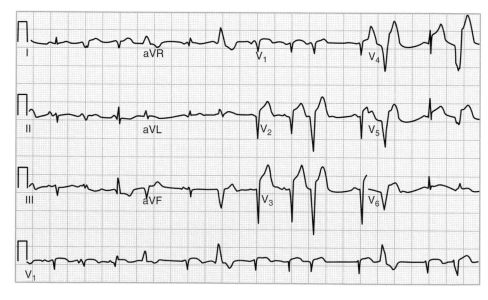

FIGURE 1-59. **ECG finding in ST elevation myocardial infarction.** Notice the ST segment elevation present in leads V_2–V_4. (Reproduced with permission from USMLERx.com.)

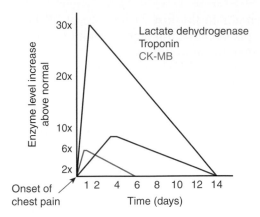

FIGURE 1-60. **Cardiac enzyme changes with myocardial infarction.** CK-MB, creatine kinase-myocardial bound fraction.

CLINICAL CORRELATION

When you see:	Think:
Coagulative necrosis	Ischemia of kidney or heart, pale tissue
Caseous necrosis	Tuberculosis, cheesy appearance
Liquefaction necrosis	Tissue softening in brain or spinal cord
Fat necrosis	Trauma
Gangrenous necrosis	Foul-smelling black tissue, superinfection, limbs

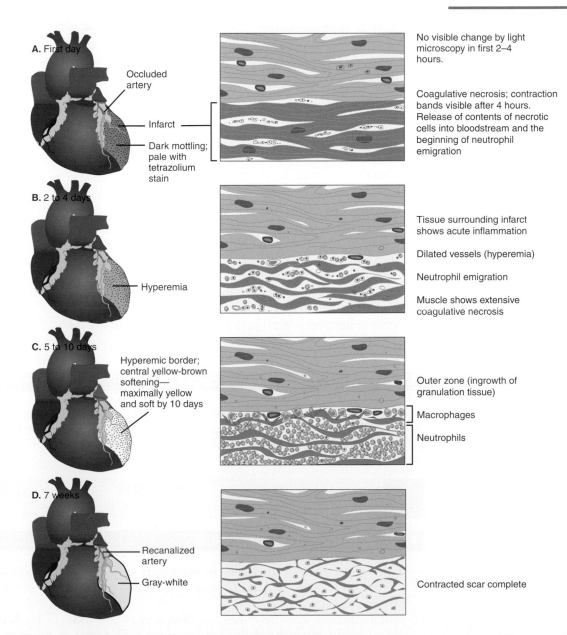

A. First day
Occluded artery
Infarct
Dark mottling; pale with tetrazolium stain

No visible change by light microscopy in first 2–4 hours.

Coagulative necrosis; contraction bands visible after 4 hours. Release of contents of necrotic cells into bloodstream and the beginning of neutrophil emigration

B. 2 to 4 days
Hyperemia

Tissue surrounding infarct shows acute inflammation

Dilated vessels (hyperemia)

Neutrophil emigration

Muscle shows extensive coagulative necrosis

C. 5 to 10 days
Hyperemic border; central yellow-brown softening— maximally yellow and soft by 10 days

Outer zone (ingrowth of granulation tissue)

Macrophages

Neutrophils

D. 7 weeks
Recanalized artery
Gray-white

Contracted scar complete

FIGURE 1-61. **Evolution of myocardial infarction.** (Modified with permission from Chandrasoma P. *Pathology Notes.* South Norwalk, CT: Appleton & Lange, 1991: 224.)

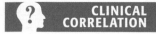

CLINICAL CORRELATION

At 7–10 days there is an increased chance of ventricular aneurysms or rupture of the papillary wall due to the central softening.

MNEMONIC

To remember when the enzymes peak—

1/2 T-CAL 123
Troponin: day **0.5**
CK-MB: day **1**
AST: day **2**
LDH: day **3**

KEY FACT

Pericarditis presents with a friction rub on auscultation.

is the test of choice in the first 24 hours post-MI because if it disappears and a second spike occurs, this signals another MI is occurring (troponin would be elevated the entire time).

■ Lactate dehydrogenase (LDH) is not used as frequently. It is elevated 12 hours after the pain starts and remains elevated for up to 2 weeks. Normally LDH-2 is greater than LDH-1, but in acute MI there is an "LDH 1-2 flip" and LDH-1 becomes elevated.

■ Serum aspartate aminotransferase (AST) begins to increase after 12 hours and lasts from 3–5 days. It is nonspecific, as it can be found in liver, cardiac, and skeletal muscle.

PROGNOSIS

■ Arrhythmia is a common cause of death within hours of an MI.
■ Sudden cardiac death.
■ Heart block.
■ Cardiogenic shock and CHF.
■ Mural thrombus and systemic embolism.
■ **Cardiac rupture,** resulting in cardiac tamponade, often 3–7 days after an MI (LAD infarct most common).
■ Posterior leaflet rupture (RCA).
■ Aneurysm.
■ **Pericarditis** is often seen 2–3 days post-MI but can occur later (at roughly 7 weeks = Dressler syndrome).
■ Silent MI occurs in the elderly diabetics who have a neuropathy that reduces sensory input.

TREATMENT

■ Acute treatment (MONA): **M**orphine, **O**xygen, **N**itroglycerin, and **A**spirin.
■ Aspirin therapy: Antiplatelet therapy decreases post-MI mortality.
■ Angioplasty is of more benefit than thrombolytics if it is readily available; however, if delayed its benefit is greatly reduced.
■ Thrombolytics: Tissue plasminogen activator or streptokinase can be given within 12 hours unless contraindicated.
■ β-Blockers have been shown to decrease mortality rates post-MI.
■ Analgesics.
■ Nitrates have no proven benefit in reducing mortality rates.
■ Heparin.

CHRONIC ISCHEMIC HEART DISEASE (CIHD)

Ischemic heart damage causes CHF that can lead to CIHD. Often found in the elderly, infarction leads to cardiac hypertrophy and decompensation. Typically, the patient has no history of angina.

Imaging

RADIOGRAPHY

■ X-ray penetration is inversely proportional to tissue density. Less X-ray absorption leads to a blacker image. Therefore, air is seen as black, while bone or metal is seen as white.
■ Posteroanterior view describes the direction of the beam. The X-rays are transmitted from behind the patient onto a film placed anterior to the patient's chest.

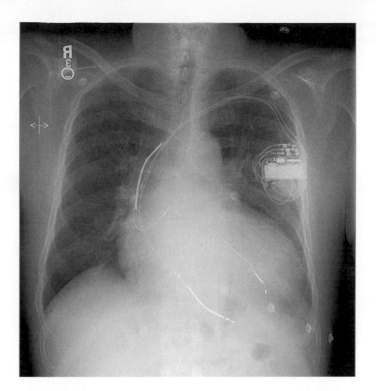

FIGURE 1-62.   Cardiomegaly. Notice the enlarged cardiac silhouette. (Reproduced with permission from USMLERx.com.)

- The normal cardiac silhouette occupies ≤ 50% of the width of the thorax. Cardiomegaly is apparent when the silhouette occupies > 50% of the width of the thorax (Figure 1-62).
- Increased pulmonary vasculature can be a sign of heart failure (Figure 1-63).
- It is imperative to be able to visualize both heart borders, as infection can blur the border lines.

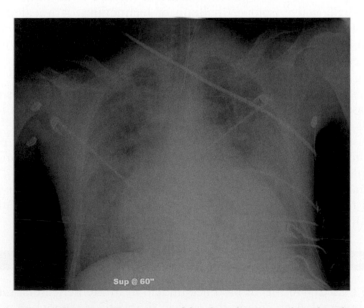

FIGURE 1-63.   Pulmonary edema. X-ray of the chest shows an enlarged cardiac silhouette, increased interstitial markings, Kerley B lines in the lateral right lower lung and perihilar alveolar infiltrates compatible with pulmonary edema in a patient with congestive heart failure. (Reproduced with permission from USMLERx.com.)

ECHOCARDIOGRAPHY

- A safe, noninvasive imaging modality using ultrasound.
- Can be used with Doppler to help evaluate blood flow, direction, turbulence, and estimation of pressure gradients.
- Can be transthoracic or transesophageal.
- Is used to evaluate fluid, ventricular function, valvular abnormalities, pericardial disease, cardiomyopathies, or CAD.

CARDIAC CATHETERIZATION

- Used for pressure measurement and contrast angiography.
- Right-sided pressures are normally measured by inserting a catheter through the femoral, brachial, or jugular vein, whereas left-sided pressures are measured through the brachial or femoral artery.
- Normal pressures are as follows:
  - RA: 0–8 mm Hg
  - RV: 15–30/0–8 mm Hg
  - Pulmonary artery: 15–30/4–12 mm Hg
  - PCWP: 1–10 mm Hg
  - LA: 1–10 mm Hg
  - LV: 100–140/3–12 mm Hg
  - Aorta: 100–140/60–90 mm Hg

NUCLEAR IMAGING

- Used to evaluate myocardial perfusion and viability.
- Uses ^{99m}Tc-labeled compounds or thallium-201.

STRESS TESTING

- Can employ exercise or drugs.
- In a nuclear stress test a patient is asked to exercise to maximum level and then a radioactive isotope (thallium or technetium) is injected into the bloodstream. The isotope enters the coronary arteries that supply the myocardium. Any area that does not receive adequate blood flow receives fewer isotopes, which is evident on the images. Stress images are compared with resting images.
- If a patient is unable to exercise, dipyridamole or adenosine is given to increase cardiac blood flow or dobutamine is given to utilize its inotropic effects.
- Abnormal results can signify CAD. The test can also be used for prognosis of patients post-MI and to determine the causes of chest pain in low-risk patients.
- Contraindications include acute MI within 2 days, severe aortic stenosis, acute myocarditis/pericarditis, acute pulmonary embolus, or acute aortic dissection.

PERICARDIOCENTESIS

- More than 20–30 mL of fluid accumulation in the pericardial sac is usually abnormal. A change in the cardiac silhouette is seen when > 250 mL of fluid accumulates.
- Indications include pericardial tamponade, symptomatic pericardial effusion, to obtain pericardial biopsy, and possible purulent pericarditis.

- Parasternal pericardiocentesis (the more common procedure) requires the needle to pass through the skin, superficial and deep fascia, pectoralis major muscle, external intercostal membrane, internal intercostal membrane, transversus thoracis muscle, fibrous pericardium, and the parietal layer of the serous pericardium.
- Subcostal pericardiocentesis requires the needle to pass through skin, superficial fascia, deep fascia, outer layer of the rectus sheath, rectus abdominis muscle, posterior layer of the rectus sheath, fibers of the diaphragm at its attachment to the costal margin, endothoracic fascia of the diaphragm, fibrous pericardium, and serous parietal pericardium.

Pharmacology

ANTIHYPERTENSIVE AGENTS

Hypertension is a common and serious disease with many sequelae, including MI, stroke, systemic vascular disease, and renal disease. Several classes of drugs are used to treat hypertension.

Diuretics

Diuretics act on the kidney with the primary purpose of reducing blood volume by increasing the rate of urine excretion. Reduction of blood volume leads to a decrease in BP. There are several types of diuretics, and they can be divided into separate classes based on their mechanism and site of action. Figure 1-64 serves as a review of the major diuretics and their mechanism of action in the kidney.

OSMOTIC DIURETICS (EG, MANNITOL)

MECHANISM. **Increase kidney tubular fluid osmolarity.** The drug is filtered through the glomerulus into the kidney tubule, where it pulls water from the interstitial space into the tubules via osmosis. This process results in **more water excreted** into the urine and less water reabsorbed into the circulation.

SITE OF ACTION. In the kidney at the proximal tubule (site of major water permeability) (Figure 1-65).

USES. Rarely used for hypertension. More commonly used for patients with increased intracranial pressure (ICP) or increased intraocular pressure (IOP).

SIDE EFFECTS. Can cause major problems if the drug cannot be filtered through the glomerulus (eg, in anuria). In this situation, the drug remains in the circulation and pulls water from the interstitial tissues into the blood. This results in increased blood volume (the exact opposite of its intended effect), leading to peripheral and/or pulmonary edema.

CARBONIC ANHYDRASE INHIBITORS (EG, ACETAZOLAMIDE)

MECHANISM. Prevent the conversion of bicarbonate (HCO_3^-) into CO_2 (mediated by carbonic anhydrase primarily at the brush border of proximal tubule cells), which is necessary for the reabsorption of HCO_3^-. This inhibition results in **excretion of HCO_3^- along with water** into the urine.

SITE OF ACTION. In the kidney at the proximal convoluted tubule (see Figure 1-65).

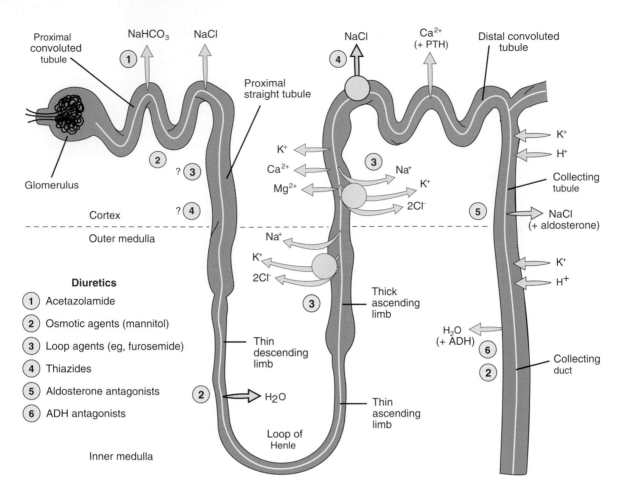

FIGURE 1-64. **Overview of sites of action of various diuretics.** ADH, antidiuretic hormone; PTH, parathyroid hormone. (Modified with permission from Katzung BG. *Basic and Clinical Pharmacology*, 10th ed. New York: McGraw-Hill, 2007: 237.)

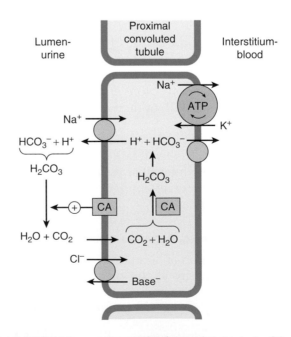

FIGURE 1-65. **Ion physiology at the proximal convoluted tubule.** CA, carbonic anhydrase. (Modified with permission from Katzung BG. *Basic and Clinical Pharmacology*, 10th ed. New York: McGraw-Hill, 2007: 239.)

USES. Rarely used for hypertension. More commonly used for patients with metabolic alkalosis, altitude sickness, glaucoma, or intracranial hypertension (pseudotumor cerebri).

SIDE EFFECTS. **Metabolic acidosis** due to increased excretion of HCO_3^-. The loss of this major source of alkalinity causes a rise in urinary pH and a drop in blood pH. In addition, acetazolamide contains a sulfa group, which causes allergic reactions in some patients.

LOOP DIURETICS (EG, FUROSEMIDE, ETHACRYNIC ACID, BUMETANIDE)

MECHANISM. **Inhibit Na^+-K^+-$2Cl^-$ channel** in the thick ascending limb of the loop of Henle. By preventing Na^+ and K^+ reabsorption into the renal medulla, they abolish the hypertonicity of the medulla (so urine cannot be concentrated in the collecting ducts). This results in marked diuresis. They also **increase Ca^{2+} excretion** because they reduce the lumen positive potential in the loop of Henle.

SITE OF ACTION. Thick ascending limb of loop of Henle (Figure 1-66).

USES. **The most efficacious diuretics,** used for edema (CHF, cirrhosis, nephrotic syndrome, and pulmonary edema), moderate to severe hypertension, and hypercalcemia.

SIDE EFFECTS. Ototoxicity, **hypokalemia,** hypercalciuria, hypocalcemia, dehydration, allergy to sulfa (furosemide, not ethacrynic acid), nephritis, gout.

THIAZIDE DIURETICS (EG, HYDROCHLOROTHIAZIDE, METOLAZONE)

MECHANISM. **Inhibit Na^+-Cl^- symporter,** thereby blocking Na^+ and Cl^- reabsorption in the distal convoluted tubule. NaCl is excreted along with water into the urine. They also increase Ca^{2+} reabsorption.

SITE OF ACTION. Early distal convoluted tubule (Figure 1-67).

USES. Mild to moderate hypertension, mild CHF, nephrogenic diabetes insipidus, idiopathic hypercalciuria.

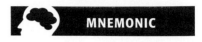

ACIDazolamide causes **ACID**osis.

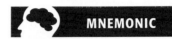

Loop diuretics—

OH DANG!
Ototoxicity
Hypokalemia, **H**ypercalciuria
Dehydration
Allergy to sulfa (furosemide)
Nephritis
Gout

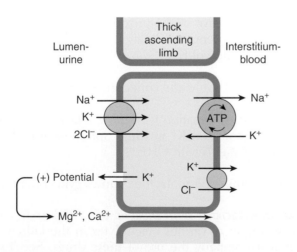

FIGURE 1-66. **Ion physiology at the loop of Henle.** (Modified with permission from Katzung BG. *Basic and Clinical Pharmacology,* 10th ed. New York: McGraw-Hill, 2007: 239.)

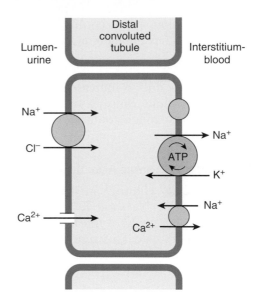

FIGURE 1-67. **Ion physiology at the distal convoluted tubule.** (Modified with permission from Katzung BG. *Basic and Clinical Pharmacology*, 10th ed. New York: McGraw-Hill, 2007: 239.)

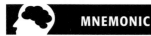

Thiazides—

HyperGLUC
Hyper**G**lycemia
Hyper**L**ipidemia
Hyper**U**ricemia
Hyper**C**alcemia

The K⁺ **STA**ys
Spironolactone
Triamterene
Amiloride

SIDE EFFECTS. Hyperglycemia, hyperlipidemia, hyperuricemia, **hypercalcemia,** sulfa allergy (hydrochlorothiazide).

POTASSIUM-SPARING DIURETICS (EG, SPIRONOLACTONE, TRIAMTERENE, AMILORIDE)

MECHANISM

- **Spironolactone: Competitive antagonist at the aldosterone receptor** in the collecting tubule (indirectly inhibits Na⁺ reabsorption).
- **Triamterene and amiloride:** Directly block Na⁺ channels in the collecting tubule.

Reasons for the K-sparing properties of this class:

- Less K⁺ secretion occurs due to inhibition of Na⁺ reabsorption in the distal tubule (Na⁺ reabsorption and K⁺ secretion are coupled in this segment of the nephron).
- Because they are not active in the proximal portions of the tubules, these agents do not greatly increase tubular flow (high flow rates through the tubules increase secretion of K⁺).

SITE OF ACTION. Collecting tubule and collecting duct (Figure 1-68).

USES. Primarily used in combination with more efficacious diuretics (eg, loop diuretics) to **prevent associated K⁺ wasting.** Spironolactone has been proven to increase survival in patients with CHF.

SIDE EFFECTS. Hyperkalemia, spironolactone causes gynecomastia.

ELECTROLYTE CHANGES ASSOCIATED WITH DIURETIC USE. All diuretics affect the reabsorption and/or secretion of various electrolytes in the kidney, so electrolyte abnormalities may accompany the use of these drugs. See Table 1-33 for a review of some alterations in electrolytes in the urine and blood for various diuretics.

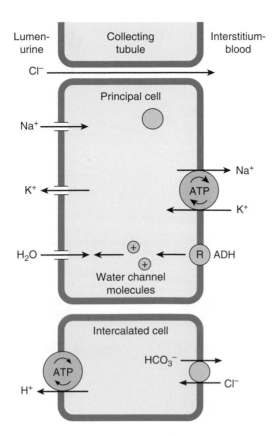

FIGURE 1-68. Ion physiology at the collecting tubule and collecting duct. (Modified with permission from Katzung BG. *Basic and Clinical Pharmacology*, 10th ed. New York: McGraw-Hill, 2007: 240.)

Sympatholytics

FUNCTION OF SYMPATHETIC RECEPTORS

Sympatholytic, or sympathoplegic, drugs reduce the effects of the sympathetic nervous system (SNS) on the CV system (Figure 1-69). Recall that arterial BP = cardiac output × systemic vascular resistance (SVR). Cardiac output is the product of HR and SV.

TABLE 1-33. Electrolyte Changes With Various Diuretics

DRUG	URINE NaCl	URINE K+	URINE Ca+	URINE HCO3−	BLOOD pH
Osmotic diuretics	↑↑	↑	↑	↑	NC
Carbonic anhydrase inhibitors	↑	↑↑	NC	↑↑	↓
Loop diuretics	↑↑↑	↑↑	↑↑	NC	↑
Thiazide diuretics	↑	↑↑	↓	NC	↑
Potassium-sparing diuretics	↑	↓	NC	NC	↓

NC = no change.

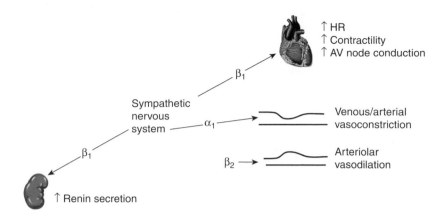

FIGURE 1-69. End-organ effects of sympathetic nervous system activity relating to blood pressure control. AV = atrioventricular; HR = heart rate.

Since multiple factors contribute to BP control, pharmacologic agents that target different parameters can be used to decrease BP.

Sympathetic activity increases BP by increasing all of the following:

- HR
- Cardiac contractility
- Venous return to the heart (preload)
- SVR (or afterload)
- Renin production in the juxtaglomerular cells of the kidney

Drugs that inhibit sympathetic activity reduce some or all of these parameters and thus lower BP. (Review the major functions of the sympathetic receptor subtypes in Table 1-34.)

CENTRALLY ACTING SYMPATHOLYTICS (EG, METHYLDOPA, CLONIDINE)

MECHANISM. Selective α_2-agonists. By activating α_2-receptors in the brain stem, these agents reduce central sympathetic outflow. The result is decreased cardiac output and SVR.

SITE OF ACTION. Brain stem.

USES. Rarely used for hypertension due to poor side effect profile, but methyldopa is traditionally considered the drug of choice for hypertension in pregnant patients.

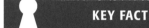

KEY FACT

Methyldopa is the drug of choice to lower BP in pregnant patients.

TABLE 1-34. Function of Sympathetic Receptors Within the Cardiovascular System

RECEPTOR	MAJOR EFFECTS ON CV SYSTEM
α_1	Vasoconstriction
α_2	- Central receptors: ↓ sympathetic outflow - Peripheral receptors: arterial vasodilation
β_1	↑ Heart rate, ↑ cardiac contractility, ↑ renin release
β_2	Vasodilation

SIDE EFFECTS

- Methyldopa: Sedation, **positive Coombs test** in 10% of patients (reversible upon discontinuation of drug).
- Clonidine: Sedation, dry mouth, **severe rebound hypertension** with abrupt discontinuation (should not be used in patients who may have difficulty obtaining/taking medication as directed).

α-ADRENERGIC RECEPTOR ANTAGONISTS (α-BLOCKERS; EG, PRAZOSIN, DOXAZOSIN, TERAZOSIN)

MECHANISM. Selective α_1-receptor antagonists; α_1-blockade decreases SVR by preventing arteriolar vasoconstriction. The result is decreased BP.

SITE OF ACTION. Primarily α_1-receptors on arterioles. Of note, also blocks α_1-receptors at the bladder sphincter (see later discussion for clinical uses).

USES. Mild to moderate hypertension. Most common use of α_1-blockers is to treat urinary hesitancy for patients with prostatic hypertrophy (by preventing bladder sphincter contraction).

SIDE EFFECTS. First-dose hypotension, reflex tachycardia, secondary Na^+ retention in kidney (use in combination with diuretic).

β-ADRENERGIC RECEPTOR ANTAGONISTS (β-BLOCKERS; EG, PROPRANOLOL, ATENOLOL, METOPROLOL, ESMOLOL, CARVEDILOL)

MECHANISM

- Nonselective β-receptor (β_1 and β_2) antagonists (propranolol):
  - Reduce HR by blocking β_1 effects.
  - Reduce contractility by blocking β_1 effects.
  - Inhibit renin production by blocking β_1 effects.
  - More side effects because of their action on β_2-receptors (see Side Effects section).
- Selective β_1-receptor antagonists (atenolol, metoprolol, esmolol):
  - Same as above due to β_1-blockade
  - Fewer side effects
- Mixed α- and β-receptor antagonists (carvedilol):
  - Same as above due to β_1-blockade
  - Plus decreased SVR due to α-blockade

SITE OF ACTION. β_1-Receptors on heart and kidney, β_2-receptors on arterioles.

USES. Hypertension, angina, patients with previous MI, CHF. Esmolol is an ultra-short-acting agent used in acute hypertensive emergencies.

SIDE EFFECTS

- **Bradycardia:** Important to remember when checking vital signs on patients who are taking β-blockers.
- **Bronchoconstriction** and asthma exacerbation (especially nonselective agents with β_2 antagonism).
- Blunted response to hypoglycemia. May be especially **dangerous in diabetics** on insulin therapy. Hypoglycemic episodes are marked by pallor, trembling, diaphoresis, and tachycardia (all mediated by increased β-receptor activity). With β-blockade, these important clues of hypoglycemia may be absent.

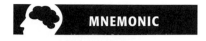

MNEMONIC

α-Blockers end in **-OSIN.**

MNEMONIC

Drugs with β-blocking action end in **-OLOL.**
Drugs with both α- and β-blocking action end in either **-ILOL** or **-ALOL.**

KEY FACT

β_2-receptors in the lung mediate bronchodilation. β_2-Blockade can impair breathing in patients with asthma or chronic obstructive pulmonary disease (COPD), so avoid nonspecific β-blocker use in these patients.

Calcium Channel Blockers and Other Vasodilators

Vasodilators **decrease SVR** by relaxing smooth muscle in arteriole walls through a number of different mechanisms. The result is the same, however—by increasing arteriolar diameter, SVR (also known as afterload) is reduced, which also reduces BP (remember, BP = cardiac output × SVR).

CALCIUM CHANNEL BLOCKERS (EG, NIFEDIPINE, AMLODIPINE, VERAPAMIL, DILTIAZEM)

MECHANISM. Block L-type Ca^{2+} channels, inhibiting entry of Ca^{2+} into arteriolar smooth muscle; this action results in arteriole dilation and reduced SVR.

SITE OF ACTION

- **Vasoselective agents** work predominantly at the arteriolar smooth muscle. The most commonly used class is the **dihydropyridines** (including nifedipine and amlodipine).
- **Nonselective agents** act equally on the heart and the arterioles. Their vasodilating action is not as potent as that of the dihydropyridines, but they also reduce cardiac contractility. Examples are **verapamil** and **diltiazem.**

USES. Mild to moderate hypertension.

SIDE EFFECTS. Constipation, bradycardia, AV block.

NITRIC OXIDE RELEASERS (EG, NITROPRUSSIDE)

MECHANISM. Spontaneously releases nitric oxide, causing relaxation of both arterial and venule smooth muscle. This action results in rapid reduction of SVR and BP.

SITE OF ACTION. Arteriolar > venule smooth muscle.

USES. Hypertensive emergencies (given in IV form).

SIDE EFFECTS. By-products of metabolism include cyanide and thiocyanate, which can be harmful to patients with poor renal function. Other side effects include excessive hypotension and reflex tachycardia.

Other Vasodilators (eg, Hydralazine, Minoxidil)

HYDRALAZINE

MECHANISM. Exact mechanism unknown.

SITE OF ACTION. Arteriolar smooth muscle.

USES. Mild to moderate hypertension.

SIDE EFFECTS. May cause **drug-induced lupus;** reflex tachycardia, and sodium retention (therefore, it is given in combination with a β-blocker and a diuretic).

MINOXIDIL

MECHANISM. Opens K^+ channels, causing hyperpolarization of smooth muscle cells and arteriolar dilation.

SITE OF ACTION. Arteriolar smooth muscle.

USES. Mild to moderate hypertension and baldness (see following section).

KEY FACT

Dihydropyridines are more active at the arterioles than the heart. Their names end in **-PINE.**

KEY FACT

Nitroprusside is a rapid-acting IV vasodilator for hypertensive emergencies.

Side Effects. Hirsutism, or excessive hairiness (minoxidil is the main ingredient in Rogaine, which is used for the treatment of alopecia, or hair loss); also reflex tachycardia and sodium retention (also given in combination with a β-blocker and a diuretic).

Angiotensin Inhibitors

The RAAS plays an intricate role in BP regulation. Two classes of drugs are used to alter this system and thereby reduce BP. Both classes reduce the action of angiotensin II, which is a molecule that increases SVR by directly causing vasoconstriction. Angiotensin II also increases Na^+ and water reabsorption in the kidney (via aldosterone). The RAAS is shown in Figure 1-70.

ANGIOTENSIN-CONVERTING ENZYME (ACE) INHIBITORS (EG, CAPTOPRIL, LISINOPRIL, ENALAPRIL)

Mechanism. These drugs **block ACEs,** thus preventing conversion of angiotensin I to angiotensin II. They also inhibit degradation of bradykinin (an intrinsic vasodilator). This action results in **decreased SVR and decreased Na^+ and water reabsorption (via reduced aldosterone).**

Site of Action. The active site of the enzyme (found on the endothelial membrane and in plasma).

Uses. **Mild to moderate hypertension, heart failure, diabetic renal disease** (usually first-line treatment for diabetics with hypertension).

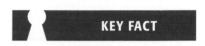

MNEMONIC

All ACE inhibitors end in **-PRIL.**

KEY FACT

Angiotensin II is an enzyme responsible for aldosterone synthesis in the adrenal cortex and is also a direct vasoconstrictor.

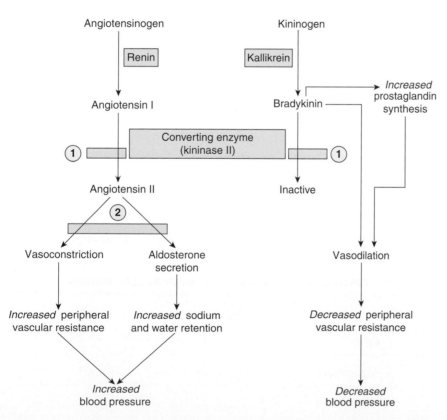

FIGURE 1-70.   Renin-angiotensin-aldosterone pathway and sites of action of ACE inhibitors and angiotensin receptor blockers. ①, ACE inhibitors; ②, angiotensin receptor blockers. (Reproduced with permission from Katzung BG. *Basic and Clinical Pharmacology,* 10th ed. New York: McGraw-Hill, 2007: 176.)

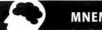

MNEMONIC

CAPTOPRIL
Cough
Angioedema
Proteinuria
Taste changes
HypOtension
Pregnancy problems
Rash
Increased renin
Lower angiotensin II

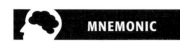

MNEMONIC

All ARBs end in **-ARTAN.**

SIDE EFFECTS. Cough, hyperkalemia, angioedema, proteinuria, taste changes, hypotension, fetal renal problems, rash.

ANGIOTENSIN II RECEPTOR ANTAGONISTS (ALSO CALLED ANGIOTENSIN RECEPTOR BLOCKERS [ARBs]; EG, LOSARTAN, VALSARTAN)

MECHANISM. Blockade of angiotensin II receptors, producing similar downstream effects as ACE inhibitors (namely, decreased SVR).

SITE OF ACTION. Heart, kidney, adrenal cortex.

USES. Mainly used in patients who cannot tolerate ACE inhibitors.

SIDE EFFECTS. Less cough than ACE inhibitors, fetal renal damage.

ACE inhibitors and ARBs affect levels of various products within the RAAS (see Figure 1-70 and Table 1-35).

ANTIANGINAL THERAPY

Angina is chest pain resulting from myocardial ischemia. Ischemia occurs when the demand of the heart exceeds that supplied by the coronary arteries. Therefore, **reducing O$_2$ demand of the heart is the goal of treatment** so that supply is greater than demand. Some of the important factors that contribute to O$_2$ demand include **preload, afterload, HR,** and **cardiac contractility.** The major agents used to alter these parameters are nitrates, β-blockers, and calcium channel blockers. After reviewing the drugs, see Table 1-36 for a recap on how the drugs affect myocardial O$_2$ demand.

Types of Angina

There are three major forms of angina:

- **Stable (effort) angina:** Due to fixed narrowing of coronary arteries.
  - Occurs with increased activity.
  - Is relieved by rest.
- **Unstable angina:** Due to **acute formation of thrombus** on atherosclerotic plaque.
  - Not associated with activity.
  - Is not relieved by rest.
  - More likely to progress to MI.
- **Variant (Prinzmetal) angina:** Due to **coronary artery vasospasm.**

TABLE 1-35. **Effects of ACE Inhibitors and Angiotensin Receptor Blockers**

	ACE INHIBITORS	ARBs
Renin	↑	↑
Angiotensin I	↑	↑
Angiotensin II	↓	↑
Aldosterone	↓	↓
Bradykinin	↑	↔

↑ = increases; ↓ = decreases; ↔ = no significant change.

TABLE 1-36. **Effects of Antianginal Agents on Parameters That Determine Myocardial O$_2$ Demand**

PARAMETER	NITRATES	β-BLOCKERS/CALCIUM CHANNEL BLOCKERS	NITRATE + β-BLOCKER/ CALCIUM CHANNEL BLOCKER
Preload	↓	↑	↔
Afterload	↓	↓	↓
Contractility	↑ (reflex)	↓	↔
Heart rate	↑ (reflex)	↓	↓
O$_2$ demand	↓	↓	↓↓

↑ = increases; ↓ = decreases; ↔ = no significant change.

Nitrates (eg, Nitroglycerin, Isosorbide Dinitrate)

MECHANISM. Vasodilates via release of nitric oxide; major effect is preload reduction (veins dilate, blood pools in veins, and venous return to the heart decreases), resulting in decreased O$_2$ demand. May cause some afterload reduction also.

USES. Stable angina, unstable angina, and variant angina.

SIDE EFFECTS. Tachycardia, orthostatic hypotension, headache.

β-Blockers (eg, Metoprolol, Atenolol, Propranolol)

MECHANISM. Reduce O$_2$ demand by reducing HR and cardiac contractility.

USES. Stable angina, **not variant angina** (because β-blockade can disrupt the balance of α and β effects and worsen vasospasms).

SIDE EFFECTS. Bradycardia, AV block.

Calcium Channel Blockers (eg, Verapamil, Diltiazem, Nifedipine)

MECHANISM. Decrease O$_2$ demand:

- Verapamil, diltiazem: Decrease HR and contractility (like β-blockers).
- Nifedipine: Decreases afterload via vasodilation.

USES. Stable angina and variant angina (calcium channel blockers are the drugs of choice).

SIDE EFFECTS. Nifedipine may cause reflex tachycardia (increased O$_2$ demand); verapamil and diltiazem can cause constipation, bradycardia, and AV block.

KEY FACT

Remember, **nitroglycerin** dilates **VEINS** >> arteries.

KEY FACT

Calcium channel blockers are the drugs of choice for variant (Prinzmetal's) angina.

DRUGS USED IN HEART FAILURE

Heart failure is defined as cardiac output insufficient for the **O$_2$ demands of the body.** It can be thought of as a chronic disease with intermittent acute exacerbations. Heart failure is characterized by poor cardiac output, and the response is to increase SNS tone and increase retention of sodium and water.

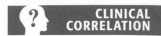

NYHA Classes of CHF
I. No limitation of activities
II. Mild limitation of activities
III. Marked limitation of activities
IV. Symptoms present at rest

The goals of therapy are to increase cardiac output and also inhibit unwanted responses. Several drugs used in heart failure have been discussed previously. These include diuretics (eg, furosemide, spironolactone), β-blockers (eg, metoprolol, carvedilol), ACE inhibitors (eg, captopril), ARBs (eg, losartan), and vasodilators (eg, nitroprusside, nitroglycerin). Review these drugs in the previous sections and study Table 1-37 for their benefits in heart failure. Other drugs used to treat heart failure include agents that directly increase cardiac output such as β-agonists, cardiac glycosides, and phosphodiesterase inhibitors.

β-Agonists (eg, Dobutamine)

MECHANISM

Selective β_1-agonist; this action increases HR and cardiac contractility, leading to an increase in cardiac output.

SITE OF ACTION

Primarily the heart.

USES

Acute exacerbations of heart failure (given IV and has a very short half-life).

SIDE EFFECTS

Angina (due to increased myocardial O_2 demand), tachycardia, arrhythmias.

TABLE 1-37.   Drugs Used in the Treatment of Heart Failure

DRUG CLASS	EXAMPLES	BENEFITS IN HEART FAILURE
Diuretics	Furosemide, spironolactone	Reduced sodium/water retention → reduced preload and afterload; spironolactone prevents detrimental effects of aldosterone (myocardial fibrosis).
β-Blockers	Metoprolol, carvedilol	Reduced sympathetic tone → reduced afterload.
ACE inhibitors/ ARBs	Captopril, losartan	Reduced sympathetic tone → reduced afterload.
Vasodilators	Nitroglycerin, nitroprusside	Vasodilation → reduced preload and reduced afterload.
Cardiac glycosides	Digoxin	Increased cardiac contractility → increased cardiac output.
β_1-Agonists	Dobutamine	Increased cardiac contractility → increased cardiac output.
Phosphodiesterase inhibitors	Milrinone, inamrinone	Increased cardiac contractility → increased cardiac output.

Cardiac Glycosides (eg, Digoxin)

MECHANISM

Blocks Na^+-K^+ ATPase, resulting in increased intracellular Na^+. The high levels of intracellular Na^+ reduce the activity of the Na^+-Ca^{2+} exchanger and more Ca^{2+} remains intracellular. This high level of intracellular Ca^{2+} improves cardiac contractility (leading to higher cardiac output). Digoxin also has some parasympathetic activity and decreases AV nodal conduction velocity.

SITE OF ACTION

Membrane of cardiac myocytes.

USES

Chronic heart failure, also atrial fibrillation.

SIDE EFFECTS

Arrhythmias, blurry yellow vision. Toxicities are highly increased with hypokalemia (important because many patients taking digoxin also take furosemide, a major cause of hypokalemia).

Phosphodiesterase Inhibitors (eg, Inamrinone, Milrinone)

MECHANISM

Block the action of phosphodiesterase, leading to increased levels of cAMP and increased Ca^{2+} flow into the cardiac myocyte. The result is increased cardiac contractility and cardiac output. Also cause some vasodilation.

USES

Acute exacerbations of heart failure.

SIDE EFFECTS

Arrhythmias.

ANTIARRHYTHMICS

Pharmacotherapy of arrhythmias is very complex (Table 1-38).

TABLE 1-38. Overview of Drugs Used to Treat Arrhythmias

CLASS	EXAMPLE(S)	MECHANISM	CLINICAL USE	SIDE EFFECTS
I (Na⁺ channel blockers)				
IA	Quinidine, procainamide, disopyramide	Decrease ventricular conduction (increased QRS interval on ECG); prolong ventricular action potential **(increased QT interval on ECG).**	Atrial and ventricular arrhythmias.	Quinidine: cinchonism (headache, tinnitus) and **torsades de pointes (due to increased QT interval);** procainamide: **drug-induced lupus**.
IB	Lidocaine	Slow conduction and increased threshold for firing of abnormal cells.	Acute ventricular arrhythmias.	CV and CNS depression with overdose.
IC	Flecainide, propafenone	Decrease ventricular conduction (increased QRS interval on ECG).	Ventricular arrhythmias.	Can cause arrhythmias (especially in post–MI patients).
II (β-Blockers)	Esmolol (IV, rapid acting), metoprolol, propranolol	Decrease AV nodal conduction (increased PR interval on ECG).	Ventricular and supraventricular arrhythmias.	Bradycardia, AV block.
III (K⁺ channel blockers)	Amiodarone, sotalol	Prolong ventricular action potential **(increased QT interval on ECG).**	Treatment and prevention of ventricular arrhythmias.	Amiodarone: pulmonary fibrosis, hepatotoxicity, thyroid disease.
IV (Ca²⁺ channel blockers)	Verapamil, diltiazem	Decrease AV nodal conduction.	Supraventricular arrhythmias.	Constipation, bradycardia, AV block.
Other	Adenosine	Decrease AV nodal conduction.	Supraventricular arrhythmias.	Flushing, hypotension, chest pain.
	Magnesium (Mg²⁺)	Unknown.	Torsades de pointes.	Respiratory depression.

AV = atrioventricular; CNS = central nervous system; CV = cardiovascular; MI = myocardial infarction.

LIPID-LOWERING AGENTS

Hyperlipidemia refers to increases in blood levels of lipoproteins or triglycerides or both. It is a major risk factor for CV diseases such as angina, MI, and stroke. Several pharmacologic agents are used to treat hyperlipidemia, and it is important to understand the key differences between the major classes of lipid-lowering agents (Table 1-39 and Figure 1-71).

TABLE 1-39. **Commonly Used Lipid-Lowering Agents**

Drug Class	Example(s)	Mechanism	LDL	HDL	TGs	Side Effects
HMG-CoA reductase inhibitors ("statins")	Lovastatin, pravastatin, simvastatin, atorvastatin	Inhibit rate-determining step in cholesterol synthesis.	↓↓↓	↑	↓	Increased LFTs, myositis
Bile acid resins	Cholestyramine, colestipol	Bind bile salts in the intestine thus preventing their reabsorption (along with cholesterol) in the intestine.	↓↓	–	↑	Bad taste, bloating, constipation, impaired absorption of fat-soluble vitamins
Cholesterol absorption inhibitors	Ezetimibe	Block absorption of cholesterol in the small intestine.	↓↓	–	–	Rarely increased LFTs
Fibrates	Gemfibrozil, fenofibrate, clofibrate	Increase synthesis of lipoprotein lipase via activation of peroxisome proliferator-activated receptor-α (PPAR-α).	↓	↑	↓↓↓	Myositis, increased LFTs
Other	Niacin (nicotinic acid, vitamin B_3)	Decreases formation and secretion of VLDL resulting in less formation of LDL.	↓↓	↑↑	↓	Flushed face (can be prevented by aspirin)

HMG-CoA = 3-hydroxy-3-methylglutaryl coenzyme A; LDL = low-density lipoprotein; LFTs = liver function tests; VLDL = very low-density lipoprotein.

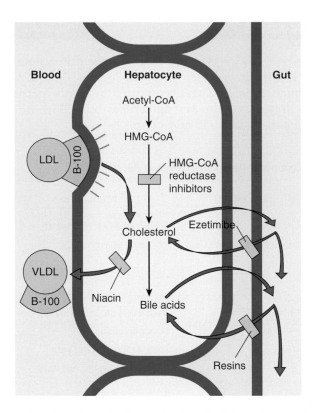

FIGURE 1-71. **Overview of mechanisms of various lipid-lowering agents.** HMG-CoA, 3-hydroxy-3-methylglutaryl coenzyme A; LDL, low-density lipoprotein; VLDL, very low-density lipoprotein. (Modified with permission from Katzung BG. *Basic and Clinical Pharmacology*, 9th ed. New York: McGraw-Hill, 2004: 239.)

ANTICOAGULANTS

Anticoagulants are used for the treatment and prevention of unwanted blood clotting. Examples include DVT, PE, and embolic stroke. They prevent clot formation by interrupting either the intrinsic (heparin) or extrinsic (warfarin) coagulation cascade. It is very important to understand the similarities of and differences between heparin and warfarin (Table 1-40).

Heparin

MECHANISM

Catalyzes the activation of antithrombin III, thus decreasing the activity of thrombin (factor IIa) and factor Xa. Heparin activity is monitored with the **partial thromboplastin time (PTT)** because of its effects on the **intrinsic coagulation pathway.** Newer low-molecular-weight heparins (eg, enoxaparin) do not have to be monitored by laboratory tests.

SITE OF ACTION

Blood.

USES

Immediate anticoagulation for DVT, PE, MI.

SIDE EFFECTS

Bleeding. Action of heparin is reversed with **protamine sulfate** (binds heparin and inactivates it). Rarely causes heparin-induced thrombocytopenia (HIT).

KEY FACT

The treatment for heparin overdose is protamine.

TABLE 1-40. Comparison of Heparin and Warfarin

DRUG	HEPARIN	WARFARIN
Structure	Large anionic polymer	Small lipid-soluble molecule
Route of administration	IV, SC	Oral
Site of action	Blood	Liver
Onset of action	Rapid (seconds)	Slow, dependent on half-life of clotting factors
Mechanism of action	Activates antithrombin III, reduces action of thrombin and Xa	Vitamin K antagonist (impairs synthesis of factors II, VII, IX, and X)
Duration of action	Acute (hours)	Chronic (weeks)
Treatment of overdose	Protamine	Fresh frozen plasma
Method of monitoring	PTT (intrinsic pathway)	PT (extrinsic pathway)

IV = intravenous; PT = prothrombin time; PTT = partial thromboplastin time; SC = subcutaneous.

Warfarin

MECHANISM

Inhibits γ carboxylation of vitamin K-dependent clotting factors (factors II, VII, IX, and X, and proteins C and S). Warfarin affects the **extrinsic coagulation pathway** and is monitored clinically with the **prothrombin time (PT)**.

SITE OF ACTION

Liver (site of synthesis of clotting factors).

USES

Chronic anticoagulation (eg, DVT prophylaxis and in atrial fibrillation for stroke prophylaxis).

SIDE EFFECTS

Bleeding. Also, warfarin crosses the placenta, so it is **contraindicated in pregnancy** (heparin is used instead). Overdose is treated with fresh frozen plasma (to supply fresh clotting factors).

ANTIPLATELET AGENTS

Drugs that have antiplatelet activity either inhibit platelet adherence to the vascular endothelium (adhesion) or platelet adherence to other platelets (aggregation). Several agents are used currently. Their major applications are to prevent MI and stroke (see Figure 1-72 for an overview of platelet activation).

MNEMONIC

To remember that warfarin activity (affecting the extrinsic pathway) is measured with PT, think **WEPT (Warfarin, Extrinsic, PT)**

CLINICAL CORRELATION

Patients on warfarin with international normalized ratio (INR) values outside of the desired range can sometimes be reversed using vitamin K supplements.

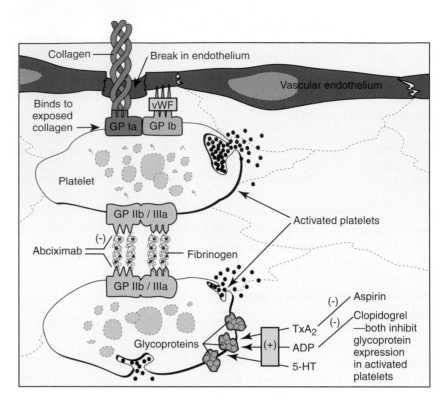

FIGURE 1-72. **Factors influencing platelet activation.** ADP, adenosine diphosphate; GP, glycoprotein; 5-HT, 5-hydroxytryptamine (serotonin); TxA_2, thromboxane A_2; vWF, von Willebrand factor.

Aspirin

MECHANISM

Acetylates and irreversibly inhibits cyclooxygenase (COX-1 and COX-2). This action prevents conversion of arachidonic acid to prostaglandins and thromboxane A_2. The result is decreased platelet aggregation.

SITE OF ACTION

In the platelet.

USES

Prevention of MI.

SIDE EFFECTS

Gastric ulcers, bleeding, Reye syndrome in children, tinnitus at very high doses.

Clopidogrel and Ticlopidine

MECHANISM

Irreversibly blocks ADP receptors on platelet membranes, thereby inhibiting platelet aggregation.

SITE OF ACTION

Platelet membrane.

USES

Prevention of thrombosis following coronary artery stent placement; stroke prevention.

SIDE EFFECTS

Bleeding. Ticlopidine can cause severe neutropenia.

Dipyridamole

MECHANISM

Inhibits adenosine uptake by the platelet (secondary to blocking intraplatelet phosphodiesterase and increasing cAMP levels). The result is decreased platelet aggregation.

SITE OF ACTION

In the platelet.

USES

In combination with aspirin to prevent stroke.

SIDE EFFECTS

Bleeding.

Abciximab

MECHANISM

Binds to glycoprotein IIb/IIIa receptor on platelets and prevents interaction between fibrinogen and IIb/IIIa receptor. The result is decreased platelet aggregation.

SITE OF ACTION

Platelet membrane.

USES

Prevention of thrombosis during coronary artery angioplasty and stenting.

SIDE EFFECTS

Bleeding, thrombocytopenia.

THROMBOLYTICS

Thrombolytics are used to lyse active clots in the circulation. Their basic mechanism is to increase formation of plasmin, the intrinsic enzyme responsible for degrading fibrin clots. The two most common applications for thrombolytic agents are early MI and early thromboembolic (ischemic) stroke.

Streptokinase

MECHANISM

Indirectly activates plasminogen. Streptokinase first binds plasminogen, forming a 1:1 complex. This complex then catalyzes the formation of plasmin from another molecule of plasminogen. Streptokinase is **not fibrin-specific** (it activates free plasminogen that is not bound to fibrin clots).

SITE OF ACTION

Free plasminogen and fibrin-bound plasminogen.

USES

Acute MI, stroke, PE.

SIDE EFFECTS

Bleeding (contraindicated in patients with active bleeding, recent surgery, or history of intracranial bleeds); **allergic response** (since it is isolated from bacteria); it also loses efficacy after initial administration because patients become sensitized; a repeat dose is much less effective than the initial dose.

Tissue Plasminogen Activator (tPA)

MECHANISM

In contrast to streptokinase, **tPA is fibrin-specific.** Therefore it only activates plasminogen molecules that are bound to fibrin clots. It directly activates plasminogen.

SITE OF ACTION

Plasminogen bound to fibrin clots.

USES

Acute MI, stroke, PE.

SIDE EFFECTS

Bleeding; does not lose efficacy after initial dose (in contrast to streptokinase). **Note:** Fibrinolysis can be reversed with **aminocaproic acid.**

CLINICAL CORRELATION

There is a 3-hour window in patients with suspected ischemic stroke in which tPA can be administered. Hemorrhagic stroke must first be ruled out with a CT scan before tPA is given.

Endocrine

Hypothalamus and Pituitary

HORMONE BASICS

The endocrine system maintains many complex communication systems between cells, tissues, and organ systems. These interactions take place locally or at a distance and are mediated by peptides, amines, and steroids called hormones.

Site of Action

Endocrine signals can be characterized by the relationship between the site of secretion and the relative location of target receptors:

- **Autocrine secretion:** Released signal affects the cell from which it was secreted (eg, neoplastic growth advanced by growth factors [GFs] released by and acting on tumor).
- **Paracrine secretion:** Released signal acts on neighboring cells that have the appropriate receptors (eg, when exposed to an allergen, mast cells release histamine, which acts on vascular smooth muscle to induce vasodilation).
- **Endocrine secretion:** Released signal enters the **bloodstream** and acts on distant receptors (eg, follicle-stimulating hormone [FSH] is secreted from the anterior pituitary and acts on granulosa cells of the ovary).
- **Exocrine secretion:** Released signal enters a **duct** and acts on epithelial surface of the skin/gut (eg, pancreas releases amylase into the duodenum).
- **Multifunctional signals:** Signals can produce different effects depending on the mode of action and the target tissue. For example, testosterone released by Leydig cells in the testes acts on muscles to stimulate growth (endocrine) but also acts on seminiferous tubules to promote spermatogenesis (paracrine).

Types of Hormones by Mechanism of Action

Hormones fall into three classes of molecules: peptides, steroids, and amines. Each class differs in precursors, site of synthesis, plasma transport, and mode of action (Table 2-1).

- **Peptides and proteins:** Preprohormone typically synthesized by rough endoplasmic reticulum (RER) → signal peptide cleavage in RER produces prohormone.
    - Transport within the Golgi apparatus results in further processing and final active hormone structure.
    - Stored in secretory vesicles and released via exocytosis into the bloodstream (water-soluble).
    - Act on cell surface receptors and second-messenger systems of target tissues (fast-acting effects).
- **Steroids:** Synthesized from cholesterol on demand (not stored) → lipid solubility allows for rapid diffusion across membrane.
    - Transported in blood bound to plasma carrier proteins due to limited solubility.
    - Diffuse across target cell membrane and bind to intracytoplasmic protein receptors.
    - Resultant steroid hormone–receptor complex enters nucleus and activates transcription of specific genes for new protein synthesis (slow-acting effects).

KEY FACT

The pancreas has both endocrine and exocrine functions. Its exocrine role includes facilitating the chemical digestion of food; the endocrine pancreas regulates glucose metabolism.

TABLE 2-1. Peptide and Steroid Hormones

	PEPTIDE/PROTEIN HORMONES	STEROID
Precursors	Amino acids	Cholesterol
Site of synthesis	Rough ER	Smooth ER
Storage	Yes (stored in vesicles)	No (produced on demand)
Carrier proteins	No (majority soluble in blood)	Yes (bound to carrier proteins)
Location of receptors	Target cell membrane	Intracytoplasmic, transported into nucleus
Signal propagation	Via second messengers	Via new gene transcription
Kinetics	Fast acting ± long-term actions	Slow-acting
Examples	ACTH, LH, insulin	Estrogen, testosterone

ACTH = adrenocorticotropic hormone; ER = endoplasmic reticulum; LH = luteinizing hormone.

■ **Amines:** Synthesized from tyrosine precursors. Examples of amine hormones include thyroid hormone, epinephrine, and norepinephrine. Epinephrine and norepinephrine are synthesized, stored, released, and act on targets in a manner similar to peptide hormones. Thyroid hormone exhibits aspects of both peptide and steroid hormones.

Plasma Transport of Lipid-Soluble Hormones

Most steroid hormones (and thyroid hormones) are hydrophobic. Plasma proteins bind to these hormones to enable them to circulate in the bloodstream. These carrier proteins, produced by the liver, may either be nonspecific or specialized for a given hormone.

Example: Corticosteroid-binding globulin has a greater affinity for cortisol and aldosterone than for other steroid hormones. Conversely, albumin is rel-

TABLE 2-2. Hormone Transport Proteins

CARRIER PROTEIN	HORMONE TRANSPORTED	SERUM CONCENTRATIONS
Corticosteroid-binding globulin (CBG)	Cortisol, aldosterone	↓ in cirrhosis, nephrotic syndrome, and hypothyroidism.
Sex hormone–binding globulin (SHBG)	Estrogen, testosterone	↑ by estrogen, OCPs, and exogenous thyroid hormone.
Thyroxine-binding globulin (TBG)	Thyroxine (T_4), triiodothyronine (T_3)	↑ by estrogen, pregnancy, and OCPs.
Serum albumin	Nonspecific steroid transporter, T_4, and T_3	↓ in cirrhosis, nephrotic syndrome, and protein malnutrition.

OCPs = oral contraceptive pills.

KEY FACT

In men, increased sex hormone-binding globulin (SHBG) → decreased free testosterone → increased risk of unopposed estrogen activity → gynecomastia

KEY FACT

The vasodilators atrial natriuretic peptide (ANP) and nitric oxide (NO) utilize extracellular and intracellular **guanylate** cyclase signaling pathways, respectively.

atively nonspecific, binding a variety of steroid hormones with equal affinity (Table 2-2).

Carrier proteins allow for another level of control within the signaling network, as hormone-protein complexes are unable to diffuse across membranes and activate target cells. Instead, free and bound forms of hormone exist in equilibrium. Only free hormone is biologically active. Therefore, the amount of free hormone in plasma determines how much hormone is available to target tissues.

Peptide Hormones: Second-Messenger Pathways

Peptide/protein hormones stimulate membrane-bound receptors on target cells, generating conformational changes in the receptors. The intracellular propagation of the signal proceeds via the action of second messengers (Table 2-3, Figure 2-1). The major second-messenger systems include:

- **Adenylate cyclase mechanism:** Hormone binds G protein-coupled receptor (GPCR) → activated G protein (G$_s$) stimulates adenylate cyclase (AC).
  - AC catalyzes formation of cAMP.
  - cAMP activates protein kinase A (PKA).
  - PKA exerts downstream effects via phosphorylation of other proteins.
  - Other hormones inhibit adenylate cyclase through a separate GPCR, using an inhibitory G protein (G$_i$).
  - cAMP is inactivated by the enzyme phosphodiesterase (PDE).

TABLE 2-3. **Hormone Signal Propagation Mechanisms**

ADENYLATE CYCLASE	INOSITOL TRIPHOSPHATE (IP$_3$)	RTK	JAK/STAT	INTRACELLULAR RECEPTOR
FSH	**G**nRH	Insulin	Growth hormone	Aldosterone
LH	**G**HRH	VEGF	Prolactin	Estrogen
ACTH	**O**xytocin	PDGF	Leptin	Testosterone
TSH	**A**DH (V$_1$ receptor)	EGF	Erythropoetin	Progesterone
CRH	**T**RH	FGF	Thrombopoetin	Vitamin D
hCG		IGF-1	GM-CSF	Triiodothyronine
ADH (V$_2$ receptor)			Interferons	
MSH			Most interleukins	
PTH				
Calcitonin				
Glucagwon				
("FLAT CHAMP")	**("GGOAT")**			

ACTH = adrenocorticotropic hormone; ADH = antidiuretic hormone; CRH = corticotropin-releasing hormone; EGF = epidermal growth factor; FGF = fibroblast growth factor; FSH = follicle-stimulating hormone; GHRH = growth hormone-releasing hormone; GM-CSF = granulocyte-macrophage colony-stimulating factor; GnRH = gonadotropin-releasing hormone; hCG = human chorionic gonadotropin; IGF-1 = insulin-like growth factor 1; JAK/STAT = Janus kinase/signal transducer and activator; MSH = melanocyte-stimulating hormone; PDGF = platelet-derived growth factor; PTH = parathyroid hormone; RTK = receptor tyrosine kinase; TRH = thyrotropin-releasing hormone; TSH = thyroid-stimulating hormone; VEGF = vascular endothelial growth factor.

- **Inositol triphosphate (IP_3) mechanism:** Hormone binds GPCR → activated G protein (G_q) stimulates phospholipase C.
  - Phospholipase C cleaves phosphatidylinositol 4,5-bisphosphate (PIP_2), a membrane lipid, producing IP_3 and diacylglycerol (DAG).
  - IP_3 opens calcium channels in endoplasmic reticulum, releasing calcium into cytoplasm.
  - DAG and calcium facilitate activation of protein kinase C (PKC).
  - PKC exerts downstream effects via phosphorylation of other proteins.
- **Receptor tyrosine kinase (RTK) mechanism:** Hormone binds two adjacent cell membrane receptors → activated receptor dimer with tyrosine kinase activity.
  - Intracytoplasmic ends cross-phosphorylate each other as well as other proteins.
  - Many of these other proteins are also tyrosine kinases, which continue to phosphorylate other proteins and transcription factors.
- **Janus kinase/signal transducer and activator (JAK/STAT) mechanism:** Hormone binds two identical cell membrane receptors → activated JAKs on cytoplasmic ends.
  - JAKs phosphorylate tyrosine residues on receptors.
  - JAKs then recruit and phosphorylate STATs.
  - Activated STATs dimerize and translocate to nucleus to modify gene expression.

> **KEY FACT**
>
> Hypothalamic and posterior pituitary hormones use IP_3 (exception: corticotropin-releasing hormone [CRH]), whereas anterior pituitary hormones use cAMP. Antidiuretic hormone (ADH) uses both mechanisms.

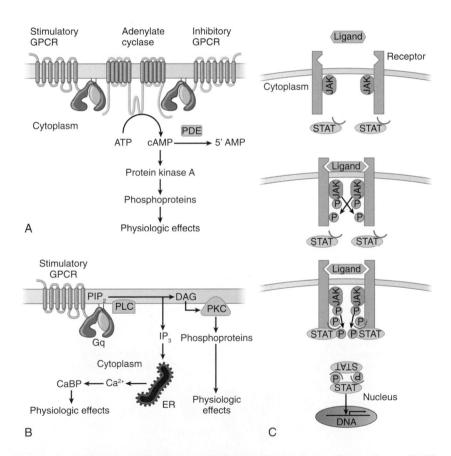

FIGURE 2-1. **Signal propagation mechanisms.** (A) Adenylate cyclase pathway. (B) Phospholipase C pathway. (C) JAK/STAT pathway. CaBP, calcium-binding protein; DAG, diacylglycerol; ER, endoplasmic reticulum; Gq and Gs, G proteins; IP_3, inositol 1,4,5-triphosphate; JAK/STAT, Janus kinase/signal transducer and activator; P, phosphate; PDE, PiP_2, phosphatidyl inositol 4,5 bisphosphate; PKC, protein kinase C; PLC, phospholipase C. (Modified with permission from Barrett KE, Barman SM, Boitano S, Brooks H. Ganong's *Review of Medical Physiology*, 23rd ed. New York: McGraw-Hill, 2010: Figures 2-26, 2-28, 2-31.)

Regulatory Control

- **Receptor up- and downregulation:** Target cells can upregulate/downregulate the number of receptors or receptor affinity for their ligands.
- **Negative feedback:** A hormone (or product of hormone signaling) acts upstream along its endocrine axis to increase or decrease its release toward the normal range.
- **Positive feedback:** Instead of maintaining homeostasis, a hormone can perpetuate an increase or decrease of its own release away from the normal range via reinforcement along its endocrine axis.
  - Feedback can occur via alterations in gene transcription, posttranslational processing, or hormone release.
  - Hormones may exhibit both positive and negative feedback controls (eg, estrogen inhibits luteinizing hormone [LH] release during the follicular phase of the menstrual cycle [negative feedback] but at midcycle promotes the LH surge and ovulation [positive feedback]).

HYPOTHALAMIC-PITUITARY AXIS

Hypothalamus

The hypothalamus is located below the thalamus and above the pituitary gland (which sits in the sella turcica). Each of its nuclei contributes to maintaining homeostasis: water balance, body temperature, hunger, thirst, and even emotions. The hypothalamus links the nervous system to the endocrine system, primarily through the pituitary gland (Figure 2-2). It does so by regulating the timing and amount of pituitary hormones secreted.

The hypothalamus exerts direct control over anterior pituitary hormone secretion via releasing/inhibiting factors (Table 2-4). These factors are synthesized by neural cell bodies in the hypothalamus, stored in granules at axon terminals, and released into the hypothalamo-hypophyseal circulation.

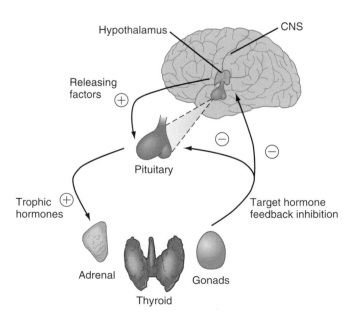

FIGURE 2-2. **Feedback regulation.** CNS, central nervous system. (Modified with permission from Kasper DL, Braunwald E, Fauci AS, et al. *Harrison's Principles of Internal Medicine,* 16th ed. New York: McGraw-Hill, 2005: 2072.)

TABLE 2-4. Overview of Hypothalamic Hormones

HORMONE	STRUCTURE	ACTIONS	REGULATION
Corticotropin-releasing hormone (CRH)	Peptide	Induces release of ACTH	Cortisol (–)
Gonadotropin-releasing hormone (GnRH)	Peptide	Induces release of LH and FSH	Testosterone (–), progesterone (–), prolactin (–)
Growth hormone-releasing hormone (GHRH)	Peptide	Induces release of GH	GHRH (–)
Somatostatin (growth hormone–inhibitory hormone)	Peptide	Inhibits release of GH and TSH	Somatomedins (+), GH (+)
Dopamine (prolactin-inhibiting factor)	Amine	Inhibits release of prolactin	Prolactin (+)
Thyrotropin-releasing hormone (TRH)	Peptide	Induces release of TSH and prolactin	

ACTH = adrenocorticotropic hormone; FSH = follicle-stimulating hormone; GH = growth hormone; LH = luteinizing hormone; TSH = thyroid-stimulating hormone.

Pituitary

The pituitary, or hypophysis, is composed of two embryologically and morphologically distinct glands (anterior and posterior) connected to the hypothalamus by the pituitary stalk. The gland rests in a bony cavity at the base of the skull called the sella turcica (Figure 2-3).

ANTERIOR PITUITARY (ADENOHYPOPHYSIS)

The anterior pituitary forms from the embryonic invagination of pharyngeal epithelium (**oral ectoderm**) called the pouch of Rathke. It is composed of five different hormone-producing cell populations, all of which are regulated by hypothalamic releasing and inhibiting hormones. The neurons that secrete these releasing hormones converge in the median eminence of the hypothalamus and act on the anterior pituitary via the hypophyseal circulation (a portal system).

POSTERIOR PITUITARY (NEUROHYPOPHYSIS)

The posterior pituitary forms from **neuroectoderm** derived from the hypothalamus. During development, it fuses with the pouch of Rathke. The posterior pituitary, composed of neural tissue, releases hormones in response to neurotransmission (not circulating hormones).

Anterior Pituitary Cell Types and Regulation

The adenohypophysis is composed of five major cell types, each of which produces one or more peptide hormones (Table 2-5).

Cell populations of the anterior pituitary can be further generalized according to reactions to histochemical stains. Periodic acid-Schiff (PAS) stain identifies

KEY FACT

Empty sella syndrome (ESS); In primary ESS, increased pressure in the sella turcica flattens the pituitary along the walls of the cavity. Secondary ESS is the regression of the pituitary secondary to injury or radiation. Both give the impression of an empty sella on imaging. This syndrome occasionally results in endocrine dysfunction.

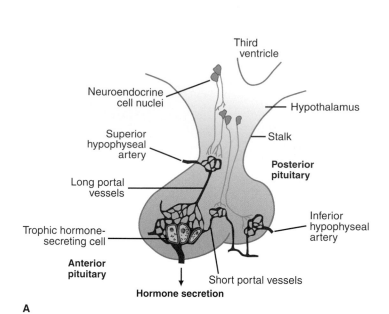

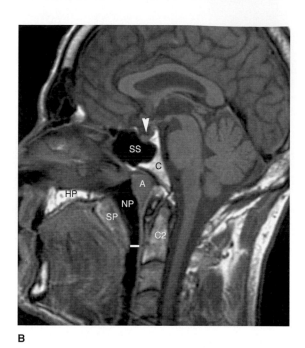

A   B

FIGURE 2-3.   (A) Schematic of pituitary gland and (B) T1-weighted MRI of pituitary gland *(white arrowhead)* **in sella turcica.**
A, adenoid; C, clivus; C2, dens of C2; HP, hard palate; NP, nasopharynx; SP, soft palate; SS, sphenoid sinus. (Part A modified with permission from Kasper DL, Braunwald E, Fauci AS, et al. *Harrison's Principles of Internal Medicine*, 16th ed. New York: McGraw-Hill, 2005: 2072. Part B reproduced with permission from Lalwani AK: *Current Diagnosis & Treatment in Otolaryngology—Head and Neck Surgery.* New York: McGraw-Hill, 2004: 45.)

three groups: Acidophils (stain orange), basophils (stain purple), and chromophobes (no stain reaction).

- **Acidophils:** Somatotropes (GH), lactotropes (prolactin)
- **Basophils:** Gonadotropes (FSH, LH), corticotropes (ACTH), thyrotropes (TSH) ("B-FLAT")
- **Chromophobes:** "Empty" cells (lack cytoplasmic granules); former acidophils or basophils after release of hormone-containing granules

TABLE 2-5.   Summary of Anterior Pituitary Hormone Function and Regulation

HORMONE	STRUCTURE	ACTIONS	REGULATION
Adrenocorticotropic hormone (ACTH)	Peptide	Induces synthesis of adrenal cortical hormones (cortisol, androgens, aldosterone).	Cortisol (−)
Follicle-stimulating hormone (FSH)	Peptide	Stimulates follicle growth in ovaries and spermatogenesis in testes.	Inhibin (−), estrogen (−), progesterone (−)
Luteinizing hormone (LH)	Peptide	Promotes testosterone synthesis in testes; promotes estrogen/progesterone synthesis in ovaries; surge causes ovulation and maintains the corpus luteum.	Testosterone (−), estrogen (+/−), progesterone (−)
Growth hormone (GH)	Peptide	Promotes protein synthesis and tissue growth.	Somatomedins (−)
Thyroid-stimulating hormone (TSH)	Peptide	Stimulates growth of thyroid gland and synthesis and secretion of thyroid hormones.	Thyroid hormones (−)
Prolactin	Peptide	Stimulates enlargement of breast tissue and milk production.	Dopamine (−), TRH (+)

Anterior Pituitary Hormones

PROLACTIN (PRL)

PRL is structurally homologous to growth hormone (GH) and human placental lactogen (HPL). All three hormones are synthesized in the RER.

- Suckling stimulates PRL secretion.
- Dopamine tonically inhibits PRL secretion.
- PRL promotes additional breast development during pregnancy (in concert with other hormones) in preparation for milk production. It also stimulates lactation (primary role) and inhibits ovulation through its effects on GnRH. PRL levels rise throughout the course of pregnancy, but their effects on lactation are inhibited by placental progesterone until birth (Figure 2-4).

GROWTH HORMONE

Growth hormone (GH) is a polypeptide hormone whose main function is to promote linear growth.

- GH may also be referred to as somatotropic hormone, or somatotropin.
- GH release is under hypothalamic regulation: Growth hormone-releasing hormone (GHRH) promotes and somatostatin inhibits GH release.
- GH also responds to exercise, trauma, and acute hypoglycemia (Figure 2-5).
- GH acts directly on tissues; its growth-promoting effect is primarily mediated via **insulin-like growth factor-1 (IGF-1)**, formerly known as somatomedin.
  - IGF-1 is produced by the liver in response to GH.
  - The metabolic effects of GH and IGF-1 include increased protein synthesis and fat utilization and decreased glucose uptake into tissues (Table 2-6).
- GH is secreted in a pulsatile pattern; at any moment in time, serum GH concentrations are usually low. After adolescence, overall production decreases and continues at a lower rate during adult life.

KEY FACT

Damage to the pituitary stalk can lead to decreased secretion of pituitary hormones secondary to disruption of the hypophyseal portal system (anterior pituitary) and hypothalamic neurons (posterior pituitary). The exception is prolactin (PRL) secretion, which is increased due to this same disruption.

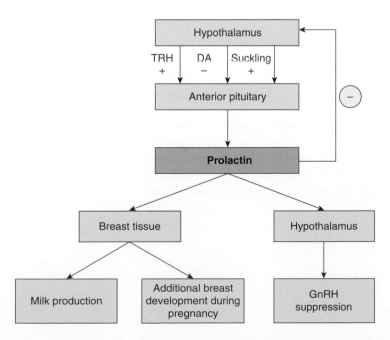

FIGURE 2-4. **Regulation of prolactin.** DA, dopamine GnRH, gonadotropin-releasing hormone; TRH, thyroid-releasing hormone.

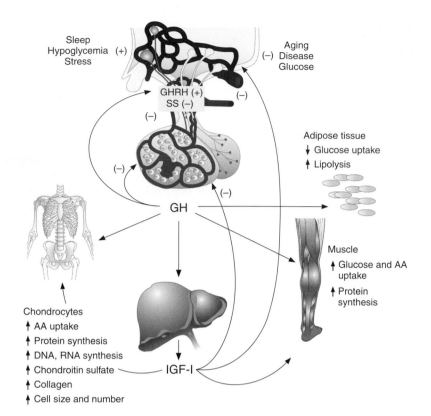

FIGURE 2-5. **GH regulation.** Factors that inhibit growth hormone (GH) secretion are insulin-like growth factor-1 (IGF-1), and somatostatin (SS). Factors that promote GH secretion are growth hormone-releasing hormone (GHRH), hypoglycemia, exercise, stress, sleep, and amino acids (AA: arginine and leucine). (Modified with permission from Molina PE. *Lange Endocrine Physiology*, 2nd ed. New York: McGraw-Hill, 2006: 56.)

TABLE 2-6. **Effects of Growth Hormone and Insulin-like Growth Factor-1**

DIRECT EFFECTS OF **GH**	INDIRECT EFFECTS OF **GH** (THROUGH **IGF-1**)
Decreases glucose uptake (counterregulatory effects).	Stimulates protein synthesis at the organ level.
Mobilizes fatty acids.	Increases protein synthesis in chondrocytes (promotes linear growth).
Stimulates protein synthesis in muscle.	Stimulates protein synthesis in muscle.
Increases lean body mass.	Increases lean body mass.

IGF-1 = insulin-like growth factor 1; GH = growth hormone.

■ GH, like glucagon, cortisol, and epinephrine, is a counterregulatory hormone that is released in response to hypoglycemia. Counterregulatory hormones increase serum glucose levels by promoting glycogenolysis, gluconeogenesis, lipolysis, and ketogenesis.

ADRENOCORTICOTROPIC HORMONE

ACTH is a polypeptide hormone that stimulates corticosteroid production by the adrenal cortex.

■ Synthesized by corticotropes in the anterior pituitary gland in response to stimulation by corticotropin-releasing hormone (CRH).
■ Synthesized from a larger precursor, proopiomelanocortin (POMC); β-lipotropin and β-endorphin are also derived from POMC (Figure 2-6).
■ A bioactive moiety, α-MSH (melanocyte-stimulating hormone), is present on the N-terminal end of ACTH.
■ ACTH regulates the size, integrity, and synthetic function of the adrenal cortex.

ANTERIOR PITUITARY HORMONE HOMOLOGY

The anterior pituitary gland produces six major hormones that can be classified into three groups based on structural homology.

■ **Glycoproteins:** FSH, LH, and TSH are each composed of α- and β-subunits. They share an identical α-subunit, but each has a unique β-subunit.
■ **Somatomammotropins:** GH and PRL are structurally related peptide hormones that belong to the same cytokine-hematopoietin family.
■ **ACTH-related peptides:** ACTH, MSH, and lipotropin are formed by cleavage of a single large precursor molecule (POMC).

FLASH FORWARD

Secondary and tertiary adrenal insufficiency (caused by pituitary or hypothalamic damage, respectively) cause cortisol deficiency but do not cause hyperpigmentation (decreased ACTH and thus decreased MSH). Because aldosterone secretion is primarily regulated by the renin-angiotensin system (RAS), these patients do not typically have hypovolemia, hypotension, hyponatremia, or hyperkalemia.

KEY FACT

Human chorionic gonadotropin (hCG) shares the same alpha subunit as FSH, LH, and TSH.

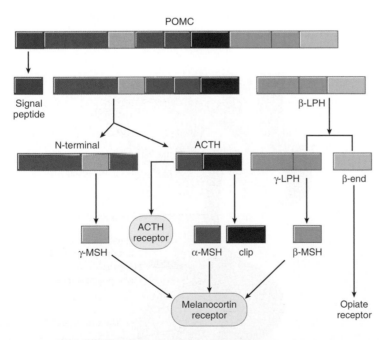

FIGURE 2-6. **Composition of proopiomelanocortin (POMC).** ACTH, adrenocorticotropic hormone; end, endorphin; LPH, lipotropic hormone; MSH, melanocyte-stimulating hormone. (Modified with permission from Molina PE. *Endocrine Physiology*, 3rd ed. New York: McGraw-Hill, 2010: Figure 3-4.)

Posterior Pituitary

Hormones of the posterior pituitary are synthesized in hypothalamic neurons (named **magnocellular neurons** because of their large cell bodies) and transported via axoplasmic flow to axon terminals in the posterior lobe of the pituitary. These hormones include oxytocin and antidiuretic hormone (ADH; a.k.a. vasopressin). The hypothalamic nuclei responsible for hormone production are the paraventricular nucleus and supraoptic nucleus (Figure 2-7).

Oxytocin and ADH are synthesized from larger precursors (prohormones) which are enzymatically cleaved within vesicles to produce active hormone. Release of oxytocin or ADH-containing granules is regulated by exogenous and endogenous stimuli, which are transformed into CNS signals.

OXYTOCIN

Two main actions (Figure 2-8):

- Promotes contractions of the uterine myometrium during labor.
- Stimulates contraction of myoepithelial cells in the breast, facilitating milk letdown to suckling infant.

Exogenous stimuli drive oxytocin secretion; signals include suckling of infant on breast and dilation of cervix (as in childbirth).

ANTIDIURETIC HORMONE

ADH plays a central role in osmoregulation.

- The osmotic concentration of extracellular fluid (ECF) is sensed by specialized neurons within or adjacent to the hypothalamus. The size of these neurons changes with extracellular osmolality, resulting in nerve signals increasing or decreasing ADH secretion as appropriate.
- ADH secretion increases in hyperosmolar conditions.

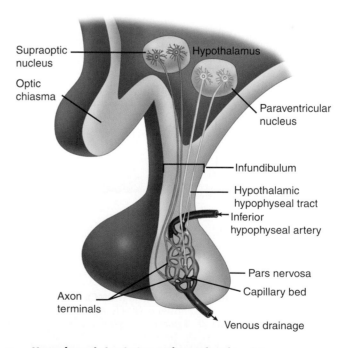

FIGURE 2-7. **Hypophyseal circulation and associated nuclei.**

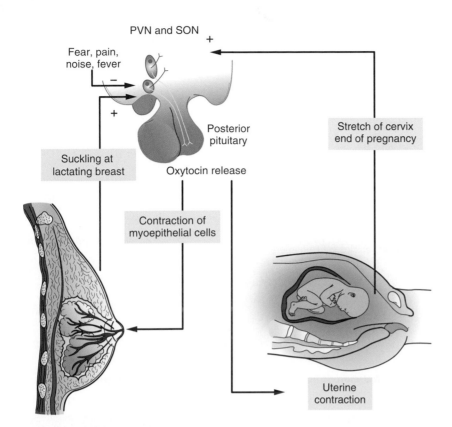

FIGURE 2-8. Oxytocin effects and regulation. PVN, paraventricular nuclei; SON, supraoptic nuclei. (Modified with permission from Molina PE. *Lange Endocrine Physiology*, 2nd ed. New York: McGraw-Hill, 2006: 35.)

- ADH increases permeability to water in the distal tubules and collecting ducts of the kidney, thereby increasing water reabsorption and decreasing plasma osmolality. It stimulates membrane-bound V_2 receptors, triggering an increase in intracellular cAMP. Special vesicles containing aquaporins (permeable water pores) are inserted into the luminal aspect of the cell membrane. Free diffusion of water occurs from tubule to peritubular fluid, decreasing ECF osmolality (Figure 2-9).
- At high concentrations, ADH constricts arterioles through the V_1 receptor. Consequently, ADH is also referred to as arginine vasopressin.
- In addition, ADH is secreted in response to large decreases (> 10%) in blood volume (Table 2-7). Secretion is stimulated by signals from atrial stretch receptors and baroreceptors.
  - Hypovolemia with resultant reduced atrial stretch results in decreased secretion of atrial natriuretic peptide (ANP). Low levels of ANP support increased secretion of ADH.
  - Baroreceptors of the aortic arch and carotid sinus sense decreased arterial pressure due to hypovolemia, resulting in decreased afferent signals to the medulla and consequent increase in ADH secretion and sympathetic stimulation.
- Unlike the RAS, which responds to subtle variations in circulating volumes, ADH secretion responds only to large decreases in blood volume.

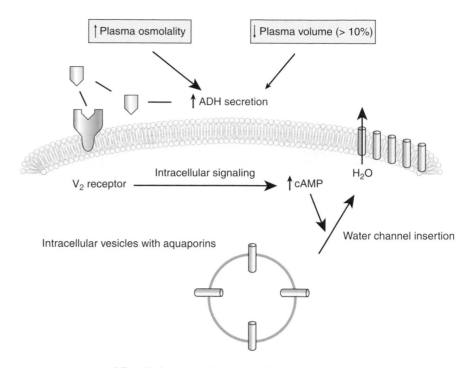

FIGURE 2-9. **Antidiuretic hormone (ADH) signaling and aquaporin insertion.**

ANTERIOR PITUITARY DISEASE

Pituitary Tumors

The most common pituitary tumor is a nonfunctioning, nonsecretory adenoma. Signs and symptoms of a pituitary tumor can be due to the effect of excess hormone if present, suppression of other hormone production due to mechanical compression, and/or elevated intracranial pressure due to mass effect.

PROLACTINOMA

The average age of onset is 20–40 years. This is the most common functioning pituitary tumor and is characterized by hypersecretion of PRL. The elevated PRL characteristically induces lactation, but PRL also inhibits GnRH. Decreased GnRH leads to decreased FSH and LH, which in turn decreases levels of progesterone and estrogen (testosterone in males), causing amenorrhea/impotence.

TABLE 2-7. **Factors Affecting Secretion of Antidiuretic Hormone**

INCREASE ADH SECRETION	DECREASE ADH SECRETION
↑ Plasma osmolality	↓ Plasma osmolality
↓ Plasma volume[a]	↑ Plasma volume[a]
↓ BP	↑ BP

ADH = antidiuretic hormone; BP = blood pressure.

[a]ADH secretion is affected by large changes in plasma volume.

DIFFERENTIAL

Dopamine tonically inhibits PRL secretion, so its depletion or pharmacologic antagonism disinhibits the anterior pituitary and PRL production. Excess PRL can arise from drugs that deplete or inhibit the synthesis/action of dopamine (reserpine, methyldopa, antipsychotics). In hypothyroidism, elevated TRH stimulates the anterior pituitary to upregulate PRL production.

PRESENTATION

- Amenorrhea, infertility, galactorrhea; decreased libido and osteopenia due to decreased estrogen in women; impotence and gynecomastia in men.
- Bitemporal hemianopsia due to superior growth of tumor, leading to compression of the optic chiasm.

DIAGNOSIS

- Serum chemistry: Elevated PRL. Rule out secondary causes by screening for hypothyrodism, pregnancy, confounding antiemetic/antipsychotic medications, renal failure, and cirrhosis. Marked psychological stress can also elevate PRL levels.
- Once secondary causes have been ruled out, MRI (or CT scan) to identify mass lesions.

TREATMENT

- **Dopamine agonists (bromocriptine, cabergoline)** are first-line treatment for any patient with hyperprolactinemia and are known to reduce the size and secretion of more than 90% of lactotroph adenomas.
- **Transsphenoidal surgery** is performed when dopamine agonists are ineffective in decreasing serum PRL concentration or the size of the adenoma or if the patient is pregnant and is suffering mass effect from the tumor.
- Asymptomatic patients without hypogonadism can be followed with **serial PRL levels.**

Gigantism and Acromegaly

This disorder of excessive GH secretion presents as gigantism in children, in whom the epiphyses have not yet closed, or as acromegaly in adults. **Gigantism** refers to excess linear height of more than 2 SD above the mean for a person's age, sex, and Tanner stage, which can occur in the setting of excess GH acting on the epiphyseal growth plates. **Acromegaly** is a related disorder resulting from GH acting on fused growth plate cartilage in adults.

DIFFERENTIAL

GH excess is most commonly caused by a pituitary adenoma composed of somatotroph cells. Less common causes include hypothalamic GHRH secretion or disruption of somatostatin tone. Gigantism can be a secondary feature of McCune-Albright syndrome and multiple endocrine neoplasia syndrome type I. Precocious puberty, normal genetics, and hyperthyroidism should be ruled out.

PRESENTATION

- Musculoskeletal and visceral overgrowth and deformity (gigantism) in children.
- Acromegaly (enlarged jaw, hands, feet, coarsening facial features, prognathism).
- Enlarged liver and heart (cardiomyopathy).

- Peripheral neuropathies such as carpal tunnel syndrome secondary to nerve compression.
- Glucose intolerance and diabetes mellitus in one-sixth of cases; also amenorrhea and impotence.
- Headache due to mass effect, and bitemporal hemianopsia due to superior growth of tumor leading to compression of the optic chiasm.
- Mean age of onset for acromegaly is in the third decade. The onset of acromegaly is insidious, as opposed to the dramatic presentation of gigantism.

DIAGNOSIS

- Elevated serum IGF-1 (sensitive screening test).
- Oral glucose tolerance test (OGTT): Administer 100 g of glucose to suppress GH, and then measure GH levels. Failure to suppress GH to < 5 ng/dL within 3 h is diagnostic.
- MRI scans to localize the tumor after a positive OGTT.

TREATMENT

- **Transsphenoidal surgery** is the treatment of choice. Can be accompanied by radiotherapy.
- **Octreotide** is a long-acting somatostatin analog that can lower GH levels to normal.
- Bromocriptine, a dopamine agonist, can work synergistically with octreotide therapy.
- Pegvisomant (GH-receptor antagonist).

PROGNOSIS

Cardiac failure is the most common cause of death in acromegalic patients. They also suffer an increased risk of colon cancer and pituitary insufficiency.

Panhypopituitarism

KEY FACT

Ischemic necrosis of the pituitary **(Sheehan syndrome):** Postpartum hemorrhage causing hypovolemic shock results in ischemic necrosis of the pituitary. This is due to the increase in size and blood demand of the pituitary during pregnancy.

This reduction in the release of all pituitary hormones may result from both primary and secondary causes. Primary causes directly affect the pituitary and include surgery, radiation, tumors, apoplexy (sudden hemorrhage into the gland, usually from adenoma), infection, infiltration by sarcoidosis or hemochromatosis, ischemia (Sheehan syndrome), carotid aneurysm, cavernous sinus thrombosis, and trauma. Secondary causes disrupt the hypothalamus or pituitary stalk and include hypothalamic tumors, hypothalamic hormone deficiency, surgery, infection, infiltration, and trauma.

PRESENTATION

Patients can present with signs and symptoms of any or all pituitary deficiencies. The most life-threatening pituitary deficiency is ACTH, followed by TSH, then FSH/LH, and lastly GH (Table 2-8).

DIAGNOSIS

Low or inappropriately normal levels of specific pituitary hormones in the setting of low target gland hormones. If neoplastic in etiology, MRI of the brain may localize the tumor for preoperative planning.

TREATMENT

Replacement of the missing hormones is required, with the most important being cortisol. Because most of the anterior pituitary hormones are proteins or glycoproteins that induce the secretion of other hormones, the target gland hormone is often used as replacement rather than the pituitary hormone (ie,

TABLE 2-8. **Clinical Findings With Hypopituitarism**

HORMONE	NORMAL FUNCTION	CLINICAL FINDINGS IN HORMONE DEFICIENCY
GH	Growth and glucose homeostasis	Children: growth failure, dwarfism. Adults: fatigue, osteoporosis, hypoglycemia ($\uparrow$ insulin sensitivity), $\uparrow$ LDL, $\uparrow$ fat mass, $\downarrow$ muscle mass, $\uparrow$ risk of cardiovascular disease.
Gonadotropin (LH/FSH)	Menstrual cycle and reproduction	Amenorrhea, impotence, genital atrophy, infertility, $\downarrow$ libido, $\downarrow$ axillary/pubic hair.
TSH	Stimulates T_4 production from the thyroid gland	Resembles primary hypothyroidism without goiter (cold intolerance, lethargy); TSH inappropriately low in the setting of low T_4.
ACTH	Stimulates glucocorticoid production from the adrenal gland	Resembles primary adrenal insufficiency but **without** skin hyperpigmentation from MSH or volume depletion, hypokalemia, and salt craving due to intact RAAS.

ACTH = adrenocorticotropic hormone; FSH = follicle-stimulating hormone; GH = growth hormone; LDL = low-density lipoprotein; LH = luteinizing hormone; MSH = melanocyte-stimulating hormone; RAAS = renin-angiotensin-aldosterone system; T_4 = thyroxine; TSH = thyroid-stimulating hormone.

TSH replaced with T_4, ACTH replaced with hydrocortisone or another glucocorticoid, LH and FSH replaced with testosterone, estrogen, or progestin).

POSTERIOR PITUITARY DISEASE

Diabetes Insipidus

Diabetes insipidus (DI) is characterized by an ineffective ADH axis, resulting in inappropriately dilute urine. Vasopressin (ADH), which is synthesized by the supraoptic nucleus and stored in the axon terminals of the posterior pituitary, functions to concentrate urine and conserve water. There are two types of DI.

- Central DI is due to absent or insufficient release of ADH from the posterior pituitary.
- Nephrogenic DI has normal ADH secretion, but the kidneys are unresponsive (renal resistance to the ADH). Causes are listed in Table 2-9.
- Primary polydipsia is a condition characterized by a marked increase in water intake, often seen in patients with psychiatric comorbidities, such as schizophrenia. It can also develop in patients with lesions affecting the hypothalamic thirst center.

PRESENTATION

Excessive urination and thirst. In children, DI can present with fever, vomiting, and diarrhea.

- The high serum osmolality stimulates thirst, causing patients to drink large amounts of water.
- Hypernatremia is usually not significant if the patient has free access to water, but is often a problem in hospitalized or debilitated patients with unrecognized DI and reduced access to water.

TABLE 2-9. Causes of Diabetes Insipidus

Central DI	■ Idiopathic (50% of cases)
	■ Trauma, surgery
	■ Tumors, sarcoidosis, TB
	■ Hand-Schüller-Christian disease
Nephrogenic DI	■ Hypercalcemia, hypokalemia
	■ Medications: Lithium, demeclocycline
	■ Pyelonephritis
	■ Aquaporin or vasopressin V$_2$ receptor gene mutations

DI = diabetes insipidus; TB = tuberculosis.

DIAGNOSIS

■ **Vasopressin challenge:** Complete fluid restriction + injection of vasopressin → increased urine osmolality (U$_{Osm}$) in central DI, but not nephrogenic DI (Table 2-10).
■ Urinalysis: Low U$_{Osm}$ and high plasma osmolality (P$_{Osm}$) in both central and nephrogenic DI, because the kidneys either do not receive ADH or cannot respond to ADH.
■ Meanwhile, U$_{Osm}$ and P$_{Osm}$ are both low in primary polydipsia, since the medullary gradient of the kidneys is washed out and dilute urine is produced.

TREATMENT

■ Vasopressin (subcutaneously, orally, or intranasally) for central DI.
■ Chlorpropamide increases the release of ADH in partial ADH deficiency.
■ For nephrogenic DI, thiazide diuretics (eg, hydrochlorothiazide [HCTZ]) or indomethacin (a nonsteroidal anti-inflammatory drug [NSAID]) can be used.

PROGNOSIS

Patients who have access to water can usually keep up with the large urinary losses. When water is not readily available, the rising serum sodium concentration can cause weakness, fever, obtundation, and eventually death.

Syndrome of Inappropriate Secretion of Antidiuretic Hormone

In syndrome of inappropriate secretion of antidiuretic hormone (SIADH), excess ADH in the absence of hyperosmolarity leads to an inability to dilute

TABLE 2-10. Differentiating Between Central and Nephrogenic Diabetes Insipidus

	INCREASE IN U$_{Osm}$ WITH WATER DEPRIVATION?	RESPONSE TO INJECTION OF ADH?
Central DI	No	Yes
Nephrogenic DI	No	No
Primary polydipsia	Yes	Yes

ADH = antidiuretic hormone; DI = diabetes insipidus; U$_{Osm}$ = urine osmolality.

urine. There is a net gain in free water over sodium, resulting in euvolemic hyponatremia. Common causes of SIADH include CNS disease; pulmonary diseases; endocrinopathies; and drugs including NSAIDs, antidepressants, chemotherapeutics, diuretics, phenothiazines, and hypoglycemics. This is summarized in Table 2-11.

MNEMONIC

SIADH = **S**odium **I**s **A**lways **D**own **H**ere

PRESENTATION

- Patients are often asymptomatic if SIADH is chronic. If onset is acute, brain swelling can result, leading to lethargy, weakness, seizures, and coma/death.
- SIADH causes volume expansion, but edema and hypertension are usually not present because of natriuresis (excreting excess sodium in urine).

DIAGNOSIS

SIADH exhibits hypotonic hyponatremia ($\downarrow$ serum Na and P_{Osm}) in the presence of increased U_{Osm} (> 300 mOsm/L).

- Blood urea nitrogen (BUN) and uric acid are also decreased, reflecting diluted fluid stores. Plasma creatinine (Cr) remains relatively normal.
- Need to rule out hypothyroidism ($\downarrow$ cardiac output, glomerular filtration rate [GFR]) and adrenal insufficiency ($\uparrow$ CRH and ADH).

KEY FACT

Hyponatremia must not be corrected too quickly because this can result in central pontine myelinolysis.

TREATMENT

Fluid restriction in mild cases of SIADH. When fluid restriction is not feasible or not working, use **conivaptan** (a V_2 receptor antagonist) or **demeclocycline** (acts on collecting tubule to limit response to ADH). Hypertonic saline may be used if cerebral edema, convulsions, or coma develops.

PITUITARY/HYPOTHALAMIC PHARMACOLOGY

Leuprolide

MECHANISM

GnRH agonist: GnRH is normally secreted in a pulsatile fashion by the hypothalamus and stimulates the release of FSH and LH from the anterior pitu-

TABLE 2-11. Common Causes of SIADH

Neoplasms with ectopic ADH secretion	- Small-cell lung carcinoma
	- Thymoma
Pulmonary diseases	- TB
	- Lung abscesses
	- Pneumonia
CNS disorders	- Skull fractures/trauma
	- Subdural hematoma
Drugs	- Chlorpropamide
	- Vincristine, vinblastine
	- Cyclophosphamide
	- Carbamazepine

ADH = antidiuretic hormone; CNS = central nervous system; TB = tuberculosis.

itary. Leuprolide is a GnRH analog that has a longer half-life; it can be used in a pulsatile fashion to increase LH/FSH or continuously to suppress LH/FSH.

USES

When given in a pulsatile fashion, it is used to treat women with amenorrhea who desire fertility. When given in a continuous fashion, leuprolide suppresses the growth of prostate cancer, leiomyomas, and endometriosis, and also halts precocious puberty.

SIDE EFFECTS

Bone pain, feet/ankle swelling.

Somatotropin

MECHANISM

GH analog: Increases lean muscle mass.

USES

Dwarfism; treats wasting associated with AIDS or malignancy.

SIDE EFFECTS

Hand/foot edema, thickening of bones/jaw, carpal tunnel syndrome, increased organ growth, decreased insulin sensitivity, hyperglycemia.

Octreotide

MECHANISM

Somatostatin analog: Somatostatin is a hypothalamic hormone that normally inhibits the release of GH, glucagon, insulin, gastrin, and vasoactive intestinal peptide (VIP). Octreotide has a longer half-life than somatostatin itself.

USES

Esophageal varices, VIPomas, carcinoid syndrome, acromegaly, Zollinger-Ellison syndrome.

SIDE EFFECTS

Gallbladder disease, pancreatitis, hypo- or hyperthyroidism, cardiac arrhythmias.

Dopamine Agonists (Bromocriptine, Cabergoline)

MECHANISM

Dopamine receptor agonists. PRL secretion is normally inhibited by dopamine from the hypothalamus.

USES

Prolactinomas, Parkinson disease (high doses required).

SIDE EFFECTS

Psychotic symptoms, dizziness, headache, nausea, lightheadedness, confusion.

Desmopressin

MECHANISM

Vasopressin analog (ADH): Has minimal V_1 activity (minimal action on vascular smooth muscle). More effect on V_2 receptors, which act on the renal collecting tubules to increase water reabsorption. Also stimulates release of von Willebrand factor (vWF) from the endothelium in platelet dysfunction disorders.

USES

Central DI, von Willebrand disease.

SIDE EFFECTS

Hyponatremia, transient headache, flushing.

Oxytocin

MECHANISM

Posterior pituitary hormone that stimulates milk secretion and induces uterine contractions during labor.

USES

Induces labor; decreases postpartum bleeding by inducing contractions. Also used to stimulate breast milk letdown in new mothers.

SIDE EFFECTS

Chest pain, confusion, excessive vaginal bleeding, palpitations, seizures.

Thyroid and Parathyroid

THYROID

The thyroid gland regulates growth and metabolic rate through the actions of its two major hormones, **thyroxine (T_4)** and **triiodothyronine (T_3)**. Also, the parafollicular (C) cells of the thyroid gland produce **calcitonin,** a hormone that lowers serum calcium levels; however, in humans, it is not usually significant in maintaining calcium homeostasis.

Anatomy

Situated anterior to the trachea, the thyroid is a butterfly-shaped structure below the larynx extending from C5 to T1. It is composed of a right and left lobe united by a thin strip of thyroid tissue called the isthmus (Figure 2-10).

The thyroid is among the largest endocrine organs, weighing 10–20 g. It receives a disproportionately large share of cardiac output per gram of tissue. The rich blood supply of the thyroid is derived from two pairs of vessels: the superior and inferior thyroid arteries.

- **Superior thyroid artery:** This first branch off the external carotid artery supplies the superior half of the thyroid.
- **Inferior thyroid artery:** Stems from the thyrocervical trunk, which is a branch of the subclavian artery.

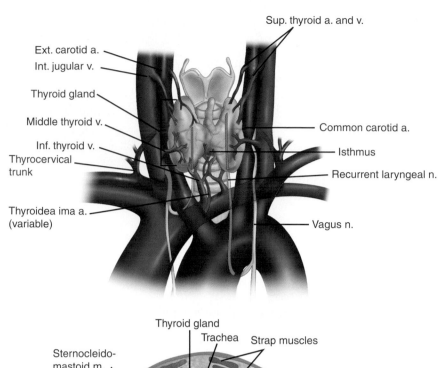

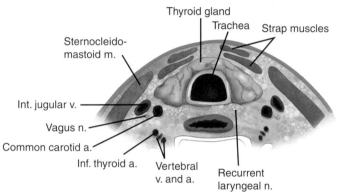

FIGURE 2-10.   Anatomy of the thyroid gland.

- Three sets of veins drain the thyroid: **Superior, middle, and inferior thyroid veins.** The superior and middle veins drain into the internal jugular veins, whereas the inferior thyroid veins empty into the brachiocephalic veins.

Embryology

The thyroid is formed from an epithelial outpouching, the **thyroid diverticulum,** which develops in the floor of the foregut at 3–4 weeks of gestation. The thyroglossal duct progenitor migrates caudally, and the thyroid gland eventually assumes its normal position below the larynx unless migration is disrupted. This duct remains patent during development, maintaining a connection between the foregut and thyroid. Ultimately, the thyroglossal duct closes, leaving the **foramen cecum** as an adult remnant. The thyroid begins secreting hormone as early as the 18th week of fetal development.

Histology

At the microscopic level, the thyroid gland is made up of spherical, closed follicles that are lined with cuboidal epithelial cells.

- The basal surfaces of follicular cells are in contact with a rich blood supply that allows for the absorption of iodide to be used in hormone production.

KEY FACT

A **thyroglossal duct cyst** develops when the thyroglossal duct does not close, persisting in the midline near the hyoid bone or at the base of the tongue. **Ectopic thyroid tissue** is most commonly found at the base of the tongue.

- The apical membranes of follicular cells face a lumen filled with a secretory substance referred to as colloid. The major constituent of colloid is the glycoprotein **thyroglobulin,** which stores iodine and is a precursor of the thyroid hormones (Figure 2-11).
- Interspersed within the walls of thyroid follicles are small collections of parafollicular C cells that synthesize and secrete calcitonin.

Thyroid Hormone Synthesis

IODIDE EXTRACTION

The thyroid acquires iodide, a necessary factor for hormone synthesis, from the circulation. The following numbered steps (1–9) refer to Figure 2-12.

1. Follicular cells possess a sodium-iodide symporter on their basal surfaces that **actively transports** iodide out of the blood and into the cytosol of follicular cells. This process of intracellular accumulation is known as **iodide trapping.**
2. Intracellular iodide rapidly diffuses across the apical membranes of follicular cells and into the colloidal lumen. Here, it binds to tyrosine residues on thyroglobulin. TSH facilitates iodide transport. Bromide, thiocyanate, and perchlorate inhibit this process.

THYROGLOBULIN SYNTHESIS AND SECRETION

Thyroglobulin is a large glycoprotein produced by the thyroid that plays an important role in thyroid hormone synthesis. Thyroid hormones are synthesized from tyrosine residues in the protein structure of thyroglobulin. It serves as both a precursor and a storage form of thyroid hormone.

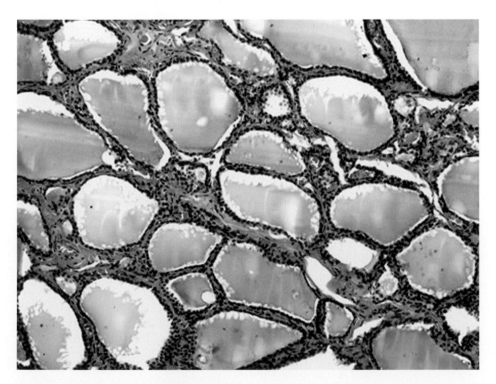

FIGURE 2-11. **Thyroid follicular cells.** (Reprinted with permission from Brunicardi F, Andersen D, Billiar T, et al. *Schwartz's Principles of Surgery,* 9th ed. New York: McGraw-Hill, 2009: Figure 38-7.)

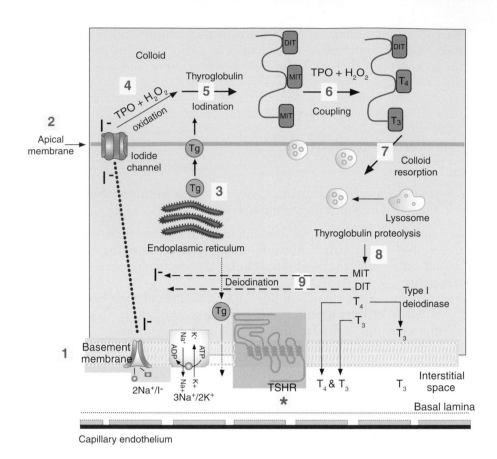

FIGURE 2-12. **Thyroid hormone biosynthesis.** DIT, diiodotyrosine; MIT, monoiodotyrosine; TG, thyroglobulin; TPO, thyroid peroxidase. TSHR, thyroid-stimulating hormone receptor. (Modified with permission from Molina PE. *Lange Endocrine Physiology*, 2nd ed. New York: McGraw-Hill, 2006: 78.)

3. Thyroglobulin is synthesized by thyroid follicular cells and is secreted across the apical membrane. Thyroglobulin is the principal component of colloid.

OXIDATION AND ORGANIFICATION

Following thyroglobulin synthesis and iodide uptake, the next step in thyroid hormone synthesis is iodination of thyroglobulin, a process that requires oxidation and organification reactions.

4. **Thyroid peroxidase,** an apical membrane enzyme, binds an iodide atom and a tyrosine moiety, brings them into close apposition, and promotes **oxidation** of iodide and tyrosine. This leads to the generation of short-lived free radicals that enable the reaction between iodide and tyrosine residues on thyroglobulin.

5. In the process of **organification,** these free radicals (ie, iodine and tyrosine moieties) undergo an additional reaction to form monoiodotyrosine (MIT). A second organification reaction can take place, adding iodine to an MIT molecule to form diiodotyrosine (DIT).

COUPLING

The final step in thyroid hormone synthesis is the coupling of two iodotyrosine residues (MIT or DIT) to form iodothyronine.

6. With MIT and DIT still bound to thyroglobulin, they undergo **coupling** reactions to form T_4 and T_3. T_4 and T_3 remain attached to thyroglobulin

as stored hormone awaiting TSH stimulation. Coupling, like oxidation, is performed by thyroid peroxidase.

- T_3 is formed by the coupling of one MIT and one DIT moiety.
- T_4 is formed by the coupling of two DIT moieties. T_4 makes up a majority of thyroid hormone synthesized in this process.

THYROID HORMONE RELEASE

TSH binds to surface receptors on thyroid epithelial cells and serves as the chief stimulus for hormone release (see * in Figure 2-12).

7. TSH-mediated stimulation of the thyroid gland results in pinocytosis of luminal colloid.
8. Within the follicular cells, lysosomes fuse with pinocytic vesicles, and thyroglobulin is proteolytically digested. Products of protein breakdown include T_4 and T_3, both of which are transported across the basal membrane and into the circulation.
9. Continued cleavage of thyroglobulin produces a large proportion of MIT and DIT molecules within follicular cells. **Deiodinase** mediates iodine moiety cleavage from MIT/DIT and recycling for future thyroid hormone synthesis.

Thyroid Hormone Transport and Metabolism

T_4 and T_3 are principally bound to thyroxine-binding globulin (TBG), a protein secreted by the liver.

- **TBG** slows metabolic inactivation and urinary excretion of thyroid hormones, thereby extending their half-lives. T_4 is the major hormone secreted by the thyroid and carried in the circulation; however, T_3 is the physiologically active form of the hormone.
- **Activation:** 5'-Deiodinase catalyzes the conversion of T_4 to T_3 by the removal of an iodine atom. 5'-Deiodinase is present in the liver, kidneys, thyroid, and target organs.
- **Inactivation:** A separate deiodinase enzyme targets another site on the T_4 molecule, forming biologically inactive **reverse T_3 (rT_3)**. Enzymatic inactivation of T_3 occurs primarily in the liver and kidneys (Figure 2-13).

>
>
> **KEY FACT**
>
> Changes in TBG levels can alter the total levels of T_3 and T_4 but **will not change free, active T_3 and T_4 levels.** Thus, patients are euthyroid and do not show signs of hypo- or hyperthyroidism.

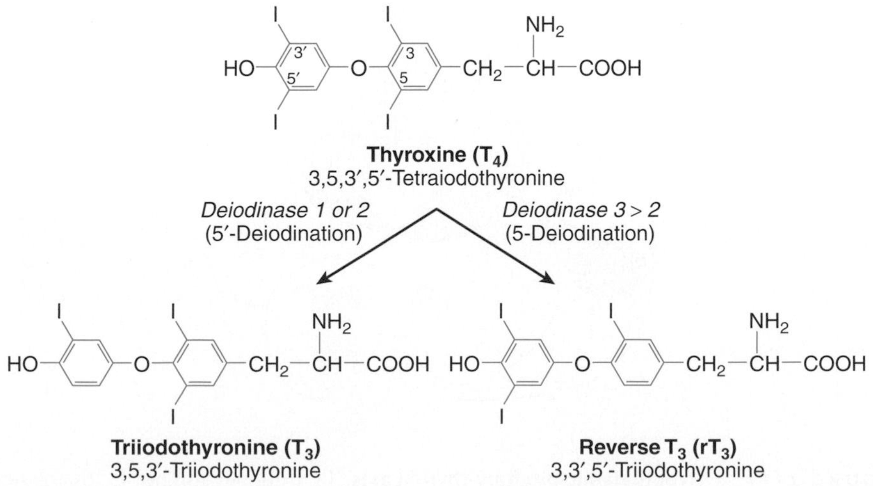

HO—⬡—O—⬡—CH_2—$\overset{NH_2}{CH}$—COOH

Thyroxine (T_4)
3,5,3',5'-Tetraiodothyronine

Deiodinase 1 or 2
(5'-Deiodination)

Deiodinase 3 > 2
(5-Deiodination)

HO—⬡—O—⬡—CH_2—$\overset{NH_2}{CH}$—COOH   HO—⬡—O—⬡—CH_2—$\overset{NH_2}{CH}$—COOH

Triiodothyronine (T_3)
3,5,3'-Triiodothyronine

Reverse T_3 (rT_3)
3,3',5'-Triiodothyronine

FIGURE 2-13. **Thyroid hormone structure.** (Modified with permission from Kasper DL, Braunwald E, Fauci AS, et al. *Harrison's Principles of Internal Medicine*, 16th ed. New York: McGraw-Hill, 2005: 2072.)

Deiodination is a major mechanism by which thyroid hormone activity is enhanced or reduced, depending on whether active hormone (T_3) or inactive hormone (rT_3) is produced.

Thyroid Hormone Regulation

The hypothalamic-pituitary axis responds to changes in the levels of **free** T_4 and T_3 in the serum (Figure 2-14).

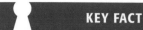

KEY FACT

The Wolff-Chaikoff effect is a protective downregulation of thyroid hormone production in the presence of large amounts of iodine (seen with cardiac catheterization and CT with contrast).

In contrast, the **Jod-Basedow effect** is the overproduction of thyroid hormone, causing overt hyperthyroidism in the presence of large amounts of iodine in persons who fail to manifest the Wolff-Chaikoff effect.

- Low levels of free thyroid hormone stimulate the release of TRH from the hypothalamus and TSH from thyrotropes in the pituitary gland.
- TRH enters the hypophyseal circulation and stimulates more release of TSH into the systemic circulation.
- TSH promotes increased thyroid hormone synthesis and secretion by upregulating the processes of iodide uptake, organification, coupling, and pinocytosis of colloid material.
- TSH also exerts trophic effects on the thyroid gland, increasing its size through continued protein synthesis.

Downstream Effects

Thyroid hormone contributes to growth, development, and metabolism.

- **Bone growth:** Thyroid hormone facilitates growth by stimulating GH gene expression in somatotrophs of the anterior pituitary. Thyroid hormone also stimulates calcification and closure of cartilaginous growth plates throughout the body.
- **CNS maturation:** Thyroid hormone is vital for CNS development during the prenatal period and for the first three years of life. As part of normal development, neuroblasts proliferate into the second trimester, after which they begin to differentiate into neurons. Thyroid hormone promotes this transition to neuronal differentiation and, ultimately, synapse formation.

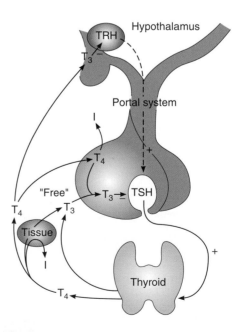

FIGURE 2-14. Hypothalamic-pituitary-thyroid axis. T_3, triiodothyronine; T_4, thyroxine; TRH, thyroid-releasing hormone; TSH, thyroid-stimulating hormone. (Modified with permission from Gardner DG, Shoback D. *Greenspan's Basic & Clinical Endocrinology*, 8th ed. New York: McGraw-Hill, 2007: 232.)

- **Adrenergic effects:** Thyroid hormone renders β_1-adrenergic receptors in the heart more responsive to signaling molecules. Contractility, stroke volume, and heart rate are all increased, thereby increasing cardiac output.
- **Basal metabolic rate (BMR):** Thyroid hormone promotes the synthesis of cytochromes, cytochrome oxidase, and Na^+–K^+ ATPase, while also increasing the number and activity of mitochondria. These actions ultimately increase O_2 consumption, the BMR, and body temperature.
- **Intermediary metabolism:** Thyroid hormone stimulates fuel mobilization and catabolism to support the body's increased BMR. Gluconeogenesis, glycogenolysis, and lipolysis are all enhanced to this end.

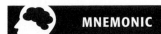 **MNEMONIC**

T_3 functions—

4 B's:
Brain maturation
Bone growth
Beta-adrenergic effects
Basal metabolic rate increases

DISORDERS OF THE THYROID

Hyperthyroidism

Hyperthyroidism causes **thyrotoxicosis;** elevated thyroid hormones in the blood. Graves disease causes the majority of cases of hyperthyroidism. Other cases are due to miscellaneous causes, including thyroiditis, toxic thyroid adenomas, and, rarely, TSH-secreting pituitary tumors, struma ovarii, and hCG-secreting tumors. See Table 2-12 for causes and their unique presentations.

PRESENTATION

- Tremor, weight loss despite robust appetite, irritability, restlessness, insomnia, heat intolerance, diaphoresis, increased frequency of bowel movements or frank diarrhea, and tachycardia/palpitations.
- Warm and moist skin due to peripheral vasodilatation and excessive sweating.
- Increased risk of atrial fibrillation, isolated systolic hypertension, and high-output cardiac failure.

 KEY FACT

Thyroid storm is a life-threatening form of thyrotoxicosis characterized by high fever, tachyarrhythmia, psychosis, confusion, diarrhea, and liver dysfunction. It is managed with intensive care unit-level support, antithyroid medications, and β-adrenergic blockers.

TABLE 2-12.   Causes of Hyperthyroidism

CAUSE	ETIOLOGY	CLINICAL MANIFESTATIONS
Graves disease	• Thyroid-stimulating immunoglobulin (TSI) binds TSH receptor on thyroid gland → ↑ T_3/T_4 (diffuse uptake on thyroid scan). Type II hypersensitivity. • Can be associated with other autoimmune disorders.	• Diffuse nontender goiter with or without bruit. • Infiltrative ophthalmopathy (exophthalmos, extraocular muscle dysfunction). • Pretibial myxedema.
Toxic multinodular goiter (Plummer disease)	• Hyperfunctioning areas that make ↑ T_3/T_4 (patchy uptake on thyroid scan). • Due to a mutation in the TSH receptor. • More common in the elderly.	• Similar to Graves disease, but less severe.
Subacute thyroiditis (de Quervain thyroiditis)	• Inflammation of thyroid gland → spilling of preformed thyroid hormones → transient hyperthyroidism. Pituitary inhibition causes transient hypothyroidism before return to euthyroid state. • Usually preceded by upper respiratory infection.	• Thyroid gland firm, painful, tender. • Fever. • ↑ ESR. • Pain radiating to ears, neck, and arm.
Struma ovarii	This is a very rare condition in which ectopic thyroid tissue develops as part of an ovarian tumor, causing hyperthyroidism.	

CHF = congestive heart failure; ESR = erythrocyte sedimentation rate; TSH = thyroid-stimulating hormone.

DIAGNOSIS

- Increased T_3 and T_4.
- Decreased TSH (except in TSH-secreting tumors).
- Anti-TSH receptor antibodies for Graves disease (thyroid-stimulating immunoglobulins).
- Radioactive iodine uptake (RAIU) scan: Localized uptake (toxic adenoma, multinodular thyroid), generalized uptake (Graves disease), or no uptake (thyroiditis, struma ovarii).

TREATMENT

- **Propylthiouracil (PTU)** and **methimazole:** Inhibit thyroid hormone synthesis by inhibiting the organification of iodine; PTU also inhibits the peripheral conversion of $T_4 \rightarrow T_3$.
- **Radioactive iodine ablation:** To destroy the thyroid follicular cells. Radioiodine is contraindicated for treatment of hyperthyroidism during pregnancy because it can cross the placenta and destroy the infant's thyroid gland, leading to hypothyroidism and its morbid sequelae.
- **β-Blockers** such as propranolol: Control of adrenergic symptoms (sweating, tachycardia, tremor).

KEY FACT

A **goiter** is an enlarged thyroid gland due to any cause, such as inflammation, tumor, or autoimmune disease. Endemic goiter, caused by iodine deficiency, is the most common cause of goiter worldwide.

Hypothyroidism

Over 95% of cases of hypothyroidism result from failure of the thyroid gland itself (primary hypothyroidism). The most common cause of primary hypothyroidism in the United States is **Hashimoto thyroiditis** (in the developing world, iodine deficiency is most common). Other causes can be seen in Table 2-13.

PRESENTATION (TABLE 2-14)

- Lethargy, fatigue, muscle weakness.
- Cold intolerance, constipation, weight gain, coarse/dry skin, macroglossia.

TABLE 2-13. Common Causes of Hypothyroidism

PRIMARY CAUSES	
Hashimoto thyroiditis	Autoimmune in origin (HLA-DR5). Antithyroid peroxidase antibodies confirm the diagnosis. Lymphocytic infiltrate with germinal centers seen on histology, as well as Hurthle cells.
Subacute (de Quervain) thyroiditis	Self-limited hypothyroidism following a flu-like illness. May have elevated ESR, jaw pain, and a tender thyroid gland. Histology shows granulomatous inflammation. Hyperthyroid earlier in course.
Iodine deficiency	Most common cause in the developing world.
Riedel thyroiditis	Rare disease in which thyroid tissue is chronically replaced by fibrosis. Rock-hard, fixed, painless goiter.
Lithium	Lithium toxicity may cause hypothyroidism.
Surgical resection and ^{131}I treatment	Surgical removal or radioactive iodine ablation may cause hypothyroidism.
SECONDARY CAUSE	
Sheehan syndrome	Postpartum pituitary necrosis secondary to postpartum hemorrhage. Decreased TSH.

ESR = erythrocyte sedimentation rate; TSH = thyroid-stimulating hormone.

TABLE 2-14. **Signs and Symptoms of Abnormal Thyroid Hormone Levels**

	HYPERTHYROIDISM	**HYPOTHYROIDISM**
Symptoms	Hyperactivity, irritability	Mental sluggishness
	Heat intolerance, sweating	Cold intolerance
	Palpitations	Dyspnea
	Fatigue, weakness	Fatigue, weakness
	Diarrhea	Constipation
	Hair loss, oily skin	Hair loss, dry skin
	Oligomenorrhea, loss of libido	Menorrhagia, loss of libido
	Weight loss, robust appetite	Weight gain, poor appetite
	Polyuria	Paresthesias
Signs	Tachycardia	Bradycardia
	Tremor	Delayed deep tendon reflex relaxation phase
	Goiter	Goiter
	Warm, moist skin	Dry, doughy skin
	Proximal muscle weakness	Carpal tunnel syndrome
	Exophthalmos	Periorbital edema
	Lid retraction, lid lag	Puffy face, hands, and feet (myxedema)
		Peripheral edema

- Delayed recovery phase of deep tendon reflexes.
- Slow mentation.
- Diastolic hypertension.
- **Myxedema coma:** Stupor, coma, and hypoventilation coupled with hypothermia, bradycardia, and hypotension. A life-threatening hypothyroid condition that results from long-standing, untreated hypothyroidism. Triggered by trauma, infections, and cold exposure. Treatment is with hormone replacement and supportive measures; mortality is high.

DIAGNOSIS

- $T_3/T_4/TSH/TRH$: May be helpful for diagnosing and distinguishing among primary, secondary, and tertiary causes.
- Chemistries: Mild normocytic anemia, hyponatremia, hypoglycemia.
- Immunology: Antithyroid peroxidase antibody test for Hashimoto thyroiditis.
- Imaging: Pituitary or pelvic imaging for tumor, if evidence of TSH-producing tumor or struma ovarii is discovered.

TREATMENT

Hypothyroidism is treated with **levothyroxine (T_4)** replacement.

Thyroid Neoplasms

Thyroid cancer is the most common endocrine malignancy in the United States, with an annual incidence of approximately 2 cases per 100,000. Risk factors include childhood head and neck radiation exposure, male gender, young age, and positive family history.

KEY FACT

In newborns, hypothyroidism causes **cretinism** (mental retardation, short stature, coarse features, umbilical hernia). Thyroid hormone deficiency during fetal development may be due to a failure of thyroid gland formation, inability to synthesize hormone (T_3/T_4), lack of iodine, radioiodine taken by the mother, or untreated hypothyroidism in the mother.

PRESENTATION

Typically presents as a solitary nodule. Dyspnea, coughing/choking spells, dysphagia, and hoarseness may occur due to compression of the trachea or esophagus.

DIAGNOSIS

- **Chemistries:** TSH (usually normal).
- **Thyroid ultrasound:** Large size (> 1–1.5 cm), irregular borders, hypoechogenicity, intranodular hypervascularity, and intranodular microcalcifications indicate increased risk for malignancy. Radioactive iodine thyroid scintiscanning is not used to determine whether a nodule should be biopsied.
- **Fine-needle aspiration:** Provides cytopathologic diagnosis of four varieties of cancer (Table 2-15). Fifteen percent of nodules are suspicious or malignant, yet most biopsies are benign or indeterminate.

TREATMENT

Thyroidectomy for all thyroid cancers except anaplastic carcinoma.

Multiple Endocrine Neoplasia

All the multiple endocrine neoplasia (MEN) syndromes are inherited in an autosomal dominant fashion. They are divided into three categories based on the oncogene and endocrine glands involved:

- **MEN 1 (Wermer syndrome):** Tumors of the **p**ancreas, **p**ituitary, and **p**arathyroid (the **3 Ps**). May present with kidney stones secondary to hyperparathyroidism and GI ulcers secondary to gastrin-producing pancreatic adenomas (gastrinomas), which cause Zollinger-Ellison syndrome.

KEY FACT

Other thyroid neoplasms include **thyroid lymphoma** (rare, history of Hashimoto thyroiditis) and **benign thyroid adenoma** (solitary nodule, may lead to hyperthyroidism).

TABLE 2-15. **Types of Thyroid Cancer**

TYPE	PREVALENCE (%)	CHARACTERISTICS	TREATMENT
Papillary carcinoma	70–80%	■ History of radiation exposure increases risk. ■ Slow-growing, spreads by lymphatics in the neck. ■ "Orphan Annie" nuclei (cells in papillary cancer have dispersed chromatin, giving appearance of empty nuclei). ■ Psammoma bodies (concentric calcification of individual necrotic tumor cells).	Lobectomy or total thyroidectomy ± radioiodine
Follicular carcinoma	10–20%	■ More aggressive than papillary carcinomas. ■ Tends to invade into blood vessels → spreads to bone, lung, and liver (lymph node involvement rare).	Total thyroidectomy + postoperative iodine ablation
Medullary carcinoma	5%	■ Arises from parafollicular "C" cells of thyroid. ■ Produces calcitonin (can be used as tumor marker). ■ Amyloid deposits (derived from altered calcitonin molecules). ■ Associated with the MEN 2A and MEN 2B syndromes.	Total thyroidectomy
Anaplastic carcinoma	5%	■ Older patients. ■ Highly aggressive. Poor prognosis (death within a few months).	Chemotherapy and radiation

MEN = multiple endocrine neoplasia.

- **MEN 2A (Sipple syndrome):** Medullary thyroid carcinoma, pheochromocytoma, and parathyroid adenoma.
- **MEN 2B:** Medullary thyroid carcinoma, pheochromocytoma, and oral/GI ganglioneuromatosis (associated with marfanoid habitus).

DRUGS FOR HYPOTHYROIDISM

Levothyroxine (T_4) is the principal pharmacologic agent used for hypothyroidism. Liothyronine (T_3) is not used routinely for the treatment of hypothyroidism because it is arrhythmogenic and can precipitate heart failure, although it may be used to treat myxedema coma.

Levothyroxine

MECHANISM

T_4 analog, binds to nuclear receptors. Leads to increased protein synthesis, increased metabolic rate, and increased β-receptors → increased sensitivity to catecholamines.

USES

Hypothyroidism.

SIDE EFFECTS

Signs and symptoms of hyperthyroidism (ie, tachycardia, heart failure, sweating, tremor, diarrhea).

ANTITHYROID DRUGS

Two main classes of drugs are used to treat hyperthyroidism: thionamides and iodine. Thionamides inhibit thyroid hormone synthesis. Excess iodine reduces thyroid synthesis and release (via the Wolff-Chaikoff effect) and radioiodine ablates cells that make thyroid hormone.

Thionamides (Methimazole, PTU)

MECHANISM

Inhibit the enzyme **thyroid peroxidase,** which catalyzes the oxidation and organification of iodine in thyroid hormone synthesis; propylthiouracil (PTU) also inhibits peripheral conversion of T_4 to T_3.

USES

Hyperthyroidism; PTU should be avoided as a first-line agent due to the potential for severe liver failure. In pregnant patients, PTU is used during the first trimester only. Methimazole is used during the second and third trimesters to reduce potential teratogenic effects.

SIDE EFFECTS

Rash, urticaria, fever, nausea; major effects include agranulocytosis, thrombocytopenia, acute hepatic necrosis, and vasculitis.

Iodine (Iodide and Radioiodine)

MECHANISM

Iodide is selectively concentrated in the thyroid gland for hormone synthesis; when given in large doses, it inhibits thyroid hormone release. Radioiodine

KEY FACT

MEN 1 arises from mutations in the self-named *men1* oncogene, whereas MEN 2A and 2B stem from mutations in the *ret* oncogene.

(^{131}I) is also concentrated in the thyroid gland and emits beta and gamma radiation.

USES

Large doses of iodide are used for thyroid storm and before thyroidectomy (to prevent thyroid storm). Radioiodine is used for hyperthyroidism and adjunctive treatment for some thyroid cancers.

SIDE EFFECTS

Metallic taste, excessive salivation, diarrhea, rash.

PARATHYROID GLAND

The parathyroid glands play an important role in calcium homeostasis and bone health, predominantly through involvement in calcium and phosphate metabolism.

- The main hormone that mediates these effects is **parathyroid hormone (PTH),** which acts on the kidneys and bone. PTH increases serum calcium while decreasing serum phosphate concentrations.
- **Vitamin D** and **calcitonin** also play important roles in calcium homeostasis, as discussed later.

Anatomy

The parathyroid glands are four small, pea-sized structures attached to the posterior aspect of the thyroid gland, external to the fibrous thyroid capsule (Figure 2-15). The glands are anatomically separated into two superior and two inferior parathyroids. Both sets are supplied by the inferior thyroid arteries with venous drainage through the thyroid plexus of veins.

Embryology

The parathyroid glands are derived from pharyngeal (branchial) pouch endoderm. Four pharyngeal pouches exist during development, each contributing

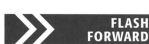

FLASH FORWARD

DiGeorge syndrome is a consequence of abnormal development of pharyngeal pouches 3 and 4 due to chromosome 22q11.2 deletion. Clinical manifestations include hypocalcemia secondary to absence of the parathyroid glands, immune deficiency secondary to absence of thymic tissue leading to abnormal T-cell maturation, and congenital cardiac malformations.

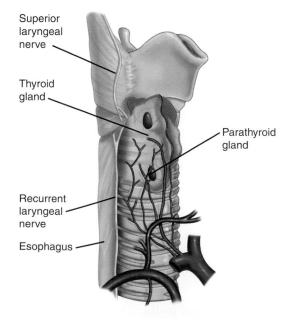

Superior laryngeal nerve

Thyroid gland

Parathyroid gland

Recurrent laryngeal nerve

Esophagus

FIGURE 2-15. **Lateral view of trachea, thyroid gland, and parathyroids.**

TABLE 2-16. Branchial Pouch Derivatives

BRANCHIAL POUCH	DERIVATIVES
First pouch	Middle ear cavity (+ Eustachian tube), mastoid air cells.
Second pouch	Epithelial lining of palatine tonsil.
Third pouch (dorsal wing)	Inferior parathyroids.
Third pouch (ventral wing)	Thymus.
Fourth pouch	Superior parathyroids, thyroid gland C cells (derived from ultimobranchial body).

KEY FACT

Branchial cysts are lesions found *lateral* to the midline of the neck. They result from failed obliteration of the temporary cervical sinuses. In contrast, **thyroglossal duct cysts,** found *medially,* result from failed obliteration of the thyroglossal duct as the thyroid gland migrates inferiorly during development.

to the formation of important structures of the head and neck (Tables 2-16 through 2-18 provide an overview of pharyngeal pouches, clefts, and arches). Each pouch represents an invagination of endodermal tissue within the foregut.

- Differentiation of the third branchial pouch takes place in the fifth and sixth weeks of gestation.
- The ventral wing of the third pouch gives rise to the thymus.
- The dorsal wing ultimately becomes the inferior parathyroids.
- By the seventh week of gestation, the third branchial pouch diverticulum elongates, ultimately allowing the developing thymus and inferior parathyroids to separate from the pharynx (Figure 2-16).
- The thymus migrates medially and caudally, pulling the inferior parathyroids until the thymus and parathyroids lose their connections to one another.
- The inferior parathyroids ultimately attach to the dorsal surface of the thyroid.
- The fourth branchial pouch, which gives rise to the superior parathyroids, follows a similar developmental course and timeline.
- The developing superior parathyroids do not migrate with another structure (ie, thymus), but rather travel a shorter distance before attaching to the dorsal surface of the thyroid.

KEY FACT

The **inferior** parathyroids are derived from the *third* branchial pouch, whereas the **superior** parathyroids are derived from the *fourth* branchial pouch, an apparent reversal of the rostrocaudal arrangement of these structures during development. This is due to the paired migration of the inferior parathyroids with the thymus, which facilitates enhanced caudal migration.

FLASH FORWARD

Ectopic parathyroid tissue results from abnormal migration. Ectopic parathyroids can be found in the anterior/posterior mediastinum, retroesophageal space, or even within the thyroid or thymus. Despite abnormal migration, the parathyroids typically remain symmetrical from side to side.

TABLE 2-17. Pharyngeal Clefts and Membranes

BRANCHIAL CLEFT	DERIVATIVES
First cleft	External auditory meatus
Second, third, and fourth clefts	Temporary cervical sinuses (normally obliterated)

BRANCHIAL MEMBRANE	DERIVATIVES
First membrane	Tympanic membrane
Second, third, and fourth membranes	Temporary structures (normally obliterated)

TABLE 2-18.   **Branchial Arches**

BRANCHIAL ARCH	DERIVATIVES (CARTILAGE)	DERIVATIVES (MUSCLE)	INNERVATION
1	Mandible, malleus, incus, sphenomandibular ligament	Muscles of mastication (temporalis, masseter, lateral/medial pterygoids), mylohyoid, anterior belly of the digastric, tensor tympani, tensor veli palatini, anterior two-thirds of the tongue.	CN V3 (mandibular nerve)
2	Stapes, styloid process, lesser horn of the hyoid, stylohyoid ligament	Stapedius, stylohyoid, posterior belly of the digastric, muscles of facial expression ("smilers").	CN VII
3	Greater ("important"?) horn of the hyoid	Stylopharyngeus, posterior one-third of the tongue.	CN IX
4	Thyroid, cricoid, arytenoids, corniculate, cuneiform	Cricothyroid, levator veli palatini, pharyngeal constrictors.	CN X (superior laryngeal branch)
5	No major developmental contributions		
6	Thyroid, cricoid, arytenoids, corniculate, cuneiform	All intrinsic muscles of larynx except the cricothyroid.	CN X (recurrent laryngeal branch)

CN = cranial nerve.

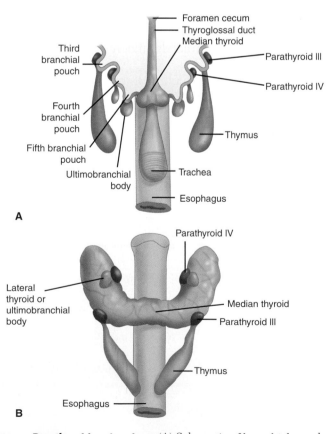

FIGURE 2-16.   **Parathyroid embryology.** (A) Schematic of branchial pouches with associated derivatives. (B) Migration of the inferior parathyroids.

Histology

The parathyroid glands are connective tissue–encapsulated structures that contain two populations of cells: **chief cells** and **oxyphil cells.**

■ Chief cells are predominant. They are small, polygonal cells with secretory granules containing PTH, arranged into curvilinear cords separated by capillaries (Figure 2-17).

■ Oxyphil cells, which have an unknown function, are large cells containing abundant acidophilic mitochondria.

CALCIUM AND PHOSPHATE HOMEOSTASIS

Calcium plays an important role in numerous physiologic processes, ranging from muscle contraction to neuronal impulse transmission. Extracellular calcium concentrations are tightly regulated to protect against large fluctuations. Only 0.1% of total body calcium is found in the extracellular fluid (ECF). The vast majority of the remaining calcium, approximately 99%, is stored within bone (Figure 2-18).

■ Forty percent of serum calcium is bound to plasma proteins.

■ Ten percent of serum calcium is complexed with anions such as phosphate and citrate.

■ Fifty percent of serum calcium is in a free, ionized form.

Only free calcium is biologically active.

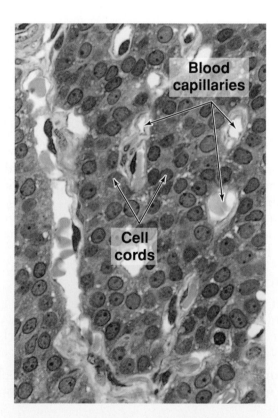

FIGURE 2-17.   Section of parathyroid gland demonstrating chief cells arranged in cords separated by capillaries. (Reproduced with permission from Junqueira LC, Carneiro J. *Basic Histology: Text & Atlas*, 11th ed. New York: McGraw-Hill, 2005: 416.)

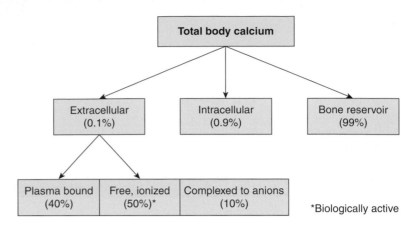

FIGURE 2-18. **Distribution of total body calcium.** Like calcium, phosphate is involved in a range of physiologic processes. A very small quantity (1%) of total body phosphate is found in the extracellular space; most phosphate is in bone.

Calcium and phosphate homeostasis are regulated through the coordinated actions of three hormones: PTH, vitamin D, and calcitonin. These hormones control calcium and phosphate by acting on bone, intestine, and kidney.

Parathyroid Hormone

PTH is a polypeptide hormone synthesized and secreted by the parathyroid **chief cells.**

PTH is initially synthesized as a larger, inactive preprohormone. Proteolytic processing produces a final active hormone that is stored in secretory granules of chief cells. Despite rapid metabolism of PTH by the kidneys after secretion, smaller peptide fragments of the hormone retain full biological activity for hours.

PTH REGULATION

The stimuli for PTH release include serum calcium and magnesium levels.

- PTH secretion is inversely proportional to serum ionized calcium levels. Low serum calcium stimulates increased PTH secretion, whereas high serum calcium levels inhibit secretion.
- Reductions in serum magnesium also affect PTH secretion. Mild decreases in magnesium stimulate PTH secretion. Severe hypomagnesemia, however, inhibits PTH secretion.

MECHANISMS OF ACTION

In order to affect serum calcium and phosphate levels, PTH alters bone turnover, renal tubule reabsorption, and vitamin D activation. Through these direct and indirect actions, PTH raises serum calcium levels and decreases serum phosphate levels (Figures 2-19 and 2-20). The specific actions include:

- **Increased bone resorption:** PTH stimulates both osteoclasts and osteoblasts (bone resorption > bone formation), leading to increased calcium and phosphate levels.
    - PTH enhances the activity of existing osteoclasts and also promotes the differentiation of new osteoclasts from progenitor cells.
    - Increased resorption from bone mineral leads to the release of both calcium and phosphate into the extracellular space.

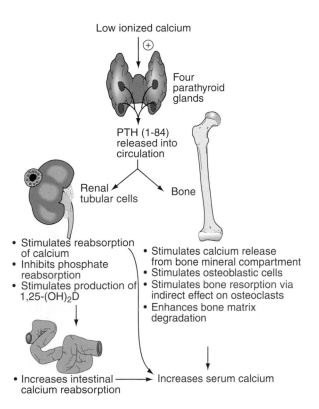

FIGURE 2-19. **Actions of PTH and 1,25-(OH)$_2$D in the maintenance of free, ionized calcium in the serum.** PTH, parathyroid hormone.

■ **Increased renal calcium reabsorption:** PTH stimulates the distal renal tubule to increase reabsorption of calcium, effectively raising serum calcium levels.

■ **Increased phosphate excretion:** In the proximal renal tubule, PTH inhibits phosphate reabsorption, leading to enhanced phosphate excretion. The reduction in serum phosphate reduces the quantity of complexed calcium in the circulation (phosphate and calcium bind in serum), thereby raising the amount of extracellular free calcium.

■ **Increased vitamin D activity increases intestinal Ca^{2+} absorption:** PTH increases the activity of 1α-hydroxylase in the kidney. This results in increased levels of 1,25-(OH)$_2$ vitamin D (calcitriol). Calcitriol affects

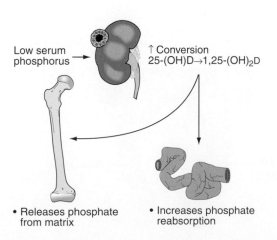

FIGURE 2-20. **Action of 1,25-(OH)$_2$D in the maintenance of serum phosphate.**

intestinal absorption of calcium and bone resorption (see next section). Thus, PTH, via its activation of vitamin D, has an indirect effect on serum calcium levels.

Vitamin D

The chief forms of vitamin D are **ergocalciferol (vitamin D$_2$)** and **cholecalciferol (vitamin D$_3$).**

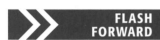

- Vitamin D$_2$ is produced by plant and fungal sources. It is not synthesized within the human body.
- Vitamin D$_3$ is produced by animal sources. Endogenous production also takes place in the skin. Specific wavelengths of UV light react with 7-dehydrocholesterol to produce vitamin D$_3$. Thus, sun exposure may help prevent vitamin D deficiency in certain individuals.

ACTIVATION

Following synthesis in the skin, cholecalciferol (vitamin D$_3$) is initially inactive. It must undergo a series of additional reactions in the liver and kidney to become biologically active (Figure 2-22).

- Cholecalciferol is first transported to the liver, where it undergoes a hydroxylation reaction to form **25-hydroxycholecalciferol.** This is the storage form of vitamin D. It is also the level measured in clinical lab tests. 25-Hydroxycholecalciferol exerts negative feedback on this reaction in the liver.
- In the kidney, 25-hydroxycholecalciferol undergoes a second hydroxylation reaction catalyzed by **1α-hydroxylase.** The product of this reaction, **1,25-dihydroxycholecalciferol [1,25-(OH)$_2$ vitamin D],** is the active form of vitamin D, also referred to as **calcitriol.** 1α-hydroxylase activity is upregulated by PTH. Therefore, increased PTH activity leads to increased vitamin D activity.

FLASH FORWARD

Vitamin D deficiency in children causes **rickets,** which is characterized by the inability to calcify newly formed bone matrix (osteoid) with consequent malformation (bowing) of long bones (Figure 2-21).

FLASH FORWARD

Vitamin D deficiency in adults results in **osteomalacia.** Like rickets, this condition is characterized by defective mineralization of bone. Osteomalacia causes pain, proximal muscle weakness, and bony deformities. It is treated with vitamin D replacement.

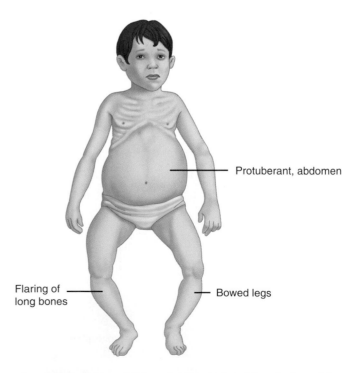

Protuberant, abdomen

Flaring of long bones

Bowed legs

FIGURE 2-21. **Clinical signs of rickets in a young boy.** Note the bowed legs, protuberant abdomen, and flaring of long bones.

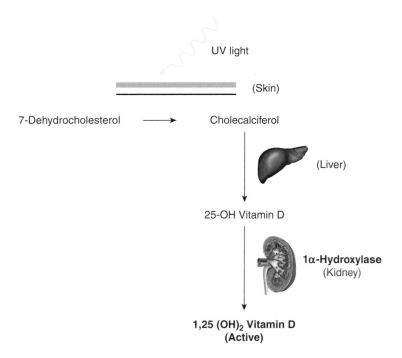

UV light

(Skin)

7-Dehydrocholesterol $\longrightarrow$ Cholecalciferol

(Liver)

25-OH Vitamin D

 1α-Hydroxylase
(Kidney)

1,25 (OH)$_2$ Vitamin D
(Active)

FIGURE 2-22. **Activation of vitamin D.**

- PTH increases 1,25-(OH)$_2$ vitamin D formation.
- Low calcium increases 1,25-(OH)$_2$ vitamin D formation.
- Low phosphate increases 1,25-(OH)$_2$ vitamin D formation.

ACTIONS

The active form of vitamin D (calcitriol) raises extracellular levels of calcium and phosphate and promotes the mineralization of bone. These metabolic changes are the result of effects on the intestine, kidneys, and bone:

- **Increases intestinal calcium and phosphate absorption:** 1,25-(OH)$_2$ vitamin D upregulates gene transcription of a calcium-binding protein (calbindin D-28K) in the intestinal brush border. This protein increases the absorption of dietary calcium.
- **Increases bone resorption of calcium and phosphate:** 1,25-(OH)$_2$ vitamin D is important for PTH-induced bone resorption. It is thought to facilitate this process by increasing calcium transport across membranes (similar to the mechanism in the intestine). Thus, at the level of bone, 1,25-(OH)$_2$ vitamin D promotes resorption of calcium and phosphate so they can be used for the mineralization of new bone.
- **Increases renal reabsorption of calcium and phosphate (minor effect):** 1,25-(OH)$_2$ vitamin D promotes increased reabsorption of both ions by the renal tubules. This effect is relatively minor and contributes little to the overall concentrations of extracellular calcium and phosphate.

Calcitonin

Calcitonin is a polypeptide secreted by the parafollicular, or C, cells of the thyroid gland. Although it promotes reduction in extracellular calcium through anti-PTH-like effects, calcitonin is not necessary for the maintenance of calcium homeostasis. Patients who have had their thyroid removed (eg, as treatment for thyroid cancer) show no changes in serum calcium concentrations despite the complete absence of calcitonin.

KEY FACT

Vitamin D and PTH act to increase resorption of old bone in order to free up calcium and phosphate for the mineralization of new bone. Although this may be counterintuitive, this process of **bone remodeling** is essential to both the maintenance of healthy bone and the recovery of bone from injury.

ACTIONS

Calcitonin is secreted in response to high serum calcium levels. It acts primarily on bone, decreasing the resorptive activity of osteoclasts. Calcitonin also has minor effects on the intestines and renal tubules aimed at decreasing extracellular calcium.

CALCIUM DISORDERS

Primary Hyperparathyroidism

In primary hyperparathyroidism, excess secretion of PTH causes hypercalcemia. A benign parathyroid adenoma is responsible for 80% of cases, and parathyroid gland hyperplasia accounts for the remaining 20% of cases.

PRESENTATION

Usually asymptomatic. Incidentally discovered based on elevated calcium levels. When symptomatic, patient presents with renal, GI, or neurologic symptoms.

MNEMONIC

Patients with hypercalcemia: "Stones, bones, groans, and psychiatric overtones."

- **Renal:** Polyuria, hypercalciuria, renal calculi (calcium oxalate). If chronic, can lead to nephrocalcinosis, decreased GFR, and eventually renal failure.
- **Skeletal:** Bone pain. Increased PTH leads to increased osteoclastic activity → increased bone resorption and decreased bone mineral density.
- **GI:** Nausea, vomiting, weight loss, constipation, anorexia, peptic ulcer disease, acute pancreatitis.
- **Neurologic:** Mental status changes, depression, fatigue.

In hypercalcemic crisis: Polyuria, dehydration, mental status changes.

DIAGNOSIS

- **Serum chemistry:** Increased Ca^{2+}, decreased phosphate; chloride is often elevated.
- Also check PTH-related peptide (PTHrP), vitamin D levels, alkaline phosphatase, urine calcium. See below for other causes of hypercalcemia.
- **Endocrine:** Increased or inappropriately normal PTH.
- **ECG:** Short QT interval.

MNEMONIC

Causes for hypercalcemia—

MISHAP
Malignancy
Intoxication with vitamin D
Sarcoidosis (see Chapter 5)
Hyperparathyroidism
Alkali (milk-alkali syndrome)
Paget disease (see Chapter 5)

TREATMENT

- Curative treatment is surgical exploration and parathyroidectomy of the adenomatous gland.
- Medical treatment for those who are not good surgical candidates or decline surgery includes encouragement of adequate hydration and physical activity. Can give diuretics (furosemide) to enhance calcium excretion. Avoid thiazide diuretics, as they can exacerbate hypercalcemia. Can also give bisphosphonates to inhibit bone loss, or calcitonin.

Other Causes of Hypercalcemia

- **Renal osteodystrophy** is a consequence of **secondary hyperparathyroidism** resulting from the death of proximal tubule cells in renal failure patients. Loss of these cells results in decreased vitamin D activation by 1α-hydroxylase. In response, the chief cells of the parathyroid glands produce excess PTH, resulting in excess bone resorption. Serum calcium levels are typically low or low-normal in secondary hyperparathyroidism.
- **Malignancy-induced hypercalcemia** can result from lytic bone metastases (eg, breast cancer) or tumor producing PTHrP, including squamous cell carcinoma of the lung and renal adenocarcinoma. PTH levels are low.

- **Vitamin D toxicity** secondary to granulomatous disease (sarcoidosis, tuberculosis), certain lymphomas or histoplasmosis. For example, in granulomatous disease, lymphocytes in the granulomas make 1α-hydroxylase → increased vitamin D → increased calcium resorption. PTH levels are low.
- **Familial hypocalciuric hypercalcemia (FHH):** Autosomal dominant disorder caused by a mutation in calcium-sensing receptors on the parathyroid glands → leads to inappropriate secretion of PTH → mild hypercalcemia. Unlike other causes of hypercalcemia, urinary calculi and renal failure are not seen in cases of FHH.
- **Thiazide diuretics:** Increase renal reabsorption of calcium in the distal tubule.
- **Milk-alkali syndrome:** Ingestion of excessive amounts of calcium-based antacids.

Primary Hypoparathyroidism

Causes, from most to least common: hypoparathyroidism following thyroid surgery, in which the surgeon accidentally removes or otherwise injures the parathyroid glands, autoimmune gland failure, gland infiltration, pseudohypoparathyroidism due to PTH end-organ resistance, and **DiGeorge syndrome** (failure of the third and fourth pharyngeal pouches to develop).

PRESENTATION

Neuromuscular excitability due to hypocalcemia.

- Muscle fatigue and weakness.
- Numbness and tingling around the mouth, hands, and feet.
- Tetany: **Chvostek sign** (tapping of the facial nerve in front of the ear → upper lip and facial muscles contract); **Trousseau sign** (inflation of a BP cuff to a pressure higher than systolic BP → carpal spasms).
- Laryngeal spasm.
- Basal ganglia calcifications (can cause Parkinsonian symptoms). The ocular lens can also be calcified, leading to cataracts.
- Depression, psychosis.

DIAGNOSIS

- **Serum chemistry:** Low or inappropriately normal PTH with low Ca^{2+}. Check albumin, vitamin D, Mg^{2+}, alkaline phosphatase, and urine calcium as well. See Table 2-19 for lab differential of hypocalcemia.
- **ECG:** Increased QT interval.
- **Imaging:** Basal ganglia calcifications.

TREATMENT

Calcium supplements, vitamin D supplements (calcitriol), and IV calcium gluconate for acute symptoms.

Other Causes of Hypocalcemia

- **Pseudohypoparathyroidism:** End-organ resistance to PTH (kidney and bones do not respond to PTH). Patients may have **Albright hereditary osteodystrophy,** characterized by short stature, shortening of the fourth and fifth metacarpals, and mild mental retardation.
- **Pseudopseudohypoparathyroidism.**
- **Hypoalbuminemia** causes a decrease in total calcium, but ionized calcium levels are normal. There are no clinical signs of calcium deficiency.
- **Severe hypomagnesemia** leads to decreased PTH synthesis and release, as well as end-organ resistance to PTH.

KEY FACT

In the case of parathyroid hyperplasia, the surgeon removes three of the four parathyroid glands and autotransplants (reimplants) the remaining gland into the patient's forearm to avoid hypoparathyroidism.

KEY FACT

Correcting for serum albumin is critical to interpreting total calcium levels.

$$\text{Free calcium} = 0.8 \times (4.0 - \text{serum albumin}) + \text{serum } Ca^{2+}$$

TABLE 2-19. Summary of Calcium Disorders

	SERUM CALCIUM	SERUM PHOSPHATE	PTH
Primary hyperparathyroidism	↑	↓	↑
Malignancy-induced hypercalcemia (PTHrP)	↑	↓	↓
Primary hypoparathyroidism	↓	↑	↓
Pseudohypoparathyroidism	↓	↑	↑/normal

- **Calcium sequestration:** Enzymatic fat necrosis uses up calcium. Most commonly a result of acute pancreatitis. Other conditions that lead to calcium sequestration include citrate excess after blood transfusions and acute increases in PO_4 due to rhabdomyolysis, tumor lysis, or acute renal failure.

CALCIUM DRUGS

Bisphosphonates (eg, Alendronate)

MECHANISM

Stabilizes bony matrix, coats hydroxyapatite to prevent osteoclasts from resorbing bone.

USES

Treatment of **postmenopausal osteoporosis** and in Paget disease to reduce bone turnover. Prevention of accelerated bone loss in patients on long-term, high-dose glucocorticoid therapy.

SIDE EFFECTS

Heartburn, erosive esophagitis, stomach upset, joint/back pain, osteonecrosis of the jaw.

Calcitonin

MECHANISM

Lowers serum calcium, has mild analgesic properties for bone pain.

ADMINISTRATION

Intranasal, subcutaneous.

USES

Hypercalcemic states.

SIDE EFFECTS

Runny nose, nasal discomfort, flushing.

Calcitriol

MECHANISM

Activated form of vitamin D; increases calcium absorption from intestines.

USES

Hypocalcemia, vitamin D replacement in patients with end-stage renal disease.

SIDE EFFECTS

Signs and symptoms of vitamin D intoxication include hypercalcemia, polyuria, weakness, headache, somnolence, and constipation.

Adrenal Gland

One important function of the adrenal (or suprarenal) glands is to coordinate the body's response to physiologic stress. The gland is anatomically and functionally divided into two parts: the adrenal medulla (core) and outer adrenal cortex.

The adrenal medulla is a functional extension of the sympathetic nervous system, secreting the catecholamines epinephrine and norepinephrine into systemic circulation.

In contrast, the adrenal cortex synthesizes steroid hormones, which have diverse functions, ranging from stress responses (**cortisol**) to control of water and electrolyte balance (**aldosterone**) to androgenizing effects (**testosterone, DHEA-sulfate**).

ANATOMY

The triangular-shaped adrenals sit atop the superoanterior aspects of the kidneys, where they are encased in a capsule of fat and connective tissue (Figure 2-23).

- The vascular supply to the adrenal glands consists of three sets of arteries:
  - **Superior adrenal arteries,** which are branches off the inferior phrenic artery.
  - **Middle adrenal arteries,** which originate from the abdominal aorta adjacent to the celiac trunk.
  - **Inferior adrenal arteries,** which are branches off the renal artery.

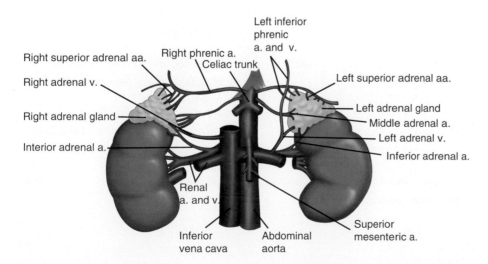

FIGURE 2-23. **Anatomy and blood supply of adrenal glands.** (Modified with permission from Brunicardi FC, et al. *Schwartz's Principles of Surgery,* 8th ed. New York: McGraw-Hill, 2005: 1450.)

FLASH FORWARD

Pheochromocytoma is a rare neoplasm formed from chromaffin cells in the adrenal medulla (90%) or extra-adrenal sites (10%). It is the most common tumor of the adrenal medulla in adults.

FLASH FORWARD

Neuroblastoma is a neoplasm formed from neural crest cells that may be found anywhere along the sympathetic chain, including the adrenal medulla. It is the most common tumor of the adrenal gland in children.

MNEMONIC

GFR (glomerulosa, fasciculata, reticularis) corresponds with **S**alt (Na⁺), **S**ugar (glucocorticoids), and **S**ex (androgens): "The deeper you go, the sweeter it gets."

- The venous drainage of the adrenal gland differs between the two sides.
  - Left adrenal → left adrenal vein → left renal vein → inferior vena cava (IVC)
  - Right adrenal → right adrenal vein → IVC

EMBRYOLOGY

The adrenal cortex and medulla differ in their embryologic origins.

- **Adrenal cortex:** Derived from mesoderm.
- **Adrenal medulla:** Derived from neural crest cells, which differentiate into chromaffin cells.

HISTOLOGY

The adrenal cortex is further divided into three distinct layers (Table 2-20).

- **Zona glomerulosa:** A relatively thin external layer (15% of the cortex) composed of cells containing the enzyme aldosterone synthase. Consequently, the zona glomerulosa is the only layer that is capable of producing appreciable quantities of the mineralocorticoid **aldosterone.**
- **Zona fasciculata:** The largest layer (75% of the cortex) composed of cells that primarily synthesize and secrete **glucocorticoids** (cortisol).
- **Zona reticularis:** The deepest layer (10% of the cortex) composed of cells that primarily synthesize adrenal **androgens** (dehydroepiandrosterone [DHEA] and androstenedione).

STEROID HORMONE SYNTHESIS

Cholesterol Acquisition

Steroid hormones of the adrenal cortex are synthesized using cholesterol as the precursor. Approximately 20% of this cholesterol is produced de novo

TABLE 2-20. **Adrenal Gland Summary**

REGION	HORMONE	CONTROLLED BY	LOSS LEADS TO...
Glomerulosa	Aldosterone	Angiotensin II, potassium	Hyponatremia, hypovolemia, hyperkalemia
Fasciculata	Cortisol	ACTH	Decreased ability to compensate for physiologic stress, decreased ability to mobilize glucose
Reticularis	Androgens	ACTH	Gynecomastia, delayed onset of puberty (in males); not a major androgen contributor

ACTH = adrenocorticotropic hormone.

within adrenal cortical cells; the remainder is acquired from circulating low-density lipoproteins (LDL). LDL molecules are internalized via endocytosis then hydrolyzed within lysosomes to produce free cholesterol within the cell.

Synthetic Pathways

Free cholesterol within adrenal cortical cells is transported to mitochondria.

- The initial step in steroid hormone synthesis is rate-limiting and conserved across all layers of adrenal cortex. In this reaction, **cholesterol desmolase** converts cholesterol to pregnenolone (Figure 2-24). ACTH and angiotensin II stimulate this conversion.
- 3-β-Hydroxysteroid dehydrogenase and 21-hydroxylase are required for the synthesis of precursors in the pathways to both aldosterone and cortisol. 11-β-Hydroxylase is required for synthesis of cortisol.
- 17-α-Hydroxylase is required to convert pregnenolone and progesterone into androstenedione and DHEA, respectively, both precursors of adrenal androgens.
- The ultimate products are aldosterone (zona glomerulosa), cortisol (zona fasciculata), and weak androgens (zona reticularis).

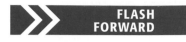

FLASH FORWARD

21-Hydroxylase deficiency, the most common form of **congenital adrenal hyperplasia** (CAH), leads to decreased levels of both glucocorticoids and mineralocorticoids with a concomitant rise in adrenal androgens. Clinically, patients show **hypo**tension, hyponatremia, **hyper**kalemia, and virilization.

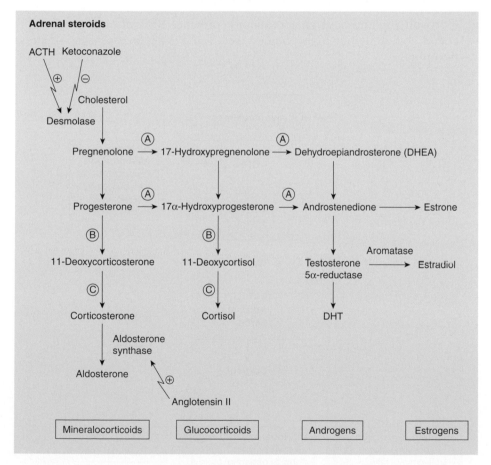

FIGURE 2-24. Steroid hormone synthetic pathways. (A), 17α-hydroxylase, (B), 21α-hydroxylase, (C), 11β-hydroxylase; ACTH, adrenocorticotropic hormone; DHT, dihydrotestosterone.

FLASH FORWARD

In **17α-hydroxylase deficiency,** individuals lack the enzyme to synthesize cortisol or androgens, resulting in the accumulation of a shared precursor, pregnenolone (see Figure 2-24). Clinically, individuals are **hyper**tensive and **hypo**kalemic, owing to shunting of pregnenolone into the synthetic pathway of aldosterone.

GLUCOCORTICOIDS

Glucocorticoid Synthesis and Regulation

The hypothalamus, anterior pituitary, and adrenal cortex interact to coordinate glucocorticoid synthesis. Hypoglycemia, trauma, illness, fever, and physical exertion trigger the hypothalamus to secrete CRH.

- CRH stimulates corticotrophs of the anterior pituitary to release ACTH (Figure 2-25).
- ACTH upregulates desmolase, the rate-limiting enzyme (RLE) in cholesterol and pregnenolone synthesis, which, in turn, makes it the RLE in cortisol synthesis. ACTH also promotes gland hypertrophy.
- While CRH and ACTH stimulate cortisol production, the system employs negative feedback to provide regulation. High levels of cortisol inhibit CRH and ACTH secretion (see Figure 2-25).

Endogenous Glucocorticoids

Glucocorticoids, so named for their effects on blood glucose levels, are now recognized for a diverse set of actions including alterations in immune function, bone turnover, and cardiovascular function.

- **Cortisol:** Predominant glucocorticoid (provides 95% of endogenous glucocorticoid activity); high potency (see Table 2-21 for overview of stress hormones).

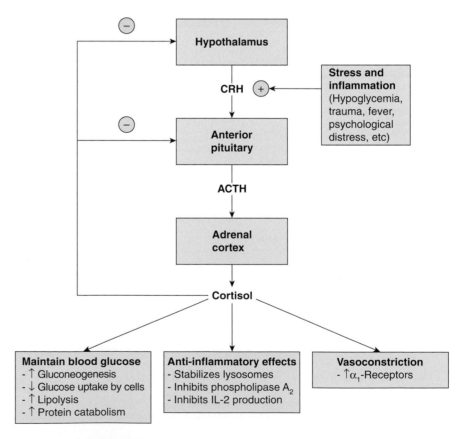

FIGURE 2-25. **Effects and regulation of cortisol.** ACTH, adrenocorticotropic hormone; CRH, corticotropic-releasing hormone; IL-2, interleukin-2.

TABLE 2-21. **Stress Hormones**

GH	▪ Increases lipolysis in adipose tissue
	▪ Promotes protein synthesis
Glucagon	▪ Increases lipolysis in adipose tissue
	▪ Stimulates glycogenolysis
	▪ Promotes gluconeogenesis
Cortisol	▪ Increases lipolysis in adipose tissue
	▪ Stimulates gluconeogenesis
	▪ Upregulates vascular adrenergic (α_1) receptors
Epinephrine	▪ Increases lipolysis in adipose tissue
	▪ Promotes glycogenolysis

GH = growth hormone.

- **11-Deoxycorticosterone:** Immediate precursor to cortisol (provides < 5% of endogenous glucocorticoid activity); low potency.
- **Synthetic (exogenous) corticosteroids:** Hydrocortisone, prednisone, methylprednisolone, and dexamethasone. Synthetic glucocorticoids with various potencies relative to cortisol.

Actions of Cortisol

Cortisol plays multiple roles in maintaining homeostasis, influencing the immune response, intermediary metabolism, vascular tone, and, to a limited extent, renal function.

- **Promotes energy mobilization via gluconeogenesis:** Cortisol effectively increases blood glucose concentration. Cortisol reduces the uptake of glucose into cells, while increasing the amount of substrate (gluconeogenic amino acids and glycerol) for gluconeogenesis in the liver. Cortisol does so by stimulating lipolysis and protein catabolism, leading to the mobilization of fatty acids and amino acids, respectively (see Figure 2-25).
- **Anti-inflammatory effects:** Cortisol both prevents inflammation and reduces existing inflammatory conditions.
- It promotes the synthesis of lipocortin, an inhibitor of phospholipase A_2. Phospholipase A_2 normally supplies arachidonic acid for the synthesis of prostaglandins and leukotrienes. Lack of these local inflammatory mediators decreases capillary permeability and the recruitment of leukocytes to the inflamed tissue.
- By stabilizing lysosomal membranes, it reduces the risk of lysosomal membrane rupture and minimizes the amount of proteolytic enzymes acting within the inflammatory milieu.
- Cortisol decreases production of inflammatory cytokines (eg, tumor necrosis factor-alpha [TNF-α]) leading to a reduction in macrophage activation.
- Cortisol also suppresses the function of the adaptive immune system by inhibiting the production of interleukin-2 (IL-2), a cytokine involved in promoting T-cell proliferation. Other cytokines are also disrupted in this process.
- Lastly, cortisol blocks the release of histamine from mast cells and serotonin from platelets, thereby inhibiting allergic reactions.

KEY FACT

Cortisol promotes gluconeogenesis and suppresses inflammation (via inhibition of phospholipase A_2 [PLA$_2$]) under conditions of physiologic stress.

- **Adrenergic receptor upregulation:** Cortisol helps smooth muscle maintain responsiveness to the vasoconstrictive effects of norepinephrine by upregulating α_1-adrenergic receptors on vascular smooth muscle cells. Cortisol also contributes to vascular tone through inhibition of nitric oxide synthase, decreasing the production of the vasodilator nitric oxide.
- **Mineralocorticoid activity:** Its mineralocorticoid effects are normally negligible relative to its marked glucocorticoid activity (because it is inactivated by renal 11-hydroxysteroid dehydrogenase); however, in disease states characterized by very high concentrations, cortisol can exert a potent mineralocorticoid effect (see Table 2-22 for an overview of abnormal cortisol states).

MINERALOCORTICOIDS

Mineralocorticoid Synthesis and Regulation

ACTH promotes aldosterone synthesis (see Figure 2-24 for its synthetic pathway); however, it has little to no effect on the rate of secretion. Only modest quantities of ACTH are necessary to initiate aldosterone synthesis. The rate of secretion is then either increased or decreased from the basal level, depending on changes in the ECF volume, sodium and potassium concentrations in the ECF, and arterial pressures. Important determinants of aldosterone secretion are:

- **High serum potassium** increases secretion.
- The **renin-angiotensin system** (RAS) increases secretion.
- **High serum sodium** decreases secretion (minimally).

Actions of Aldosterone

Aldosterone has three major and related effects: Increased sodium reabsorption, increased BP, and increased potassium excretion.

- **Increased sodium reabsorption:** Aldosterone stimulates the synthesis of new sodium channels in the principal cells of the collecting tubules. These additional sodium channels promote sodium reabsorption and reduce sodium excretion in the urine.
- **Increased arterial pressure:** Aldosterone increases total sodium reabsorption, but does not significantly alter serum sodium concentration. This is because water is also reabsorbed by the collecting tubules. The net effect is an **increase in extracellular volume,** which, over time, can cause arterial pressure to rise.

KEY FACT

Activation of the RAS and high serum potassium are the major stimuli for the release of aldosterone from the adrenal cortex.

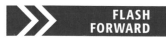

FLASH FORWARD

Cushing syndrome is characterized by a classic clinical picture: hypertension, central obesity, weight gain, moon facies, insulin resistance, skin thinning/purple striae, buffalo hump, hirsuitism, osteoporosis, and amenorrhea.

TABLE 2-22. Abnormal Cortisol States

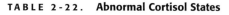

DISORDER	CORTISOL	ACTH
Primary hypercortisolism (cortisol-producing tumor)	↑	↓
Pituitary hypersecretion of ACTH (Cushing disease)	↑	↑
Primary adrenal insufficiency (Addison disease)	↓	↑
Secondary adrenal insufficiency	↓	↓

■ **Increased potassium secretion:** Aldosterone induces the opening of large numbers of sodium and potassium channels in the principal cells of the collecting ducts. Enhanced sodium reabsorption is accompanied by increased potassium secretion into the tubule lumen.

ADRENAL ANDROGENS

Adrenal androgens (androstenedione, DHEA, and dehydroepiandrosterone sulfate [DHEA-S]) play a relatively minor role in androgen homeostasis, in part because these steroid hormones are relatively weak androgens and make up a small percentage of circulating sex steroids. Nonetheless, during several periods of development, adrenal androgens take on a more important role.

■ **Fetal development:** During pregnancy, because the placenta cannot synthesize cholesterol from acetate, it is incapable of producing sex steroids de novo. Instead, it produces androgens and estrogens from precursors (eg, DHEA-S) produced by the maternal and fetal adrenal glands.
■ **Adrenarche:** Adrenarche is a stage of adrenal maturation marked by increased synthesis of androgens, resulting in pubic and axillary hair growth during puberty. The weak androgens released from the adrenals are peripherally converted to the more powerful androgens testosterone and dihydrotestosterone (DHT), which ultimately act in secondary sexual differentiation in both sexes.
■ **Menopause:** Menopause is marked by a cessation of ovarian estrogen production; however, postmenopausal women are not completely estrogen-deficient. Androstenedione produced by the adrenals and ovaries is peripherally converted to estrone by the enzyme **aromatase**. Estrone is a weaker estrogen relative to estradiol, the major premenopausal estrogen; consequently, estrone does not provide adequate protection against the long-term consequences of estrogen deficiency (eg, accelerated bone mineral density loss, vasomotor symptoms such as flushing and diaphoresis, and cardiovascular changes such as the development of hypertension).

FLASH FORWARD

Because patients with **11β-hydroxylase deficiency** lack an enzyme in the adrenal steroid synthetic pathway (see Figure 2-24), they cannot produce normal levels of cortisol and aldosterone. The steroid precursors are shunted into the production of excessive quantities of sex hormones. Consequently, patients with 11β-hydroxylase deficiency are **hypertensive,** and females are **virilized.**

DISORDERS OF THE ADRENAL GLAND

Cushing Syndrome

Cushing syndrome refers to the signs and symptoms of excess cortisol and is most commonly caused by exogenous glucocorticoid therapy. Other causes include pituitary adenomas (Cushing disease; excess ACTH from the pituitary → bilateral adrenal hyperplasia), adrenocortical tumors, and ectopic ACTH production (small-cell carcinoma of the lung, bronchial carcinoid tumors).

PRESENTATION

Patients with Cushing syndrome present with features consistent with excess cortisol (Figure 2-26).

■ Central obesity, moon facies, buffalo hump
■ Hypertension
■ Glucose intolerance (decreased peripheral glucose utilization, increased hepatic gluconeogenesis)
■ Purple striae
■ Proximal muscle wasting and weakness
■ Osteoporosis
■ Depression and mania

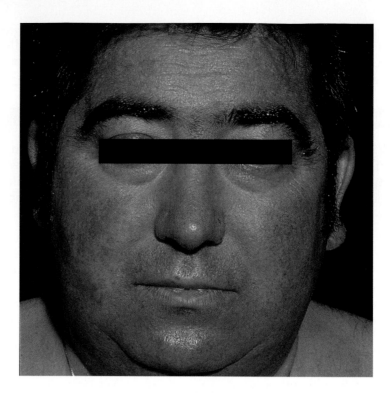

FIGURE 2-26. **Presentation of Cushing syndrome.** Note the swelling of the face into a rounded shape–Cushingoid "moon face." (Reproduced with permission from Wolff K, Johnson RA, Suurmond D. *Fitzpatrick's Color Atlas & Synopsis of Clinical Dermatology*, 5th ed. New York: McGraw-Hill, 2005: 442.)

DIAGNOSIS

The initial screen is the overnight dexamethasone (a cortisol analog) suppression test (Figure 2-27). In normal individuals, dexamethasone suppresses ACTH release from the pituitary and results in decreased cortisol release. In Cushing syndrome, cortisol levels fail to be suppressed. A 24-h urinary free

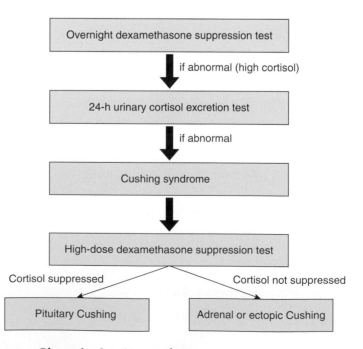

FIGURE 2-27. **Diagnosis of Cushing syndrome.**

cortisol level is the gold standard diagnostic test. Once the diagnosis is confirmed, an ACTH level is assessed. If the ACTH level is high, then the excess cortisol is ACTH-dependent and a high-dose dexamethasone suppression test is performed. Cortisol is suppressed in Cushing disease, but not with ectopic ACTH-producing tumors (Table 2-23).

Primary Hyperaldosteronism (Conn Syndrome)

Conn syndrome is caused by excess secretion of aldosterone, resulting in increased sodium reabsorption and potassium secretion. Primary aldosteronism is most commonly due to a benign adenoma in the zona glomerulosa. Secondary causes include:

- Renin-secreting tumors, renovascular disease such as renal artery stenosis, and malignant hypertension.
- Edematous state with decreased arterial volume (congestive heart failure [CHF], cirrhosis, nephrotic syndrome).
- Diuretics.
- Excess nonaldosterone mineralocorticoid due to exogenous mineralocorticoids, CAH, and excessive ingestion of licorice (leads to build-up of precursors of cortisol).

PRESENTATION

- Sodium and water retention causes hypertension. Severe hypokalemia causes symptoms of muscle weakness and can cause arrhythmia.
- Excess aldosterone causes increased Na^+ reabsorption and increased K^+ and H^+ secretion → mild hypernatremia, hypokalemia, and metabolic alkalosis.

DIAGNOSIS

Screen for hypertension.

- **Serum chemistry:** Mildly increased Na^+, decreased K^+ and increased bicarbonate.
- **Hormones:** Both aldosterone and renin are measured and the aldosterone-to-renin ratio (ARR) is calculated. Secondary to the high aldosterone levels, renin is often suppressed. An ARR > 20–30 is diagnostic.
- **Sodium suppression test:** Sodium-load patient and then measure for appropriate aldosterone suppression. Infusion of saline normally decreases aldosterone levels but does not do so in Conn syndrome.

TREATMENT

Surgery to remove the adenoma in the adrenal gland, if possible. If the patient is a poor surgical candidate or suffers from bilateral adrenal hyperplasia, medi-

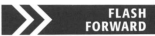

FLASH FORWARD

In **Conn syndrome,** or primary hyperaldosteronism, excessive aldosterone is produced by adrenocortical adenomas, carcinomas, or hyperplasia of the zona glomerulosa. Patients are generally **hypertensive** and **hypokalemic.**

TABLE 2-23. **Summary of Cushing Syndrome**

	SERUM/ URINE CORTISOL	ACTH	HIGH-DOSE DEXAMETHASONE TEST
Pituitary Cushing	↑	↑	Cortisol suppressed
Adrenal Cushing	↑	↓	Not performed
Ectopic Cushing	↑	↑	Cortisol not suppressed

cal management is preferred. Spironolactone inhibits aldosterone action on the kidneys. Other antihypertensives can also be used to manage the patient's high BP.

Addison Disease

Addison disease results from adrenal gland failure and is most commonly due to autoimmune destruction of the adrenal glands. Primary causes include infection (TB, cytomegalovirus, histoplasmosis, or disseminated meningococcemia in **Waterhouse-Friderichsen syndrome**), vascular disorders (hemorrhage or infarction), metastasis, infiltrative disease (hemochromatosis, amyloidosis, or sarcoidosis), and drugs such as ketoconazole and rifampin. Secondary cortisol deficiency results from abrupt withdrawal of corticosteroids or any cause of primary or secondary panhypopituitarism leading to decreased ACTH secretion.

PRESENTATION

- Most commonly manifests as weakness, fatigue, anorexia, nausea/vomiting, orthostasis, hyponatremia, and hypoglycemia, which stem from decreased cortisol and mineralocorticoid deficiency.
- Increased ACTH in primary adrenal insufficiency leads to skin hyperpigmentation (due to increased MSH) and hyperkalemia; decreased aldosterone leads to hypotension (due to salt loss), weakness, and hypoperfusion.

DIAGNOSIS

- **ACTH stimulation testing:** Administer ACTH IV to stimulate cortisol. Normally, the adrenal gland increases its production of cortisol in response to ACTH. In primary and chronic secondary adrenal insufficiency, cortisol production does not increase considerably when ACTH is given.
- **Serum chemistry:** Decreased Na^+, increased K^+, decreased glucose.
- **Endocrine:** Decreased AM cortisol levels; ACTH may be elevated (primary), or normal/decreased (secondary).

TREATMENT

Treatment for Addison disease involves replacement of glucocorticoids and mineralocorticoids. Treatment of secondary hypocortisolism requires only glucocorticoids.

Congenital Adrenal Hyperplasia

CAH is a group of autosomal recessive disorders that cause cortisol deficiency. This results in increased ACTH production and bilateral adrenal gland hyperplasia.

TREATMENT

Glucocorticoids prevent excess ACTH secretion from the pituitary gland.

Pheochromocytoma

Pheochromocytoma is a catecholamine-producing tumor that arises from chromaffin cells, which are mainly located in the adrenal medulla (10% are extra-adrenal). Pheochromocytoma may be associated with multiple endocrine neoplasia (MEN) types II and III, neurofibromatosis, and von Hippel-Lindau syndrome.

KEY FACT

CAH
Hypertension → 17α-hydroxylase deficiency
Increased sex hormones → 21-hydroxylase deficiency
Increased sex hormones and hypertension → 11β-hydroxylase deficiency
(See Figure 2-24)

PRESENTATION

Hypertension, palpitations, anxiety, weight loss, and headaches—all occurring in an episodic fashion.

DIAGNOSIS

- 24-h urinary metanephrines and catecholamines or plasma free metanephrines.
- Clonidine suppression test → if above tests are equivocal, clonidine normally decreases catecholamines, but they remain elevated in patients with pheochromocytoma.

TREATMENT

The treatment of choice is surgical removal of the pheochromocytoma. Medical therapy involves use of α-blockers (phenoxybenzamine, phentolamine) and β-blockers. α-Blockade should be achieved prior to surgery.

KEY FACT

Pheochromocytoma rule of 10s:
10% familial
10% bilateral
10% malignant
10% in children
10% extra-adrenal

Pancreas

The pancreas is a multifunctional organ of the endocrine and digestive systems. The endocrine pancreas plays a vital role in carbohydrate, lipid, and protein metabolism through the secretion of two hormones: insulin and glucagon.

ANATOMY

The pancreas is a retroperitoneal organ situated posterior to the stomach. It lies between the duodenum and spleen (Figure 2-28). It is divided into four segments: head, neck, body, and tail. The pancreatic head lies adjacent to the second segment of the duodenum, and the tail abuts the spleen. The body

FLASH FORWARD

Because of its transverse orientation anterior to the vertebral column, the pancreas is susceptible to rupture following severe abdominal trauma (eg, traffic accidents). Seat belts transmit large compressive forces on the abdomen that effectively drive the vertebral column through the body of the pancreas.

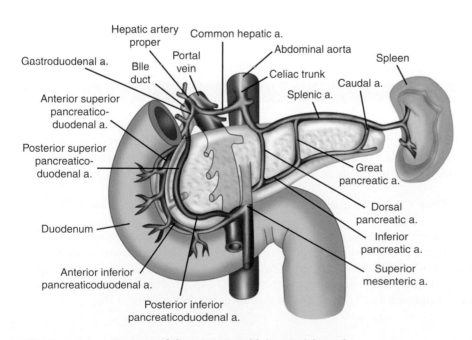

FIGURE 2-28. **Anatomy of the pancreas with its arterial supply.**

of the pancreas lies transversely across the retroperitoneum. (**The pancreatic ductal system is discussed in Chapter 3.**)

The **arterial blood supply** to the pancreas is composed of:

- **Pancreatic arteries:** Supply the body and tail of the pancreas; derived from the splenic artery.
- **Superior pancreaticoduodenal:** Supplies the head of the pancreas; derived from the gastroduodenal artery.
- **Inferior pancreaticoduodenal:** Supplies the head of the pancreas; derived from the superior mesenteric artery (SMA).

The **venous drainage** of the pancreas is provided by pancreatic veins that drain into the portal vein from tributaries of the splenic vein and superior mesenteric vein.

EMBRYOLOGY

The primitive gut is composed of the foregut, midgut, and hindgut. Foregut derivatives include the esophagus, stomach, upper duodenum, liver, gallbladder, and pancreas.

The mature pancreas develops from two separate buds of tissue off the foregut: the ventral and dorsal pancreatic buds. The ventral bud gives rise to the pancreatic head and uncinate process, and the dorsal bud forms the remaining components of the pancreas. (See Chapter 3 for more details.)

During development, the buds rotate and fuse to form a complete pancreas derived primarily from endoderm (acinar cells, islet cells, and acinar epithelium are endoderm derivatives).

Pancreatic exocrine and endocrine functions begin at different stages of development. Exocrine function does not begin until shortly after birth, whereas endocrine signaling commences at weeks 10–15 of development. The developing fetus can begin to regulate blood glucose levels relatively early in development.

HISTOLOGY

The islets of Langerhans are clusters of hormone-producing cells interspersed within pancreatic exocrine tissue. Each islet contains hundreds of endocrine cells surrounded by rich capillary networks. Approximately 1 million islets are found across the pancreas, with greater numbers located in the tail.

The three major cell populations within islets are shown in Table 2-24.

Autonomic nerve fibers innervate the blood vessels and endocrine cells of the pancreatic islets. The sympathetic and parasympathetic nervous systems influence insulin and glucagon secretion. Because nerve fibers are in close apposition with only 10% of islet endocrine cells, gap junctions between cell membranes play a role in the spread of signals to the remaining cells.

FLASH FORWARD

An **annular pancreas** develops when impaired rotation of the pancreatic buds prevents normal fusion. The buds remain wrapped around the duodenum, which typically manifests as polyhydramnios and duodenal obstruction.

FLASH FORWARD

During pregnancy, a woman with diabetes mellitus must strictly control her blood glucose levels. Maternal glucose crosses the placenta during pregnancy and causes fetal hyperinsulinemia. Hyperglycemia has adverse effects on the developing fetus, increasing the risk of fetal congenital anomalies. Following delivery, rapid withdrawal of high glucose levels in the setting of persistent hyperinsulinemia in the neonate may result in severe hypoglycemia.

FLASH FORWARD

In **type 1 diabetes mellitus (DM-1),** autoimmune destruction of pancreatic β-cells leads to insulin insufficiency.

TABLE 2-24.   Islet Cell Types and Function

CELL TYPE	QUANTITY (%)	LOCATION	HORMONE	FUNCTION
Alpha (α)	20	Peripheral	Glucagon	Increases blood glucose
Beta (β)	70	Central	Insulin	Decreases blood glucose
Delta (δ)	< 5	Variable	Somatostatin	Inhibits release of other islet cell hormones

(Adapted with permission from Junqueira LC, Carneiro J, *Basic Histology*: *Text & Atlas*, 11th ed, New York: McGraw-Hill, 2005: 408.)

INSULIN

Biosynthesis

Insulin is a small protein composed of two polypeptide chains, A and B, joined by disulfide linkages. It is synthesized as a preprohormone. A series of proteolytic reactions in the endoplasmic reticulum and Golgi complex generate the biologically active form of insulin (51 amino acids) and an inactive peptide referred to as **C-peptide** (31 amino acids). C-peptide is derived from the cleavage of proinsulin to form insulin. On stimulation of the β-cell, insulin and C-peptide are released into the circulation in equimolar quantities.

Secretion

Glucose is the most powerful stimulus for insulin release (Table 2-25). Glucose enters β-cells via the glucose transporter **GLUT 2**. This transport is by facilitated diffusion, meaning that the intracellular glucose concentration equilibrates with the serum glucose concentration. Increases in serum glucose within β-cells are shunted into the glycolytic pathway. Increased glucose catabolism leads to a rise in the intracellular ATP:ADP ratio, which causes the **ATP-sensitive potassium channel** on the surface of β-cells to close. Closure of this potassium channel leads to depolarization of the cell, resulting in opening of calcium channels. This rise in intracellular calcium facilitates insulin release from the cell (Figure 2-29).

FLASH FORWARD

In patients with hypoglycemia secondary to high circulating insulin levels, C-peptide levels help distinguish between endogenous (eg, insulinoma) and exogenous (eg, surreptitious use) sources.

C-peptide levels can also be used to assess remaining endogenous insulin production in type 2 DM.

TABLE 2-25.   Factors Affecting Insulin Release

PROMOTE INSULIN SECRETION	INHIBIT INSULIN SECRETION
Glucose	α-Adrenergic stimulation
Amino acids	Somatostatin
Vagal stimulation	Drugs: Phenytoin, vinblastine, colchicine
Sulfonylureas	
CCK, GIP, glucagon-like peptide	
Secretin, gastrin	
β-Adrenergic stimulation	

CCK = cholecystokinin; GIP = gastric inhibitory polypeptide.

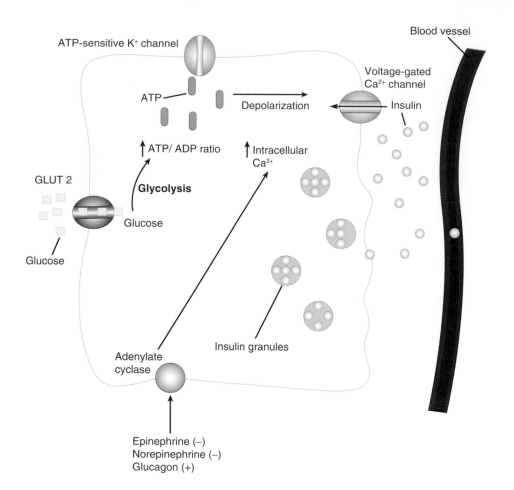

FIGURE 2-29. **Pancreatic β-cell insulin secretion.** GLUT 2, glucose transporter-2.

Another mediator of insulin release is the second messenger cAMP. Serum glucose stimulates cAMP formation within the β-cell, which mobilizes intracellular calcium stores. This calcium combines with calcium entering as a result of membrane depolarization (see earlier discussion) to increase insulin secretion.

Insulin Receptor Activation

Stimulation of the insulin receptor leads to downstream signaling cascades that result in alterations in metabolism and growth.

- The insulin receptor is a member of the tyrosine kinase superfamily of cellular receptors. It consists of two entirely extracellular α-subunits and two transmembrane β-subunits linked by disulfide bonds. The β-subunits have tyrosine kinase activity.
- Insulin binds to the α-subunits of its receptor, resulting in autophosphorylation and activation of the β subunits. The activated β-subunits recruit additional proteins to the cell membrane, including adapter molecules, kinases, and phosphatases (Figure 2-30).
- Two signaling pathways exist downstream of the activated insulin receptor:
  - **Mitogenic pathway:** Responsible for the growth-promoting effects of insulin due to activation of the mitogen-activated protein (MAP) kinase cascade.

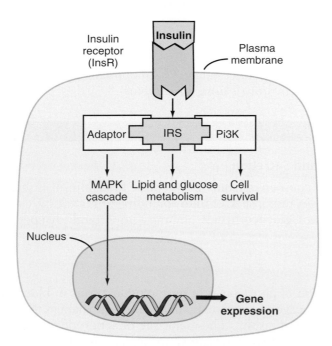

FIGURE 2-30. **Insulin receptor and downstream signaling.** IRS, insulin receptor substrate; MAPK, mitogen-activated protein kinase; Pi3K, phosphoinositide 3-kinase. (Modified with permission from Brunicardi FC. *Schwartz's Principles of Surgery*, 8th ed. New York: McGraw-Hill, 2005: 412.)

- **Metabolic pathway:** Responsible for alterations in nutrient metabolism. Activation of phosphatidylinositol-3-kinase in the metabolic pathway leads to GLUT 4 transporter insertion in the cellular membrane and stimulation of anabolic pathways.
- Insulin-bound receptors are internalized within the cell membrane following continued exposure to insulin. This downregulation desensitizes target tissues to the effects of insulin.
- In response to low insulin levels, target tissues upregulate the number of insulin receptors on their surfaces.

ACTION

Insulin's actions on carbohydrate and lipid metabolism are mediated mainly by three types of tissues: liver, muscle, and fat. The coordinated actions of insulin at these tissues promote the storage of nutrients by the body.

- Effects on the liver:
  - Stimulates glycogen formation (upregulates activity of glucokinase and glycogen synthase).
  - Inhibits glycogenolysis (↓ glycogen phosphorylase activity).
  - Inhibits gluconeogenesis (↑ phosphofructokinase-2 activity).
  - Inhibits catabolism of fatty acids and amino acids.
  - Promotes triglyceride synthesis.
- Effects on muscle:
  - Increases glucose uptake (promotes insertion of GLUT 4 on target cell membranes).
  - Stimulates glycogen formation (upregulates activity of glycogen synthase).
  - Increased amino acid uptake and protein synthesis.
  - Decreased protein degradation.

- Effects on fat:
    - Increased glucose uptake (promotes insertion of GLUT 4 on target cells).
    - Increased triglyceride storage (↑ lipoprotein lipase activity promotes triglyceride hydrolysis from lipoproteins).

GLUCAGON

Biosynthesis and Secretion

Glucagon is a counterregulatory polypeptide to insulin. It is secreted by pancreatic α-cells in response to stimuli including amino acids, catecholamines, gastric hormones, glucocorticoids, and most importantly, hypoglycemia (Table 2-26).

ACTION

The main action of glucagon is to promote elevations in blood glucose concentrations. Glucagon is a catabolic hormone that balances the energy-storing (anabolic) effects of insulin. The major site of action of glucagon is the liver. It stimulates surface-bound receptors on hepatocytes, thereby activating adenylate cyclase and raising the levels of cAMP within cells. cAMP is the second messenger responsible for mediating the downstream effects of glucagon. The major actions of glucagon are:

- **Promotes increases in serum glucose:**
    - Increased glycogenolysis (secondary to ↑ glycogen phosphorylase activity).
    - Increased gluconeogenesis (secondary to ↓ phosphofructokinase-2 activity).
    - Increased amino acid uptake by liver (provides substrate for gluconeogenesis).
- **Stimulates increases in serum fatty acids:**
    - Activates adipose cell lipase, thereby increasing serum free fatty acids.
    - Inhibits storage of triglycerides in the liver.
- **Leads to elevations in urea production:** Amino groups from catabolized amino acids are shunted into the urea cycle.

The minor actions of glucagon are:

- Increased bile secretion.
- Increased cardiac contractility.
- Decreased gastric acid secretion.
- Increased local blood flow in selected tissues.

TABLE 2-26.   Factors Affecting Glucagon Secretion

↑ GLUCAGON SECRETION	↓ GLUCAGON SECRETION
Hypoglycemia	Hyperglycemia
Norepinephrine, epinephrine	Fatty acids
Amino acids	Somatostatin
CCK, gastrin	Insulin
Glucocorticoids	

CCK = cholecystokinin.

SOMATOSTATIN

Somatostatin is a relatively small polypeptide (14 amino acids) secreted by the pancreatic δ-cells in response to high levels of blood glucose, amino acids, fatty acids, and gastric hormones. Somatostatin lengthens the period over which nutrients are incorporated into the circulation. Actions of somatostatin include:

- Decreased secretion of insulin and glucagon (paracrine effect).
- Decreased gastric, duodenal, and gallbladder motility.
- Decreased function of intestinal mucosa (decreased absorption and secretion).

DISORDERS OF THE ENDOCRINE PANCREAS

Diabetes Mellitus

Hyperglycemia is the key feature in DM, which results either from reduced insulin secretion (type 1, DM-1) or tissue resistance to insulin (type 2, DM-2) (Table 2-27). Complications of DM can be divided into neuropathy, microvascular disease (retinopathy, nephropathy), and macrovascular disease (atherosclerosis).

PRESENTATION

- Polyuria, polydipsia (glucose-induced osmotic diuresis → dehydration).
- Macrovascular complications:
  - Atherosclerosis: Advanced glycosylation end-products (AGE) produce changes in collagen composition in arterial walls and trap LDL, leading to increased lipid deposition.
  - Coronary artery disease.
  - Peripheral vascular disease.
  - Stroke—commonly due to carotid artery stenosis or arteriolosclerosis of the lenticulostriate arteries.

TABLE 2-27. DM-1 and DM-2

FEATURE	DM-1	DM-2
Percentage of DM cases	10%	90%
Prevalence	0.2–0.5%	2–4%
Age of onset	< 30	> 40
Pathogenesis	Family history uncommon; HLA-B8, -B15, -DR3, and -DR4 association; autoimmune islet β-cell destruction	Family history common (90–100% concordance rate for identical twins)
Body habitus	Thin	Obese (fat reduces number of insulin receptors)
Treatment	Insulin	Diet; oral hypoglycemic drugs; insulin
Dreaded complications	Diabetic ketoacidosis	Hyperosmolar nonketotic coma

DM = diabetes mellitus; HLA = human leukocyte antigen.

- Microvascular complications:
  - Diabetic nephropathy: Hyalinization of glomerular arterioles (Kimmel-stiel-Wilson nodules), proteinuria/microalbuminuria.
  - Diabetic retinopathy (Figure 2-31).
  - Diabetic neuropathy: Peripheral neuropathy (loss of pain and vibratory sensation in the legs—characteristic "stocking" distribution), autonomic neuropathy (sexual impotence, delayed gastric emptying).

DIAGNOSIS (TABLE 2-28)

Glycosylated hemoglobin A_{1c} (HbA_{1c}) provides a way to monitor glucose control over the preceding 2–3 months. Ideal goal is to keep $HbA_{1c} < 7\%$ (Table 2-29).

TREATMENT

Insulin is usually given by subcutaneous injection; it can also be given IV for emergency situations (DKA). All DM-1 patients need insulin. For DM-2 diabetics, diet and exercise should be the first-line therapy. Most require pharmacologic treatment, including oral hypoglycemic drugs (metformin, sulfonylurea) and some also need insulin. Complications include fungal infections, particularly *Candida albicans,* and nonhealing ulcers and wounds.

PATHOGENESIS OF DIABETIC KETOACIDOSIS

Diabetic ketoacidosis (DKA) is a complication of DM-1. Events (eg, forgetting to take insulin, infections, illnesses, excess alcohol ingestion) that decrease insulin precipitate ketoacidosis. Lack of insulin causes lipolysis and releases free fatty acids from adipose tissues. Patients present with:

- Kussmaul respirations (rapid, deep breathing)
- Acetone in breath (fruity odor)
- Dehydration, orthostatic hypotension
- Altered consciousness/coma

Decreased insulin → increased lipolysis → increased glycerol and free fatty acids → β-oxidation of free fatty acids → increased ketones.

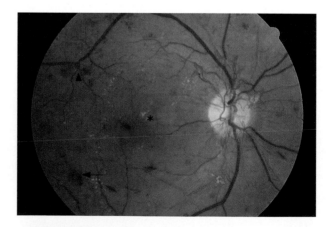

FIGURE 2-31.   Diabetic retinopathy. Shown are exudates (*), microaneurysms (*arrowhead*), and blot hemorrhages (*arrow*). (Reproduced with permission from Kasper DL, Braunwald E, Fauci AS, et al. *Harrison's Principles of Internal Medicine,* 16th ed. New York: McGraw-Hill, 2005: 2163.)

TABLE 2-28. **Diagnostic Criteria for Diabetes**

TEST	DIABETES CRITERIA
Random plasma glucose	> 200 mg/dL with symptoms
Fasting glucose	> 125 mg/dL on two occasions

Insulinoma

An uncommon cause of hypoglycemia in nondiabetics, insulinomas result from tumors of β-cells in the pancreas. Often associated with MEN I syndrome. Other causes of hypoglycemia that must be ruled out include exogenous insulin or sulfonylureas or decreased glucose production secondary to adrenal insufficiency, liver failure, alcoholism, hypopituitarism, glucagon deficiency, or sepsis.

PRESENTATION

Patients with insulinomas present with the Whipple triad:

- Fasting hypoglycemia.
- Symptoms of hypoglycemia (excessive epinephrine → sweating, tremor, tachycardia; CNS dysfunction → dizziness, headache, change in mental status).
- Relief of symptoms after IV glucose.

DIAGNOSIS

Increased insulin + C-peptide.

- Chemistries: Check glucose level and C-peptide; if increased insulin but decreased C-peptide, then it is factitious hypoglycemia (Table 2-30).
- β-Hydroxybutyrate.
- Blood urea nitrogen/creatinine, liver function tests, thyroid function tests (BUN/Cr, LFTs, TFTs).
- Insulin-like growth factor-1 (IGF-1).

TREATMENT

Surgical resection is used to treat insulinomas. For acute treatment for other causes of hypoglycemia, sugar-containing foods are given by mouth. If the patient cannot eat, either 50% dextrose in water ($D_{50}W$) is given IV or glucagon is administered IM.

Other types of tumors of the islet cells are included in Table 2-31.

KEY FACT

Causes of hypoglycemia:
- Exogenous insulin
- Insulinomas
- Ethanol ingestion
- Postoperative complication of gastric surgery
- Reactive hypoglycemia
- Liver failure

TABLE 2-29. **Interpretation of HbA₁c Levels**

> 10%	Poor control
8.5–10%	Fair control
7–8.5%	Good control
< 7%	Ideal control

HbA_{1c} = glycosylated hemoglobin A_{1c}.

TABLE 2-30. Insulinoma Versus Factitious Hypoglycemia

	INSULINOMA	FACTITIOUS HYPOGLYCEMIA
Serum insulin	↑	↑
C-peptide	↑	↓

DIABETES DRUGS

DM-1 requires insulin; DM-2 can be managed by lifestyle modifications (exercise, diet), oral hypoglycemic drugs, and/or insulin. The goals of diabetic pharmacologic therapy are to control acute symptoms and limit future complications.

Insulin

Insulin is self-administered by subcutaneous injection, typically in the abdomen, arms, or legs. It can be given IV in emergency situations (ie, DKA). Dosing depends on the type of insulin (eg, short-acting vs. long-acting) that is prescribed. New inhaled forms are also available.

MECHANISM

Supplies insulin in insulin deficiency (DM-1) or resistance (DM-2), leading to decreased plasma glucose.

USES

- DM-1, DM-2, DKA.
- Insulin comes in short-, intermediate-, and long-acting forms that affect its dosing schedule (Table 2-32).

SIDE EFFECTS

Hypoglycemia, hypokalemia (K^+-shift into intracellular compartment).

TABLE 2-31. Other Tumors of the Pancreatic Islet Cells

TUMOR	FEATURES	DIAGNOSIS
Gastrinoma (Zollinger-Ellison syndrome)	Excess gastrin release leads to ↑ acid and peptic ulcer disease.	- ↑ Basal acid output (BAO) - IV secretin test shows ↑ gastrin.
Glucagonoma	- Tumor of α-cells. - Associated with diabetes. - **Necrolytic migratory erythema** (red, scaly rash).	Glucagon levels not suppressed by glucose.
VIPoma (Verner-Morrison syndrome, pancreatic cholera)	Increase in vasoactive intestinal peptide (VIP); watery diarrhea; hypokalemia; achlorhydria.	**Clinical**

TABLE 2-32. Types of Insulin

INSULIN TYPE	ONSET OF ACTION	DURATION OF ACTION	NOTES
Ultrashort-acting ◾ Insulin lispro ◾ Insulin aspart	20 min	4 h	
Rapid acting ◾ Regular	1 h	6–8 h	Only type of insulin given IV
Intermediate-acting ◾ NPH (neutral protamine Hagedorn) ◾ Lente	2–4 h	10–18 h	Most widely used type of insulin
Long-acting ◾ Glargine ◾ Protamine zinc ◾ Ultralente	◾ 12 h ◾ 14–24 h ◾ 18–24 h	◾ 24 h ◾ 36 h ◾ 36 h	Establishes basal insulin level

ORAL HYPOGLYCEMIC DRUGS

Sulfonylureas

MECHANISM

Inhibits potassium channels on β-cells and prevents hyperpolarization, thus leading to membrane depolarization, increased calcium influx, and insulin release; increased insulin leads to decreased glucagon release from α-cells and increased tissue sensitivity to insulin.

USES

DM-2; for glucose control after failure of conservative diet and exercise regimen. Successful therapy requires ~ 30% of β-cell function (secondary failure of drug due to decreased β-cell function). Used in thin patients.

- ◾ **First-generation:** Tolbutamide (good in renal dysfunction), chlorpropamide (long-acting, may cause SIADH and disulfiram-like reactions).
- ◾ **Second-generation:** Glipizide, glyburide.

SIDE EFFECTS

Hypoglycemia, weight gain, type IV hypersensitivity reaction; hypoglycemia with cimetidine, insulin, salicylates, sulfonamides.

Metformin

MECHANISM

Decrease hepatic glucose production; increase peripheral insulin sensitivity. Exact mechanism of action unknown. Decreases postprandial glucose levels but does not cause weight gain or hypoglycemia (euglycemic).

USES

First-line treatment for obese diabetic patients; synergistic with sulfonyl-ureas, in patients without renal failure. Contraindicated in patients with renal impairment (drug excreted by kidneys) or CHF.

SIDE EFFECTS

Lactic acidosis, GI distress (nausea, diarrhea), avoid IV contrast.

Acarbose

MECHANISM

Inhibits α-glycosidase → decreased carbohydrate absorption from the GI tract → decreased insulin demand.

USES

DM-2.

SIDE EFFECTS

Flatulence, diarrhea, abdominal discomfort.

Thiazolidinediones (Rosiglitazone, Pioglitazone)

MECHANISM

Binds nuclear peroxisome proliferator-activated receptor (PPAR) to control transcription of insulin-responsive genes, leads to insulin sensitization and decreased hepatic gluconeogenesis and insulin receptor upregulation.

USES

DM-2, in the absence of liver disease, CHF or coronary artery disease.

SIDE EFFECTS

Weight gain, edema (peripheral or macular), liver function abnormalities.

Repaglinide

MECHANISM

Works like sulfonylureas by stimulating release of insulin from the pancreas.

USES

DM-2.

SIDE EFFECTS

Hypoglycemia, weight gain.

Gastrointestinal

Embryology

OVERVIEW OF GASTROINTESTINAL SYSTEM DEVELOPMENT

The development of the GI tract is divided into three main sections. These sections share common innervations and vascular supply:

- Cephalic foldings form the **foregut**: oral cavity, pharynx, esophagus, stomach, duodenum proximal to the bile duct, liver, pancreas, bile ducts, and gallbladder. Note that the cephalic foldings also give rise to the trachea and lungs, though these are not considered part of the foregut.
- Lateral foldings form the **midgut**: duodenum distal to the bile duct, jejunum, ileum, cecum, appendix, ascending colon, and proximal two-thirds of the transverse colon.
- Caudal foldings form the **hindgut**: distal third of the transverse colon, descending colon, sigmoid colon, rectum, and upper portion of the anal canal.

Fourth Week

Embryonic foldings (cephalic, lateral, and caudal) form the primitive gut tube:

- Endoderm becomes intestinal epithelium and glands.
- Mesoderm becomes connective tissue, muscle, and wall of intestine.
- Migrating neural crest cells form the autonomic nervous system innervation.

Sixth Week

The midgut loop has cranial (proximal to the superior mesenteric artery [SMA]) and caudal (distal to the SMA) limbs. The cranial loop undergoes rapid growth and is herniated out the umbilicus.

Tenth Week

The abdominal cavity enlarges and allows the herniated midgut loops to return while undergoing a counterclockwise rotation. After a total 270-degree rotation around the axis of the SMA, the organs begin to take their adult positions.

Embryologic Remnants

Postnatally, several vessels of the prenatal circulation form ligaments in the adult:

- Umbilical vein—ligamentum teres hepatis
- Umbilical arteries—medial umbilical ligaments
- Ductus venosus—ligamentum venosum
- Ductus arteriosus—ligamentum arteriosum
- Allantois–urachus—median umbilical ligament

CONGENITAL MALFORMATIONS OF THE GI TRACT

Omphalocele

Failure of herniated midgut to return to the abdominal cavity during the fifth week of embryonic development. The herniated intestine is **covered by peri-**

CLINICAL CORRELATION

The vitelline duct joins the yolk sac at the junction of the cranial and caudal limbs of the midgut loop. It persists as Meckel diverticulum in 2% of the population, making it the most common congenital anomaly of the GI tract.

CLINICAL CORRELATION

A failure of neural crest cell migration causes Hirshsprung disease—congenital megacolon. It is associated with Down syndrome and presents with failure to pass meconium, chronic constipation, and dilation of proximal colon.

MNEMONIC

- Umbi**L**ical arteries—media**L** umbilical ligaments
- Alla**N**tois–urachus—media**N** umbilical ligament
- Note there are two umbilical arteries and two medial umbilical ligaments, but only one allantois and one median umbilical ligament.

toneal membrane and is **midline** through the umbilicus (Figure 3-1A). Most commonly affects children of mothers at the extremes of reproductive age.

PRESENTATION

During the second-trimester ultrasound or when a herniated sac is found at birth. Twenty-five percent to 40% of affected infants have other birth defects, such as chromosomal abnormalities, congenital diaphragmatic hernia, or heart defects. Omphaloceles can be a part of **Beckwith-Wiedemann syndrome,** which is a collection of congenital defects that include macrosomia, macroglossia, midline abdominal wall defects (omphalocele, hernia), ear pits or creases, and hypoglycemia.

DIAGNOSIS

Herniated sac can be visualized by ultrasound in 95% of cases. Serum **α-fetoprotein (AFP)** levels are elevated in 70% of cases.

TREATMENT

Close monitoring of the fetus during pregnancy and prompt treatment following delivery, including surgical reduction of the herniated contents.

Gastroschisis

A full-thickness abdominal wall defect caused by vascular injury during development allowing small or large bowel to escape the abdominal cavity. **No protective peritoneal membrane** covers the herniated intestine, which protrudes lateral to the umbilicus (Figure 3-1B). Gastroschisis is more common in children born to women < 20 years of age.

PRESENTATION

Most often seen in the second-trimester ultrasound in combination with polyhydramnios and an elevated serum AFP. Extruded abdominal contents are noted at birth. The defect is usually to the right of the umbilicus and may be associated with intestinal atresia.

> ### ? CLINICAL CORRELATION
>
> α-Fetoprotein (AFP) is part of the triple screen exam for normal newborn development. Elevated levels are also associated with neural tube defects, gastroschisis, hepatocellular carcinoma, and yolk sac tumors.

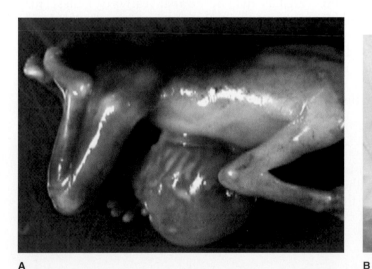

A

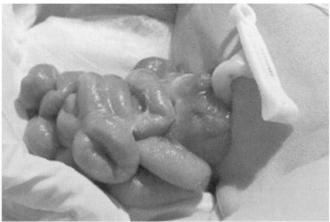

B

FIGURE 3-1.   Omphalocele and gastroschisis. (A) Omphalocele in a newborn. Note the presence of a peritoneal membrane covering the herniated bowel defect and that the defect is midline. (B) Gastroschisis. Note the absence of a peritoneal membrane covering the exposed midgut and that most defects are to the right of midline. [(A) Reproduced with permission from USMLERx.com. (B) Reproduced with permission from Brunicardi FC, Andersen DK, Billiar TR, et al. *Schwartz's Principles of Surgery*, 9th ed. New York: McGraw-Hill, 2010: Figure 39-31.]

DIAGNOSIS

Herniated bowel resembles cauliflower on ultrasound. Elevated AFP on triple screen.

TREATMENT

Surgical correction of the abdominal wall defect with return of the herniated contents to the abdomen. **Artificial covering** may be used to minimize heat/fluid loss and assist with **temperature regulation** (exposed bowel causes increased heat loss). **Nasogastric tube (decompresses the stomach), broad-spectrum antibiotics,** and **total parenteral nutrition (TPN).**

Intestinal Malrotation

Develops as a result of abnormal midgut development and rotation.

- **Cecum** remains in the right upper quadrant (RUQ) or in the left abdomen, and the **duodenojejunal** junction remains to the right of the midline.
- Peritoneal attachments to the lateral abdominal wall normally fix the cecum retroperitoneally. In malrotation, they cross over the duodenum to reach the high, malrotated cecum and are called **Ladd bands.** They can cause partial or complete obstruction of the duodenum (which can manifest from infancy to early adulthood).
- **Midgut volvulus** occurs when the malrotated intestine twists on the axis of the **SMA,** compromising intestinal blood flow.

PRESENTATION

Midgut volvulus may occur at any time, often during the first year of life, and presents with sudden onset of severe **bilious** emesis, abdominal pain and distention, and rectal bleeding. Delay in recognition and treatment can lead to significant intestinal necrosis, resulting in shock and loss of viable intestine. Resection of the small bowel may lead to **short gut syndrome.**

DIAGNOSIS

- **Abdominal plain film:** Variable; may be normal (early) or gasless, may show a "double-bubble" sign, pneumatosis intestinalis (air in the bowel wall), or free air.
- **Upper GI study:** Documents the position of the ligament of Trietz and intestinal rotation; may have a corkscrew appearance.
- **Ultrasound:** May show twisted superior mesenteric vessels ("whirlpool sign"), fixed midline bowel loops, and duodenal dilation. Near 100% sensitivity.

TREATMENT

Urgent surgery consisting of Ladd procedure: Counterclockwise volvulus reduction, lysis of adhesive bands, bowel resection if needed, appendectomy, and repositioning of the small intestine and cecum. May lead to short-bowel syndrome or death if treatment is delayed.

Duodenal Atresia

During weeks 5–8 of development, the duodenum becomes completely obstructed by proliferating endoderm. Failure of the duodenum to recanalize by week 10 results in duodenal atresia.

KEY FACT

Malrotation—Abnormality in development causing the intestines to take a different position in the abdomen than usual.

Volvulus—Twisting of a loop of bowel or other structure about its base of attachment, constricting venous outflow. The large intestine is predisposed to volvulus.

CLINICAL CORRELATION

Seventy percent of patients with malrotation have associated anomalies, including:
- Other abdominal defects: Situs inversus, septal defects, transposition of the great vessels, and anomalous systemic or pulmonary venous return.
- Asplenia or polysplenia.

KEY FACT

Bilious emesis in a neonate is presumed to be midgut volvulus until proven otherwise!

PRESENTATION

Vomiting (bilious or nonbilious) and abdominal distention appear within 48 hours of birth. If the biliary system is obstructed, physical exam may reveal an abdominal mass or jaundice. The newborn may be small for gestational age. Incidence is 1 in 2500 to 1 in 40,000 live births.

Nearly one third of affected newborns have **Down syndrome.** Of those affected, 30% also have:

- Gastroschisis.
- Imperforate anus or other intestinal atresia.
- Cardiac, renal, and vertebral malformations.

DIAGNOSIS

Duodenal atresia may be detected by prenatal ultrasound or may not become apparent until birth.

- **Prenatal ultrasound:** Polyhydramnios from inability to swallow amniotic fluid (seen in 50%) or dilated bowel.
- **Abdominal radiograph:** "Double-bubble" sign due to dilation of the stomach and proximal duodenum (Figure 3-2).

KEY FACT

Women who use vasoactive substances (eg, cigarettes or medications) during the first trimester are three times more likely to have a child with duodenal atresia.

MNEMONIC

Use **VACTERL** to remember mesodermal defects:
Vertebral defects
Anal atresia
Cardiac defects
Tracheo**E**sophageal fistula
Renal defects
Limb defects (bone and muscle)

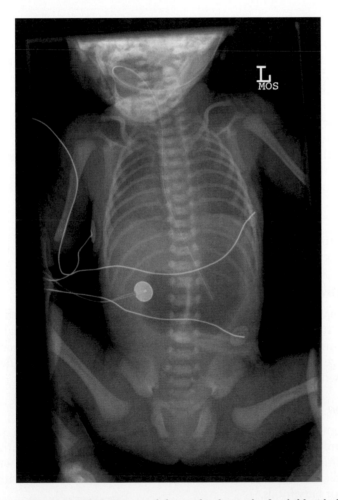

FIGURE 3-2. **Double-bubble sign.** An abdominal radiograph of a child with duodenal atresia showing dilation of the stomach and proximal duodenum. (Courtesy Dr. Evelyn Anthony, Brenner Children's Hospital, Wake Forest University Baptist Medical Center.)

TREATMENT

Definitive treatment is **duodenoduodenostomy** (anastomosis of the proximal and distal duodenum to bypass the obstruction) or **duodenojejunostomy.** Preoperative patients need a nasogastric tube, IV fluids, and correction of electrolyte abnormalities. Postoperative care may include TPN until oral feeds can be started.

Pyloric Stenosis

Pyloric stenosis is of idiopathic cause and develops as a result of congenital hypertrophy of the pylorus, which in turn results in obstruction of the gastric outlet. Incidence is 1 in 600 live births; it is most commonly seen in firstborn males.

PRESENTATION

Usually between 3–6 weeks of age, patients present with difficulty feeding followed by projectile, **nonbilious** vomiting. **Signs of illness** (fever, diarrhea) are notably absent. Affected children are often hungry after the episodes and may develop abdominal pain, belching, and weight loss. Wavelike motions may be seen over the abdomen after feeding and just before vomiting occurs.

DIAGNOSIS

- Physical exam classically demonstrates a palpable "olive" mass in the epigastric region. Lab tests may demonstrate hypochloremic, metabolic alkalosis secondary to loss of HCl in emesis, with hypokalemia late in presentation.
- **Ultrasound** shows an elongated and hypertrophic pylorus.
- Barium studies show:
  - **String sign:** Seen on barium swallow when barium moves through the pylorus.
  - **Shoulder sign:** The pylorus bulges into the antrum of the stomach.
  - **Double-tract sign:** Parallel streaks of barium seen in the narrow pylorus.

TREATMENT

Pyloromyotomy (longitudinal incision through the muscle of the pylorus with dissection to the submucosa) is definitive therapy.

Pancreas Divisum

A failure of the dorsal and ventral pancreatic buds to fuse during development. This forces the bulk of the pancreas (derived from the dorsal pancreatic bud) to drain through the minor papilla, causing a relative stenosis of pancreatic drainage (Figure 3-3). This is the **most common congenital defect of the pancreas,** with an incidence of 3–10% of live births.

PRESENTATION

Most patients are asymptomatic; however, those who develop pancreatitis (from failure of drainage through the minor papilla) present with epigastric pain radiating to the back and abdominal distention associated with nausea, vomiting, diarrhea, and jaundice. Symptoms may be worsened with ingestion of alcohol or fatty foods.

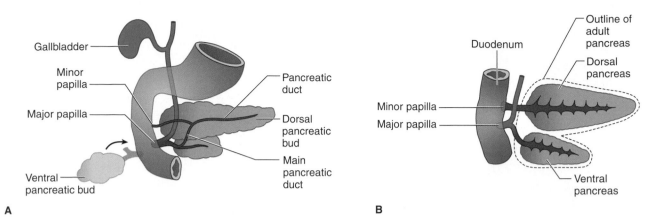

FIGURE 3-3   Pancreas divisum. (A) Note that the major papilla derives from the ventral pancreatic bud. (B) When the buds fail to fuse, pancreas divisum results, forcing the bulk of the pancreas (the dorsal pancreatic bud) to drain through the minor papilla.

DIAGNOSIS

Most patients are asymptomatic, and no diagnosis is made. Those that have episodes of pancreatitis may undergo the following workup:

- Amylase and lipase: Usually elevated in acute episodes of pancreatitis.
- Endoscopic retrograde cholangiopancreatography (ERCP): Demonstrates two separately draining pancreatic ducts. Associated risk of causing pancreatitis.
- Magnetic resonance cholangiopancreatography (MRCP): Noninvasive method that shows direct continuity of the dorsal pancreatic duct and the minor papilla.

TREATMENT

- For acute episodes of pancreatitis: Rest, gastric suction, fluid and electrolyte replacement, and pain control.
- Definitive surgical treatment is poorly established, but endoscopic options include sphincterotomy (cutting of the minor papilla during ERCP to enlarge its opening) or an ERCP-guided stent of the minor papilla.

Esophageal Atresia with Tracheoesophageal Fistula

Maldevelopment of the upper GI tract may cause the esophagus to end in a blind pouch (atresia) associated with a fistula between the trachea and distal esophagus. There are multiple less common variants of atresia and fistula formation (Figure 3-4).

PRESENTATION

Most patients present with **cyanosis** (bluish skin due to poor oxygenation), **choking and vomiting with feeding**, drooling, and **poor feeding.**

DIAGNOSIS

- Prenatal ultrasound usually shows polyhydramnios, although the diagnosis is most commonly suggested based on an infant's **difficulty with feeding.** In this case, the examiner attempts to place a feeding tube but will not be able to reach the stomach.
- Radiography: Reveals an air bubble in the proximal esophagus and air in the stomach and intestines.

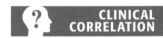

CLINICAL CORRELATION

Annular pancreas is a rare congenital anomaly (1 in 20,000 live births) in which the ventral pancreatic duct encircles the descending duodenum and fuses to the dorsal pancreatic duct, causing duodenal obstruction.

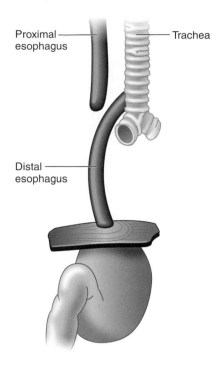

FIGURE 3-4. **Esophageal atresia with tracheoesophageal fistula.** Ninety percent of cases of tracheoesophageal fistula result in a blind pouch end of the esophagus and a fistula between the distal esophagus and trachea. This is correlated with a very high risk of aspiration and suffocation. (Modified with permission from Morgan GE, Mikhail MS, Murray MJ. *Clinical Anesthesiology*, 4th ed. New York: Lange Medical Books/McGraw-Hill, 2005: Figure 44-3.)

CLINICAL CORRELATION

TE fistula is often associated with other mesodermal anomalies (VACTERL) or the presence of a single umbilical artery. Complications include aspiration, paroxysmal suffocation, pneumonia, and severe fluid and electrolyte imbalances.

TREATMENT

Tracheoesophageal (TE) fistula is considered a surgical emergency. The esophagus must be repaired immediately to protect the newborn's airway. Preoperatively, the baby is NPO (nothing by mouth), and care is taken to prevent aspiration.

Anatomy

ABDOMINAL WALL

The abdomen is defined as the region of the trunk that lies between the diaphragm (superiorly) and the inlet of the pelvis (inferiorly).

Surface Anatomy

Landmarks of the abdominal wall are shown in Figure 3-5.

Linea Alba

A vertical fibrous band that extends from the symphysis pubis to the xiphoid process and lies in the midline. It is formed by fusion of the aponeuroses of the muscles of the anterior abdominal wall and is represented on the surface by a median groove.

Linea Semilunaris

Defines the lateral edge of the rectus abdominis muscle and crosses the costal margin at the tip of the ninth costal cartilage.

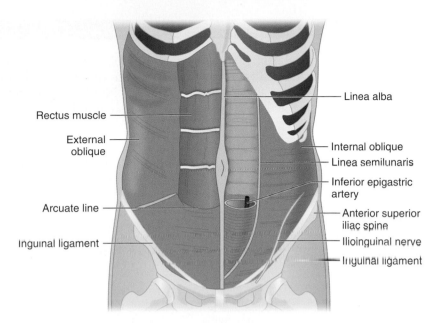

FIGURE 3-5.   **Landmarks of the abdominal wall.**

Arcuate Line

Defines the lower limit of the posterior aspect of the rectus sheath. Above the arcuate line, the aponeuroses of the internal oblique split and form a layer posterior to the rectus abdominis muscle along with the aponeuroses of the transversalis muscle (Figure 3-6). Inferiorly, the aponeuroses of the external, internal and transversalis muscles all form an anterior sheath, with only the transversalis fascia on the posterior aspect. The arcuate line usually forms one third of the distance from the umbilicus to the pubic crest and is the landmark at which the **inferior epigastric arteries perforate the rectus abdominis muscles.**

Inguinal Groove

Formed by the inguinal ligament. It lies beneath a skin crease in the groin and is formed by the rolled-under margin of the aponeurosis of the external oblique muscle.

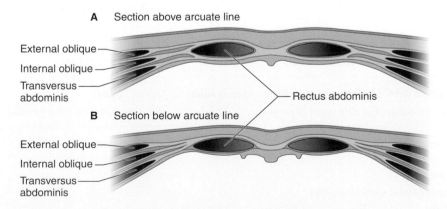

FIGURE 3-6.   **Cross-section of the anterior abdominal wall.** Note that above the arcuate line (A), the aponeurosis of the internal oblique is split around the rectus abdominis muscle whereas below the arcuate line (B), the aponeuroses of all three muscle layers gather anterior to the rectus abdominis muscle. The inferior epigastric vessels pierce the abdominal sheath at this line.

ABDOMINAL PLANES AND REGIONS

Vertical lines and horizontal planes are used to pinpoint anatomic features and help to define the sites of abnormalities and disease processes within the abdominal cavity. In this way, the abdomen is divided into four quadrants or nine regions, usually projected onto the anterior abdominal wall.

Abdominal Regions

Anatomically, there are **nine** defined regions of interest (Table 3-1 and Figure 3-7). In clinical practice, however, these regions are defined imprecisely.

Abdominal Quadrants

The abdomen can be divided into **four** quadrants (Table 3-2), using a horizontal line and a vertical line that intersect at the umbilicus.

TABLE 3-1. **Contents of the Respective Abdominal Regions**

RIGHT HYPOCHONDRIAC	EPIGASTRIC	LEFT HYPOCHONDRIAC
Liver and gallbladder	Esophagus and stomach Adrenal glands Liver	Stomach Pancreas
Right kidney	(Transverse colon)	Spleen
Colon, hepatic flexure	Abdominal aorta and vena cava Pylorus and duodenum (first part)	Left kidney Colon, splenic flexure
RIGHT LUMBAR	**UMBILICAL**	**LEFT LUMBAR**
Kidney	(Transverse colon)	Kidney
Colon (ascending) Gallbladder	Duodenum and pancreas	Colon (descending)
Small intestine	Abdominal aorta and vena cava	Pancreas
Duodenum (first part)	Small intestine Iliac vessels	Small intestine (jejunum)
RIGHT ILIAC	**HYPOGASTRIC**	**LEFT ILIAC**
Cecum Right ovary/fallopian tube (female)	Distensible pelvic organs (eg, bladder in infants or in adults when full; uterus after 12th week of pregnancy)	Sigmoid colon Left ovary/fallopian tube (female)
Appendix	Small intestine	Small intestine
Small intestine (ileum)	Iliac vessels Spermatic cords, seminal vesicles Rectum	

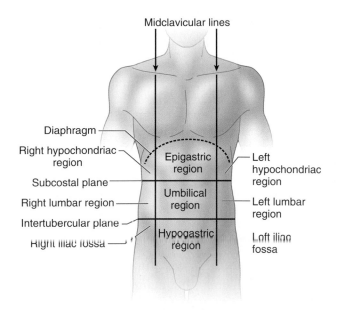

FIGURE 3-7.   Surface anatomy of the abdominal wall.

TABLE 3-2.   Abdominal Quadrants

	RIGHT	**LEFT**
Upper	Liver (right lobe)	Liver (left lobe) Stomach
	Gallbladder (fundus where the linea semilunaris crosses the costal margin)	Spleen Pancreas (body, tail)
	Kidney and suprarenal gland	Kidney and suprarenal gland
	Colon (hepatic) flexure and right transverse	Colon (splenic) flexure and left transverse
	Duodenum (parts 1–3) with pancreas (head) Small intestine Pylorus	Small intestine (jejunum and proximal ilium)
Lower	Colon (ascending)	Colon (descending and sigmoid)
	Cecum	Small intestine
	Appendix (including McBurney point)	
	Small intestine (ileum) Right ovary/Fallopian tube Right ureter	Left ovary/Fallopian tube Left ureter

MNEMONIC

To remember the fascial layers:
You go **Camp**ing **Outside**
(**Camp**er fascia is **external** to
Scarpa).

KEY FACT

During embryonic development, the
testes and spermatic cord (in males)
and the round ligament of the
uterus (in females) descend through
the inguinal canal.

**FLASH
FORWARD**

- **Direct inguinal hernia:**
  Protrudes **medial** to the
  epigastric artery and vein;
  Directly through Hesselbach
  triangle (inferior epigastric artery,
  rectus abdominis, inguinal
  ligament).
- **Indirect inguinal hernia:**
  Protrudes **lateral** to the
  epigastric artery and vein
  through the deep inguinal
  ring, often by an incomplete
  obliteration of the processus
  vaginalis.
- **Femoral hernia:** Protrudes
  below the inguinal ligament in
  the femoral triangle (sartorius,
  adductor longus, inguinal
  ligament).

**CLINICAL
CORRELATION**

Failure of the processus vaginalis to
obliterate leads to communication
between the abdominal cavity and
the scrotal sac. This allows a fluid
collection called a hydrocele to
accumulate in the scrotum.

Layers of the Abdominal Wall

The anterolateral abdominal wall is made up of (see Figures 3-5 and 3-6):

- Skin
- Superficial fascia (fatty [Camper] and membranous [Scarpa])
- Deep fascia
- Aponeuroses of the muscle layers—anterior wall
- External oblique muscle—lateral wall
- Internal oblique muscle—lateral wall
- Transversus abdominis muscle—lateral wall
- Transversalis fascia
- Extraperitoneal fat
- Parietal peritoneum

Inguinal Canal

The inguinal canal is an oblique passage through the inguinal region and a site of inguinal hernias (both direct and indirect; Figures 3-8 and 3-9).

Boundaries of the inguinal canal:

- **Deep inguinal ring:** Oval opening in the fascia transversalis lateral to the inferior epigastric vessels.
- **Superficial inguinal ring:** Triangular defect in the aponeurosis of the external oblique muscle, lateral to the pubic tubercle.
- **Anterior wall:** Aponeurosis of the external oblique muscle with some of the internal oblique aponeurosis laterally.

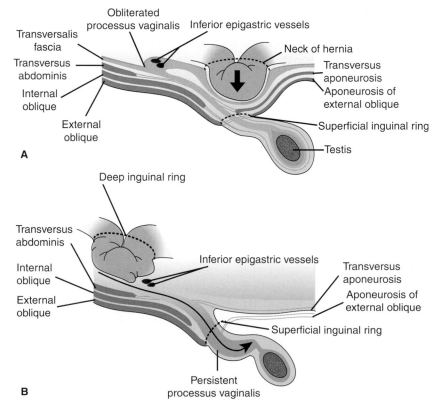

FIGURE 3-8.   Inguinal hernias. Direct (A) and indirect (B). (Modified with permission from Tintinalli JE, Kelen GD, Stapczynski JS, et al, eds. *Tintinalli's Emergency Medicine: A Comprehensive Study Guide*, 6th ed. New York: McGraw-Hill, 2004: 528.)

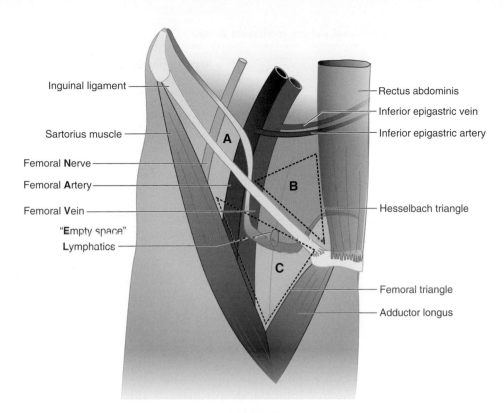

Inguinal ligament

Sartorius muscle

Femoral **N**erve

Femoral **A**rtery

Femoral **V**ein

"**E**mpty space"

Lymphatics

Rectus abdominis

Inferior epigastric vein

Inferior epigastric artery

Hesselbach triangle

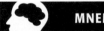

Femoral triangle

Adductor longus

FIGURE 3-9. **Femoral canal and sites of herniation.** (A) Indirect hernias pass through the deep inguinal ring which overlies the external iliac vessels just lateral to the inferior epigastric vessels. (B) Direct hernias pass through Hesselbach triangle which is defined by the inferior epigastric artery, rectus abdominis muscle, and inguinal ligament. (C) Femoral hernias pass through the femoral ring, medial to the femoral vein, and bulge out of the femoral triangle, which is bounded by the inguinal ligament, adductor longus, and sartorius.

- **Posterior wall:** Mainly transversalis fascia, with the conjoint tendon (falx inguinalis) medially. The conjoint tendon is the merger of the internal abdominal oblique and transverse abdominis aponeuroses.
- **Roof:** Internal oblique and transverse abdominal muscles.
- **Floor:** Inguinal and lacunar ligaments.

Femoral Triangle

The femoral triangle is the anatomic region of the upper inner thigh bounded by the following (see Figure 3-9):

- **Superiorly:** Inguinal ligament
- **Laterally:** Sartorius muscle
- **Medially:** Adductor longus muscle

PERITONEUM AND ABDOMINAL VISCERA

Abdominal and Pelvic Peritoneum

The peritoneum is a serous membrane that covers the abdominal organs (Table 3-3) and is composed of **two layers:** the parietal and visceral peritoneum.

MNEMONIC

Contents of the femoral triangle (from lateral to medial) include: **NAVEL**

Femoral **N**erve
Femoral **A**rtery
Femoral **V**ein
Empty space
Lymphatic
OR
Venous near the penis.
The vein is more medial than the artery.

TABLE 3-3.   Intraperitoneal and Extraperitoneal Viscera

INTRAPERITONEAL VISCERA	RETROPERITONEAL VISCERA
Stomach	Parts two, three, and four of the duodenum
First part of duodenum	Ascending and descending colon
Jejunum, ileum, cecum, appendix	Distal rectum
Transverse and sigmoid colon	Head, neck, and body of pancreas
Proximal rectum	Abdominal aorta
Liver and gallbladder	Inferior vena cava
Tail of pancreas	Kidneys, ureters, and adrenal glands
Spleen	Distal esophagus

PARIETAL PERITONEUM

- The outer membrane that lines the deep surface of the abdominal walls and the inferior surface of the diaphragm.
- The nerve supply originates from the nerves of the surrounding abdominal muscles and skin, intercostal and phrenic nerves in the abdominal region, and obturator nerve in the pelvic region.

VISCERAL PERITONEUM

The membrane that directly covers the abdominal organs. There is no somatic nerve supply to the visceral peritoneum.

PERITONEAL CAVITY

- The peritoneal cavity is a narrow, "potential" space between the opposing layers of the peritoneum, and it reflects the rotation of the GI tract during its embryonic development. Some, but not all abdominal organs are contained within the peritoneal cavity (see Table 3-3).
- **Normally, no space** exists between the parietal and visceral peritoneum (only ~50 mL of serous peritoneal fluid).
- In **pathologic conditions** (eg, ascites), more fluid can accumulate between the two layers of peritoneum. This phenomenon of extravascular fluid accumulation is known as **third spacing.**

As a "potential" space, the peritoneal cavity can be divided into the greater and lesser peritoneal sacs.

- The **lesser sac** (omental bursa) is a pouch of peritoneum that lies posterior to the stomach, liver, and lesser omentum. It communicates with the greater sac through the **epiploic foramen** (omental, or **Winslow,** foramen).
- The anterior border of Winslow foramen is the hepatoduodenal ligament, which contains the portal triad (hepatic artery, bile duct, and portal vein). It can be used surgically to control hemorrhage during a cholecystectomy.
- The **greater sac** encompasses the rest of the peritoneum and is subdivided by the transverse mesocolon into the supracolic compartment (above), and the infracolic and pelvic compartments below the mesocolon.

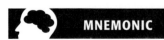

CLINICAL CORRELATION

- Ascites is an accumulation of extra fluid in the peritoneal cavity (common causes include liver failure, right-sided heart failure, ovarian cancer).
- Pneumoperitoneum is air or other gas in the peritoneal cavity (due to intestinal or stomach perforation, or intentional insufflation for laparoscopy).

KEY FACT

Remember that third spacing includes all nonintravascular space where edema and fluid can accumulate. It is not limited to the intraperitoneal space.

MNEMONIC

Retroperitoneal organs—

SAD PUCKER
Suprarenal glands
Aorta/IVC
Duodenum
Pancreas (except tail)
Ureters
Colon (ascending/descending)
Kidneys
Esophagus (distal)
Rectum

MESENTERY

Mesentery is a double layer of peritoneum that wraps around abdominal organs, contains blood vessels, and attaches the organ to its major blood supply.

ARTERIAL SUPPLY OF THE GI TRACT

The arterial blood supply of the GI tract is derived from the abdominal aorta.

Abdominal Aorta

The abdominal aorta is the portion of the descending aorta inferior to the diaphragm. It gives off **three large branches** from the anterior surface that supply blood to the GI organs (Figure 3-10 and Table 3-4):

- Celiac trunk: Supplies derivatives of the foregut (esophagus through proximal duodenum [Figure 3-11]). It is located just inferior to the diaphragm and phrenic arteries.
- Superior mesenteric artery (SMA): Supplies derivatives of the midgut (distal duodenum to splenic flexure of the colon).
- Inferior mesenteric artery (IMA): Supplies derivatives of the hindgut (splenic flexure of the colon through proximal rectum).

The abdominal aorta also gives rise to the **inferior phrenic, middle suprarenal, renal,** and **gonadal** arteries. The abdominal aorta divides into the **left** and **right common iliac** arteries, which then descend into the pelvis.

Key Anastomoses of the Abdominal Arterial System

Anastomoses are connections of two vessels that can allow collateral flow around obstructions or infarcts (eg, thromboembolism), transfer of pressure from one system to another (eg, portal hypertension), or perfusion of a region with relatively stenotic blood supply (eg, watershed infarcts). Several key anastomoses occur in the abdominal arterial system (Table 3-5).

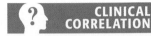

CLINICAL CORRELATION

Atherosclerosis can cause gradual occlusion at the bifurcation of the abdominal aorta, which may result in claudication and impotence.

KEY FACT

Remember the arterial branches of the abdominal aorta are paired or unpaired:

- Paired: Inferior phrenic, middle suprarenal, renal, gonadal, iliac
- Unpaired: Celiac, SMA, IMA, median sacral

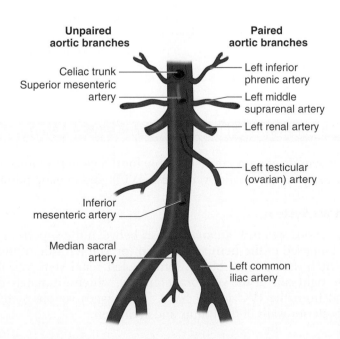

FIGURE 3-10.   **Abdominal aorta and its branches.**

TABLE 3-4. Main Branches of the Abdominal Aorta

PRIMARY BRANCHES	SECONDARY BRANCHES	ORGANS SUPPLIED
Celiac Artery		
Left gastric artery	Esophageal branch of the left gastric artery	Esophagus, stomach
Splenic artery	Dorsal pancreatic artery, short gastric arteries, left gastro-omental (gastroepiploic) artery	Stomach, pancreas, spleen[a]
Common hepatic artery	Gastroduodenal artery (then right gastro-omental and superior pancreaticoduodenal), right gastric artery, hepatic artery proper	Upper duodenum, liver, gallbladder, pancreas, stomach
Superior Mesenteric Artery		
Inferior pancreaticoduodenal arteries	Anterior and posterior inferior pancreaticoduodenal arteries	Head of the pancreas; second through fourth portions of duodenum
Middle colic artery	Marginal artery of Drummond	Transverse colon
Right colic artery		Ascending colon
Intestinal arteries (jejunal and ileal arteries)	Arterial arcades and vasa recta	Jejunum and ileum
Ileocolic artery	Colic and ileal arteries; ileal branch gives rise to the appendicular artery	Ileum, cecum, appendix
Inferior Mesenteric Artery		
Left colic artery	Marginal artery of Drummond	Descending colon
Sigmoid artery		Sigmoid colon
Superior rectal artery		Rectum (proximal portion)

[a]The spleen is not a foregut derivative. It is of mesodermal origin.

VENOUS DRAINAGE OF THE GI TRACT

Three major venous systems are responsible for the venous drainage of the GI tract are the azygos vein, inferior vena cava (IVC), and hepatic portal system.

Azygos Venous System

The azygos venous system is an anastomosis between the superior (SVC) and IVC. It is composed of the **hemiazygos vein** (on the left side of the vertebral column), which drains some blood from the left renal vein into the **azygos vein** (on the right side of the vertebral column), which ultimately drains part of the blood from the IVC to the SVC. The azygos venous system mainly drains the posterior walls of the thorax and abdomen.

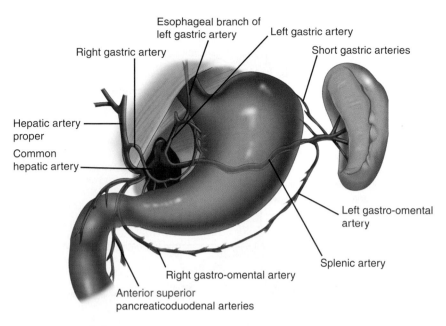

FIGURE 3-11.   Celiac trunk.

Inferior Vena Cava Venous System

The IVC venous system (Figure 3-12) is responsible for draining the blood from the lower half of the body (below the diaphragm) into the right atrium. Drainage patterns:

- Formed by the left and right common iliac veins at L5.
- The **right** gonadal and suprarenal veins drain directly into the IVC; their **left** counterparts drain into the left renal vein, which then drains into the IVC.

Portal Venous System

The portal venous system is centered on the portal vein, which drains blood from the spleen, intestine, and colon into the liver, and is formed by the **supe-**

> **CLINICAL CORRELATION**
>
> Left testicular varicocele may occur as a result of occlusion of the left renal vein (eg, compression by a left renal tumor).

TABLE 3-5.   Key Anastomoses of the Abdominal Arterial System

MAJOR ANASTOMOSES	CONNECTING ARTERIES	CLINICAL CORRELATION
Celiac trunk–SMA	Superior and inferior branches of the pancreaticoduodenal arteries	Dual supply of the pancreatic head in case of infarct
SMA–IMA	Middle colic–left colic arteries	Severe hypotension can cause relative infarction and necrosis of the splenic flexure
IMA–internal iliac	Superior rectal–middle rectal arteries	Dual supply of the proximal rectum
Subclavian/Internal thoracic–external iliac	Superior epigastric–inferior epigastric arteries	Collateral flow around an aortic stenosis (eg, coarctation of the aorta)

IMA = inferior mesenteric artery; SMA = superior mesenteric artery.

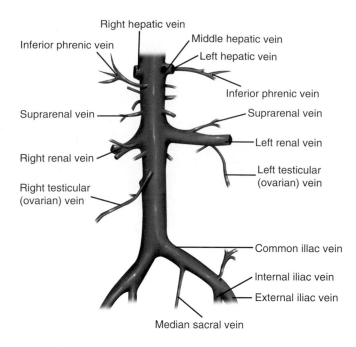

FIGURE 3-12. **Inferior vena cava.**

KEY FACT

Lymphatic drainage from organs almost always follows the arterial supply. For example, lymphatic drainage from the foregut passes through the celiac nodes (as the foregut is supplied by the celiac trunk).

rior mesenteric and splenic veins. The portal vein is situated in the hepatoduodenal ligament.

The portal vein transports nutrient- (and toxin) rich blood from the GI tract as well as products of lysed RBCs from the spleen to the sinusoids of the liver. The liver then drains through the hepatic veins into the IVC.

PORTAL TO INFERIOR VENA CAVAL ANASTOMOSES (COLLATERALS)

Pathologies that cause portal hypertension, such as cirrhosis from metabolic insults or infection, lead to collateral intra-abdominal venous flow pathways (anastomoses; [Figure 3-13 and Table 3-6]).

LYMPHATIC DRAINAGE OF THE GI TRACT

The end point of all lymphatic flow from the GI tract and its organs is the **thoracic duct,** which in turn empties into the venous system at the **junction** of the **internal jugular vein** and **left subclavian vein.**

Before passing into the thoracic duct, the lymph from the GI tract passes through the preaortic lymph nodes, which can be divided into the celiac, superior mesenteric, and inferior mesenteric nodes.

Peyer Patches

Peyer patches, known as gut-associated lymphoid tissue (GALT), are conspicuous aggregates of lymphoid tissue located throughout the lamina propria and submucosa of the digestive tract. They play a critical role in immune function by acting as the first line of defense against pathogens invading the gut. This occurs through specialized epithelium that contains microfold cells (M

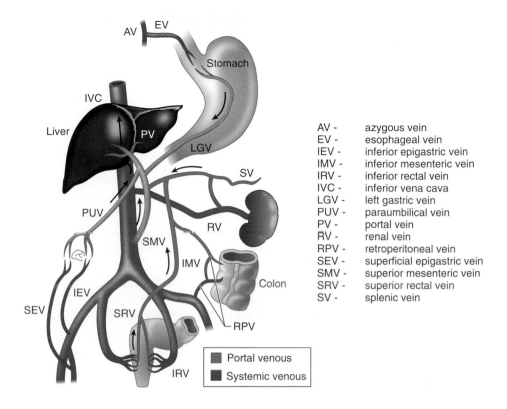

FIGURE 3-13. **Portosystemic anastomoses in portal hypertension.**

AV -   azygous vein
EV -   esophageal vein
IEV -   inferior epigastric vein
IMV -   inferior mesenteric vein
IRV -   inferior rectal vein
IVC -   inferior vena cava
LGV -   left gastric vein
PUV -   paraumbilical vein
PV -   portal vein
RV -   renal vein
RPV -   retroperitoneal vein
SEV -   superficial epigastric vein
SMV -   superior mesenteric vein
SRV -   superior rectal vein
SV -   splenic vein

 Portal venous
Systemic venous

cells), which directly sample antigen in the intestinal lumen and present it to antigen-presenting cells. Large concentrations are typically found in the ileum and, in certain pathologic states such as inflammatory bowel disease (IBD), can proliferate to the point at which they are visible to the naked eye (this may be associated with idiopathic intussusception).

- Peyer patches produce **secretory IgA** in germinal centers of B cells located in the lamina propria.
- Mucosa-associated lymphoid tissue lymphomas (MALTomas) can also arise from within Peyer patches.

KEY FACT

Lymphadenopathy is often the first sign of GI infection or neoplasia.

TABLE 3-6. **Key Portosystemic Venous Anastomoses in Portal Hypertension**

REGION	ANASTOMOSIS (PORTOSYSTEMIC)	CLINICAL SIGNIFICANCE
Esophagus	Left gastric vein–esophageal venous plexus (to azygos vein)	Esophageal varices
Umbilicus	Paraumbilical vein–superficial and inferior epigastric veins	Caput medusa (engorged veins that look like snakes around the umbilicus)
Rectum	Superior rectal vein–middle and inferior rectal veins	Enlarged internal hemorrhoids and anorectal varices
Retroperitoneal	Visceral veins of Retzius–retroperitoneal parietal veins	Ascites

NERVE SUPPLY OF THE GI TRACT

The GI tract has a rather complex nerve supply, divided into two major groups: extrinsic (parasympathetic and sympathetic innervation), and intrinsic (enteric) innervation.

Extrinsic Innervation

Extrinsic motor and sensory innervation is supplied by both sympathetic and parasympathetic nerves (Figure 3-14).

SYMPATHETIC INNERVATION

Preganglionic fibers arise at spinal cord levels **T5–L1** and synapse with the prevertebral abdominal ganglia (celiac, superior, and inferior mesenteric). The postganglionic fibers form **splanchnic nerves** to innervate the gut and communicate with the enteric nervous system.

The primary **postganglionic** neurotransmitter is **norepinephrine,** which acts as an **inhibitory neurotransmitter** in the GI tract, **decreasing motility** as well as secretory and digestive functions.

PARASYMPATHETIC INNERVATION

Supplied by the vagus and pelvic nerves:

- The **vagus** nerve (CN X) provides both **parasympathetic afferent** and **efferent** stimuli for the esophagus through the splenic flexure of the colon.

MNEMONIC

The parasympathetic system allows one to **rest** and **digest** (via the **vagus** nerve).

PARASYMPATHETIC

Neurons of the autonomic parasympathetic division project from the medulla oblongata and sacral regions of the spinal cord

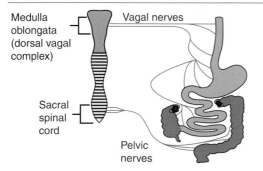

SYMPATHETIC

Neurons of the autonomic sympathetic division project to the gut from thoracic and first lumbar segments of the spinal cord

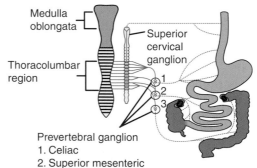

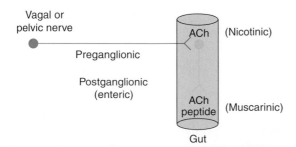

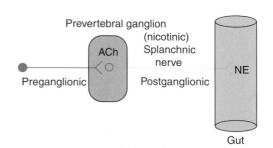

FIGURE 3-14. **Extrinsic nervous system of the GI tract.** ACh, acetylcholine; NE, norepinephrine. (Modified with permission from McPhee SJ, Ganong WF. *Pathophysiology of Disease: An Introduction to Clinical Medicine,* 5th ed. New York: McGraw-Hill, 2006: 346.)

- **Pelvic nerves** arising at S2 and S3 innervate the hindgut (splenic flexure through proximal rectum).
- Preganglionic fibers of the parasympathetic (vagus and sacral) nerves **synapse directly** in the enteric nervous system on nicotinic receptors, whereas postganglionic neurons are shorter and use muscarinic receptors.
- The parasympathetic system **increases** the activity level of the enteric nervous system.

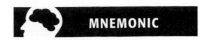

MNEMONIC

Parasympathetic **P**roduces secretions and **P**ropels food, but **S**ympathetic **S**uppresses GI function.

There are several key similarities and differences between the parasympathetic (PNS) and sympathetic (SNS) innervation of the GI tract:

- Both divisions use acetylcholine (ACh) and nicotinic receptors at the ganglion, whereas the enteric innervation by the PNS is muscarinic ACh and by the SNS is norepinephrine.
- Preganglionic neurons are shorter in the SNS and longer in the PNS, whereas postganglionic neurons are longer in the SNS and very short in the PNS.
- The PNS is PARA and originates cephalic and sacral, whereas the SNS is between in the thoracolumbar region.

Intrinsic Innervation

Also known as the **enteric nervous system,** or the "third division" of the autonomic nervous system. It is composed of a series of ganglionic nerve plexuses, contained entirely within the gut wall and running from esophagus to anus. Enteric neurons use many neurotransmitters, most notably **neuropeptides.**

The two principal components of the enteric nervous system are the **myenteric (Auerbach)** plexus and the **submucosal (Meissner)** nerve plexus (Figure 3-15):

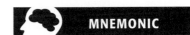

MNEMONIC

- **A**uerbach is **A**uter or **M**yenteric is between the **M**uscle.
- **M**yenteric is for **M**otility
- **S**ubmucosal makes **S**ecretions

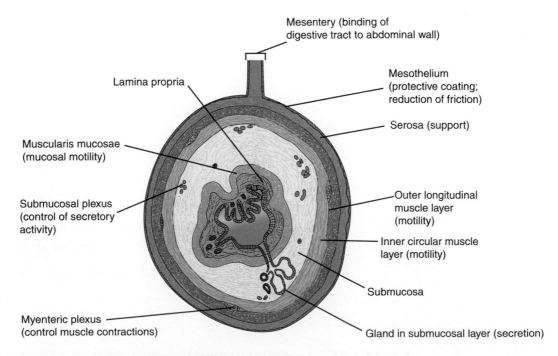

FIGURE 3-15. **Cross-section of digestive tract wall.**

CLINICAL CORRELATION

Overdistention, ischemia, and chemical and mechanical irritation are examples of noxious stimuli resulting in abnormal visceral sensation, which tends to produce dull, achy, colicky discomfort.

KEY FACT

- Visceral peritoneum has no somatic nerve supply, and pain is poorly localized.
- Parietal peritoneum shares somatic innervation with the abdominal wall. Thus, the pain is localized.

CLINICAL CORRELATION

- Appendicitis begins as dull, aching, cramping (visceral) periumbilical pain (approximately in the T10 dermatome).
- Once the appendiceal inflammation becomes transmural, the parietal peritoneum becomes inflamed, resulting in sharp pain localized in the area directly over the appendix **(McBurney point).**

- The **myenteric (Auerbach) nerve plexus** is located between the **outer longitudinal** and **inner circular muscle layers.** Its main function is to coordinate **motility** along the full length of the gut wall.
- The **submucosal (Meissner) nerve plexus** is located in the **submucosa** between the innermost mucosal layer and the inner circular layer of smooth muscle. Its main function is to **regulate secretions, blood flow, and absorption.**

Visceral Sensation

- **Normal visceral sensation,** for the most part, is not consciously perceived, except for sensations such as hunger and rectal distention.
- **Abnormal visceral sensation,** however, is perceived as diffuse **pain.**

VISCERAL VERSUS PARIETAL PAIN

- Due to the differential innervation of the viscera and the parietal peritoneum, visceral pain results in **cramping** pain, whereas parietal pain causes **sharp** pain.
- The pain fibers that originate in the **viscera** are transmitted via autonomic nerves, mainly sympathetic, **type C fibers,** which only transmit **colicky, cramping, poorly localized** types of pain.
- In contrast to the viscera and visceral peritoneum, the parietal peritoneum is innervated by extensions of the **peripheral spinal nerves,** which carry the same types of noxious pain sensations as those overlying the dermatomes. Therefore, parietal pain results in **sharp, localized** pain.
- If the pathologic process progresses from the visceral to the parietal region, the referred pain will become localized, corresponding to the dermatome overlying the affected organ.

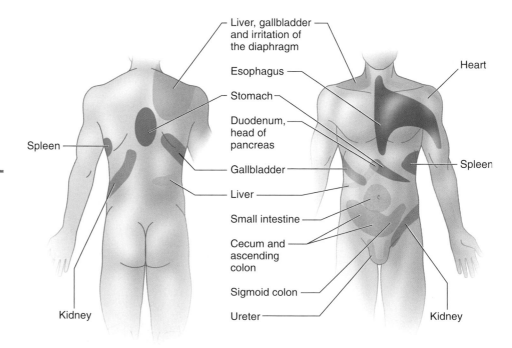

FIGURE 3-16.   **Location of pain referred from major abdominal and thoracic organs.**

REFERRED PAIN

Many organs have an embryonic origination in one location of the body and then **migrate** to another area, pulling their vascular and nervous supply with them. Thus, **visceral pain** is often **referred** to the site of embryologic origin rather than the actual location of the organ.

Example: The embryologic origin of the diaphragm and its nerves is in the neck. When the diaphragm or the surrounding abdominal structures are inflamed and cause diaphragmatic irritation (ie, cholecystitis, ruptured spleen), the patient often feel pains in the shoulder because the corresponding dermatome shares a C3–C4 nerve root with the phrenic nerve. This phenomenon is known as **referred pain**.

The same concept holds true for other abdominal and thoracic organs (Figure 3-16).

Physiology

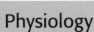
HYPOTHALAMUS

The hypothalamus controls the body's sense of hunger and fullness.

- **Lateral hypothalamic area (LHA):** Sensation of hunger (ie, stimulates feeding).
- **Ventromedial nucleus of the hypothalamus (VNH):** Sensation of fullness (ie, tells the person to stop feeding).

MOUTH

The mouth is the first site of digestion. It is the site of mechanical breakdown of the food by mastication (chewing).

- The **chewing reflex** causes the up-and-down movement of the lower jaw. This functions to mix the food bolus with lubricating saliva and salivary enzymes, as well as produce smaller particles for swallowing.
- Most of the muscles of mastication are innervated by the trigeminal nerve (CN V).

Salivary Secretions

The salivary glands produce approximately 1 L of saliva each day. Saliva helps buffer, dilute, moisten, and digest food, while also protecting the oral cavity from bacteria. Secretion is stimulated by the smell, sight, taste, or even thought of food, as well as vagal afferents.

The two major types of salivary protein secretions are **serous** (eg, α-amylase) and **mucous** (mucin).

- **Major salivary glands** include the parotid (serous), submandibular (or submaxillary; mixed serous and mucous), and sublingual glands (mixed).
- **Minor salivary glands** include a group of tiny glands located in the buccal mucosal area.

KEY FACT

Visceral sensations from the gut are vaguely localized to the median plane, regardless of the location of the viscus.

KEY FACT

Lesions of the:
LHA can cause anorexia.
- The "fat" lateral nuclei make you hungry.
VNH can cause obesity.
- The "skinny" medial nuclei make you feel full.

KEY FACT

Leptin is a protein hormone released from adipocytes. It acts on many parts of the hypothalamus, especially the arcuate and paraventricular nuclei. Leptin decreases appetite and increases metabolism.

KEY FACT

Peptide YY is produced by the small intestine and colon and reduces appetite in response to eating.

Salivary glands contain acinar cells that feed into salivary ducts. These structures are both surrounded by **myoepithelial cells,** which contract to express saliva.

KEY FACT

The salivary glands are unique because they are stimulated by both the sympathetic and parasympathetic branches of the autonomic nervous system.

- **Parasympathetic stimulation:** An **increase** in the secretion of watery saliva is mediated by **CN VII** (facial nerve) and **CN IX** (glossopharyngeal nerve) from the superior and inferior salivatory nuclei in the brain stem via **muscarinic receptors.**
- **Sympathetic stimulation** is mediated via β-adrenergic receptors and causes an **increase** in secretion of viscous saliva (via T1–T3 nerves of the superior cervical ganglion).

Composition of Saliva

- **Enzymes:**
  - α-**Amylase (ptyalin):** Begins digestion of carbohydrates, particularly starches, by hydrolyzing α-1,4 bonds. It is **inactivated** by the **low pH** of the **stomach.**
  - **Lingual lipase:** Begins digestion of lipids; breaks down triglycerides into fatty acids and monoglycerides. It is capable of continued digestion within the stomach. **In contrast to pancreatic lipase,** it can cleave fatty acids from all three positions on a triglyceride.
- **Ions:**
  - High in HCO_3^- and K^+.
  - Low in Na^+ and Cl^-.
- **Tonicity:**
  - In **low** flow rate states (< 1 mL/min), saliva is **hypotonic** relative to plasma, with low Na^+ and Cl^- and high K^+.
  - In **high** flow rate states (~ 4 mL/min), saliva is **closer to isotonic** (relative to plasma), with high Na^+ and Cl^- and low K^+.
  - Slower flow rates allow more time for ductal cells to transport ions and adjust the tonicity of the secretions (Figure 3-17). The exception to this rule is HCO_3^-, which is selectively stimulated and is secreted in proportion to flow rate.

KEY FACT

Aldosterone causes an increase in the secretion of K^+ and reabsorption of Na^+ and Cl^-, similar to its actions in the renal distal tubule.

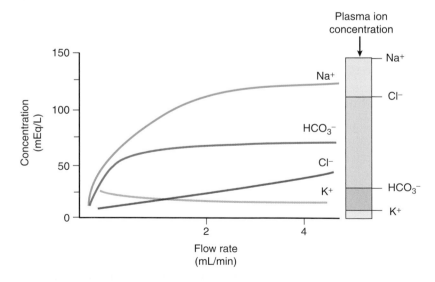

FIGURE 3-17. Salivary flow rates and secretory tonicity. Low flow rates provide more time for resorption of sodium and chloride whereas potassium is secreted slightly more, resulting in a hypotonic solution. High flow rates are nearly isotonic due to less time provided for ion exchange. Bicarbonate is selectively stimulated and therefore increases secretion in proportion to flow rate (eg, parasympathetic stimulation increases both bicarbonate secretion and flow rate).

- The **pH** is between 6 and 8.
- **Antibacterial actions:** The flow of saliva and the presence of enzymes and antibodies help to fight dental caries:
  - Lysozyme attacks bacteria and digests food particles.
  - Lactoferrin.
  - Thiocyanate ions enter bacteria and become bactericidal.
  - Antibodies (IgA).
  - Defensins.

Swallowing (Deglutition)

Deglutition is a process regulated by the **swallowing reflex,** which is **coordinated in the medulla (swallowing center).** Simply stated, swallowing is propulsion of the food bolus through the pharynx while respiration is temporarily blocked. The **three stages** of swallowing are voluntary, pharyngeal, and esophageal.

- **Voluntary (oral) stage:** The bolus is pushed to the posterior of the pharynx, which has a high concentration of somatosensory receptors, by the tongue. This triggers the involuntary stages of swallowing.
- **Pharyngeal phase:** Initiated through the epithelial swallowing receptor reflex, this phase is carried out through the following steps:
  - **Upward movement of the soft palate** to prevent reflux of food into the nasal cavities.
  - **Constriction of the palatopharyngeal folds,** which creates a small passageway that permits only properly masticated food to pass into the posterior pharynx.
  - **Tightening of the vocal cords** and upward movement of larynx causes **closure of the epiglottis,** which swings backward over the opening of the larynx to prevent food from entering the trachea.
  - The **upper esophageal sphincter (UES)** relaxes in < 1 second.
  - Peristaltic waves move the bolus from the pharynx to the esophagus.
  - During this stage, **breathing is inhibited.**
- **Esophageal phase:** Controlled by both the swallowing reflex and the enteric nervous system. It involves movement of food toward the stomach, causing **relaxation of the lower esophageal sphincter (LES)** as a result of **vagal stimulation** (peptidergic neurons releasing vasoactive intestinal peptide [VIP]).
- As food passes the UES, it contracts to prevent reflux into the pharynx.
- **Primary peristalsis** is a continuous peristaltic wave controlled by the swallowing center in the medulla. Food movement is accelerated by gravity.
- **Secondary peristalsis** is a reflexive reaction mediated by the enteric nervous system. Distention of the esophagus triggers a peristaltic contraction that clears the esophagus of remaining food.

As food passes down the esophagus, it triggers the proximal region of the stomach to relax, a phenomenon known as **receptive relaxation.**

ESOPHAGUS

The esophagus is a muscular tube lined with **nonkeratinized stratified squamous epithelium.** It connects the pharynx through the UES to the stomach via the LES.

- **Upper esophagus:** Mostly skeletal muscle; primarily controlled by the nucleus ambiguus.
- **Lower esophagus:** Predominantly smooth muscle; controlled by the dorsal nucleus of the vagus nerve.

FLASH FORWARD

Chronic gastroesophageal reflux disease (GERD) can lead to Barrett esophagus, which is metaplasia of stratified squamous epithelium of the lower esophagus into columnar epithelium similar to that of intestinal mucosa.

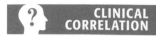

GERD has many causes, including:
- **Poor tone** of the **LES.**
- **Increased intra-abdominal pressure** (eg, morbid obesity), which overwhelms the LES.
- **Hiatal hernias.**
- Ingestion of certain foods (eg, citrus, caffeine, fatty, or spicy).

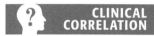

Damage to the myenteric plexus in the lower two-thirds of the esophagus causes achalasia (failure of the LES to relax).

The esophagus quickly propels food toward the stomach via **peristaltic contractions** controlled by:

- The **extrinsic nervous system:** The sympathetics and parasympathetics of the CNS.
- The **intrinsic nervous system** (enteric nervous system): Myenteric (**Auerbach**) plexus, which promotes motility of smooth muscle, and the submucosal (**Meissner**) plexus, which controls secretion and blood flow.
- The enteric nervous system uses **ACh, dopamine,** and **serotonin** as neurotransmitters.

Because the esophagus is located in the thoracic cavity, its pressure is equal to intrathoracic pressure, which is negative relative to the abdominal cavity and atmosphere. The **UES** prevents air from entering the esophagus, whereas the **LES** prevents reflux of gastric contents.

Vomiting

Vomiting (emesis) is controlled by the vomiting center of the medulla, which can be stimulated by afferents from:

- Gastric overdistention.
- Oropharyngeal stimuli.
- Chemoreceptor trigger of the area postrema of the medulla.
- Vestibular stimulus.

The vomiting reflex includes several sequential actions: reverse peristalsis (from the small intestine), relaxation of the stomach and pylorus, forced inspiration (increases abdominal pressure), relaxation of the LES, and forceful expulsion.

Retching is the initial phase of vomiting, but occurs against a closed UES. In this case, the bolus returns to the stomach through a patent LES.

STOMACH

Anatomy and Histology

The stomach functions as both a reservoir and site of digestion for the food bolus. It has three layers of smooth muscle: longitudinal, circular, and oblique. It is also organized into several different functional regions (Figure 3-18).

- Cardia: Distal to the LES; does not secrete acid.
- Fundus: Dilated region superior to a horizontal line drawn through the cardial orifice.
- Body: Between the fundus and antrum, food reservoir and major site of gastric digestion. Contains multiple cells types:
  - **Parietal cells:** Secrete hydrogen ion (H^+) and intrinsic factor (IF).
  - **Chief cells:** Secrete pepsinogen, a key enzyme in protein digestion.
- Antrum: Distal region that is highly muscular, grinds food, and regulates gastric emptying. Contains multiple cell types:
  - **Mucus-secreting cells:** Release both mucus and bicarbonate.
  - **G cells:** Secrete gastrin, which stimulates gastric acid, motility, and growth of gastric mucosa.

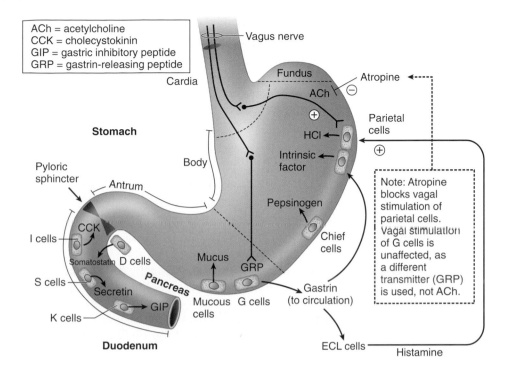

ACh = acetylcholine
CCK = cholecystokinin
GIP = gastric inhibitory peptide
GRP = gastrin-releasing peptide

Note: Atropine blocks vagal stimulation of parietal cells. Vagal stimulation of G cells is unaffected, as a different transmitter (GRP) is used, not ACh.

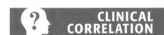

FIGURE 3-18. **Stomach anatomy, histology, and physiology.**

Mechanical Contractions

The stomach's main motor functions include storage, mixing, emptying, and hunger contractions.

Interstitial cells of Cajal (ICC) function as the pacemakers of the GI tract and generate spontaneous electrical slow waves. They also transduce signals from the enteric motor neurons through local smooth muscle to stimulate contractions. The stomach's baseline rate is 3–5 contractions per minute, also known as the **basal electrical rhythm.**

- **Parasympathetic** stimulation of the vagus nerve **increases** stomach contractions, whereas **sympathetic** stimulation via the celiac plexus **decreases** stomach contractions.
- **Migrating motility complex (MMC):** Contractions of the stomach and small intestine during fasting conditions. These contractions occur in a cyclic motor pattern and prevent bacterial overgrowth (housekeeping).
- They repeat every 90–120 minutes and are mediated by **motilin.**
- The fundus and body of the stomach undergo receptive relaxation via a vagovagal reflex caused by esophageal distension. This is augmented by cholecystokinin (CCK), which increases the stomach's distensibility.
- Food is **stored** for about 45 minutes and undergoes mixing before it is squeezed out via the pyloric sphincter. Phasic waves of contraction can narrow the pyloric sphincter and force the bolus back into the stomach for more efficient mixing; this is also known as **retropulsion.**
- **Emptying** of the stomach is enabled by an intense contraction, which pushes the food through the pyloric sphincter.

CLINICAL CORRELATION

Interstitial cells of Cajal are implicated in both gastrointestinal stromal tumors (GIST) and GI motility disorders.

FLASH BACK

Pyloric stenosis is a condition in which there is hypertrophy of the muscle of the pyloric sphincter preventing the passage of chyme, resulting in projectile vomiting. The classic physical finding is an olive-shaped mass on abdominal exam.

The **rate of stomach emptying** is controlled by the content of food.

- Hypotonic or hypertonic food delays gastric emptying.
- The presence of lipids and partially digested proteins in the food stimulates the release of CCK, which decreases gastric motility, thus delaying gastric emptying.
- Increase of H^+ in the duodenum inhibits gastric emptying via direct neural reflexes.

General Regulation of Gastric Secretions

Gastric secretion occurs in three interrelated stages: **cephalic, gastric,** and **intestinal phases.**

- **Cephalic phase:** Parasympathetic stimulation from the appetite centers of the hypothalamus and/or amygdala to the stomach produces salivary and gastric secretions due to the sight, smell, or thought of food.
- **Gastric phase:** Initiated by distention of the stomach, the gastric phase uses long vagovagal and enteric reflexes to stimulate the **release of gastrin** and increase acid production.
- **Intestinal phase:** Further release of gastrin from the duodenum as a result of the presence of protein in the upper portion of the small intestine.

The **presence of chyme** in the intestines stimulates gastric secretion in the intestinal phase. However, it also **paradoxically inhibits gastric secretion** via the **reverse enterogastric reflex,** as well as through the release of several hormones, including secretin, gastric inhibitory peptide, VIP, and somatostatin.

The inhibition of gastric secretions helps regulate the amount of chyme entering the duodenum.

The secretory products of the stomach are depicted in Table 3-7.

Mechanism of Hydrochloric Acid Secretion

Mechanism of gastric HCl secretion in parietal cells (Figure 3-19):

- $CO_2 + H_2O \rightarrow H^+ + HCO_3^-$ via the action of **carbonic anhydrase.**
- H^+–K^+ ATPase pump secretes H^+ into the stomach lumen, in exchange for K^+.
- HCO_3^- and Cl^- are exchanged at the basal aspect of the parietal cell, adding bicarbonate to the bloodstream, while Cl^- follows H^+ into the stomach lumen. This bicarbonate is eventually secreted by the pancreas into the small intestine.

This influx of HCO_3^- into the venous system is called the "alkaline tide," reflecting an acute increase in pH; this can also raise the urine pH after a large meal.

Regulation of Hydrochloric Acid Secretion

The vagal system stimulates gastric acid secretion through both direct and indirect mechanisms. The **direct mechanism** uses vagal innervation of parietal cells to stimulate **muscarinic ACh receptors;** these subsequently activate the inositol 1,4,5-triphosphate (IP_3) second-messenger system and intracellular Ca^{2+} to promote H^+ secretion.

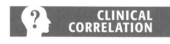
CLINICAL CORRELATION

In patients with excessive vomiting, the gastric acid does not enter the duodenum and there is no stimulation for secretion of pancreatic HCO_3^-, leaving the bloodstream at an elevated pH (metabolic alkalosis).

TABLE 3-7. **Gastric Secretions**

Product	Source	Location	Action	Regulation Stimulus	Regulation Inhibition
Gastric acid (HCl)	Parietal (oxyntic) cells	Body, fundus	Aids in digestion. Activates pepsin from pepsinogen. Kills pathogens.	Gastrin, ACh (vagus), histamine.	Low pH, prostaglandins, GIP secretion (negative feedback), somatostatin.
Intinsic factor (IF)	Parietal (oxyntic) cells	Body, fundus	Binds to vitamin B_{12}, leading to its uptake in the ileum.	Gastrin, ACh (vagus), histamine.	Low pH, prostaglandins, GIP secretion (negative feedback), somatostatin.
Pepsinogen	Chief cells	Body, fundus	Precursor for pepsin. Digests protein at a pH between 1.0 and 3.0.	ACh (vagus), increased local H^+.	Somatostatin.
Mucus	Mucous cells	Entire stomach (particularly antrum)	Protects mucosa from the acidic environment and pepsin.	ACh (vagus).	
HCO_3^-	Mucous cells	Entire stomach (particularly antrum)	Neutralizes acid.	ACh (vagus).	
Gastrin	G cells	Antrum (and duodenum)	↑ Secretion of: H^+, pepsinogen, histamine. Trophic on gastric mucosa. ↑ Gastric motility.	Small peptides, amino acids, Ca^{2+} in gastric lumen, GRP (vagus), gastric distention.	↑ H^+ in the gastric antrum.

ACh = acetylcholine; GIP = gastric inhibitory peptide; GRP = gastrin-releasing peptide.

The **indirect mechanism** functions by vagal nerve release of **gastrin-releasing peptide (GRP) at G cells** in the gastric antrum. GRP is released in response to the cephalic phase or gastric distention and stimulates the secretion of **gastrin** from G cells in both the gastric antrum and duodenum. Gastrin is secreted in response to small peptides, amino acids, or Ca^{2+} in the stomach lumen, gastric distention, and vagal stimulation. Gastrin stimulates parietal cells (H^+), chief cells (pepsinogen), enterochromaffin-like (ECL) cells (histamine), growth of gastric mucosa (trophic action), and gastric motility.

Primarily stimulated by gastrin, **histamine** is released from ECL cells in the gastric mucosa and stimulates the parietal cells through H_2 **receptors.** It is also released by vagal ACh.

Because these regulatory systems use different receptors and second messengers, they undergo **potentiation** (the response to two stimulants is greater than the sum of the two responses individually).

FLASH FORWARD

The proton pump inhibitors (PPIs, eg, omeprazole) function to inhibit gastric acid secretion at the H^+–K^+ ATPase.

H_2-receptor antagonists, such as cimetidine, decrease the secretion of histamine.

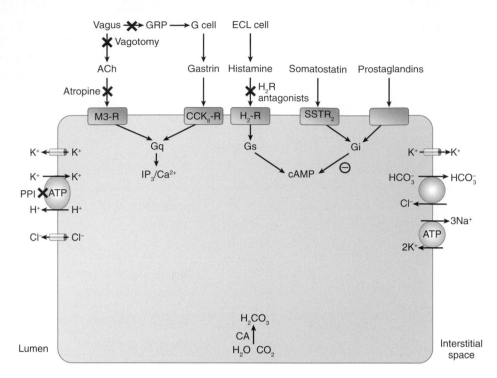

FIGURE 3-19. **Acid secretion by parietal cells.** The regulatory mechanisms of HCl secretion by parietal cells, stimulated by histamine, acetylcholine, and gastrin or inhibited by somatostatin and prostaglandins, are demonstrated. M3-R, muscarinic 3-receptor; H_2-R, histamine 2-receptor; CCK_B-R, cholecystokinin B receptor; SSTR2, somatostatin receptor type 2; GRP, gastrin-releasing peptide; ACh, acetylcholine; Gq, Gs, Gi, G proteins (stimulatory, inhibitory); IP_3, inositol triphosphate; cAMP, cyclic adenosine monophosphate; PPI, proton pump inhibitor; CA, carbonic anhydrase. (Modified with permission from McPhee SJ, Ganong WF. *Pathophysiology of Disease: An Introduction to Clinical Medicine*, 5th ed. New York: McGraw-Hill, 2006: 353.)

> **KEY FACT**
>
> Atropine can block the direct pathway (by blocking muscarinic ACh receptors).
> Vagotomy decreases acid production by blocking both the direct and indirect pathways (Figures 3-18 and 3-19).

As the food bolus passes into the duodenum, several mechanisms begin to decrease the release of gastric H^+, including:

- **pH:** The lack of food in the stomach to buffer the H^+ secretion causes a decrease in pH. Below a pH of 3.0, gastrin release is inhibited.
- Fatty acids, amino acids, and glucose in the duodenum cause the release of **gastric inhibitory peptide (GIP)** from K cells in the proximal small intestines, which inhibits acid production (and increases insulin release).

Excess H^+ in the duodenum triggers **secretin** release from S cells, which increases the release of pancreatic and biliary HCO_3^- into the duodenum.

Absorption

The stomach is capable of absorbing alcohol and lipid-soluble drugs, such as aspirin.

SMALL INTESTINE

Anatomy and Histologic Characteristics

Approximately 6 m long, the small intestine is the primary site of digestion and absorption. It is divided into three regions: the duodenum, jejunum, and ileum.

The **duodenum** is mostly retroperitoneal (second, third, and fourth portions), begins at the gastroduodenal junction at the pyloric sphincter, and is divided into four parts:

- **Superior (first portion):** The only truly peritoneal segment of the duodenum; it is attached superiorly to the hepatoduodenal ligament and inferiorly to the greater omentum.
- **Descending (second portion):** Fixed retroperitoneal location; receives both the common bile duct and the main pancreatic duct through the hepatopancreatic (Vater) ampulla.
- **Horizontal (third portion):** Fixed retroperitoneal location at the level of L3; it runs between the divergence of the SMA and the aorta.
- **Ascending (fourth portion):** Retroperitoneal; meets the jejunum at the duodenojejunal flexure, located by the suspensory muscle of the duodenum (ligament of Treitz).

Following the duodenum, the small intestine is mobile and suspended in the peritoneal cavity by mesentery.

The **jejunum** accounts for the proximal three-fifths of the remaining small intestine. The **ileum** represents the remaining distal two-fifths, ending at the **ileocecal valve,** which marks the start of the large intestine.

The plicae circulares, intestinal villi, and crypts of Lieberkühn form the major histologic features of the small intestine and are composed of multiple cell types (Figure 3-20):

- **Plicae circulares:** Circular folds of submucosa that run one-half to two-thirds of the way around the lumen. They begin in the duodenum, are most frequent in the proximal jejunum, and reduce in size and frequency toward the terminal ileum.
- **Intestinal villi:** Intraluminal projections of the lamina propria ~1 mm in height, each containing a single terminal branch of the arterial, venous, and lymphatic trees (lacteals).
- **Crypts of Lieberkühn:** Spaces between intestinal villi responsible for cell proliferation (putative multipotential stem cells in the crypts are thought to serve as progenitor cells of the four major cell types contained within the villi: enterocytes, goblet cells, enteroendocrine cells, and Paneth cells).
- **Enterocytes:** Surface epithelial cells responsible for absorption as well as secretion of some digestive enzymes (Table 3-8). Under electron microscopy, numerous microvilli are noted on each enterocyte, further increasing the absorptive surface of the intestine up to 600 times. They make up the **brush border** facing the intestinal lumen and are involved in H_2O and electrolyte balance in the small intestine.
- **Goblet cells** secrete mucus into the GI lumen; they increase in frequency from the duodenum to the terminal ilium.

KEY FACT

The superior (first) portion of the duodenum is the most common site of duodenal ulcers based on its proximity to gastric acid.

KEY FACT

The horizontal (third) portion of the duodenum is the most common site of traumatic duodenal injuries (crushed against the L3 vertebra).

KEY FACT

The plicae circulares, intestinal villi, and microvilli all function to slow the progression of the food bolus through the small intestine and significantly increase the surface area for absorption.

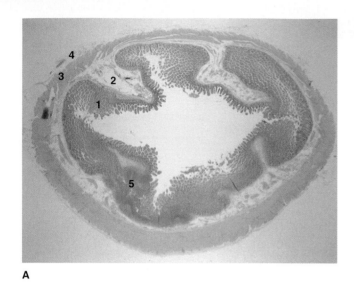

A

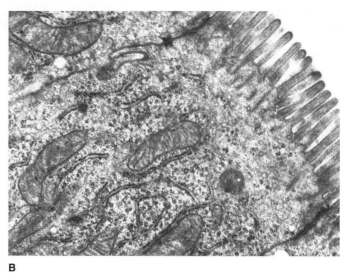

B

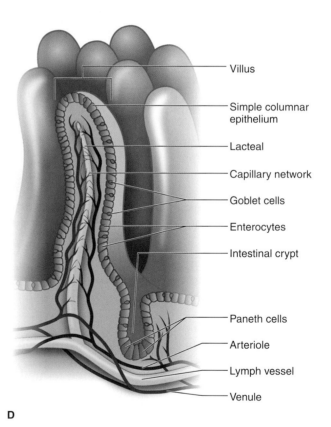

Villus

Simple columnar epithelium

Lacteal

Capillary network

Goblet cells

Enterocytes

Intestinal crypt

Paneth cells

Arteriole

Lymph vessel

Venule

C   D

FIGURE 3-20. **Small intestine anatomy and histology.** (A) Cross-section of small intestine demonstrating plicae circulares. 1, Mucosa with villi; 2, Submucosa; 3, Muscularis, circular and longitudinal; 4, Adventitia; 5, Lymphatic nodules. (B) Electron micrograph of the intestinal brush border. Note the numerous microvilli enhancing the surface area. (C) Peyer patches seen in a section of rabbit ileum. This is a major site of M cells. (D) Diagram of an intestinal villus with cell locations. Enteroendocrine cells are not shown, but migrate upward and can be found at all levels of each villus. (A, B, & C reproduced with permission from USMLERx.com. D modified with permission from Fox SI. *Human Physiology*, 10th ed. New York: McGraw-Hill, 2008.)

TABLE 3-8. **Small Intestinal Secretions**

PRODUCT	SOURCE	ACTION	REGULATION STIMULUS
Cl^-	Crypts of Lieberkühn	Makes a watery fluid for easier absorption.	CCK, secretin, enteric nervous reflexes
HCO_3^-	Crypts of Lieberkühn	Makes a watery fluid for easier absorption. Helps neutralize gastric acids.	CCK, secretin, enteric nervous reflexes
Peptidases	Brush border enterocytes	Hydrolysis of dipeptides and tripeptides into amino acids.	Enteric nervous reflexes
Sucrase	Brush border enterocytes	Hydrolysis of sucrose into fructose and glucose.	Enteric nervous reflexes
Maltase	Brush border enterocytes	Hydrolysis of maltose into two glucoses.	Enteric nervous reflexes
Isomaltase	Brush border enterocytes	Hydrolysis of saccharides not digested earlier.	Enteric nervous reflexes
Lactase	Brush border enterocytes	Hydrolysis of lactose into galactose and glucose.	Enteric nervous reflexes
α-Dextrinase	Brush border enterocytes	Hydrolysis of terminal α-1,4 bonds, to make glucose.	Enteric nervous reflexes
Intestinal lipase	Brush border enterocytes	Breakdown of neutral fats into fatty acids and glycerol.	Enteric nervous reflexes
Heavy alkaline mucus	Brunner glands	Protects duodenum from the large amount of gastric acid.	Secretin, tactile/irritating stimuli, ACh (vagus)
Mucus	Goblet cells	Lubricates and protects intestines.	Enteric nervous reflexes

ACh = acetylcholine; CCK = cholecystokinin.

- **Enteroendocrine cells** secrete endocrine (eg, CCK, secretin, GIP, motilin) and paracrine (eg, somatostatin, histamine) hormones into the bloodstream.
- **Paneth cells** secrete growth factors and antimicrobial substances (eg, lysozyme, α-defensin) into the lumen as a component of innate immunity.
- **M cells (microfold):** Modified epithelial cells that cover lymphatic nodules (ie, Peyer patches) in the lamina propria. They contain microfolds that take up microorganisms and macromolecules in endocytotic vesicles for presentation to CD4+ T lymphocytes.

The average life span of intestinal cells is 3–6 days.

Because digestive enzymes can only interact on the surface of chyme, the surface area of ingested food must be increased. The length and tubular structure of the intestines, as well as the endothelial brush border, plicae circulares, and intestinal villi increase the surface area, aiding absorption.

- The small intestine does not store food.
- Contraction waves: Initiated by ACh and substance P.
- Relaxation: Initiated by VIP and nitric oxide.

The **basal electric rhythm of the small intestine is faster** than that of the stomach: 12 waves per minute in the duodenum and 8–9 waves per minute in the ileum.

- Chyme is **mixed** via **segmental** contractions and **propelled forward** with **peristaltic** contractions (which increase with parasympathetic stimulation from the vagus nerve and decrease with sympathetic stimulation from the mesenteric ganglion).
- Fasting MMC occurs every 90 minutes.

Absorption

The primary location for absorption of nutrients is the small intestine (Table 3-9).

- **Nonfat, water-soluble** nutrients are absorbed through the small intestine into the portal vein, where they are transported to the liver for storage and processing.
- **Fat-based nutrients** enter into the mesenteric lymphatic system of the intestines via the terminal lacteals and use the thoracic duct to enter the bloodstream, bypassing the liver.

TABLE 3-9. Nutrient Digestion and Absorption

Nutrient	Absorbed Products	Mechanism	Clinical Correlation
Carbohydrates	Monosaccharides: Glucose Galactose	SGLT1 (Na^+-dependent cotransport)	4 kcal/g; transported to liver through portal vein; associated with lactose intolerance; monosaccharides exit the cell through a GLUT 2 transporter (facilitated diffusion) (Figure 3-21).
	Fructose	GLUT 5 (facilitated diffusion)	
Lipids	FFA Monoglycerides Cholesterol Lysolecithin	Diffusion (through micelles formed from bile salts)	9 kcal/g; transported to lacteals and through lymphatics to systemic circulation (bypass liver); facilitate absorption of fat-soluble vitamins (A, D, E, K); abetalipoproteinemia from lack of ApoB prevents absorption (Figure 3-22).
Protein	Di/Tripeptides	H^+-dependent di/tripeptide cotransport	4 kcal/g; transported to liver through portal vein; deficient absorption associated with pancreatic disease (eg, chronic pancreatitis, cystic fibrosis); Hartnup disease is caused by a lack of the neutral AA cotransporter.
	AA	Na^+-dependent AA cotransport	
Vitamins	Fat-soluble	In micelles with lipids	A, D, E, K are affected by anything that inhibits lipid absorption; B_{12} is absorbed by an independent mechanism involving intrinsic factor.
	Water-soluble	Na^+-dependent cotransport	
Calcium	Ca^{2+}	Calbindin-D28K (vitamin D-dependent Ca^{2+}-binding protein)	Needs active vitamin D (1,25-dihydroxycholecalciferol) from liver and kidney metabolism; deficiency of active vitamin D associated with rickets (children), osteomalacia (adults).

AA = amino acids; Apo B = apolipoprotein B; FFA = free fatty acids; GLUT = glucose transporter; SGLT = sodium-glucose transport protein.

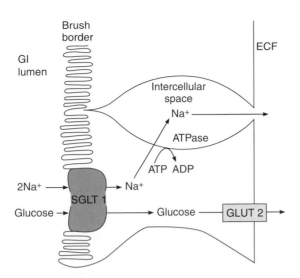

FIGURE 3-21.   Mechanism for glucose transport across intestinal epithelium. (Modified with permission from Ganong WF. *Review of Medical Physiology*, 22nd ed. New York: McGraw-Hill, 2005: 472.)

- **Water** and **ions** (ie, Na^+, Cl^-, K^+) are absorbed passively with solutes. Sodium can facilitate the absorption of other nutrients through a cotransporter, whereas a basolateral Na^+–K^+ ATPase maintains the sodium gradient.

Certain key nutrients (Fe, folate, vitamin B_{12}) have individual mechanisms and locations of absorption (Table 3-10).

FLASH BACK

Vibrio cholerae produces the cholera toxin, which causes increased secretion of chloride, leading to osmotic diarrhea.

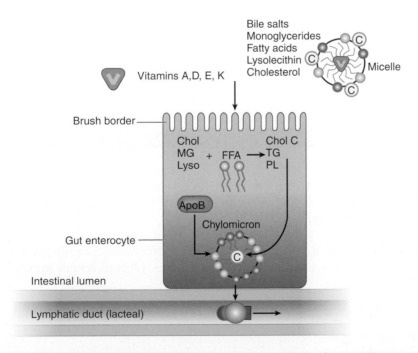

FIGURE 3-22.   Mechanism of lipid absorption. Chol C, cholesterol ester; MG, monoglyceride; Lyso, lysolecithin; FFA, free fatty acids; TG, triglycerides; PL, phospholipid; ApoB, apolipoprotein B. (Modified with permission from Brunicardi FC, Andersen DK, Billiar TR, et al. *Schwartz's Principles of Surgery*, 8th ed. New York: McGraw-Hill, 2005: 27.)

TABLE 3-10.   **Specific Nutrient Absorption**

Nutrient	Location	Mechanism	Clinical Correlation
Iron (Fe^{2+})	Duodenum	Absorbed as ferrous iron (Fe^{2+}, < 5% absorbed) or heme iron (~25%); digested in enterocytes, stored bound to ferritin and transported by transferrin.	Iron deficiency anemia (microcytic, hypochromic), Plummer-Vinson syndrome, hemosiderosis.
Folate	Proximal jejunum	Brush border splits polyglutamates into monoglutamates, which are absorbed and converted to the transport form, 5-methyltetrahydrofolate.	Neural tube defects (congenital effect of maternal deficiency), megaloblastic anemia.
Vitamin B_{12} (cobalamin)	Terminal ileum	Gastric pepsin releases B_{12} from food, binds to R-protein (salivary secretion) in stomach, pancreatic proteases degrade R-protein in duodenum, binds intrinsic factor (from parietal cells), absorbed in terminal ileum.	Associated with pernicious anemia (megaloblastic), gastrectomy (loss of parietal cells), deficiency masked by folate supplementation.

Lipids (Figure 3-22) are emulsified by bile acids in the small intestine and form micelles due to their hydrophobic nature. **Micelles** transport fatty acids, cholesterol, and monoglycerides to the brush border of the enterocytes. Glycerol is hydrophilic and is not part of the micelle body.

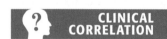
CLINICAL CORRELATION

Abetalipoproteinemia is an inability of chylomicrons to leave the enterocyte due to a lack of β-apolipoprotein.

- Within the **enterocyte,** reesterification of the fatty acids, monoglycerides, and cholesterol takes place to form triglycerides, phospholipids, and cholesterol esters.
- Triglycerides and cholesterol esters are mixed with apoproteins to form **chylomicrons.**
- Chylomicrons then enter the lymphatic system and enter the bloodstream via the thoracic duct.

Hormones and Peptides

GI hormones and peptides found in the small intestine are listed in Table 3-11.

COLON

The main function of the colon is the **reabsorption of electrolytes and water,** as well as short-term storage of undigested material (feces), followed by its excretion. The colon is larger in diameter than the small intestine and is inhabited by normal bacterial flora.

The colon is divided into several anatomic segments: the cecum and ascending, transverse, descending, and sigmoid colon. Overall length averages 1.5–1.8 m.

- In contrast to the small intestine, the colon has no villi and only a few folds.
- It contains goblet, endocrine, and absorptive cells.
- The colon is the **most efficient absorber of water** via actively transported sodium. It can also absorb chloride, potassium, and short-chain fatty acids.
- Its muscle layer has three longitudinal bands of smooth muscle (tenia coli) and typical haustrations (sacculated wall).

TABLE 3-11. **Gastrointestinal Hormones and Peptides**

Hormone/ Peptide	Source	Action	Stimulation	Inhibition
Gastrin	G cells (gastric antrum and duodenum)	Stimulates parietal cells (H+), chief cells (pepsinogen), ECL cells (histamine); trophic on gastric mucosa; increases gastric motility.	Small peptides, amino acids, or Ca^{2+} in gastric lumen, gastric distention, vagal stimulation.	Low gastric pH
CCK	I cells (duodenum and jejunum)	Stimulates pancreatic enzyme secretion (amylase, lipase, proteases) and gallbladder contraction, relaxes sphincter of Oddi, trophic on exocrine pancreas and gallbladder, inhibits gastric emptying.	Fatty acids and amino acids in the small intestine.	Secretin
Secretin	S cells (duodenum)	Stimulates pancreatic and biliary HCO_3^- secretion (neutralizes gastric acid to facilitate pancreatic enzymes) and production of bile, trophic on exocrine pancreas, inhibits gastric H+ secretion.	Decreased gastric pH, fatty acids in the duodenum.	
Somatostatin	D cells (duodenum), delta cells (pancreatic islets)	Inhibits gastric acid and pepsinogen secretion, pancreatic and small intestine secretion, gallbladder contraction, and insulin and glucagon release.	Decreased luminal pH.	Vagal stimulation
GIP	K cells (duodenum and jejunum)	Stimulates insulin release (endocrine), inhibits gastric H+ secretion (exocrine).	Amino acids, fatty acids, oral glucose.	
Pancreatic polypeptide	F cells (PP cells; pancreas and small intestines)	Inhibits pancreatic enzyme and HCO_3^- secretion.	Ingestion of carbohydrates, proteins, or lipids.	
GLP-1	L cells (small intestine)	Stimulates insulin release, inhibits gastric acid and glucagon secretion, decreased gastric motility.	Oral glucose load.	
Motilin	ECL cells (duodenum and jejunum)	Stimulates MMC in the stomach and small intestines and production of pepsin.	Released by absence of food for > 2 h.	
Histamine	ECL cells	Stimulates gastric acid secretion.	Gastrin, ACh (vagus).	
VIP	Enteric neurons and pancreas	Stimulates receptive relaxation of the stomach, relaxation of intestinal smooth muscle, intestinal secretion of water and electrolytes, and increased release of pancreatic HCO_3^-.	Intestinal distention and vagal activation.	
GRP, or bombesin	Neurons of gastric mucosa (vagus)	Increases secretion of gastrin from G cells.	Cephalic phase, gastric distention.	

ACh = acetylcholine; CCK = cholecystokinin; ECL = enterochromaffin-like; GIP = gastric-inhibitory polypeptide; GLP-1 = glucagon-like peptide-1; GRP = gastrin-releasing peptide; VIP = vasoactive intestinal peptide.

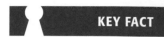

KEY FACT

No MMC occur in the colon.

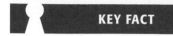

KEY FACT

The colon can secrete excess potassium in diarrhea, resulting in hypokalemia.

- The colonic bacteria synthesize **vitamin K,** B-complex vitamins, folic acid, and **short-chain fatty acids** (a preferred source of nutrition by colonocytes) and metabolize nitrogen from urea to NH_3.
- Peristaltic waves open the ileocecal valve and force chyme into the cecum. The colon has **slow waves** that slowly mix the feces, allowing fluid reabsorption in the ascending colon with **haustrations** (segmental contractions), which take about 8–15 hours and cause a net movement of feces to the transverse colon, where transit speed tends to increase.
- **Large contractions** of the colon (**mass movements**) occur one to three times per day and prepare stool to be eliminated by moving feces large distances toward the rectum. Distention of the rectum produces the urge to defecate and initiates the **rectosphincteric reflex** (both intrinsic and cord reflexes that relax the **internal anal sphincter**).
- **Contractions increase** with parasympathetic stimulation of the vagus and sacral nerves and **decrease** with sympathetic stimulation from the mesenteric ganglion.
- A full stomach can cause a parasympathetic reflex known as the **gastrocolic reflex,** which **increases** the frequency of **mass movements.**

The colon is capable of secreting **potassium** and bicarbonate.

Feces consist of water, bacteria, undigested plant products, and inorganic matter.

EXOCRINE PANCREAS

The bulk of pancreatic tissue (90%) is exocrine glandular tissue composed of acinar cells and a ductal system; approximately 2% is endocrine via the islets of Langerhans, and the remaining portion is supporting tissue. The acinar cells synthesize pancreatic enzymes in the rough endoplasmic reticulum (ER) and store the inactive enzymes, known as zymogens, in secretory vacuoles.

Pancreatic Enzymes

The pancreas secretes about 1 L per day of fluid into the duodenum. This is composed of enzymes and high concentrations of bicarbonate. These enzymes digest carbohydrates, protein, fats, and nucleic acids (Table 3-12). The bicarbonate neutralizes gastric acid to create an optimal pH for pancreatic enzymes to function.

- The **release of pancreatic secretions** is stimulated by CCK, secretin, and ACh from the vagus nerve.
- Once the inactive and active enzymes are excreted out the pancreatic duct via the ampulla of Vater, the duodenal brush border enzyme **enterokinase (enteropeptidase)** activates **trypsinogen** to **trypsin.**
- Trypsin can activate the remaining zymogens and proenzymes into their active form; it also autocatalyzes more trypsinogen to trypsin.
- The pancreas produces enzyme inhibitors to inactivate trace amounts of active enzymes within the pancreatic parenchyma.

GI hormones found in the pancreas include somatostatin, pancreatic peptide, and VIP (Table 3-11).

KEY FACT

Pancreatic insufficiency can lead to malabsorption, steatorrhea, and deficiency in fat-soluble vitamins.

TABLE 3-12. Pancreatic Enzymes

ENZYME	ZYMOGEN/PROENZYME	ENZYME CLASS	CATALYZING ACTIVITY
Pancreatic α-amylase	None (secreted as active form)	Polysaccharidase	Hydrolysis of starch to oligosaccharides and disaccharides. Hydrolysis of glycogen. Does **not** hydrolyze cellulose.
Trypsin	Trypsinogen	Protease	Activates other pancreatic zymogens. Hydrolysis of proteins into peptides.
Chymotrypsin	Chymotrypsinogen	Protease	Hydrolysis of peptides into amino acids.
Carboxypeptidase	Procarboxypeptidase	Protease	Hydrolysis of peptides into amino acids.
Elastase	Proelastase	Protease	Hydrolysis of elastin.
Pancreatic lipase	None (secreted as active form)	Lipase	Hydrolysis of neutral fats into fatty acids and monoglycerides.
Colipase	Procolipase	Lipase	Assists lipase by displacing inhibitory bile salts.
Cholesterol ester hydrolase	None (secreted as active form)	Lipase	Hydrolysis of cholesterol esters into cholesterol and fatty acids. Also hydrolyses the ester bond of triglycerides to glycerol and fatty acids.
Phospholipase A_2	Prophospholipase	Lipase	Hydrolysis of phospholipids into fatty acids and lysolecithin.
Ribonuclease	None (secreted as active form)	Nuclease	Hydrolysis of RNA into ribonucleotides.
Deoxyribonuclease	None (secreted as active form)	Nuclease	Hydrolysis of DNA into deoxyribonucleotides.

LIVER AND GALLBLADDER

Liver Overview

Located in the right upper quadrant, the liver typically spans from the fifth intercostal space in the midclavicular line to the right costal margin.

Anatomically, the liver is divided into **four lobes:** right, left, caudate, and quadrate. The **right and left lobes** are divided by the **falciform ligament,** making the right lobe significantly larger than the left.

Functionally, the liver is divided into eight segments (numbered I–VIII) based on blood supply. This division is significant for surgeons as liver resections are done based on this segmental division.

- **Hepatocytes** are polygonal epithelial cells arranged in long plates one to two cells thick, giving the histologic specimen a very uniform appearance.

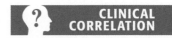

CLINICAL CORRELATION

On physical exam, the size of the liver can be determined by percussion dullness; usually it is not palpable below the costal margin.

CLINICAL CORRELATION

- Zone I of the liver lobule receives blood from the portal system first and is primarily affected by toxins; it is also the hepatic exit for bile and is most quickly affected by bile stasis.
- Zone III is located farthest from the hepatic artery and is most likely to be damaged by ischemia and fat accumulation.

KEY FACT

Functions of hepatocytes:
- Formation of bile and bile pigments
- Production of serum proteins (albumin)
- Uptake of chylomicrons
- Production of plasma lipoproteins
- Drug, vitamin, and hormone metabolism
- Vitamin and mineral storage

- **Liver sinusoids** course between these plates of hepatocytes. They are composed of fenestrated endothelial cells and are in free communication with each other throughout the liver.
- The **liver lobule** (Figure 3-23) is an anatomic and functional structure created by the radial arrangement of plates of hepatocytes and the intervening sinusoids around the central vein. The lobules are separated by connective tissue. Traveling within this connective tissue in between the lobules are the **portal triads—branches of the hepatic artery, portal vein, and bile duct.**
- Each hexagonally shaped lobule is divided into **three zones:** zone I encircles the portal triad, zone III is located around the central veins, and zone II is between the other zones (Figure 3-24).
- The **space of Disse** occurs between the endothelial cells of the sinusoids and the hepatocytes themselves.
- **Kupffer cells** are macrophages that are specific to the liver and reside in the liver sinusoids.

The liver has a dual blood supply, with 80% of the blood coming from the portal vein and the other 20% from the hepatic artery.

- The **portal venous blood** comes from the venous drainage of the GI tract; it is therefore rich in nutrients but lacks oxygen. This blood allows the liver to perform its metabolic functions.
- The **arterial supply** to the liver is responsible for oxygenating the hepatocytes and supporting liver cells.

Liver Function

- **Aids digestion:** Hepatocytes continuously secrete bile acids. Most of the **bile** produced by the liver is **recycled** through the ileum via a Na^+-dependent bile salt cotransporter and then travels up the portal vein into the liver as the **enterohepatic circulation.**
- Serves as the **first site of metabolism** of ingested substances absorbed from the small intestine.

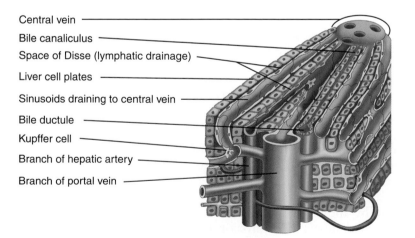

Central vein
Bile canaliculus
Space of Disse (lymphatic drainage)
Liver cell plates
Sinusoids draining to central vein
Bile ductule
Kupffer cell
Branch of hepatic artery
Branch of portal vein

FIGURE 3-23. **Detailed structure of the liver lobule.** (Modified with permission from Chandrasoma P, Taylor CE. *Concise Pathology*, 3rd ed. Originally published by Appleton & Lange. Copyright © 1998 by The McGraw-Hill Companies, Inc.)

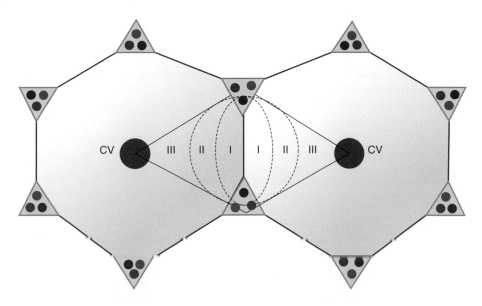

FIGURE 3-24. Histologic representation of the liver zones.

- **Maintains the body's blood chemistry:** The liver is the site of many key biochemical processes, such as gluconeogenesis and glycolysis, pharmacologic metabolism, and protein synthesis.
- **Storage:** Maintains a supply of glycogen, vitamins, iron, and copper.

Gallbladder

The main function of the gallbladder is to **store and concentrate bile.** After eating, vagal nerve stimuli cause the gallbladder to contract and the sphincter of Boyden to relax, promoting the release of bile into the common bile duct.

The gallbladder is located on the inferior surface of the liver. It is **divided into the fundus, body, and neck;** it drains through the **cystic duct** (Figure 3-25).

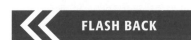

FLASH BACK

Drugs absorbed by the small intestine are subject to "first-pass metabolism" by the liver.

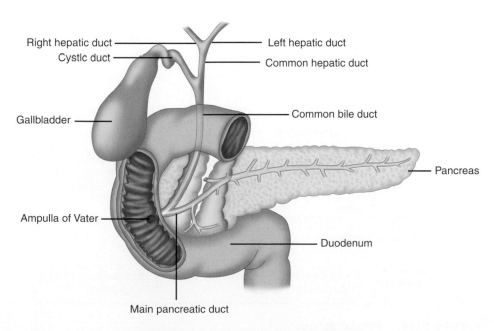

FIGURE 3-25. The gallbladder and its surrounding structures.

- The cystic duct joins with the **common hepatic duct** to form the **common bile duct.**
- The **common bile duct** descends and finally joins with the pancreatic duct at the **ampulla of Vater** to empty into the second portion of the duodenum.
- Histologically, the mucosa of the gallbladder is composed of **simple columnar epithelium** in which all of the cells are virtually identical; it resembles the small intestine and colon, but lacks goblet cells and crypts.
- The **absorptive epithelium** uses Na^+–K^+ ATPase to create electrolyte gradients that dehydrate and **concentrate the bile.**

Bilirubin

Bilirubin is a product of heme metabolism (Figure 3-26).

RETICULOENDOTHELIAL SYSTEM (RES)

The body produces approximately 250–300 mg of heme daily, chiefly from the breakdown of senescent RBCs. A smaller portion comes from turnover of hepatic heme, hemoproteins, and premature destruction of RBCs in the bone marrow (an important clinical consideration with hematologic disorders involving intramedullary hemolysis).

Normally, heme is oxidized to **biliverdin** by heme oxygenase, and then reduced to **bilirubin** by biliverdin reductase.

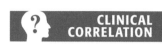

CLINICAL CORRELATION

Cholelithiasis (gallstones) is typically caused by excess cholesterol within the gallbladder. They can also result from precipitated calcium or bilirubin.

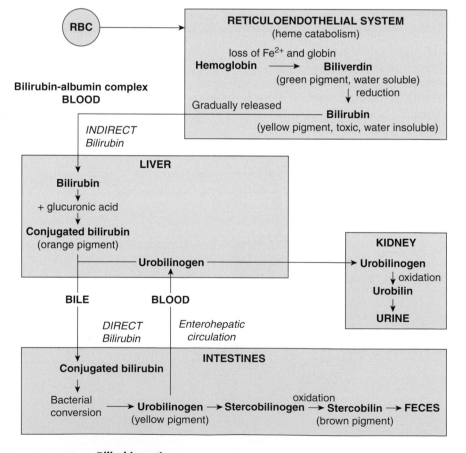

FIGURE 3-26. Bilirubin pathway.

LIVER AND GALLBLADDER

- **Unconjugated bilirubin (indirect bilirubin)** is transported to the liver in the bloodstream bound to albumin, as it is insoluble at physiologic pH.
- **In the liver,** hepatocytes take up bilirubin by carrier-mediated processes. It is then transported to the ER and **conjugated** with glucuronic acid by bilirubin uridine diphosphate (**UDP)-glucuronyltransferase.**
- Conjugated bilirubin (direct bilirubin; bilirubin glucuronide), now in a water-soluble form, is excreted into bile.

COLON

Normal gut bacteria **hydrolyze** the majority of conjugated bilirubin to an unconjugated form called **urobilinogen** (~80–90% is excreted in the stool; ~10–20% is passively absorbed in the terminal colon, where it enters the portal venous system and is recycled by the liver).

KIDNEYS

Approximately 10% of the resorbed urobilirubin is filtered and secreted by the kidney.

Bile

Produced by hepatocytes, bile is excreted into the bile canaliculi, where it travels down the bile ducts until it is either excreted or stored in the gallbladder. Bile has **two main functions:**

- Helping to **emulsify** large fats, thus aiding in their absorption by the small intestine.
- Serving as a means of excretion of excess cholesterol, bilirubin, and some pharmaceuticals. Bile salts and lecithin together increase the solubility of cholesterol several million times.

There are several steps in bile synthesis (Figure 3-27):

- **Primary bile acids** are synthesized in the liver from cholesterol.
- **Cholesterol** is first converted into **cholic acid** or **chenodeoxycholic acid** and then **conjugated** with either glycine or taurine to form bile salts.
- More than 95% of bile is **recycled in the ileum,** where it is transported back up into the hepatocytes via the **enterohepatic cycle.**
- Approximately 0.2–0.6 mg of bile is lost in feces each day; this loss is balanced by de novo production in hepatocytes.

Secondary bile acids are the result of bacterial metabolism of primary bile acids that have been recirculated via the enterohepatic cycle.

Composition of bile:

- Bile salts
- Phospholipids
- Cholesterol
- Lecithin
- Water
- Bilirubin
- Ions

FLASH FORWARD

Jaundice is a yellowing of the skin, and icterus is a yellowing of the sclerae due to elevated bilirubin levels.
Increased indirect bilirubin indicates excess hemolysis or severe liver damage.
Increased direct bilirubin may indicate a blockage of the bile ducts.

KEY FACT

Key regulatory factors:
- CCK is the primary stimulatory regulator of bile excretion.
- Somatostatin is the primary inhibitory regulator of bile excretion.
- Secretin also stimulates the liver to produce bile.

FLASH FORWARD

Bile acid sequestrants interrupt enterohepatic circulation by binding bile acids in the GI tract and preventing reabsorption; this forces increased de novo synthesis from cholesterol.

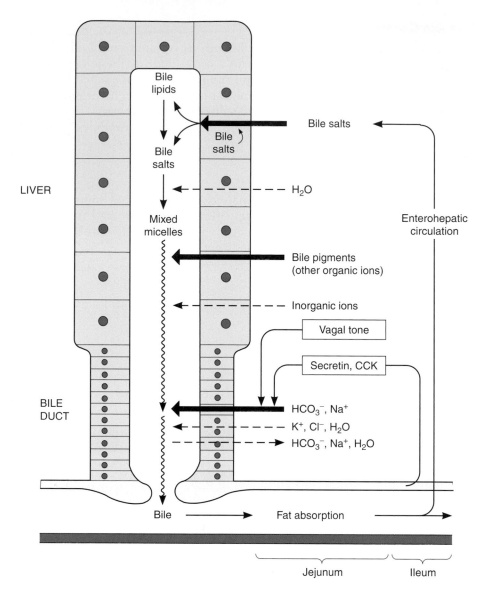

FIGURE 3-27. **Bile formation.** Solid lines into the ductular lumen indicate active transport; dotted lines represent passive diffusion. (Modified with permission from Doherty GM, Way LW. *Current Surgical Diagnosis and Treatment*, 12th ed. New York: McGraw-Hill, 2006: 576.)

Pathology

ORAL CAVITY

Mouth and Jaw

- **Lichen planus** is a self-limited, nonmalignant disease of unknown cause that results in classic Wickham striae, which are white, lace-like patterns on top of papules or plaques.
- **Oral candidiasis** (Figure 3-28) is a yeast infection in the mouth; it is commonly seen in breast-feeding infants or **immunocompromised hosts.**

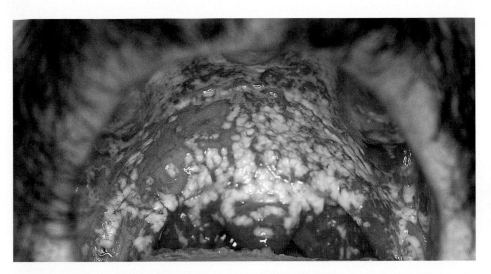

FIGURE 3-28. **Oral candidiasis (thrush).** Extensive cottage cheese-like plaques, colonies of *Candida*, on the palate and uvula of an individual with advanced HIV disease. Patches of erythema between the white plaques represent erythematous (atrophic) candidiasis. Involvement may extend into the esophagus and be associated with dysphagia. (Reproduced with permission from Wolff K, Johnson RA, Suurmond R. *Fitzpatrick's Color Atlas & Synopsis of Clinical Dermatology*, 5th ed. New York: McGraw-Hill, 2005: 723.)

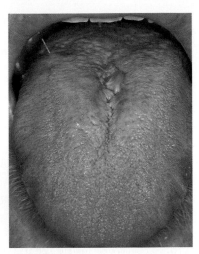

FIGURE 3-29. **Hairy tongue.** Filiform hyperkeratoses of the papillae result in a brownish coating on the dorsum of the tongue in this 31-year-old cigarette smoker. (Reproduced with permission from Wolff K, Johnson RA, Suurmond R. *Fitzpatrick's Color Atlas & Synopsis of Clinical Dermatology*, 5th ed. New York: McGraw-Hill, 2005: 1019.)

Similar to nonmalignant lesions, premalignant lesions like leukoplakia can cause white papules or plaques on the tongue. Clinically, they can be difficult to differentiate from conditions like lichen planus. Premalignant lesions are also hard to identify because they lack the classical characteristics of advanced cancer: pain, ulceration, induration, and cervical lymphadenopathy.

- **Leukoplakia** (Figure 3-29) is **squamous cell hyperplasia,** which can develop into dysplasia, carcinoma in situ, and invasive carcinoma. It can also be seen in inflammatory conditions unrelated to malignancy. **Hairy leukoplakia** is a distinct inflammatory condition affecting immunocompromised patients (**pre-AIDS–defining condition**).
- Malignant lesions are the most common pathologic finding in the mouth. Smoking is the greatest risk factor for oral cancer. **Squamous cell carcinoma (SCC)** is the most common oral cancer. Risk factors include chronic cigarette smoking and alcohol use.

Characteristic pathologic findings and treatments are described in Table 3-13.

Salivary Glands

Sjögren syndrome, an autoimmune condition, is the most notable disease affecting the salivary glands. Other important conditions include salivary stones, benign and malignant tumors, and infections such as mumps (described in Table 3-14).

SJÖGREN SYNDROME (XEROSTOMIA; KERATOCONJUNCTIVITIS SICCA)

Can occur independently or in conjunction with another autoimmune condition, such as rheumatoid arthritis or systemic lupus erythematosus (SLE).

FLASH BACK

Centers for Disease Control and Prevention (CDC) category "B," pre-AIDS–defining conditions seen in the mouth:

- Hairy leukoplakia, an inflammatory condition caused by Epstein-Barr virus.
- Oral thrush.
- Herpetic stomatitis and herpes esophagitis; caused by herpes simplex virus.

TABLE 3-13. **Most Common Pathologies Affecting the Mouth and Jaw**

	PRESENTATION	DIAGNOSIS	TREATMENT	PROGNOSIS
SCC	Persistent papules, plaques, erosions, ulcers.	Biopsy with TNM staging.	Combination of surgery, radiation, and chemotherapy, depending on stage.	Related to stage; often diagnosed at a late stage and frequently recurs, even if caught early.
Melanoma	Oral lesion with asymmetry, irregular borders, color changes, increasing diameter.	Biopsy.	Surgical resection with negative margins; radiation if negative margins are not obtained.	Depends on stage, including tumor thickness and ulceration.
Leukoplakia	White patches or plaques on oral mucosa.	Biopsy.	Surgery, cryotherapy ablation, carbon dioxide laser ablation.	1–20% of lesions progress to malignancy in 10 years.
HSV-1 herpetic stomatitis	Vesicular lesions with erythematous bases.	Multinucleated giant cells on Tzanck smear.	Acyclovir, pain management, fluids.	Recurs; some patients have success with chronic suppression.
Aphthous ulcers	Localized, shallow, round ulcers with gray bases that heal in 7–14 days.	Clinical presentation.	Symptomatic relief with oral analgesics.	Some patients have recurrent aphthous stomatitis.
Oral candidiasis (thrush)	White plaques that **cannot be scraped off.**	KOH prep.	Nystatin mouthwash for 7–10 days.	Can be recurrent if patient immunocompromised.

HSV = herpes simplex virus; SCC = squamous cell carcinoma; TNM = tumor, nodes, metastasis.

KEY FACT

Hallmarks of Sjögren syndrome are dry eyes (keratoconjunctivitis sicca) and dry mouth (xerostomia) along with multisystem involvement, including skin, lung, heart, and kidney.

The hallmark of this syndrome is an abnormal lymphocytic infiltration of exocrine glands, most notably the salivary and lacrimal glands, resulting in the classic findings of dry mouth and dry eyes. This abnormal lymphocyte activity also leads to an increased risk of **lymphoma.**

DIAGNOSIS

The presence of **anti-Ro/SSA** or **anti-La/SSB antibodies** is indicative of Sjögren syndrome. Additionally, the following tests may be used.

- **Schirmer test** is a measure of tear production.
- **Rose Bengal stain** can show areas of corneal or conjunctival epithelial cell damage.
- A **salivary gland biopsy** sample from the lip may show focal collections of lymphocytes.

TREATMENT

- **Symptomatic:** Eye drops for keratoconjunctivitis sicca and the use of sugarless candy or lozenges containing malic acid to stimulate the production of saliva.
- **Good oral hygiene and dental care** is important because of an increased risk of dental caries, gum disease, and halitosis due to decreased saliva

TABLE 3-14. Most Common Diseases of Salivary Glands

	CAUSE/PRESENTATION	DIAGNOSIS	TREATMENT	PROGNOSIS
Mumps	Paramyxovirus (parotitis, fever, myalgias, headache, anorexia, orchitis).	Positive IgM mumps antibody, rise in IgG titers, isolation of mumps virus.	Symptomatic: analgesics and antipyretics.	Vaccination has decreased the incidence of mumps infections.
Hypertrophy	Can be caused by eating disorders (bulimia), kwashiorkor, alcoholism, and metabolic disease.	Clinical observation.	Treat underlying disease.	
Sialolithiasis (salivary stones)	▪ Submandibular glands; more common in men. ▪ Forms when saliva rich in calcium is stagnant. ▪ Some association with gout and nephrolithiasis.	Palpation of salivary ducts or imaging studies if not palpable.	Conservative therapy. Hydration (and sucking on candy to increase salivation), moist heat, massaging the gland, and milking the duct.	Secondary infection; chronic sialolithiasis may indicate dysfunctional gland.
Salivary gland tumors	▪ Risk factors: radiation and EBV. ▪ Smoking has not been connected to malignant tumors, but is linked to benign papillary cystadenoma lymphomatosum. ▪ Most common tumor is pleomorphic **adenoma** (mixed tumor), affecting parotid glands.	Fine-needle aspiration with TNM staging biopsy, CT, MRI.	▪ Benign: surgical excision. ▪ Malignant: Wide margin surgical excision with or without chemo- or radiation therapy.	High rate of recurrence.

EBV = Epstein-Barr virus; Ig = immunoglobulin; TNM = tumor, nodes, metastasis.

production. May also help to prevent salivary calculi, dysphagia, and oral candidiasis.

▪ More severe cases may require **pilocarpine,** a muscarinic agonist that stimulates salivation and has side effects of sweating, abdominal cramping, and flushing.

ESOPHAGUS

Esophageal Atresia and Tracheoesophageal Fistula

The most common congenital anomaly of the esophagus, often associated with tracheoesophageal fistula (TEF) (connection between the trachea and esophagus).

There are several forms of esophageal atresia (EA), many with TEF (Figure 3-30). Each type depends on the anatomy of the esophagus and the presence or absence of a fistula.

KEY FACT

Patients with Sjögren syndrome have an increased risk of lymphoma.

KEY FACT

In the most common form of EA/TEF, (type III; see Figure 3-30C), the proximal esophagus ends in a blind pouch, and the distal esophageal segment demonstrates a proximal TEF.

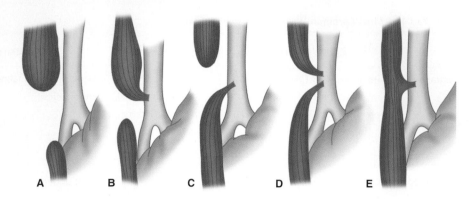

FIGURE 3-30. **The five varieties of esophageal atresia and tracheoesophageal fistula.** (A) Isolated esophageal atresia (EA). (B) EA with tracheoesophageal fistula (TEF) between proximal segments of esophagus and trachea. (C) EA with TEF between distal esophagus and trachea. (D) EA with TEF between both proximal and distal ends of esophagus and trachea. (E) TEF without EA (H-type fistula). (Modified with permission from Brunicardi FC, Andersen DK, Billiar TR. *Schwartz's Principles of Surgery*, 8th ed. New York: McGraw-Hill, 2005: 1481.)

PRESENTATION

Depends on the type of EA/TEF:

- Neonates typically present very early with frothing and bubbling at the nose and mouth as well as coughing, cyanosis, and respiratory distress exacerbated by feeding.
- Children who have TEF but no EA can present later in life with recurrent pneumonia from the aspiration of gastric contents.

DIAGNOSIS

- The diagnosis is confirmed by trying to pass a nasogastric tube into the stomach. If it does not pass easily, an anteroposterior chest radiograph will show the catheter coiled in the blind pouch.
- **Distal TEF** can be diagnosed by a gas-filled GI tract on plain film.

TREATMENT

Surgical correction.

Esophageal Diverticula

Saccular outpouchings that can be found in the esophagus just as they are found in the colon.

- **False (pulsion) diverticula:** Mucosal layers protruding through the muscularis; most common type.
- **True (traction) diverticula:** Contains all layers of the esophageal wall; less common type.

The three characteristic locations of the diverticula:

- **Pharyngoesophageal (Zenker, pulsion) diverticulum** (Figure 3-31): Located immediately above the cricopharyngeus muscle of the upper esophageal sphincter (UES).

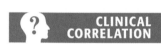

CLINICAL CORRELATION

Maternal polyhydramnios: Develops as a consequence of EA. Also found in duodenal atresia and Down syndrome.

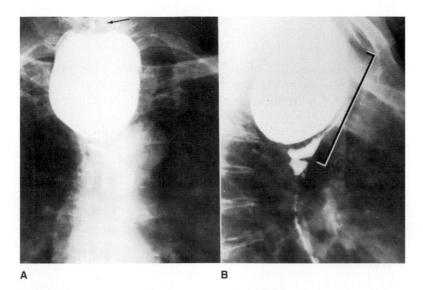

A   B

FIGURE 3-31.   **Large pharyngoesophageal diverticulum.** (A) Note origin in the midline (*arrow*) and (B) compression of esophagus (*bracket*). (Reproduced with permission from Doherty GM, Way LW. *Current Surgical Diagnosis and Treatment*, 12th ed. New York: McGraw-Hill, 2006: 460.)

- **Midesophageal (traction) diverticula:** Usually located in the middle third of the esophagus. Typically associated with inflammatory conditions such as tuberculosis (TB).
- **Epiphrenic (pulsion) diverticula:** Located in the distal esophagus in the region of the lower esophageal sphincter (LES).

DIAGNOSIS

Patients typically present in their 60s. The earliest sign is transient dysphagia. As the pouch enlarges, more debris is retained and patients can aspirate, complain of gurgling or **regurgitating undigested food,** or have a mass in the neck. The best diagnostic technique is a barium swallow.

TREATMENT

Surgical treatment depends on type and location.

- Traction diverticula rarely require surgical treatment.
- Zenker diverticula require division of the cricopharyngeus muscle without diverticulectomy (relaxation of the muscle corrects for the defect).
- Epiphrenic diverticula require distal esophageal myotomy with diverticulectomy.

Esophageal Varices

Develops as a consequence of portal hypertension resulting in increased pressure in the left gastric vein. Veins have thinner walls in the distal esophagus and are thus more prone to dilation and bleeding. Variceal bleeding is often a cause of upper GI bleeds in alcoholic and cirrhotic patients.

DIAGNOSIS

Via endoscopy; sometimes difficult to detect during active variceal hemorrhage.

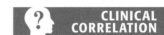

CLINICAL CORRELATION

Zenker and epiphrenic types of diverticula are commonly associated with motor abnormalities of the esophagus, such as spasm, achalasia, and UES/LES hyperactivity.

TREATMENT

Medications can aid in stopping an acute bleed but are not curative.

- **Vasopressin:** Vasoconstriction of mesenteric vessels, which decreases portal venous flow.
- **Somatostatin** or **octreotide:** Inhibits release of vasodilating hormones, indirectly causing vasoconstriction.
- **Endoscopy:** Definitive treatment, either sclerotherapy or variceal band ligation.
- **Balloon tamponade** can provide short-term hemostasis.
- Transjugular intrahepatic portosystemic shunt (**TIPS procedure**—an artificial shunt from the portal vein to the hepatic vein, which reduces the pressure).
- **Beta-blockers** are drug of choice for prophylaxis.

Mallory-Weiss Tear

Longitudinal tears in the esophagus at the esophagogastric junction. Associated with severe retching (alcohol intoxication). Accounts for 5–10% of upper GI bleeds.

Boerhaave Syndrome

Occurs in the setting of spontaneous esophageal rupture with exit of gastric contents into the mediastinum. Associated with overindulgence in food and alcohol. High mortality rate.

Achalasia

Defined as "**failure to relax,**" achalasia is characterized by:

- Aperistalsis (required for diagnosis).
- Increased resting tone of the LES and incomplete relaxation of LES when swallowing.

Achalasia can be due to primary (most common) or secondary causes.

- **Primary/embryologic achalasia** develops as a result of the failed **migration of ganglionic cells** to the myenteric plexus; these cells are required for LES relaxation.
- **Secondary achalasia** occurs from any pathologic process that impairs esophageal motility. **Chagas disease** (principal cause of achalasia in South America) develops as a result of infestation with *Trypanosoma cruzi*, which destroys the myenteric plexus of the esophagus, duodenum, colon, and ureter.
- **Achalasia-like conditions** can occur with amyloidosis, sarcoidosis, or carcinoma.
- In achalasia, the dilated portion of the esophagus lacks ganglia, but the narrowed portion is structurally normal.

Always consider esophageal cancer in patients with swallowing difficulties and **systemic signs.** Endoscopy is warranted if cancer is considered.

PRESENTATION

Presents with progressive dysphagia beginning with solid foods and progressing to liquids, as well as with frequent nocturnal regurgitation and/or aspiration of undigested food.

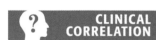

CLINICAL CORRELATION

Difficulty in swallowing both solid and liquid food indicates a motility (neuromuscular) problem.
Difficulty in swallowing solid food only indicates an anatomic (mechanical) problem.
Difficulty in swallowing liquids only indicates esophagitis.

DIAGNOSIS

- Manometry shows normal or elevated resting LES pressure, decreased LES relaxation, and absence of peristalsis.
- Barium swallow classically shows a dilated esophagus with a distal "**bird-beak**" narrowing (Figure 3-32).

TREATMENT

Surgical treatment is curative, balloon dilation, and calcium channel blockers can be used for systematic treatment.

Hiatial Hernia

Herniation of part of the stomach into the thoracic cavity. Associated conditions include reflux, ulceration, bleeding, and perforation.

- **Sliding hernia (95%):** Protrusion of the stomach above the diaphragm, creating a bell-shaped dilation. GERD may be a manifestation. Treatment is the same for GERD (see following section).
- **Paraesophageal hernia:** Part of the greater curvature protrudes through the esophageal hiatus, next to the esophagus. More prone to strangulation than a sliding hernia. Treatment is surgical correction to prevent strangulation.

Gastroesophageal Reflux Disease

Gastroesophageal reflux disease (GERD) develops as a result of abnormal relaxation of the LES and/or delayed gastric emptying with increased pressure in the stomach (eg, hiatal hernia or pregnancy). These abnormalities allow gastric contents to reflux into the esophagus, thus leading to esophageal injury, and if left untreated, chronic inflammation.

PRESENTATION

Symptoms of GERD include heartburn, water brash (an acidic taste in the mouth), dysphagia, hoarseness, globus sensation (lump in the throat), chronic cough (especially at night), and regurgitation.

DIAGNOSIS

Definitive diagnosis is established with endoscopic observation of mucosal changes. For some patients, pH monitoring may be helpful. A **triad of histologic features** indicative of mucosal inflammation is key to a GERD diagnosis:

- Eosinophils (advanced cases show neutrophils)
- Basal zone hyperplasia
- Elongation of the lamina propria papillae

TREATMENT

Lifestyle and diet changes (smoking cessation; avoidance of alcohol and caffeine, fatty foods, acidic foods, spicy foods, and chocolate), antacids, and over-the-counter histamine H_2-blockers for heartburn. More advanced disease requires pharmacologic acid suppression with histamine blockers or proton pump inhibitors. GERD that is incompletely controlled by medication and lifestyle changes can be treated surgically with gastroesophageal fundoplication (Nissen fundoplication).

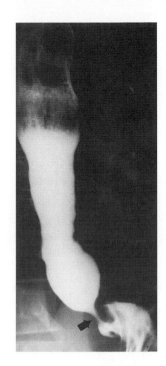

FIGURE 3-32. Bird-beak esophagus typical of achalasia. Aperistalsis of the esophagus associated with smooth narrowing at the lower end of the esophagus (*arrow*), suggesting achalasia of the esophagus. (Reproduced with permission from Chen MYM, Pope TL, Ott DJ. *Basic Radiology.* New York: McGraw-Hill, 2004: 258.)

PROGNOSIS

Long-standing reflux can predispose to Barrett esophagus, which can ultimately develop into adenocarcinoma of the esophagus (Figure 3-33).

Barrett Esophagus

A precancerous lesion of the distal esophagus and a complication of long-standing GERD. It occurs when esophageal mucosa undergoes intestinal metaplasia from squamous to specialized columnar cells containing goblet cells (Figure 3-34). Gastric-type columnar cells may be present.

PRESENTATION

Long-standing GERD. Advanced cases may present with progressive (weeks to months) dysphagia for solids, weight loss, cough, and/or regurgitation/aspiration (worse at night).

DIAGNOSIS

- **Endoscopy:** Red, velvety GI mucosa extending upward from the gastroesophageal junction, in contrast to the normal pale pink squamous epithelial mucosa of the esophagus.
- **Biopsy:** Intestinal-type goblet cells in the columnar mucosa of the esophagus.

TREATMENT

Regular endoscopic surveillance for at-risk patients to ensure Barrett has not progressed to esophageal cancer, along with aggressive medical or surgical treatment of GERD. Due to the high risk of esophageal cancer, patients with Barrett esophagus and high-grade dysplasia typically undergo esophagectomy.

PROGNOSIS

Complications of Barrett esophagus include strictures, peptic ulceration, and the potential for malignant transformation into adenocarcinoma.

Esophageal Cancer

The incidence varies greatly, depending on geographic region, suggesting environmental causative factors. In the United States, it is more common in

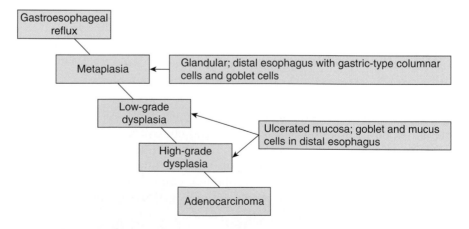

FIGURE 3-33. **Progression from gastroesophageal reflux disease to Barrett esophagus and adenocarcinoma.**

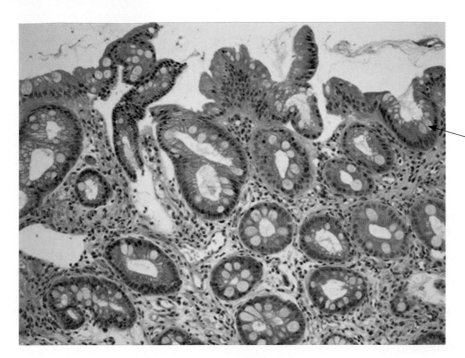

FIGURE 3-34. **Histology of Barrett esophagus.** Histopathologic findings in nondysplastic Barrett esophagus. Note the glandular epithelium containing goblet cells (*arrow*). (Reproduced with permission from Greenberger NJ, Burakoff R. *Current Diagnosis and Treatment: Gastroenterology, Hepatology, and Endoscopy.* New York: McGraw-Hill, 2009: Plate 11.)

African Americans, males, and those with lower socioeconomic status. There are two major types:

- **SCC:** Linked to smoking, alcohol consumption (liquor > beer), nitrites, smoked opiates, fungal toxins, radiation, and lye exposure.
- **Adenocarcinoma:** A result of chronic GERD leading to intestinal metaplasia of stratified nonkeratinized esophageal epithelium (Barrett esophagus), which leads to dysplastic changes in the columnar epithelium and adenocarcinoma.

PRESENTATION

Typically, SCC appears in the upper and middle esophagus, whereas adenocarcinoma appears in the lower esophagus. Most common presenting symptoms are dysphagia and weight loss. The disease is usually incurable once dysphagia is present, as > 60% of the esophageal circumference is involved. Other symptoms include odynophagia, emesis, and aspiration secondary to TEF formation.

Unlike most cancers that spread hematogenously, esophageal cancer **typically spreads locally** to surrounding tissue, lymph nodes, lungs, liver, and pleura.

DIAGNOSIS

- Periodic screening endoscopy is recommended in high-risk patients with biopsy of suggestive lesions.
- **Contrast radiography:** Identifies esophageal strictures, ulcerations, and mucosal abnormalities with a ragged, ulcerated appearance. However, only high-grade lesions are seen with this approach.

TREATMENT

Esophagectomy for potentially curable lesions with or without preoperative chemotherapy and radiation therapy. Palliative treatment for symptomatic advanced-stage lesions (stricture balloon dilation and esophageal stent placement).

PROGNOSIS

Tumor resection, chemotherapy, and radiation therapy are used in some patients to reduce tumor burden, but these are rarely curative. Survival rate 5 years after diagnosis is around 25%.

STOMACH

Gastritis

Gastritis is an inflammation of the gastric mucosa. Depending on the cause, type, and duration of inflammation, it can be subdivided into acute and chronic types.

ACUTE GASTRITIS

Acute, transient mucosal damage with mucosal edema and inflammation (Figure 3-35). The injury can erode the mucosa and affect underlying epithelium, in which case **hemorrhagic gastritis** develops. Most common causes include:

- Nonsteroidal anti-inflammatory drug (NSAID) overuse
- Alcohol consumption
- **Cushing ulcers** associated with head trauma
- **Curling ulcers** associated with burns
- Uremia
- **Stress-induced gastritis:** Hemoccult-positive stools and visible changes on endoscopic examination of the stomach

CHRONIC (ATROPHIC) GASTRITIS

Continuous inflammation of the gastric mucosa leads to mucosal atrophy and epithelial metaplasia (hence "chronic" and "atrophic"). Based on the location of the injury and the causative agent, chronic gastritis is divided into **types A** and **B**.

- **Type A:** Affects the fundus and body of the stomach and spares the antrum. Typically secondary to pernicious anemia (also known as autoimmune gastritis). It is associated with antibodies to parietal cells (specifically targeting the H^+–K^+ ATPase) and to the intrinsic factor (IF). It leads to achlorhydria with consequent hypergastrinemia.
- **Type B:** Antral-predominant, sparing the fundus and body. Typically secondary to chronic *Helicobacter pylori* infection.

PRESENTATION

Abdominal pain, dyspepsia, and visual changes noted on endoscopic inspection **do not reliably correlate** with the histopathologic diagnosis of gastritis.

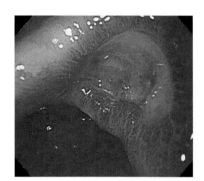

FIGURE 3-35. **Gastric ulcer.** Note sharply demarcated edges, clean base, and minimal elevation of the edges. (Reproduced with permission from Fauci AS, Kasper DL, Braunwald E, et al. *Harrison's Principles of Internal Medicine*, 17th ed. New York: McGraw-Hill, 2008: Figure 285-2.)

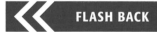

FLASH BACK

Mucosal damage in type B gastritis develops due to the erosive nature of ammonia, which is a product of urea degraded by the *H pylori* urease.

DIAGNOSIS

Can be confirmed only histologically (biopsy).

- Diagnosis of *H pylori* infection is based on biopsy (specimen shows gram-negative rods), **urease breath test,** and **stool and serum antigens** (see the section on peptic ulcer disease [PUD] for further discussion).
- Pernicious anemia is always suspected in patients with megaloblastic anemia, chronic neurologic changes, and an **abnormal Schilling test.**

TREATMENT

- For treatment of *H pylori*, see the section on PUD.
- Patients with pernicious anemia need **parenteral** vitamin B_{12} supplementation.
- Proton pump inhibitors are normally given to patients in the ICU or those who have suffered head trauma or burns as prophylaxis against acute erosive gastritis.

PROGNOSIS

All forms of gastritis have the potential to lead to adenocarcinoma of the stomach. Type B gastritis can lead to MALTomas as well.

Ménétrier Disease

Hyperplasia of mucus-secreting cells resulting in rugal hypertrophy and **hypoproteinemia.** Also causes atrophy of parietal cells, thus resulting in achlorhydria. Patients are at risk for adenocarcinoma.

Peptic Ulcer Disease (PUD)

Ulcer formation in the stomach or the first part of the duodenum. Gastric mucosal cells secrete mucus with large quantities of **bicarbonate** in order to maintain a **pH of 6–7 around the epithelial cells,** in contrast to the pH of **1–2** in the **gastric lumen.** When the mucus layer is breached, by drugs, bacteria, or systemic disorders, epithelial injury occurs, and ulcers can form.

Gastric Ulcers

Less common and occur later in life. Typically develop along the lesser curvature, in the **antral** and **prepyloric** regions. Malignant transformation is **more common** than with duodenal ulcers. They are primarily caused by *H pylori.* Basal and nocturnal acid secretion is typically normal to **decreased.**

Duodenal Ulcers

More than 95% occur in the first portion of the duodenum. Ulcers are typically > 1 cm in size, and **malignancy is extremely rare.** Basal and nocturnal acid secretion tends to be **increased.** NSAIDs and *H pylori* are also associated risk factors.

PRESENTATION

Burning, gnawing epigastric pain is typical but not specific for this diagnosis (Table 3-15).

- Patients with **duodenal ulcers** tend to give a history of pain **2–3 hours after meals** that is **relieved with food.**
- Patients with **gastric ulcers** have increased **pain with food,** as well as nausea and weight loss.

TABLE 3-15.   The Most Common Characteristics of Peptic Ulcer Disease

	GASTRIC ULCER	DUODENAL ULCER
Percentage	25%.	75%.
Common causes	*Helicobacter pylori* (~80%), NSAID use.	*H pylori* (90–95%), NSAID use.
Presenting symptoms	Pain with food.	Pain 2–3 h after meals and relieved by food.
Complications	Perforation, bleeding, malignancy, gastric outlet obstruction.	Perforation, bleeding, gastric outlet obstruction, pancreatitis.
Malignancy	10%.	Rare.
Location	Type-dependent; typically lesser curvature.	First portion of duodenum.

On physical exam, patients can have tenderness to palpation in the epigastric region. Abdominal rigidity and peritoneal signs are concerning for perforation (most common with duodenal ulcers), which can lead to peritonitis. The most common complication is **upper GI bleeding**, which presents as melena or hematemesis.

DIAGNOSIS

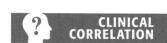

CLINICAL CORRELATION

Patients with perforated duodenal ulcer often present with epigastric pain radiating to the left shoulder as well as with air under the diaphragm on chest film.

- **Contrast radiography** can show defects in the gastric and duodenal epithelium caused by ulcers, although small erosions are typically missed.
- *H pylori* infection must also be excluded, as a large number of cases are secondary to this common bacterium. Tests include serum antibodies (**not useful in confirming successful treatment**), stool antigen (**useful in confirming eradication**), urease breath test, and biopsy of tissue via esophagogastroduodenoscopy.
- On endoscopy, the gross appearance is a clean, sharply demarcated ulceration; **unlike ulcerated cancers**, the edges are only slightly elevated.

TREATMENT

If secondary to chronic NSAID use, the medication should be discontinued or limited. Misoprostol can be added to protect the mucosa if NSAIDs cannot be stopped. Lifestyle changes such as discontinuing alcohol and tobacco are also helpful if these are thought to contribute. Antibiotics should be administered if the patient is found to be infected with *H pylori*.

- One well-accepted current treatment recommendation is **clarithromycin + amoxicillin + proton pump inhibitor ± bismuth subsalicylate for 10–14 days.**
- For gastric ulcer, biopsy should be performed at the margin of the ulcer to rule out malignancy.

Zollinger-Ellison Syndrome

This syndrome is associated with multiple peptic ulcerations in the stomach and duodenum due to excess gastrin secretion by a gastrinoma, leading to excess gastric acid production.

Gastric Cancer

Gastric cancer is a malignant tumor that is the second most common cause of cancer-related death worldwide. Histologically, about 85% are adenocarcinomas, and the remaining 15% are lymphomas and leiomyosarcomas.

ADENOCARCINOMA

There are two types of gastric adenocarcinoma:

- **Intestinal type:** Thought to arise from the intestinal metaplasia of gastric mucosal cells. Lesions are typically ulcerative and occur in the antrum and lesser curvature (Figure 3-36). Risk factors are a diet high in salt and nitrates, *H pylori* colonization, and chronic gastritis.
- **Diffuse type:** Cells lack normal cohesion, resulting in an infiltrating, discrete mass in the stomach wall. They are more common in younger patients, involve all portions of the stomach, and result in decreased motility, hence, the term **linitis plastica**, or **"leather bottle,"** appearance.

PRIMARY GASTRIC LYMPHOMA

The stomach is the most common extranodal site for lymphoma formation, often associated with *H pylori* infection. Histology ranges from low-grade (mucosal-associated lymphoid tissue [MALT] lymphomas) to high-grade large-cell non-Hodgkin lymphomas.

PRESENTATION

- Asymptomatic until metastasis or incurable extensive growth has occurred. Patients with **advanced cancer** present with insidious upper abdominal pain, postprandial fullness, early satiety, weight loss, and nausea.
- Typically spreads locally to adjacent organs (direct extension to porta hepatis and transverse colon) and peritoneum.
- Metastases to the left supraclavicular lymph node produces palpable lymphadenopathy (**node of Virchow**).
- Hematogenous dissemination to the ovaries (**Krukenberg tumor:** Figure 3-37).

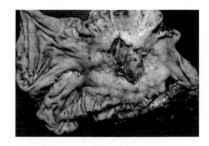

FIGURE 3-36. Gastric adenocarcinoma. Irregular ulcer with thickened rolled borders. (Reproduced with permission from USMLERx. com.)

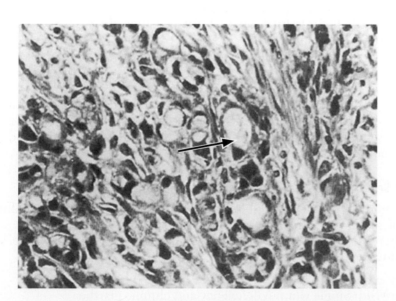

FIGURE 3-37. Primary "signet ring neoplasm" (*arrow* is pointing at classic signet ring cell) in mucosa. (Reproduced with permission from DeCherney AH, Nathan L. *Current Diagnosis & Treatment Obstetrics & Gynecology*, 10th ed. New York: McGraw-Hill, 2007: Figure 52-8.)

- **Sister Mary Joseph sign:** Metastatic mass that protrudes into the umbilicus producing a bulging palpable nodule.
- **Leser-Trélat sign:** Multiple outcroppings of seborrheic keratosis.

DIAGNOSIS

Double-contrast radiographic examination and CT scan imaging can identify very small lesions. Lack of distention is also a clue to diffuse-type gastric cancer. Definitive diagnosis is established based on biopsy.

TREATMENT

- Surgical resection of involved gastric tissue and adjacent lymph nodes, along with radiation and chemotherapy.
- *H pylori* antibiotic therapy is often enough to treat MALT lymphomas, but subtotal gastrectomy with chemotherapy and radiation is used for higher-grade lymphomas.

PROGNOSIS

- Prognosis for patients with **adenocarcinoma** is poor (5-year survival rate is 10–20%).
- Prognosis for patients with **primary gastric lymphoma** is somewhat better (5-year survival rate is 40–60%).

SMALL AND LARGE INTESTINE

Malabsorption Syndromes

This group of disorders is characterized by **decreased absorption,** most often in the small bowel, of essential nutrients. Patients can present with **chronic diarrhea** and/or **steatorrhea** (fatty stool) as well as with systemic effects, such as weight loss and specific vitamin and mineral deficiencies, particularly the **lipid-soluble vitamins A, D, E, and K.**

Underlying pathophysiologies include:

- Pancreatic insufficiency (exocrine deficiencies).
- Damage to the intestinal mucosal surface (surgical resection or pathologic insult to the intestinal villi).
- Liver deficiencies (inadequate bile salt production, abetalipoproteinemia).
- Decreased intestinal transit time (eg, after bariatric surgery).

The spectrum of malabsorption syndromes includes celiac sprue, lactate deficiency, Whipple disease, tropical sprue, short bowel syndrome, bacterial overgrowth syndrome, protein-losing enteropathy, pancreatic failure, and pernicious anemia.

CELIAC SPRUE (GLUTEN-SENSITIVE ENTEROPATHY)

Autoimmune entity with antibodies against the water-insoluble **gliadin** fraction of **gluten,** a protein found in wheat, barley, rye, and oats. Age at presentation varies, but it classically occurs in infants during the time of **cereal introduction.**

- Symptoms can be:
  - **Mild:** Single vitamin deficiency and chronic diarrhea.
  - **Severe:** Characteristic **chronic diarrhea** with steatorrhea and pale, bulky, foul-smelling stools; multiple vitamin and mineral deficiencies; weight loss; **growth retardation;** and **failure to thrive.**

- Associated with **dermatitis herpetiformis** (Figure 3-38).
- In 80–90% of cases, association with the human leukocyte antigens **(HLA)-B8** or **HLA-DW3.**
- **Classic pathohistologic findings:** Mucosal inflammation, villous atrophy (flattening), and crypt hyperplasia (Figure 3-39). Primarily affects the duodenum and jejunum.
- Can be diagnosed by identifying **antigliadin, antiendomysial,** or **anti–tissue transglutaminase** antibodies as well as a confirmatory small-bowel biopsy.
- **Treatment:** Elimination of gluten-containing foods from the diet is curative in 90% of cases. Remaining patients can be treated with steroids, which typically improve symptoms.

DISACCHARIDASE DEFICIENCY

- The most common entity involves **lactase (a brush border enzyme)** deficiency and presents as dairy intolerance. It is rare as an inborn error but is common during adulthood as the lactase present in the immature brush border disappears, thus causing **acquired lactose intolerance.** There are no intestinal changes.
- **Treatment:** Avoidance of offending disaccharide or administration of oral enzyme supplements such as lactase.

Whipple Disease

Malabsorptive syndrome with associated systemic symptoms secondary to infection by the gram-positive organism *Tropheryma whippelii.*

- **Symptoms:** Typical malabsorptive symptoms, such as weight loss and diarrhea, along with systemic signs of infection with fever, polyarthralgias, and abdominal pain. Can affect multiple organ systems, including the CNS.
- **Pathohistologic findings:** Distended lamina propria of the small intestine filled with distinctive **periodic acid-Schiff (PAS)-positive** macrophages with pale, foamy cytoplasm.
- *T whippelii* is best visualized with electron microscopy.
- **Treatment:** Antibiotics are necessary to eradicate the bacterial source. Drug of choice is ceftriaxone followed by oral double-strength **trimethoprim-sulfamethoxazole** for 1 year.

Other malabsorption syndromes (Table 3-16) include but are not limited to tropical sprue, **abetalipoproteinemia,** and **intestinal lymphangiectasia.**

Diverticular Disease

Diverticula can be either **congenital** (involving the entire thickness of the involved segment) or **acquired** (mucosal herniation through the muscular layer).

- **Diverticulosis** is the condition of having diverticula, typically implied as being colonic.
- **Diverticulitis** results when the diverticula in question become inflamed.

Meckel Diverticulum

Congenital true diverticulum (Figure 3-40) of the terminal ileum that results from incomplete closure of the **omphalomesenteric duct,** found in approximately 2% of the population, ~60 cm (2 ft) from the ileocecal valve, and normally 2 inches long. Mucosa can be ileal (50% of cases), **gastric,** pancreatic, duodenal, or colonic.

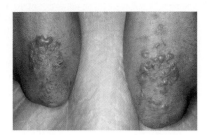

FIGURE 3-38. **Dermatitis herpetiformis seen in celiac sprue, manifested by pruritic, grouped vesicles in a typical location.** The vesicles are often excoriated and may occur on the knees, buttocks, and posterior scalp. (Reproduced with permission from Kasper DL, Braunwald E, Fauci AS, et al, eds. *Harrison's Principles of Internal Medicine,* 16th ed. New York: McGraw-Hill, 2005: 287.)

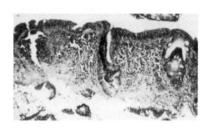

FIGURE 3-39. **Total villous atrophy in a case of celiac disease.** Note the flat surface epithelium without villi. The surface epithelium also appears more cuboidal, with less cytoplasmic mucin than is normal. The hypercellular appearance of the surface epithelium is due to the presence of numerous intraepithelial lymphocytes (visible only at higher magnification). (Reproduced with permission from Chandrasoma P, Taylor CR. *Concise Pathology,* 3rd ed. New York: McGraw-Hill, 2004.)

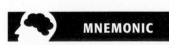

MNEMONIC

For Meckel diverticulum, remember the rule of 2s:
2 inches long
2% of the population
2 feet from the ileocecal valve
2% are symptomatic

TABLE 3-16. Overview of Malabsorption Syndromes

Syndrome	Morphology	Clinical Manifestations	Treatment
Celiac sprue	▪ Gluten-sensitive enteropathy. ▪ Biopsy: Mucosal. ▪ Inflammation, villous atrophy, and crypt hyperplasia. ▪ Can be diagnosed with anti-gliadin, anti-endomysial, or anti-tissue transglutaminase antibodies, as well as with biopsy.	Diarrhea, vitamin/mineral deficiency, **dermatitis herpetiformis** rash.	▪ Avoid gluten-containing foods such as wheat, barley, rye, and oats. ▪ Steroids (in ~10% of patients).
Tropical sprue	▪ Unknown occult tropical bacteria.	Diarrhea, steatorrhea, weight loss, **folate deficiency.**	**Tetracycline** for 6 months. Folic acid replacement.
Whipple disease	▪ Caused by gram-positive bacterium **Tropheryma whippelii.** ▪ Flat, blunt villi. ▪ Foamy **macrophages (PAS-positive),** found in lamina propria.	Fever, polyarthralgias, weight loss, diarrhea, abdominal pain.	**Trimethoprim-sulfamethoxazole** for 1 year.
Disaccharidase deficiency	Enzyme deficiency that causes malabsorption.	Chronic diarrhea.	Avoid offending foods.
Abetalipoproteinemia	Congenital lack of apolipoprotein-B; autosomal recessive.	Steatorrhea, acanthotic erythrocytes, serum lipid abnormalities, ataxia, atypical retinitis pigmentosa.	Medium-chain triglycerides, vitamin E and fat-soluble vitamins.
Intestinal lymphangiectasia	Ectatic lymphatics; either sporadic or secondary to cardiac disease.	▪ Nausea, vomiting, intermittent diarrhea, and occasionally steatorrhea. ▪ Peripheral edema from hypoalbuminemia.	Low-fat, high-protein, medium-chain triglyceride diet.

PAS = periodic acid-Schiff.

PRESENTATION

▪ Typically asymptomatic and discovered incidentally (patients are typically < 5 years of age).
▪ Patients can present with endocrine dysfunction due to gastric or pancreatic tissue hormonal production found in the Meckel diverticula.

DIAGNOSIS

▪ Abdominal pain and intestinal obstruction can result from intussusception or volvulus.
▪ **Bleeding** may result from mucosal ulcer formation in those with ectopic gastric tissue.
▪ If gastric mucosa is present, a **Meckel scan** may be performed by IV injection of **technetium-99** (^{99}Tc), which is taken up by parietal cells of the ectopic gastric mucosa.

TREATMENT

Once symptoms occur, surgical excision is curative.

Diverticulosis

Multiple acquired (**pulsion**) diverticula (Figure 3-41) found at the origin of a mesenchymal feeder artery and typically located in the sigmoid colon. It is thought to related to a low-fiber diet, which results in increased luminal pressure due to increased colonic muscular contractions required to move stool. Incidence increases with age in Western populations, occurring in almost 50% of adults > 50 years of age.

PRESENTATION

- Typically asymptomatic and discovered incidentally on colonoscopy, abdominal CT scan, or barium enema.
- Symptomatic patients can present with rectal bleeding or with anemia due to blood loss.

DIAGNOSIS

- Often discovered incidentally on colonoscopy.
- If patient presents with rectal bleeding or anemia, barium enema can be useful for diagnosis.

TREATMENT

- **High-fiber diets** are typically suggested in order to increase stool bulk and decrease colonic intraluminal pressure.

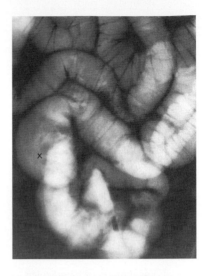

FIGURE 3-40. Smooth, saccular structure of the distal small bowel consistent with a Meckel diverticulum (x shows the diverticulum). Differential diagnosis: Benign ulcers of the small bowel are rare, and ulcerated malignancies are usually irregular in appearance. (Reproduced with permission from Chen MYM, Pope TL, Ott DJ. *Basic Radiology*. New York: McGraw-Hill, 2004: 266.)

> **KEY FACT**
>
> Diverticulosis is the most common cause of painless hematochezia in patients > 60 years old.

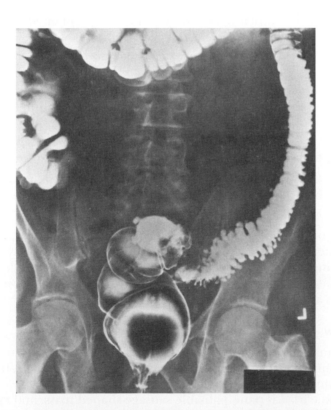

FIGURE 3-41. Diverticulosis of sigmoid colon on barium enema. (Reproduced with permission from Brunicardi FC, Andersen DK, Billiar TR, et al. *Schwartz's Principles of Surgery*, 8th ed. New York: McGraw-Hill, 2005: 1082.)

- Diverticular bleeding is managed with fluid repletion and transfusion as necessary. With most mild to moderate cases, bleeding resolves spontaneously (~80% of cases).
- Severe cases can be treated with vessel cauterization or clipping during colonoscopic visualization.
- **Mesenteric angiography** is both **diagnostic and therapeutic,** as vasoconstriction and artificial blood clot formation can be induced.

Diverticulitis

Most common complication of diverticulosis, due to infection thought to be secondary to an impacted **fecalith,** resulting in lymphatic obstruction and localized ischemia, which can lead to bacterial overgrowth. Abscess formation and perforation with peritonitis are serious complications of diverticulitis.

PRESENTATION

Patients with diverticulitis typically present with LLQ abdominal pain, guarding, or peritoneal signs (rebound tenderness), as well as **leukocytosis,** fecal leukocytes, and fever. Constipation or obstruction may develop secondary to localized swelling.

DIAGNOSIS

Care must be taken when obtaining imaging studies due to the risk of diverticular perforation during acute infection. Therefore, **barium enema** and **colonoscopy** are **contraindicated.**

- **Abdominal CT** scan can be used to assess for diverticular inflammation as well as pericolic abscess formation.
- An **upright abdominal plain film** should also be obtained to rule out free peritoneal air, which would suggest perforation.

TREATMENT

When there are no signs of perforation, treatment is bowel rest, pain management, fluid resuscitation, and **broad-spectrum antibiotics.** Surgery is required for signs of perforation as well as for drainage of large abscesses.

Intussusception

A condition that typically develops in children < 2 years of age as a result of distal "telescoping" of a portion of the proximal bowel into a more distal one (Figure 3-42). Most common at the **ileocecal junction.**

- The majority of pediatric cases are idiopathic, although there is a seasonal and clinical relationship to certain viral infections, particularly **rotavirus.**
- Remaining cases are secondary and occur when a proximal "lead point" is pulled into the distal segment by peristaltic contractions; most commonly found in adults, in which case cancer must be ruled out.

PRESENTATION

- Symptoms consist of sudden onset of episodic, crampy, severe abdominal pain lasting 10–20 minutes, followed by relatively symptom-free periods. Emesis and nausea can occur during these episodes.
- The classic triad is **pain, palpable sausage-shaped mass,** and **currant-jelly stools,** although all three symptoms are not typically present at the same time.

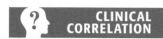

CLINICAL CORRELATION

Typical presentation of diverticulitis is similar to the symptoms of "left-sided appendicitis."

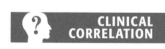

CLINICAL CORRELATION

Secondary causes of intussusception:
- Intestinal lymphomas
- Meckel diverticulum
- Vascular malformations
- Intestinal polyps

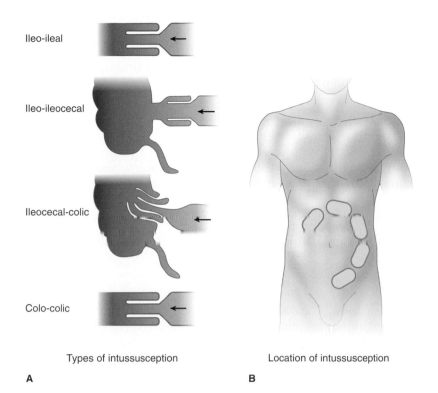

Ileo-ileal

Ileo-ileocecal

Ileocecal-colic

Colo-colic

Types of intussusception   Location of intussusception

A   B

FIGURE 3-42.   Diagram of the different possible types of intussusception. (A) The four types of intussusception: The enfolding of the lumen is in the direction of fecal flow, as shown by the arrows. (B) Locations: The usual sites of palpable masses are shown as sausage-shaped outlines; these are usually in the colon. (Reproduced with permission from LeBlond RF, Ge-Gowin RL, Brown DD. *DeGowin's Diagnostic Examination*, 9th ed. New York: McGraw-Hill, Figure 9-33.)

DIAGNOSIS

- Air contrast enemas are both **diagnostic and therapeutic** in most cases.
- On abdominal plain film, a filling defect in the large colon is diagnostic.
- Abdominal ultrasound can also be used to visualize the intussusception, revealing a **bull's-eye** or **coiled-spring** pattern due to invagination of the proximal segment.

TREATMENT

As mentioned, nonsurgical means are attempted first (**air contrast enema**). Surgery is indicated if enema fails or if perforation occurs.

Hirschsprung Disease (Congenital Megacolon)

Hirschsprung disease (HD) is characterized by **complete functional obstruction** of the large bowel due to the **absence of ganglion cells** of both the submucosal and myenteric neural plexuses.

- Aganglionic bowel **always** involves the **anus** and then progresses proximally to varying degrees (the most severe disease involves the entire colon and even some small intestine).
- Obstruction leads to the characteristic **dilation** of normal bowel proximal to the aganglionic segment, hence, the name **congenital megacolon.**
- Several **genetic mutations** have been associated with HD, the most common of which is the *RET* proto-oncogene.
- HD has also been associated with Down syndrome, Waardenburg syndrome, cardiac defects, and several other congenital conditions. HD occurs in about 1:5000 live births, with a male:female ratio of 3:1 or 4:1.

CLINICAL CORRELATION

Early differential diagnosis of HD includes cystic fibrosis, which may present similarly.

PRESENTATION

Typically manifests in a newborn as a **failure to pass meconium** within the first 48 hours of life. Other symptoms of bowel obstruction can be present, such as bilious vomiting and abdominal distention.

DIAGNOSIS

- Rectal biopsy is considered the gold standard for diagnosis and reveals the absence of ganglion cells in the rectal tissue.
- Barium enema can suggest the diagnosis and shows severe dilation of the proximal colon that abruptly narrows into the aganglionic distal colon.

TREATMENT

Surgical correction. The aganglionic section is resected, and the normal bowel is connected to the anus.

Omphalocele

Defect of the periumbilical abdominal wall allowing protrusion of a **membranous sac** of peritoneum into which the intestines herniate. The defect is **midline.** Associated with other congenital malformations (see Figure 3-1A).

TREATMENT

Surgery.

Gastroschisis

Defect of the abdominal wall **lateral of midline** that is **not covered** with peritoneum. Usually an isolated congenital defect (see Figure 3-1B).

TREATMENT

Surgery.

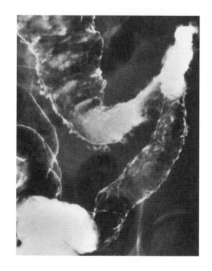

FIGURE 3-43.   Crohn disease. Segmental Crohn disease of the transverse and descending portions of the colon, showing multiple deep ulcers projecting from the margins of the affected colon, and small aphthoid ulcers appearing like erosions seen in the upper GI tract. (Reproduced with permission from Chen MYM, Pope TL, Ott DJ. *Basic Radiology.* New York: McGraw-Hill, 2004: 275.)

INFLAMMATORY DISEASES OF THE COLON

By definition, *colitis* is an inflammation of the colon. There are several causes; the most common are discussed below.

Crohn Disease (CD) and Ulcerative Colitis (UC)

These are two major idiopathic types of inflammatory bowel disease (IBD) (Figures 3-43 and 3-44).

PRESENTATION

UC and CD share many features resulting from bowel inflammation, including **diarrhea with blood or mucus, crampy abdominal pain,** fever, tenesmus, weight loss, and blood loss; however, they also differ in important ways, as listed in Table 3-17. Consider IBD or colon cancer in any patient with rectal bleeding and systemic signs.

DIAGNOSIS

Diagnosis is made by colonoscopy with biopsy specimen showing characteristic histologic findings.

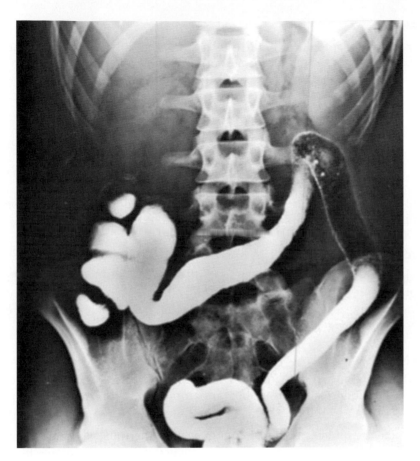

FIGURE 3-44. **Ulcerative colitis.** "Lead pipe" appearance on barium enema. (Reproduced with permission from George J. Chang, Andrew A. Shelton, Mark L. Welton. *Current Diagnosis and Treatment: Surgery*, 13th ed. New York: McGraw-Hill, 2010: Figure 30-17.)

TABLE 3-17. **Clinical and Pathologic Features of Crohn Disease and Ulcerative Colitis**

	CROHN DISEASE	**ULCERATIVE COLITIS**
POSSIBLE CAUSE	**INFECTIOUS**	**AUTOIMMUNE**
Location	May involve **any portion** of the GI tract (from mouth to anus), usually the terminal ileum and colon; **skip lesions,** with **rectal** sparing.	**Colitis** only occurs in the **large intestine; continuous lesions,** always with rectal involvement.
Gross morphology	**Transmural inflammation; cobblestone-like** mucosa, **creeping fat,** bowel wall thickening ("string sign" on barium swallow), linear ulcers, fissures, fistulas.	Mucosal and submucosal inflammation only; friable mucosal pseudopoylps with freely hanging mesentery.
Microscopic morphology	**Noncaseating granulomas** and lymphoid aggregates.	Crypt abscesses and ulcers, bleeding, **no granulomas.**
Complications	Strictures, fistulas, perianal disease, malabsorption, nutritional depletion.	Severe stenosis, toxic megacolon, **colorectal carcinoma.**
Extraintestinal manifestations	Migratory polyarthritis, erythema nodosum, ankylosing spondylitis, uveitis, immunologic disorders.	Pyoderma gangrenosum, primary sclerosing cholangitis.

TREATMENT

The medical treatment for both IBDs is similar and includes **anti-inflammatory** (sulfasalazine for milder forms; corticosteroids and azathioprine for more severe cases), **antidiarrheal,** and **antibiotic** medications.

PROGNOSIS

Surgical therapy (**colectomy**):

- In patients with uncontrolled UC, colectomy is **curative.**
- In patients with CD, surgery is **not curative** but is required to manage complications in 70% of patients.
- Both types of IBD are associated with an increased risk of colon cancer; this risk is higher in UC.

Pseudomembranous Colitis

Pseudomembranous colitis is an acute inflammation of the colon mediated by overgrowth of *Clostridium difficile.* Typically, this is precipitated by a course of antibiotics (classically, ampicillin, clindamycin, or a cephalosporin) that clears the normal colonic bacterial flora (*E coli* and *Bacteroides fragilis*).

PRESENTATION

Symptoms are due to the *C difficile* toxins. A and B toxins attack the colonic mucosa, leading to hypermotility, inflammation, and increased capillary permeability.

- Typical symptoms include frequent watery diarrhea, abdominal pain or cramping, and fever. It can also be associated with occult colonic bleeding.
- In severe cases, the colonic mucosa becomes covered with yellow or gray exudates, hence the term **pseudomembranous colitis** (Figure 3-45). This can lead to toxic megacolon, volvulus, or colonic perforation, all of which can be life threatening.

DIAGNOSIS

A stool sample is tested for the A and B toxins of *C difficile.*

TREATMENT

The first step in treating pseudomembranous colitis is stopping the inciting antibiotic.

- **Antidiarrheal agents** such as loperamide are **contraindicated,** as they will prolong production of toxins in the colon, thus worsening the condition.
- *C difficile* infection can be treated with metronidazole (first-line) or oral vancomycin.

Infectious Colitis

Infectious causes of colitis can be viral, bacterial, or parasitic. Patients with infectious colitis typically present with severe diarrhea, fever, leukocytosis, and abdominal pain. Clues in the history may include travel, recent antibiotic use, specific food consumption, and immunodeficiency. Review specific organisms in the microbiology section. (See Table 3-18 for common causes of infective diarrhea).

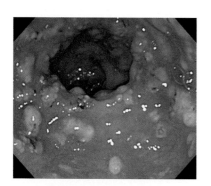

FIGURE 3-45. Pseudomembranous colitis with yellow pseudomembranes. (Image courtesy of Samir.)

TABLE 3-18. Causes of Diarrhea

CAUSES OF BLOODY DIARRHEA	CAUSES OF WATERY DIARRHEA
Campylobacter	Vibrio cholerae
Salmonella	Clostridium perfringens
Shigella	Giardia
Enterohemorrhagic Escherichia coli (EHEC)	Cryptosporidium (in immunocompromised)
Enteroinvasive E coli (EIEC)	Enterotoxigenic E coli (ETEC)
Yersinia	Viruses (rotavirus, Norwalk, adenovirus)
C difficile	
Entamoeba histolytica	

Typhoid Fever

Salmonella typhi is the agent responsible for typhoid fever, the symptoms of which include bacteremia, splenomegaly, and even liver necrosis, as well as ulceration of Peyer patches with intestinal bleeding and ulceration. If the gallbladder is colonized, the individual becomes a carrier. **Rose spots,** a classic rash on the skin, are pathognomonic.

Entamoeba histolytica

Entamoeba histolytica is a dysentery-causing protozoan parasite (Figure 3-46). Amebae invade the crypts of colonic glands and burrow down into the submucosa. The organisms fan out laterally, creating **flask-shaped ulcers.** They can penetrate the portal venous system and spread to the liver, where they may form abscesses. Diagnosis is by stool ova and parasites or stool *E histolytica* antigen.

Giardia lamblia

Giardia lamblia is an intestinal protozoan that attaches to the small intestinal mucosa but does not appear to invade. Therefore, fecal leukocyte tests are negative. Associated with greasy, fatty stools and foul-smelling flatulence. Diagnosis is by *Giardia* antigen stool testing. Treatment is metronidazole.

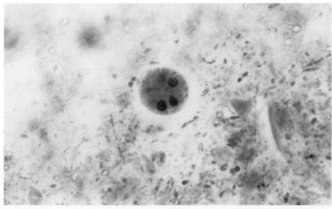
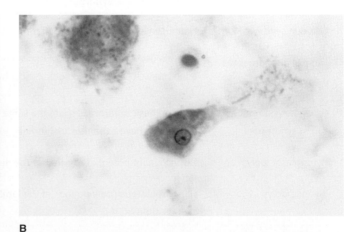

A   B

FIGURE 3-46. ***Entamoeba histolytica* cyst (A) showing three of the four nuclei, and trophozoite (B) demonstrating a single nucleus with a central, dot-like nucleolus.** (Reproduced with permission from Fauci AS, Braunwald E, Kasper DL, et al, eds. *Harrison's Principles of Internal Medicine,* 17th ed. New York: McGraw-Hill, 2008: 1215.)

Cryptosporidia

Cryptosporidiosis leads to diarrhea in immunocompromised people and is a potentially fatal complication of AIDS.

TUMORS OF THE COLON

Benign Polyps

These polyps are common after the age of 40 and have extremely low potential for malignancy (see Table 3-19 for types of polyps).

- **Hyperplastic polyps** are the most common type of benign polyp.
- **Juvenile polyps** are hamartomatous proliferations of the lamina propria enclosing widely spaced, dilated cystic glands. Usually seen in children < 5 years old but can be diagnosed at any age.
- **Other types** include mucosal polyps, submucosal polyps, inflammatory pseudopolyps, and other types of hamartomatous polyps.

Adenomatous Polyps

By definition, adenomatous polyps are dysplastic and therefore are potentially malignant. There are three subtypes:

- **Tubular** adenomas are the most common of the three. On gross examination, they have a stalk connected to the bowel and a head that is free in the lumen.
- **Tubulovillous** polyps are so named because they have characteristics of both tubular and villous adenomas; they have an intermediate rate of malignant conversion.
- **Villous** adenomas have the **highest rate of malignant conversion.** Histologically, they have a cauliflower-like appearance with fingerlike villi extending down into the center of the polyp.

Multiple Polyposis Syndromes

Several genetic disorders can cause multiple colonic polyps, usually at young ages. Polyps and tumors typically arise in the proximal (right-sided) colon.

TABLE 3-19. Types of Colonic Polyps and Syndromes

Cowden syndrome	Hamartomatous polyps in the GI tract. Increased risk of neoplasms of the thyroid, breast, uterus, and skin.
Familial adenomatous polyposis (FAP)	Patients develop 500–2500 colonic adenomas that carpet the mucosal surface. Most polyps are tubular adenomas. 100% risk of colonic cancer by midlife. Increased risk of duodenal cancer.
Gardner syndrome and Turcot syndrome	Both of these syndromes share the same APC genetic defect as FAP, but differ in one regard: these two syndromes have extraintestinal tumors, whereas FAP does not.
Hyperplastic polyp	No malignant potential. Formed as the result of abnormal mucosal maturation, inflammation, or architecture.
Juvenile polyp	Hamartomatous proliferations of the lamina propria enclosing widely spaced, dilated cystic glands. Usually seen in children < 5 y.
Peutz-Jeghers syndrome	Hamartomatous polyps and melanotic mucosal and cutaneous pigmentation.

APC = adematous polyposis coli.

FAMILIAL ADENOMATOUS POLYPOSIS (FAP)

Autosomal dominant genetic disorder caused by a mutation in the adenomatous polyposis coli (APC) gene. Those affected have numerous precancerous and cancerous colon polyps (Figure 3-47) in the second or third decade of life; the diagnosis is confirmed if more than 100 colorectal polyps are found. Virtually 100% of affected patients develop colorectal cancer. Prophylactic total colectomy is therefore indicated even during childhood or early adulthood.

GARDNER SYNDROME

Autosomal dominant genetic disorder characterized by multiple adenomatous colon polyps in conjunction with other extraintestinal tumors, including osteomas, hepatoblastomas, papillary thyroid carcinoma, and periampullary adenomas.

TURCOT SYNDROME

Autosomal recessive disorder that causes colonic polyps and tumors of the central nervous system, especially glioblastoma multiforme and medulloblastoma.

HEREDITARY NONPOLYPOSIS COLORECTAL CANCER (HNPCC)

Autosomal dominant disorder that causes colorectal adenomas and colorectal cancer. A mutation in a **DNA mismatch repair gene (*hMLH1* or *hMSH2*)** is thought to be the cause of the disease. HNPCC has also been classified as part of Lynch I or Lynch II syndrome. Lynch II syndrome is also associated with extracolonic tumors (endometrium, ovary, and pancreas).

PEUTZ-JEGHERS SYNDROME

Autosomal dominant disorder characterized by a combination of hamartomatous colon polyps and **mucocutaneous hyperpigmented lesions** on the lips (Figure 3-48), oral mucosa, hands, and genitals. The colon polyps rarely become cancerous, but they can cause symptoms such as obstruction, pain, and bleeding. Those affected have a higher likelihood of cancer in the stomach, breast, and ovaries.

Colorectal Cancer

Histologically, colorectal cancer is **adenocarcinoma of the large intestine or rectum (or both)**. It is the third most common cancer, as well as the second leading cause of cancer-related death in both men and women in the United States.

- **Risk factors** include advanced age, family history, low-fiber diet, villous adenomas, IBD (especially UC), FAP, Peutz-Jeghers syndrome, juvenile nonpolyposis, and HNPCC.
- **Screening** should start at age 50 with colonoscopy every 10 years and fecal occult blood with rectal exam testing every year. Flexible sigmoidoscopy can be used instead of colonoscopy but must be done at least every 5 years.
- Colon cancer typically arises from dysplastic adenomas in the colon. Research shows that, over time, underlying genetic mutations along with environmental influences **(two-hit hypothesis)** lead to the stepwise conversion of normal colonic epithelium to dysplastic adenomas and, finally, to malignant adenocarcinoma **(adenoma-carcinoma sequence;** Figure 3-49).

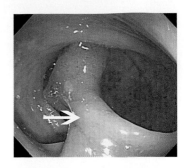

FIGURE 3-47. Pedunculated colon polyp on a thick stalk covered with normal mucosa (*arrow*). (Reproduced with permission from Fauci AS, Kasper DL, Braunwald E, et al, eds. *Harrison's Principles of Internal Medicine*, 17th ed. New York: McGraw-Hill, 2008: Figure 285-5.)

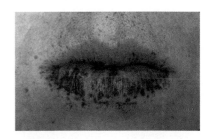

FIGURE 3-48. Peutz-Jehgers syndrome. (Image courtesy of Uniformed Services University of the Health Sciences.)

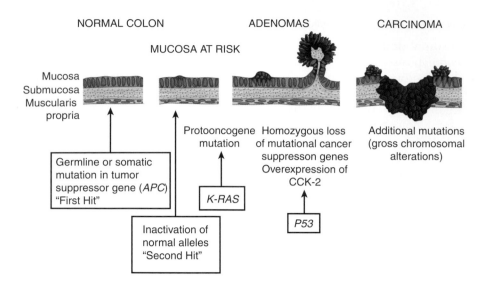

FIGURE 3-49. **Adenoma-carcinoma sequence.** The development of carcinoma from adenomatous lesions is referred to as the adenoma-carcinoma sequence.

KEY FACT

Mutated *RAS* remains in an activated state, continuously delivering mitotic signals and thus preventing apoptosis.

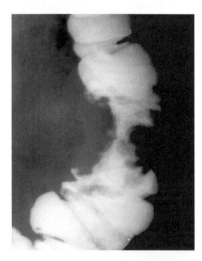

FIGURE 3-50. **Annular, constricting adenocarcinoma of the descending colon.** This radiographic appearance is referred to as an "apple-core" lesion and is always highly suggestive of malignancy. (Reproduced with permission from Kasper DL, Braunwald E, Fauci AS, eds. *Harrison's Principles of Internal Medicine*, 16th ed. New York: McGraw-Hill, 2005: 530.)

- The most common mutations are in the **APC** gene, which occur **early** in the development of colon cancer, and in the *p53* gene, which occur **later**. Many other gene mutations, including of the **K-RAS** gene, have been implicated and occur at various stages in the development of cancer.

PRESENTATION

Colon cancer typically occurs in adults > 50.

- **Left-sided (sigmoid) colon cancer:**
  - **Early** symptoms of **obstruction** (the left side has a narrower lumen).
  - Tumors produce a **"napkin-ring,"** or **"apple-core"** constriction (encircling annular growth; Figure 3-50).
  - May complain of a change in bowel habits.
- **Right-sided colon cancer:**
  - **Anemia,** weight loss, and abdominal **pain.**
  - Tumors look like **cauliflower** (polypoid or fungating appearance).
  - Stool is watery in the right colon; thus, obstruction seldom occurs.
- **Either side:**
  - Stool changes (melena, hematochezia, pencil-thin-caliber stools).
  - Abdominal discomfort.
  - Constitutional symptoms such as weight loss, night sweats, fever.
  - Unexplained anemia in men and postmenopausal women—think colon cancer.

DIAGNOSIS

- Colonoscopy with tissue biopsy revealing adenocarcinoma is the gold standard for diagnosis. Once the diagnosis is made, CT scans are done to look for metastases.
- **Carcinoembryonic antigen (CEA)** is not recommended as a diagnostic serum marker for colon cancer; however, it can be very useful in evaluating the success of surgical resection, as well as in monitoring the growth or recurrence of the cancer.

TREATMENT

Surgical resection and chemotherapy (usually involving fluorouracil) are the most common treatments.

- Colon cancer can **metastasize hematogenously** as well as through the **lymphatics.**
- The most common sites of **metastasis** are the regional lymph nodes, **liver,** lungs, and peritoneum; other possible sites for metastases are the bones and brain.

PROGNOSIS

Depends on the stage of the tumor at diagnosis. Favorable when the cancer is detected early, before metastasis has occurred. Once widespread, the 5-year survival rate drops to < 10%.

Carcinoid Tumors

Small, slow-growing neoplasm arising from neuroendocrine cells along the GI tract, which release a variety of humoral substances. This can result in carcinoid syndrome if the tumor metastasizes to or past the liver (the liver can no longer clear the hormones if this occurs).

PRESENTATION

Carcinoid syndrome: Wheezing, flushing, diarrhea, and right-sided valvular lesions.

DIAGNOSIS

High urine levels of 5-HIAA (serotonin metabolite).

TREATMENT

Surgical excision is curative if tumor is small. Octreotide can be used for symptomatic treatment.

APPENDICITIS

Appendicitis is the most common indication for emergency abdominal surgery in children, but it can occur in all age groups, with peak ages 15–30 years.

PRESENTATION

Classic presentation is fever and periumbilical abdominal pain, later localizing to the right lower quadrant (**McBurney point**), accompanied by signs of peritoneal irritation (rebound tenderness, rigidity, guarding). Anorexia, vomiting, constipation, and diarrhea may also be present.

DIAGNOSIS

Diagnosis is **clinical.** It is better to take out a healthy appendix than to let one rupture. Testing is only done on stable patients with a questionable diagnosis.

- Leukocytosis, pyuria, and fecal leukocytes are the most common laboratory findings. Pregnancy testing is helpful on premenopausal women to rule out ectopic pregnancy.
- Abdominal CT is generally diagnostic and should be performed in equivocal cases.

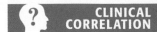

CLINICAL CORRELATION

CEA can be elevated in other conditions:

- **Malignant:** Cancers of the pancreas, stomach, breast, lung, and certain types of thyroid and ovarian cancers.
- **Other:** Chemotherapy and radiation therapy may lead to temporary elevation of CEA (massive death of tumor cells releases CEA into the circulation).

FLASH BACK

McBurney point is located two-thirds of the distance from the anterior superior iliac spine to the umbilicus.

TREATMENT

Surgical appendectomy is necessary and curative. There is a 40% rate of perforation in the pediatric population, but the mortality rate is < 1%.

ABDOMINAL HERNIAS

Hernias are abnormal protrusions of the abdominal contents through a defect in the abdominal wall.

The **hernial mass** consists of three parts: covering tissues (formed by layers of the abdominal wall), a peritoneal sac, and any structure (including viscera) contained within the abdominal cavity.

Hernias are described as reducible, irreducible, or strangulated (Table 3-20).

- **Reducible:** Most common type, usually painless. The abdominal contents can be easily returned to the abdomen.
- **Irreducible (incarcerated):** Difficult to return the contents to the abdominal cavity. Can become painful if bowel is obstructed or incarcerated.
- **Strangulated:** The entrapped organ (usually bowel, sometimes fat) becomes incarcerated in the fascial defect, resulting in compromised blood supply. Strangulated hernias are intensely painful and very dangerous due to bowel obstruction and possible necrosis. They require immediate surgical repair.

PRESENTATION

- **Inguinal hernias:** Most common type; more often seen in **men.** With a direct hernia, there is herniation of abdominal contents through floor of Hesselbach triangle. With indirect hernias, there is herniation of abdominal contents through the internal and then external inguinal rings. Treatment is surgical. Patients may complain of a painless bulge in the inguinal region that is exacerbated by increased intra-abdominal pressure (ie, coughing, straining with defecation, lifting weight). Patients may also have a feeling of heaviness in the groin.
- **Femoral hernias:** More often seen in **women.** Patients frequently present with a palpable lump medial to the femoral pulse and inferior to the ingui-

> **KEY FACT**
>
> Hesselbach (inguinal) triangle: A site of direct inguinal hernias:
> - Rectus abdominis muscle (medial)
> - Inguinal ligament (inferior)
> - Inferior epigastric blood vessels (superior and lateral)

TABLE 3-20. Causes of the Most Common Abdominal Hernias

HERNIA TYPE	CAUSE	LOCATION
Indirect inguinal hernia	Congenital weakness in the fascial margin of the internal inguinal ring (patent processus vaginalis).	Originate lateral to the inferior epigastric vessels.
Direct inguinal hernia	Congenital or acquired weakness in the fascia of the inguinal canal floor.	Originate medial to the inferior epigastric vessels (above and medial to the pubic tubercle).
Femoral hernia	Weakness of the femoral septum, allowing protrusion of the hernial sac through the femoral canal within the femoral sheath.	Originate below and lateral to the pubic tubercle.
Umbilical	Congenital (eg, infants) or acquired (eg, multiparous women) abnormality in the musculature around the umbilical cord.	Originate at the umbilicus.
Incisional	Acquired as a postoperative complication.	Originate at surgical incision sites.

nal ligament. These hernias have a tendency to become incarcerated or strangulated because of the relatively small area of the femoral ring and the presence of unyielding anatomic structures (eg, sharp free edge of the lacunar ligament). Consequently, these hernias can be painful and require prompt surgical repair.

- **Umbilical hernias:** Often present in **infants** or **children** due to congenital defects in the abdominal wall at the umbilicus. In adults, umbilical hernias are more common in multiparous women and patients with comorbid medical conditions that cause chronically increased abdominal pressure (ie, chronic cough, chronic obstructive pulmonary disease [COPD], ascites). Patients usually complain of a bulge at the umbilicus that worsens on Valsalva maneuver. Pain may be present if bowel becomes incarcerated or strangulated. Severe pain and erythema of the skin suggest necrosis of underlying bowel and warrants immediate surgical repair.

DIAGNOSIS

Based on clinical symptoms and physical exam.

- A **direct inguinal** hernia bulge should be felt on either side of the finger, and the **indirect inguinal** hernia bulge should be felt on the tip of the finger.
- **Femoral** hernias can often be palpated medial to the femoral pulse and inferior to the inguinal ring.
- CT scan or ultrasound may be necessary with patients who have hernias that are not easily palpable (ie, obese patients).

TREATMENT

Surgical repair (herniorraphy).

HEPATOBILIARY SYSTEM

Jaundice

Patients with jaundice often present with yellowed skin or sclera that represents an underlying increase in serum bilirubin (Table 3-21).

- **Physiologic jaundice:** Extremely common (50% of newborns). A condition in **neonates** that results from the relative deficiency in glucuronyl transferase in the immature liver in newborns. They also have a large red cell mass with a shorter cellular life span.
- **Hemolysis** resulting from mild trauma during the birth process can exacerbate the condition by increasing bilirubin production.
- **Adult jaundice:** A pathologic process due to overproduction (eg, hemolysis) or impaired excretion (eg, bile duct obstruction, hepatocellular dysfunction) of bilirubin.

PRESENTATION

- Scleral icterus typically appears first, generally at serum bilirubin levels > 3 mg/dL. Yellowing of the skin is seen at even higher levels of serum bilirubin.
- **Newborns:** Jaundice present **at birth** is **pathologic and is often due to an inherited hyperbilirubinemia.** In contrast, **physiologic jaundice** of the newborn is clinically benign and occurs **48–72 hours following birth.** Bilirubin levels rise at < 5 mg/dL/day and peak at < 15 mg/dL. Direct bilirubin comprises < 10% of the total.

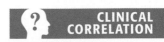

MNEMONIC

Both indirect and direct hernias occur in the inguinal canal.
INdirect hernias are **IN** the **IN**ternal ring and spermatic cord and commonly occur in **IN**fants.

CLINICAL CORRELATION

By far, the most common cause of jaundice in adults is choledocholithiasis, gallstones lodged in the biliary tree.

TABLE 3-21.   Jaundice: Underlying Causes

JAUNDICE	DISEASES	SERUM BILIRUBIN	URINE BILIRUBIN	URINE UROBILINOGEN

Conjugated	Hepatocellular disease:
	  Dubin-Johnson syndrome: Inherited defect in liver excretion of
	    bilirubin that leads to a glossy black liver
	  Rotor syndrome: Defect in hepatic storage of conjugated
	    bilirubin, without a black liver
	Physical obstruction of the bile duct by:
	  Gallstones
	  Tumors, especially pancreatic tumors
	  Primary sclerosing cholangitis (PSC)
	  Parasites
		↑ Direct bilirubin
		(> 15%)
			↑	Normal

Unconjugated	Hemolytic diseases:
	  Sickle cell
	  Glucose-6-phosphate dehydrogenase deficiency
	  Spherocytosis
	  Microangiopathic hemolytic anemia
	  Paroxysmal nocturnal hemoglobinuria
	  ABO/Rh isoimmunization
	  Autoimmune hemolytic anemia (warm and cold)
	Inherited hepatocellular diseases:
	  Crigler-Najjar type 1: Absent UDP-glucuronyl transferase
	  Crigler-Najjar type 2: Less severe and responds to
	    phenobarbital, which induces hepatic enzymes, including
	    UDP-glucuronyl transferase
	  Gilbert syndrome: Transient decrease in the activity of UDP
	    glucuronyl transferase, which causes asymptomatic rise in
	    indirect bilirubin, associated with stress; common, affecting
	    about 5% of the population
	Acquired hepatocellular disease:
	  Cirrhosis
	  Hepatitis
	  Drugs (ie, steroids, rifampin, probenecid, ribavirin)
	  Liver failure (ie, sepsis)
		↑ Indirect
		bilirubin
			Absent
			(acholuria)
				↑ (from heme
				metabolism)

UDP = uridine diphosphate.

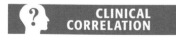

CLINICAL CORRELATION

Other common clinical entities are tumors (especially pancreatic) and liver failure.

DIAGNOSIS

The **most important step** in diagnosis is determining if the jaundice is secondary to conjugated (direct) or unconjugated (indirect) hyperbilirubinemia (Figure 3-51).

- **Direct** hyperbilirubinemia is always pathologic.
- **Indirect** hyperbilirubinemia may be physiologic or pathologic.

TREATMENT

Address the underlying condition. Physiologic jaundice of the newborn typically resolves with normal maturation and breast-feeding/hydration within 1–2

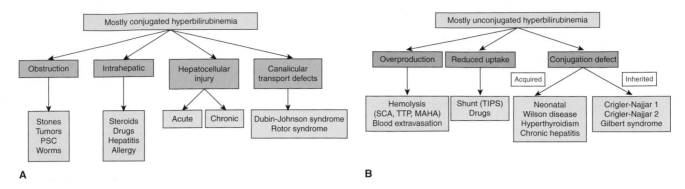

FIGURE 3-51. **Differential diagnosis for elevation of (A) direct and (B) indirect bilirubin.** PSC, primary sclerosing cholangitis; MAHA, microangiopathic hemolytic anemia; TIPS, transjugular intrahepatic portosystemic shunt; TTP, thrombotic thrombocytopenic purpura; SCA, sickle cell anemia.

weeks. More severe cases of unconjugated hyperbilirubinemia in the newborn can be treated with phototherapy, or exposure to blue-green light. The light converts bilirubin to its photoisomer, which is water-soluble and therefore easier to excrete. Prior to development of phototherapy, newborns with severe unconjugated hyperbilirubinemia were at risk of developing **kernicterus,** permanent neurologic damage from bilirubin crossing the blood-brain barrier, which is not yet fully formed in neonates.

Hereditary Hyperbilirubinemias

Rare conditions that can be differentiated by the predominant form of bile acids (conjugated or unconjugated) present in the bloodstream.

Hereditary Causes of Direct (Conjugated) Hyperbilirubinemia

DUBIN-JOHNSON SYNDROME

Rare inherited **autosomal recessive** condition caused by impaired intrahepatic bilirubin secretion.

- The absence of the canalicular protein **multidrug-resistant protein 2 (MRP-2)** impairs transport of conjugated bilirubin and other non–bile acid organic anions into the bile canaliculus.
- Grossly, the **liver** appears **pigmented and often enlarged,** but is functionally normal.

PRESENTATION

Mostly asymptomatic, but may present with chronic or recurrent jaundice of varying intensity.

DIAGNOSIS

- Elevated serum direct bilirubin
- Normal CBC
- Normal liver enzymes
- Grossly black liver on biopsy

TREATMENT

No treatment is usually necessary. Individuals with this disorder have a normal life expectancy.

ROTOR SYNDROME

Similar to Dubin-Johnson syndrome, but now known to be a separate disorder. In Rotor syndrome, defects occur in the hepatic storage of conjugated bilirubin, which causes it to leak out. Grossly, however, the **liver appears normal.**

Hereditary Causes of Indirect (Unconjugated) Hyperbilirubinemia

GILBERT SYNDROME

- Benign inherited condition causing mild, intermittent indirect hyperbilirubinemia. Present in approximately 5% of the population.
- Caused by transient reduction in hepatic glucuronyl transferase activity to about one-third normal levels, leading to a decrease in bile conjugation.

PRESENTATION

Usually an incidental finding in an otherwise healthy adolescent or young adult male (male-to-female predominance 2–7:1); manifests as **mild jaundice** during **periods of stress,** such as concurrent illness, strenuous exercise, or fasting.

DIAGNOSIS

- Elevated serum indirect bilirubin (usually two to three times normal, almost always < 6 mg/dL).
- Normal CBC.
- Normal liver enzymes.

TREATMENT

No treatment necessary; reassurance only.

CRIGLER-NAJJAR SYNDROME (TYPE 1)

Rare autosomal recessive genetic condition. Type 1 is the more severe form and is caused by a **complete lack of hepatic glucuronyl transferase, the enzyme responsible for conjugation of indirect to direct bilirubin.** On gross inspection, the liver appears normal.

PRESENTATION

Suspect in **neonates** presenting with severe **jaundice at birth.** Due to the complete lack of glucuronyl transferase, bile is colorless and contains only traces of unconjugated bilirubin.

DIAGNOSIS

Severe jaundice and icterus in a newborn with severely elevated serum indirect bilirubin (> **30 times normal values).**

TREATMENT

- Aggressive treatment with phototherapy and exchange transfusions in the immediate neonatal period.
- Heme oxygenase inhibitors, which inhibit the breakdown of heme, and cholestyramine.
- Liver transplant prior to onset of brain damage.
- Patients **do not** respond to **phenobarbital.**
- Fatal within 18 months after birth if untreated (due to severe kernicterus).

CRIGLER-NAJJAR SYNDROME (TYPE 2)

Less severe than type 1, a nonfatal disorder caused by a **partial lack of hepatic glucuronyl transferase.** As with type 1, the liver is morphologically normal.

PRESENTATION

Suspect in **neonates** presenting with severe **jaundice at birth.** Babies have strikingly yellow skin due to high levels of unconjugated bilirubin.

DIAGNOSIS

Severe jaundice in a newborn and severely elevated serum indirect bilirubin.

TREATMENT

Phototherapy; patients respond to phenobarbital.

PROGNOSIS

Can lead to neurologic damage due to kernicterus if untreated. Excellent prognosis if treated; patients develop normally.

Infectious Hepatitis

Infectious hepatitis is caused by five distinct viruses. They cause a range of illnesses, from benign, self-limited disease to fulminant liver failure to chronic infections that progress to cirrhosis and death. See Table 3-22 for further information.

Alcoholic Hepatitis

Alcoholic hepatitis is due to reversible inflammatory liver damage caused by a high level of alcohol consumption over time and is the most common cause of cirrhotic liver disease in most Western countries. Genetic and environmental factors both play an important role in the pathophysiology of this disease.

TABLE 3-22. **Types of Viral Hepatitis**

	ROUTE OF TRANSMISSION	PROGNOSIS	UNIQUE CHARACTERISTICS
Hepatitis A	Contaminated food/water (fecal-oral)	Self-limited illness, usually benign.	Does not cause a carrier state.
Hepatitis B	All bodily fluids apart from stool (parenteral)	Acute illness with possible fulminant liver failure, can progress to a chronic symptomatic or asymptomatic state.	Can be transmitted from mother to child.
Hepatitis C	Blood transfusions, occupational exposure, IV drug use (parenteral), sexual transmission (rare)	Can progress to chronic infection and cirrhosis.	Concurrent alcohol use accelerates the progression of disease.
Hepatitis D	Must be encapsulated with the hepatitis B surface antigen to replicate (parenteral)		In the United States, mostly found among IV drug users.
Hepatitis E	Contaminated water (fecal-oral)		A high rate of mortality among pregnant women.

Direct toxicity from ethanol and its metabolites, in addition to oxidative damage, disrupt the function of cell and mitochondrial membranes, thus leading to lipid accumulation.

PRESENTATION

Can be asymptomatic in its mildest form or can present with fulminant hepatic failure and death in its most severe form.

- **Classic presentation:** Nausea, malaise, tachycardia, and low-grade fever in an individual with a history of heavy alcohol use.
- **Patients with concomitant hepatic failure or portal hypertension:** Ascites, significant hematemesis from ruptured esophageal varices, especially with a history of vomiting, or evidence of encephalopathy, such as asterixis and altered mental status. Right upper quadrant (RUQ) tenderness and hepatomegaly may be noted on physical exam.

DIAGNOSIS

Clinical diagnosis can be made based on presentation and history of alcohol abuse.

- **Lab tests** reveal elevated aspartate aminotransferase (AST) and alanine aminotransferase (ALT) in a ratio of 2:1, elevated alkaline phosphatase (ALP), and prolonged prothrombin time (PT).
- **Histology** (Figure 3-52): Steatosis, neutrophilic infiltrate, centrilobular balloon necrosis of hepatocytes, and eosinophilic inclusion bodies known as Mallory bodies. Eventually, alcoholic hepatitis leads to irreversible fibrosis.

TREATMENT

Alcoholic steatosis and hepatitis can be reversible if the patient is able to achieve abstinence from alcohol, the most important goal of treatment.

- **Immediate treatment** should include nutritional support with calories, fluids, vitamins (especially thiamine and folate) and minerals as well as close monitoring for signs of alcohol withdrawal. Seizures and other symptoms of withdrawal can be fatal if left untreated.
- **Vitamin K** should be given to reverse the coagulopathy that may result from underproduction of clotting factors in liver failure.
- A 4-week course of **prednisolone** may benefit patients with severe forms of the disease.

PROGNOSIS

If alcohol abuse continues, the patient risks progression to cirrhosis, which carries a much poorer prognosis.

Reye Syndrome

Reye syndrome is a rare childhood hepatoencephalopathy. The pathogenesis is thought to be damage to mitochondria caused by **salicylate (aspirin)** metabolites or some other toxin in the milieu of a viral infection or underlying mitochondrial polymorphism, although cases also occur in the absence of salicylate use.

Mitochondrial dysfunction leads to elevation of short-chain fatty acids and hyperammonemia as well as cerebral edema.

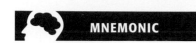

MNEMONIC

A Scotch and Tonic:
Alcoholic hepatitis: **AST** >> ALT
Viral hepatitis: **AST** << ALT

KEY FACT

A mildly elevated AST may be the only laboratory abnormality in mild cases.

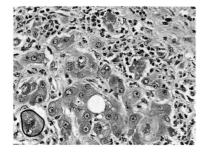

FIGURE 3-52. Microscopic features of alcoholic hepatitis. Alcoholic hepatitis characterized by single or focal cell swelling (*ballooning, outlined cell*) and cellular necrosis, as well as the presence of eosinophilic cytoplasmic inclusions known as Mallory bodies (*asterisk*). (Reproduced with permission from USMLERx. com.)

PRESENTATION

Vomiting, lethargy, drowsiness, and progressive stupor, often preceded by upper respiratory infection (eg, influenza A or B or varicella) combined with **salicylate** use. Signs of increased intracranial pressure, such as hypercapnea, irregular respirations, and sluggish pupils, may also be present.

DIAGNOSIS

- Lab findings reflect liver damage and include:
  - Elevated **AST**
  - **Hyperammonemia**
  - Normal or slightly elevated **bilirubin**
  - Prolonged **PT**
- Histology of the liver shows diffuse microvesicular steatosis (nucleus is not dislocated) with **large, pleomorphic mitochondria.**

TREATMENT

Generally supportive. If cerebral edema is controlled, the liver usually is able to regenerate. **Intracranial pressure** is managed with hyperventilation, mannitol, and barbiturates.

PROGNOSIS

At least 70% of patients survive, and the prognosis is related to the depth of coma and peak ammonia levels. Patients should be screened for fatty acid metabolism defects and should not be given aspirin.

Cirrhosis and Portal Hypertension

Cirrhosis is an **irreversible scarring** of the liver that occurs after years of chronic insult. In essence, cirrhosis is **chronic liver damage,** characterized by complete disarray of the hepatic cytoarchitecture, with progressive scarring (generalized fibrosis) and typical "regenerative" nodule formation. Morphologically (Figure 3-53), it can be divided into:

- **Micronodular cirrhosis:** Nodules < 3 mm, uniform in size.
- **Macronodular cirrhosis:** Nodules > 3 mm, with increased risk of hepatocellular carcinoma (HCC), usually due to significant liver injury leading to hepatic necrosis (postinfectious, or drug-induced).
- **Mixed: Macromicronodular** form.

Many etiologic agents are involved in the development of cirrhosis (Table 3-23). They are generally divided into four major groups:

- Infectious.
- Inherited/metabolic disorders.
- Drugs/toxins affecting the liver.
- Other causes: Underlying primary diseases that ultimately affect the liver.

Cirrhosis is a major risk factor for the development of HCC. Alcoholism is the most common cause of cirrhosis in the United States.

KEY FACT

AST is located in the mitochondria; thus, mitochondrial damage results in elevated AST (seen in both Reye syndrome and alcoholic hepatitis).

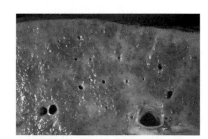

FIGURE 3-53. Liver with end-stage cirrhosis. (Reproduced from the Centers for Disease Control and Prevention, Public Health Image Library [PHIL] ID #71. Courtesy of Dr. Edwin P. Ewing, Jr.)

TABLE 3-23. Causes of Cirrhosis

TYPE OF CIRRHOSIS	CAUSES
Infectious	**Viral hepatitis,** brucellosis, capillariasis, echinococcosis, schistosomiasis, toxoplasmosis.
Inherited/metabolic disorders	AAT, Alagille syndrome, biliary atresia, Fanconi syndrome, **hemochromatosis, Wilson disease,** glycogen storage diseases.
Drugs/toxins	**Alcohol,** amiodarone, arsenic, oral contraceptive pills.
Other	**Heart failure** with long-standing congestion of the liver, **biliary obstruction,** CF, graft-versus-host disease, nonalcoholic steatohepatitis (NASH), **primary sclerosing cholangitis,** sarcoidosis.

AAT = α_1-antitrypsin; CF = cystic fibrosis.

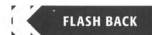
FLASH BACK

Hepatic portal vein to inferior vena cava (IVC) anastomoses (collaterals):

- Esophagus: Left gastric vein to azygos vein leads to esophageal varices.
- Umbilicus: Paraumbilical vein to superficial and inferior epigastric veins leads to caput medusae.
- Rectum: Superior rectal vein to middle and inferior rectal veins leads to hemorrhoids.

FLASH BACK

Portal hypertension in the context of congestive heart failure (CHF):

- Prolonged right-sided failure with retrograde transmission of venous pressure via the IVC.
- Liver sinusoids dilated/engorged with blood, leading to liver swelling and centrilobular fibrosis/alternating congestion ("nutmeg liver").
- Hepatic failure, pulsatile liver.
- Firm, enlarged liver with signs of chronic liver disease in patients with CHF.

PRESENTATION

Cirrhosis has a variety of manifestations:

- **Clinical presentation:** Complex, resulting from severely impaired liver function (hepatocellular damage), consequences of diffuse hepatic tissue scarring with portal hypertension, or a combination of both.
- **Jaundice** and **pruritus** resulting from the inability of the liver to conjugate bilirubin.
- **Hypoalbuminemia** as a result of impaired albumin synthesis.
- **Hyperestrogenism,** which causes **spider hemangiomas, palmar erythema, gynecomastia (in males),** and **hypogonadism.**
- **Anemia** (multifactorial, folate deficiency can contribute).
- **Coagulopathies** from decreased production of clotting factors.
- **Portal hypertension,** leading to esophageal varices, caput medusae, and hemorrhoids as described earlier (Figure 3-54).
- **Splenomegaly** resulting in **thrombocytopenia.**

Additional sequelae include ascites, peripheral edema, and/or hydrothorax (Figure 3-55):

- **Hypoalbuminemia** leads to decreased intravascular oncotic pressure and, along with **portal hypertension,** contributes to the formation of **ascites.** Ascitic fluid can become infected, causing **spontaneous bacterial peritonitis.**
- **Hepatic encephalopathy:** Severe loss of hepatic function leads to **shunting** of blood around the liver, leading to accumulation of toxic metabolites in the blood (**ammonemia**) and causing brain toxicity.
- **Hepatorenal syndrome:** Increased portal venous pressure leads to decreased effective intravascular volume and decreased renal perfusion pressure (due to intrarenal redistribution of blood flow). Renal failure can thus develop in the presence of liver failure without intrinsic renal problems.

PATHOHISTOLOGY

Bridging fibrosis and small **regenerative nodules** (Figure 3-56).

- Represent hepatocytic reaction to injury.
- Lack of normal liver cytoarchitecture (no portal triads and sinusoids).
- Contribute to increased intrasinusoidal pressure (intrasinusoidal hypertension).

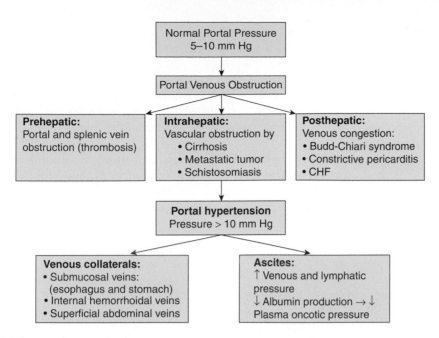

FIGURE 3-54. **Pathophysiology of portal hypertension.** CHF, congestive heart failure.

CLINICAL CORRELATION

Cirrhosis leads to a complete disarray of liver function, and thus elevated ALP, bilirubin, γ-glutamyl transferase, and PT, as well as anemia, thrombocytopenia, hypoalbuminemia, and hyponatremia.

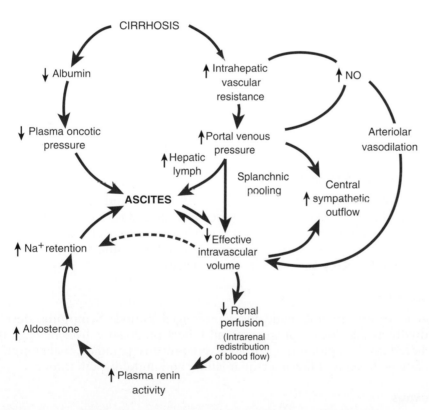

FIGURE 3-55. **Multiple factors involved in the development of ascites.** NO, nitric oxide. (Modified with permission from Kasper DL, Braunwald E, Fauci AS, et al, eds. *Harrison's Principles of Internal Medicine*, 16th ed. New York: McGraw-Hill, 2005: 1865.)

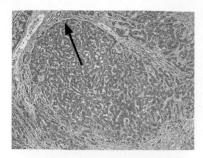

FIGURE 3-56. Histologic features of cirrhosis. Liver cell nodules of varying sizes are trapped in fibrous bands of tissue. Reactive bile duct proliferation is shown in the fibrous septae (*arrow*), with macrovesicular fatty change present in the hepatocytes. (Reproduced with permission from USMLERx. com.)

KEY FACT

AST:ALT ratio of > 2.0 (cutoff > 1.5) is highly suggestive of alcoholic cirrhosis.

CLINICAL CORRELATION

Suspect PBC in women with a history of Sjögren syndrome, Raynaud disease, or scleroderma.

KEY FACT

Circulating antimitochondrial antibody is detected in > 90% of PBC cases.

DIAGNOSIS

- **Physical exam** may reveal any of the signs and symptoms mentioned above as evidence of liver disease.
- The **damaged liver** may be enlarged and tender.
- A **cirrhotic liver** is shrunken, firm, and nodular.
- **Lab tests** may reveal elevated AST and ALT, but normal values do not rule out cirrhosis, as these values return to normal as the hepatocytes "burn out."
- Although not used for diagnosis, **RUQ ultrasound** shows the nodules characteristic of cirrhosis. Ultrasound can also be used to evaluate for splenomegaly, ascites, portal vein thrombosis, and HCC.
- The **gold standard** for diagnosing cirrhosis remains **tissue biopsy.** However, biopsy is not necessary if the patient's presentation and workup are both consistent with cirrhosis.

TREATMENT

- For complications of cirrhosis: Sclerotherapy or banding for symptomatic esophageal varices, drainage of excess peritoneal fluid for ascites (called **paracentesis**), nutritional support.
- Treatment of hepatic encephalopathy: lactulose (reduces the ammonia production of colonic bacteria), neomycin (decrease the colonic concentration of ammoniagenic bacteria).
- Procedures, such as portocaval shunting (more invasive) and transjugular intrahepatic portosystemic shunting (less invasive), that allow blood to bypass the portal venous system are also used, thus relieving the symptoms and complications of portal hypertension. However, these do not address the issue of hyperammonemia and are typically used only as a bridge to liver transplantation.

PROGNOSIS

Can be fatal if it progresses to liver failure or HCC. Cirrhosis is not uniformly fatal.

Primary Biliary Cirrhosis (PBC)

PBC is characterized by destruction of the small- and medium-sized bile ducts in the liver, resulting in **intrahepatic cholestasis.** PBC has a poorly understood pathophysiology; however, it is frequently associated with a variety of autoimmune disorders, thus suggesting an autoimmune cause. It primarily affects middle-aged women (35–60 years of age).

PRESENTATION

Most cases are asymptomatic for a prolonged period. **Symptoms develop gradually** as the disease progresses and reflect progressive liver damage due to cholestasis. Symptoms range from severe pruritus, jaundice, malabsorption, and fatigue to signs of hepatocellular failure and portal hypertension.

DIAGNOSIS

The **most classic lab abnormality** is an **extreme elevation in ALP,** along with elevated AST and ALT, cholesterol (especially HDL), **IgM,** and cryoglobulins. **Antimitochondrial antibodies** are highly specific for this disease.

Liver biopsy confirms the diagnosis; positive findings include lymphocytic infiltrates in the portal regions, granulomas, and loss of bile ductules in the liver parenchyma (Figure 3-57).

TREATMENT

No therapies can halt or reverse PBC; it is possible only to provide symptomatic relief and slow the progression of disease. The most common drug used is ursodiol in an attempt to reduce cholestasis; whether it improves prognosis is controversial. Liver transplantation is the only life-saving treatment currently available.

PROGNOSIS

Progressive disease that ultimately leads to cirrhosis of the liver.

INBORN ERRORS OF METABOLISM

Hemochromatosis

- An inherited, **autosomal recessive,** male-predominant metabolic disorder of iron storage, characterized by increased intestinal iron absorption.
- Excessive serum levels of iron lead to deposition in and damage to several major organs, including the liver, pancreas, heart, joints, and pituitary gland.

PRESENTATION

Organ damage usually does not become apparent until patients are at least 40 years of age. Early signs include weakness, weight loss, abdominal pain, and loss of libido.

- **Cirrhosis** with iron deposits (Figure 3-58) affecting the hepatocytes and resulting in hepatomegaly and symptoms of chronic liver disease.
- Iron deposition in **pancreatic islet cells** can lead to type 1 diabetes mellitus (DM-1).
- **Iron deposition** in the skin and **increased melanin production** cause bronze skin discoloration (hence, the name **bronze diabetes**).
- Significant risk of **heart failure.**

DIAGNOSIS

- Clinical presentation.
- Elevated percentage of transferrin saturation (> 50%).
- Elevated serum iron and ferritin.
- Iron:total iron-binding capacity ratio > 50%.
- Urinary iron.
- Confirm with liver biopsy.

TREATMENT

- Intermittent phlebotomy to remove excess body iron
- Chelating agents (deferoxamine)
- Abstinence from alcohol consumption (increases iron absorption)
- Supportive treatment of common complications (ie, diabetes, CHF)

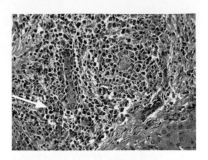

FIGURE 3-57. Histologic features of primary biliary cirrhosis. This slide shows a granuloma, a common feature of primary biliary cirrhosis, as well as inflammatory cells (*arrow*) attacking the bile ducts. (Reproduced with permission from USMLERx. com.)

KEY FACT

- Clinical symptoms of hemochromatosis: Males >> females; partly because menses causes loss of iron.
- Females are clinically affected after menopause.

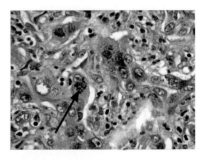

FIGURE 3-58. Hemosiderin-laden hepatocytes (*arrow*) indicative of hemochromatosis. (Reproduced with permission from USMLERx. com.)

CLINICAL CORRELATION

Distinguish between:
Hemo*chromatosis* = Inherited disorder.
Hemo*siderosis* = Acquired disorder of iron overload (eg, due to repeated blood transfusions in patients with thalassemia).

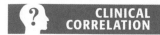

High levels of copper in serum are a result of inadequate copper excretion in the liver.

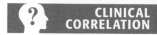

In Wilson disease, copper fails to enter the circulation as ceruloplasmin, which leads to low levels of ceruloplasmin in serum.

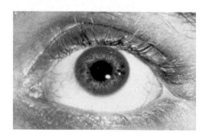

FIGURE 3-59. Kayser-Fleischer ring of Wilson disease. (Reproduced with permission from Fauci AS, Kasper DL, Braunwald E, et al, eds. *Harrison's Principles of Internal Medicine,* 17th ed. New York: McGraw-Hill, 2008: Figure 354-1.)

 KEY FACT

Hepatic adenoma: Linked to hormonal influence; oral contraceptives are thought to play an etiologic role.

Wilson Disease (Hepatolenticular Degeneration)

An inherited **autosomal recessive** metabolic disorder characterized by excessive serum levels of **copper** with deposition in major organs (primarily the liver, brain, kidneys, and corneas).

Wilson disease develops as a result of a mutation in the *ATP7B* **gene** on **chromosome 13 (13q14.3),** which codes for a **P-type ATPase** that transports copper into bile and incorporates it into ceruloplasmin. The mutant form of *ATP7B* inhibits the release of copper into bile.

PRESENTATION

Suspect Wilson disease in **young adult patients** who present with stigmata of liver disease along with neurologic changes.

- Classically, patients have **Kayser-Fleischer rings** (deposits of copper on the outer edges of the corneas; Figure 3-59) on **slit-lamp** examination.
- Liver disease can present in the form of hepatitis, cirrhosis, or decompensation.
- Neurologic changes resulting from copper accumulation in the brain.

DIAGNOSIS

- Decreased serum ceruloplasmin levels.
- Increased serum and urine copper levels.
- Confirm with liver biopsy.

TREATMENT

- Avoid copper-rich foods.
- Copper **chelators,** primarily **penicillamine.** Alternative agents include potassium sulfide, pyridoxine, and zinc acetate.

PROGNOSIS

Wilson disease is a chronic illness that can be fatal without treatment.

HEPATIC TUMORS

Hepatic tumors can be either primary tumors (derived from liver cells) or metastatic tumors. **The most common tumors of the liver are metastatic (ie, colon cancer).**

Benign Liver Tumors

The most common benign tumors include hepatic adenoma (HA) and focal nodular hyperplasia (FNH).

HEPATIC ADENOMA

Seen predominantly in women in the third and fourth decades. Risk factors include: the use of **oral contraceptives,** use of anabolic steroids, and type I glycogen storage diseases. Usually benign but they do have premalignant potential, and large adenomas can rupture.

FOCAL NODULAR HYPERPLASIA

As with HA, **FNH** also occurs primarily in women but is **not associated** with the use of oral contraceptives.

PRESENTATION

- **HA:** Primarily in the right liver lobe and often large (> 10 cm). Clinical features include pain and palpable mass or signs of intratumor hemorrhage.
- **FNH:** Generally asymptomatic and incidental finding on imaging studies as a solid tumor in the right lobe consisting of a fibrous core with stellate projections.

HISTOLOGY

Both tumors consist of normal or slightly atypical hepatocytes; however, FNH also contains **biliary epithelium** and **Kupffer cells.** Hepatocytes contain increased glycogen, appearing paler and larger than normal.

DIAGNOSIS

CT, MRI, and selective hepatic angiography are used to make the diagnosis.

- Hypervascular appearance on angiography.
- Technetium scans typically show **uptake in FNH** due to the presence of Kupffer cells but lack of uptake in HA.

TREATMENT

Imaging to follow progression of small tumors. If the lesion is > 8–10 cm, near the surface, and resectable, then surgical removal may be appropriate.

- Patients with HA should stop taking oral contraceptives.
- Pregnancy increases the risk of hemorrhage in HA due to hormonal influence; women with large adenomas should be counseled to avoid pregnancy.

PROGNOSIS

In HA, the risk of malignant change is small, although it is increased with multiple tumors and tumors > 10 cm. In FNH, there is no evidence for malignant transformation.

Malignant Liver Tumors

The two most common types of liver carcinoma are primary HCC and metastatic carcinoma.

HEPATOCELLULAR CARCINOMA

HCC is one of the most common tumors in the world, with the highest prevalence in Asia and sub-Saharan Africa due to the high prevalence of **hepatitis B and C**; it is less common in the United States and Western Europe. It is four times more common in men.

PRESENTATION

Symptoms are similar to those of chronic liver disease. The most common presenting symptoms are pain or mass in the RUQ. **Physical exam** may reveal friction rub or bruit over the liver. **Elevations of AFP and ALP** are common.

DIAGNOSIS

Based on imaging (Figure 3-60), and elevated serum AFP levels. A workup for HCC should be done on any solitary nodule seen on CT in a patient with cirrhosis.

KEY FACT

Kupffer cells are characteristically absent in HA.

KEY FACT

Risk factors for hepatocellular carcinoma: Anything that causes chronic liver disease can lead to HCC:

- Hepatitis B
- Hepatitis C
- Aflatoxin B1, which is found in peanuts affected by *Aspergillus;* common in China and Africa
- Hemochromatosis
- Tyrosinemia
- Cirrhosis
- α_1-Antitrypsin deficiency
- Long-term androgenic steroid use

CLINICAL CORRELATION

Maintain a high index of suspicion with cirrhotic patients who exhibit clinical changes, such as new-onset encephalopathy, ascites, jaundice, or variceal bleeding.

KEY FACT

High levels of AFP (> 500–1000 µg/L) in an adult with liver disease and no obvious GI tumor strongly suggest HCC.

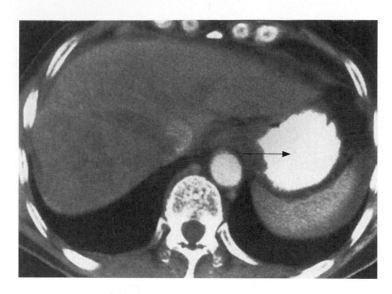

FIGURE 3-60. **Focal lesion within the right lobe of the liver.** This lesion (*arrow*) is associated with a clot entering the hepatic vein and even the inferior vena cava, findings typical of hepatocellular carcinoma. (Reproduced with permission from Chen MYM, Pope TL Jr, Ott DJ. *Basic Radiology.* New York: McGraw-Hill, 2004: 293.)

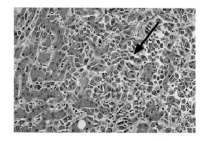

FIGURE 3-61. **Photomicrograph with standard hematoxylin and eosin stain of hepatocellular carcinoma cells (*arrow*) in hepatic parenchyma.** (Reproduced with permission from Kantarjian HM, Wolff RA, Koller CA. *Anderson Manual of Medical Oncology.* New York: McGraw-Hill, 2006.)

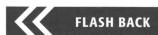

FLASH BACK

The liver is the most common site of metastasis for GI (and other) tumors due to its size, high rate of blood flow, unique dual blood supply, and cytoarchitecture.

Liver biopsy may be performed but diagnosis can usually be made based on imaging. **Histologically,** tumors can range from well differentiated (Figure 3-61) to poorly differentiated. Central areas of necrosis may exist in large tumors. Bile globules and acidophilic inclusions are sometimes present.

TREATMENT

Depending on tumor, node, metastasis (TNM) classification, treatment options include partial hepatectomy, liver transplantation, radiofrequency ablation, or percutaneous acetic acid or ethanol ablation.

PROGNOSIS

Usually diagnosed late, when distant metastases (lung, brain, bone, and adrenal) have already occurred. The median life expectancy after diagnosis is 6–20 months.

METASTATIC TUMORS

In the United States, the incidence of metastatic carcinoma is at least **20 times greater** than that of primary HCC. The most common metastases include tumors from the **GI tract, the lungs, the breast,** and from metastatic **melanoma.**

PRESENTATION

Most symptoms can be attributed to the primary tumor; however, patients may also present with nonspecific symptoms of weakness, weight loss, fever, sweating, and loss of appetite. Liver biochemical tests are often abnormal, but mildly elevated and nonspecific.

DIAGNOSIS

Evidence of metastatic disease to the liver should be sought for any patient with primary malignancy, especially of the lung, GI tract, or breast.

TREATMENT

Most metastatic carcinomas respond poorly to all forms of treatment, which is usually only palliative. The exception is metastatic colon cancer, which has a 5-year survival rate of at least 25% after resection.

Other Liver Tumors

- **Hemangioma:** Benign and generally left untreated.
- **Cholangiocarcinoma:** Increased risk associated with liver flukes (*Clonorchis sinensis*), often seen in immigrants.
- **Angiosarcoma:** Associated with vinyl chloride use.
- **Hepatoblastoma:** Main primary liver tumor in **children.**

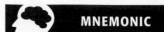

MNEMONIC

Metastases >> Primary liver tumors
  Cancer **S**ometimes **P**enetrates
  Benign **L**iver
(**C**olon > **S**tomach > **P**ancreas >
  Breast > **L**ung)

GALLBLADDER DISEASE

Cholelithiasis

Gallstones are a common cause of RUQ pain and are classically found in patients who are overweight, middle-aged, and female. About 10–20% of Americans have gallstones, and about 50% of these people eventually have symptoms.

There are three types of stones, namely cholesterol, mixed, and pigment (bilirubin) (Table 3-24).

Stones form when there is a disruption in cholesterol transport from the liver into the bile; this process is coupled with a simultaneous secretion of phospholipid and bile salts. Disruption of the **cholesterol:bile salt ratio** leads to cholesterol precipitation in the gallbladder, thus enabling the formation of stones.

- **Cholesterol load > bile salts:** Bile salts and lecithin are unable to solubilize the cholesterol.
- **Disrupted bile salt production** (decreased bile acid absorption from the intestine or hepatic failure) leads to increased cholesterol:bile salt ratio.

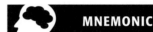

MNEMONIC

Risk factors for gallstones (4 Fs)
Fat
Fertile
Female
Forties

TABLE 3-24. Types of Gallstones and Typical Findings

	COMPONENTS	RISK FACTORS	RADIOGRAPHY
Cholesterol stones	Cholesterol	Crohn disease (inhibits bile acid recycling in the terminal ileum), CF, clofibrate (decreases bile acid secretion), estrogen, multiparity, rapid weight loss, Native American heritage, advanced age.	Mostly **radiolucent** (cannot be seen); **10–20%** are **opaque** due to calcifications.
Mixed stones, most common types	Cholesterol and pigment	Most common.	Radiolucent.
Pigment	Pigment (bilirubin)	Chronic RBC hemolysis, alcoholic cirrhosis, advanced age, biliary infection.	**Radiopaque** (seen on radiograph).

CF = cystic fibrosis.

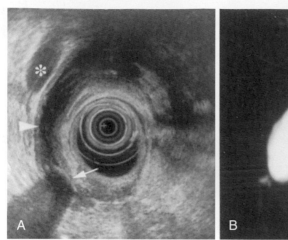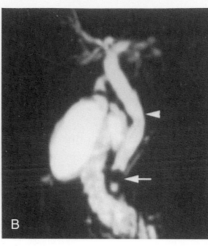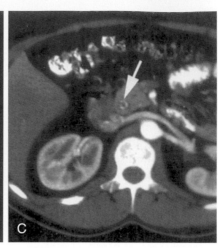

FIGURE 3-62. **Methods of bile duct imaging.** Arrows mark bile duct stones. Arrowheads indicate the common bile duct, and the asterisk marks the portal vein. (A) Endoscopic retrograde cholangiopancreatography (ERCP). (B) Magnetic resonance cholangiography (MRCP). (C) Helical computed tomography. (Reproduced with permission from Kasper DL, Braunwald E, Fauci AS, et al, eds. *Harrison's Principles of Internal Medicine*, 16th ed. New York: McGraw-Hill, 2005: 1736.)

PRESENTATION

Gallstones are strongly suggested by RUQ pain, which occasionally radiates to the right shoulder. The pain is usually worse after meals (**postprandial pain**) and can be associated with nausea/vomiting and fatty food intolerance.

DIAGNOSIS

Ultrasound is the best way to visualize gallstones. **Radiography** can be deceiving because most gallstones are radiolucent and may not appear on abdominal plain film. Endoscopic retrograde cholangiopancreatography (**ERCP**) is both a diagnostic and therapeutic procedure that can visualize gallstones in the common bile duct (Figure 3-62) and remove them.

TREATMENT

Elective cholecystectomy (removal of the gallbladder) in symptomatic patients. Some patients may not require surgery but should modify their diet and avoid fatty food.

PROGNOSIS

The prognosis is good, but there are many potential complications:

- Recurrent biliary colic (intermittent pain).
- Acute cholecystitis (prolonged blockage of the cystic duct, causing gallbladder inflammation or infection).
- Choledocholithiasis (gallstone obstructing the common bile duct).
- Acute cholangitis (bacterial infection of the biliary tree).
- Gallstone ileus and gallstone pancreatitis.

Cholecystitis

Inflammation of the gallbladder is a common complication of cholelithiasis (Figure 3-63).

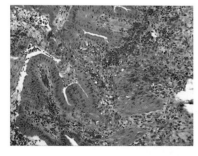

FIGURE 3-63. **Acute cholecystitis.** Neutrophilic and lymphocytic infiltrates (*arrow*) can be seen within the epithelium and muscular wall of the gallbladder. (Reproduced with permission from USMLERx.com.)

PRESENTATION

Very similar to that of cholelithiasis: Postprandial colicky RUQ pain radiating to the right scapula, as a result of intermittent blockage of the common bile duct. Nausea/vomiting and bloating can also be present.

- Jaundice may occur as a result of complete blockage of the common bile duct (choledocholithiasis), leading to infection or **cholangitis.**
- **Charcot triad:** Epigastric/RUQ pain, fever, and jaundice may indicate the presence of cholangitis.

DIAGNOSIS

- Classic physical exam feature is the **Murphy sign.**
  - **Elicitation:** Palpate the right subcostal area (gallbladder fossa) while the patient inspires deeply; the gallbladder descends toward the examiner's fingers.
  - **Positive response:** The patient feels increased discomfort and/or pain with this maneuver and will have disruption of deep inspiration.
- Ultrasound exam can show stones in the gallbladder, thickening of the gallbladder wall, and edema. Hepatobiliary iminodiacetic acid (HIDA) scan (**cholescintigraphy**) is more sensitive for cholecystitis and can confirm the diagnosis.

TREATMENT

Start antibiotics (usually against gram-negative bacteria, such as *E coli* and *Klebsiella*, empirically), and perform cholecystectomy once the patient is stable.

Gallbladder Carcinoma

Tumors of the gallbladder itself are much more common than tumors arising from within the bile ducts. They usually manifest in the seventh decade of life and are more common in women than in men. Gallstones are present 60–90% of the time. The 5-year survival is < 1%, as the tumor has often already invaded the liver at the time of diagnosis.

Primary Sclerosing Cholangitis

Chronic cholestatic liver disease characterized by inflammation, fibrosis, and irregular dilation of obstructed intrahepatic and extrahepatic bile ducts.

PRESENTATION

Usually diagnosed in the context of IBD, although it can also present with abnormal liver function tests, pruritus, RUQ pain, and fatigue.

DIAGNOSIS

Elevated alkaline phosphatase. MRCP shows multiple strictures and dilation of the intra- and extrahepatic bile ducts.

EXOCRINE PANCREAS

Acute Pancreatitis

Caused by activation of pancreatic enzymes, which leads to **pancreatic autodigestion** with **hemorrhagic fat necrosis.**

CLINICAL CORRELATION

Charcot triad (cholangitis): RUQ pain, fever, jaundice
Reynolds pentad = Charcot triad + Shock and altered mental status

KEY FACT

"Sonographic" Murphy sign when it occurs during ultrasound examination.

KEY FACT

Positive HIDA scan = obstruction in passage (cystic duct) = nonvisualization of gallbladder confirms diagnosis.

KEY FACT

Primary sclerosing cholangitis is often associated with IBD, especially ulcerative colitis.

MNEMONIC

Causes of acute pancreatitis—

I GET SMASHED
Idiopathic
Gallstones
Ethanol
Trauma
Steroids
Mumps
Autoimmune disease
Scorpion sting
Hypercalcemia/Hyperlipidemia
ERCP
Drugs

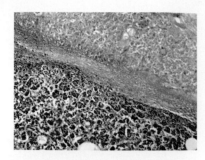

FIGURE 3-64. **Acute pancreatitis with extensive necrosis.** (The entire upper portion of this photomicrograph shows extensive parenchymal necrosis, whereas the lower portion is relatively spared. (Reproduced with permission from USMLERx.com.)

KEY FACT

Dideoxyinosine can cause fatal pancreatitis!

FLASH BACK

Morphine may cause spasm of the sphincter of Oddi and worsen pain.
Meperidine is the preferred analgesic for treating the pain of acute pancreatitis because it does not cause spasm of the sphincter of Oddi.

KEY FACT

The primary defect resulting from chronic pancreatitis may be digestive enzymes trapped in the ducts, leading to ductal obstruction and ductal dilation, diffuse atrophy of acinar cells, fibrosis, and eventual calcification that leads to chronic pain and pancreatic insufficiency.

PRESENTATION

Classically presents as sudden-onset epigastric abdominal pain radiating to the back and flanks accompanied by anorexia and nausea. May occur following a large meal or drinking binge.

DIAGNOSIS

Clinical symptoms and imaging:

- Leukocytosis and elevated serum amylase (> 3 times upper limit of normal) and lipase (more specific, persists longer) should be expected.
- **Histology:** Fat necrosis with pale basophilic calcium soaps, hemorrhage, necrotic debris, and inflammatory response (Figure 3-64).
- Abdominal plain film may show localized ileus (**sentinel loop**) in C-loop of duodenum.
- Contrast-enhanced CT is recommended for severe pancreatitis in order to rule out pseudocyst and fully visualize the extent of disease.

TREATMENT

- Rest, gastric suction, fluid and electrolyte replacement, and pain control with opioids (**meperidine**).
- Surgical treatment is only for trauma, ductal stones, obstructive lesions, and infected pancreatic necrosis.

PROGNOSIS

- About 20–30% of patients may have complications of necrosis, organ failure, or both, including disseminated intravascular coagulation (DIC), acute respiratory distress syndrome (ARDS), diffuse fat necrosis, hypocalcemia, pseudocyst formation, hemorrhage, and infection.
- About 10% of patients with pancreatic cancer present with acute pancreatitis. Suspect it in older patients with no other risk factors.

Chronic Pancreatitis

Chronic pancreatitis may present as episodes of acute inflammation in a previously injured pancreas or as chronic damage with persistent pain or malabsorption. The causes are similar to those of acute pancreatitis.

- In the United States, **alcoholism** is the most common cause in **adults.**
- **Cystic fibrosis (CF)** is the most common cause in **children.**

PRESENTATION

- Epigastric pain radiating to the back is often absent in chronic disease.
- More common type of pain is persistent, deep-seated, and unresponsive to antacids; worsened by ingestion of fatty foods or alcohol.
- Symptoms of **pancreatic insufficiency** include **steatorrhea,** weight loss, and deficiencies of fat-soluble vitamins (**A, D, E,** and **K**).

DIAGNOSIS

- In **contrast to acute pancreatitis,** serum amylase and lipase are usually not elevated. The classic triad includes progressive parenchymal fibrosis with **pancreatic calcification, steatorrhea, and DM.**
- Radiographic hallmark is the presence of scattered calcifications (Figure 3-65).

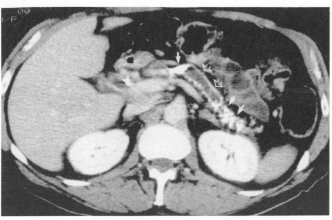

A

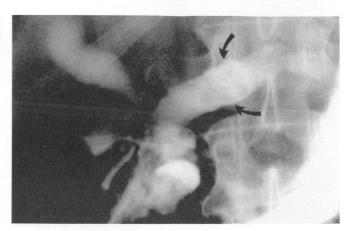

B

FIGURE 3-65. **Chronic pancreatitis and pancreatic calculi.** CT scan and endoscopic retrograde cholangiopancreatography (ERCP) appearance. (A) There is evidence of an atrophic pancreas with multiple calcifications (*arrows*). Note the markedly dilated pancreatic duct seen in this section through the body and tail (*open arrows*). (B) ERCP in the same patient demonstrates the dilated pancreatic duct as well as an intrapancreatic duct calculus (*curved arrows*). (Reproduced with permission from Fauci AS, Kasper DL, Braunwald E, et al, eds. *Harrison's Principles of Internal Medicine*, 17th ed. New York: McGraw-Hill, 2008: Figure 307-4.)

TREATMENT

Address the two major problems: **pain and malabsorption.**

- **Pain:** Avoid alcohol and large meals. Use of narcotics can often lead to opiate addiction and has led to the use of palliative procedures (resection of strictures, stent placement, and ductal decompression).
- **Malabsorption:** Enzyme replacement and dietary fat restriction.

PROGNOSIS

Patients who abstain from alcohol and use vigorous replacement therapy do reasonably well.

Pancreatic Adenocarcinoma

- Pancreatic adenocarcinoma is a malignancy of the exocrine portion of the pancreas; it is one of the most deadly cancers (5-year survival rate of < 5%).
- **Risk factors:** Age, smoking, family history, and chronic pancreatitis associated with alcohol abuse.

PRESENTATION

Tumors are located in the head of the pancreas 75% of the time, giving the classic presentation of **painless obstructive jaundice,** and are silent until late in disease progression. Common signs and symptoms include unexplained weight loss, malaise, epigastric pain that radiates to the middle of the back, and signs of obstructive jaundice. Other signs include **migratory phlebitis (Trousseau sign)** and, occasionally, the onset of DM.

DIAGNOSIS

- No lab test is specific for pancreatic cancer, although elevated bilirubin and ALP confirm biliary obstruction.
- The best tumor marker for pancreatic cancer is **CA 19-9;** it is not diagnostic but can be used to monitor progression of the disease.
- CT scan is the most common imaging study used for diagnosing pancreatic cancer (Figure 3-66). Other studies include ERCP (during which a biopsy can be taken), MRI, and endoscopic ultrasound.

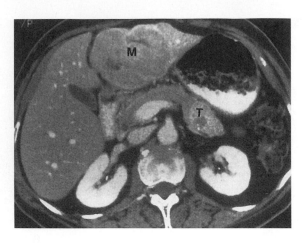

FIGURE 3-66.   **Focal lesion occupying the left lobe of the liver (M) and a focal-enhancing mass in the pancreatic tail (T), representing a pancreatic neoplasm metastatic to the liver.** (Reproduced with permission from Chen MYM, Pope TL, Ott DJ. *Basic Radiology.* New York: McGraw-Hill, 2004: 293.)

TREATMENT

Surgical resection, called a pancreaticoduodenectomy (Whipple operation), is the only treatment that has had any success in prolonging survival. Chemotherapy and radiation have had minimal success.

PROGNOSIS

Pancreatic cancer has a dismal prognosis, with death usually occurring within 1 year of diagnosis.

ENZYME MARKERS OF GI PATHOLOGY

Commonly used laboratory assays (Table 3-25) available in most clinical practices include serum **AST, ALT, γ-glutamyl transferase,** bilirubin, **ALP, amylase, lipase,** and **PT.** Other, more specialized markers (ie, **ceruloplasmin** with Wilson disease) are used when rare conditions are suspected.

Many of these enzyme markers can be affected by pathologies outside the gut. Therefore, the differential diagnosis must include both extrinsic (outside the GI tract) and intrinsic (within the GI tract) pathologies.

Aspartate Aminotransferase (AST)

ANATOMIC SIGNIFICANCE

Intracellular (**cytosol and mitochondria**) enzyme found in liver cells, but also in skeletal muscle, heart, brain, and RBCs.

PHYSIOLOGIC ACTION

Catalyzes the transfer of amino groups to form pyruvate.

LAB TEST INTERPRETATION

Increased concentration in the bloodstream with **tissue** (especially liver) **damage.** Tissue damage may occur with liver damage, or with cor pulmonale (right heart failure), myocardial ischemia, and extensive trauma.

TABLE 3-25. Key Enzyme Markers of GI Pathologies

Enzyme Marker	Range of Normal Values	Key Pathologies Indicated by Abnormality
AST	0–35 IU/L	Increased in liver damage (any cause).
ALT	0–35 IU/L	Increased in liver damage (any cause).
GGT	9–85 IU/L	Increase specific for liver disease (any cause).
Bilirubin		
Direct	0.1–0.4 mg/dL	
Indirect	0.2–0.7 mg/dL	
Total	0.1–1.2 mg/dL	
Alkaline phosphatase	41–133 IU/L	Nonspecific indicator of tissue damage (liver, bone, or intestinal); also increased in pregnancy.
Amylase	20–110 IU/L	Increased in pancreatic pathologies, intestinal disease, and ruptured ectopic pregnancy.
Lipase	0–160 IU/L	Increased in pancreatitis (acute and chronic); also increased in other pancreatic pathologies.
PT	11–15 s	Increased in liver disease and warfarin therapy.
Ceruloplasmin	20–35 mg/dL	Decreased in Wilson disease (hepatolenticular degeneration).

ALT = alanine aminotransferase; AST = aspartate aminotransferase; GGT = γ-glutamyltransferase; PT = prothrombin time.

Alanine Aminotransferase (ALT)

ANATOMIC SIGNIFICANCE

Intracellular (**cytosol**) enzyme; relatively specific to the liver. Also found in kidney cells, skeletal muscle, and cardiac tissue.

PHYSIOLOGIC ACTION

Catalyzes the transfer of amino groups to form oxaloacetate.

LAB TEST INTERPRETATION

Increased along with AST in the bloodstream with **tissue** (especially liver) **damage.** Levels approximate the magnitude of liver damage. Also increased with right heart failure, myocardial ischemia, and extensive trauma.

AST AND ALT ELEVATIONS

Individually, abnormal values of AST or ALT are relatively nonspecific measures of liver damage. Certain characteristics in the pattern of elevation and the ratio of AST to ALT, however, enable clinical correlations to be made (Table 3-26).

TABLE 3-26. Level of AST and ALT Elevations

MILD AST AND ALT ELEVATION (< 5× UPPER NORMAL LIMIT)	SEVERE AST AND ALT ELEVATION (> 15 × UPPER NORMAL LIMIT)	EXTREME AST AND ALT ELEVATION (AST AND ALT ≥ 5000)	NONHEPATIC CAUSES OF AST:ALT ABNORMALITIES
Wilson disease	Wilson disease	Acute viral hepatitis (with unusual viruses such as herpes simplex virus)	Drugs (ie, statins) Pregnancy
Chronic hepatitis (viral, alcoholic, etc)	Acute viral hepatitis	Acute toxic injury (ie, acetaminophen poisoning)	
Ethanol α_1-antitrypsin deficiency Toxins/drugs	Ischemic injury Toxins/drugs Budd-Chiari syndrome Autoimmune hepatitis Hepatic artery ligation	Acute ischemic injury	Myocardial infarct Muscle disorders

KEY FACT

Check for γ-glutamyl transpeptidase (specific to the hepatobiliary system) to differentiate hepatobiliary involvement from other pathologies.

γ-Glutamyl Transferase

ANATOMIC SIGNIFICANCE

Present in hepatic and biliary epithelial cells.

PHYSIOLOGIC ACTION

Induced by alcoholic intake.

LAB TEST INTERPRETATION

Increased in liver disease. γ-Glutamyl transferase is sensitive but **not specific** for liver disease. Best tool to assess recent alcohol use.

Alkaline Phosphatase

ANATOMIC SIGNIFICANCE

Synthesized in liver, bone, intestine, and placenta.

PHYSIOLOGIC ACTION

Nonspecific indicator of tissue damage (liver, bone, intestine, and/or placenta).

LAB TEST INTERPRETATION

Increased in **obstructive hepatobiliary disease.** Also increased in bone disease (ie, Paget disease, bone metastases), hyperparathyroidism, **pregnancy (third trimester),** and GI disease (ie, perforated ulcer).

Amylase

ANATOMIC SIGNIFICANCE

Synthesized primarily in the pancreas and salivary glands; however, also produced by the ovaries, intestines, and skeletal muscle.

PHYSIOLOGIC ACTION

Hydrolyzes complex carbohydrates.

LAB TEST INTERPRETATION

Increased in **pancreatic disease** (pancreatitis, pseudocyst, pancreatic duct obstruction, malignancy), **bowel obstruction or infarction, mumps, parotitis, peritonitis, and ruptured ectopic pregnancy. Decreased in pancreatic insufficiency and CF.**

Lipase

ANATOMIC SIGNIFICANCE

Synthesized in the pancreas, liver, intestine, stomach, tongue, and other cells throughout the body.

PHYSIOLOGIC ACTION

Hydrolysis of glycerol esters and long-chain fatty acids.

LAB TEST INTERPRETATION

Increased in **pancreatic pathologies** (including acute/chronic pancreatitis, pseudocyst, and malignancy), **CF, intestinal malignancy, IBD, peritonitis, biliary disease, and liver disease.**

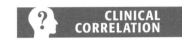

CLINICAL CORRELATION

Measuring lipase levels is the most specific test to detect pancreatitis.

Prothrombin Time

ANATOMIC SIGNIFICANCE

Measures activity of clotting factors synthesized in the liver.

PHYSIOLOGIC ACTION

Screening test used to evaluate the extrinsic pathway of the coagulation system and monitor warfarin therapy. Also a relatively rapid and sensitive indicator of hepatic capacity for protein synthesis, since the half-lives of factors II and VII are relatively short (hours).

LAB TEST INTERPRETATION

Increased with **liver disease, warfarin therapy, vitamin K deficiency, and DIC.**

Ceruloplasmin

ANATOMIC SIGNIFICANCE

Synthesized in the liver.

PHYSIOLOGIC ACTION

Main copper-carrying protein in serum.

LAB TEST INTERPRETATION

Decreased in **Wilson disease,** malnutrition, nephrotic syndrome, and Menkes disease (X-linked disorder of copper deficiency).

Pharmacology

This section describes the drugs used to treat the most common GI pathologies. Figure 3-67 summarizes the physiology of gastric secretions and the mechanism of action of respective compounds used in the treatment of certain GI diseases.

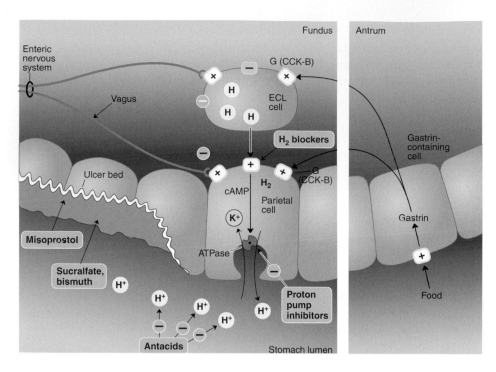

FIGURE 3-67. **Summary of gastrointestinal therapies.** CCK-B, cholecystokinin-B; G, gastrin receptor; H_2, histamine receptor. (Modified with permission from Katzung BG, Trevor AJ. *USMLE Road Map: Pharmacology.* New York: McGraw-Hill, 2003: 159.)

KEY FACT

Cimetidine can increase blood levels of other drugs cleared by the P450 system (eg, selective serotonin reuptake inhibitors [SSRIs], tricyclic antidepressants [TCAs], phenytoin, and calcium channel blockers). Caution should be taken when using these drugs simultaneously.

HISTAMINE BLOCKERS

KEY DRUGS

Cimetidine, ranitidine, famotidine, nizatidine.

MECHANISM

Reversibly blocks the histamine H_2 receptors responsible for stimulating the stomach parietal cells, leading to decreased H^+ secretion by these cells.

USES

Treatment and maintenance therapy of PUD, GERD, and dyspepsia.

SIDE EFFECTS

Cimetidine is a potent inhibitor of the cytochrome P450 system. It is also a potent antiandrogenic and can lead to decreased renal creatinine clearance. Ranitidine also inhibits the P450 system, although to a lesser degree than cimetidine. The other H_2 blockers are relatively free of these side effects.

PROTON PUMP INHIBITORS (PPIs)

KEY DRUGS

Omeprazole, lansoprazole, rabeprazole, esoprazole.

MECHANISM

Irreversibly inhibits the H^+–K^+ ATPase pump in the stomach parietal cells.

USES

PUD, gastritis, GERD, Barrett esophagus, and Zollinger-Ellison syndrome.

SIDE EFFECTS

Generally mild and include headache, nausea, and diarrhea. Patients taking PPIs for long periods are also at increased risk of fractures.

BISMUTH AND SUCRALFATE

MECHANISM

Bind to the ulcer base, providing a protective layer for the stomach, as well as allowing HCO_3^- secretion to restore the pH gradient in the mucus layer. Sucralfate suppresses *H pylori* and inhibits acid secretion in infected patients with duodenal ulcers. Bismuth lacks antiacidic properties.

USES

Binding agents commonly used to aid in ulcer healing as well as to treat traveler's diarrhea.

SIDE EFFECTS

Sucralfate has minimal adverse side effects other than possible aluminum toxicity. Bismuth toxicity can occur in patients with renal failure.

MISOPROSTOL

MECHANISM

Prostaglandin E_1 analog. Increases the production and secretion of the gastric mucus barrier and decreases acid production.

USES

The main GI indication is the prevention of NSAID-induced peptic ulcers. Commonly used in the maintenance of a patent ductus arteriosus (PDA) and in the induction of labor.

SIDE EFFECTS

Diarrhea and crampy abdominal pain. Contraindicated in women of childbearing age due to its abortifacient properties.

INFLIXIMAB

MECHANISM

IgG1 monoclonal antibody with a high specificity and affinity for tumor necrosis factor alpha (TNF-α). Infliximab most likely works by destroying activated TNF-α cells through apoptosis or complement-mediated actions. TNF-α is found in the stool of patients with Crohn disease and may be correlated with disease severity.

USES

Indicated for severe or fistulizing Crohn disease that is refractory to corticosteroids and other therapies such as mesalamine. Also used in a variety of rheumatologic conditions, including ankylosing spondylitis, psoriatic arthritis, rheumatoid arthritis, and ulcerative colitis.

KEY FACT

PPIs must be "turned on" by an acidic environment in the parietal cell compartment. Therefore, PPIs work poorly in patients with concomitant use of antisecretory agents (H_2 blockers).

KEY FACT

Triple therapy for *H pylori* ulcers: a PPI, clarithromycin, and amoxicillin. Quadruple therapy also includes bismuth.

SIDE EFFECTS

Infusion reactions, such as shortness of breath, hypotension, fever/chills, and urticaria, can occur. Delayed hypersensitivity reactions are marked by myalgia, fever, and rash.

SULFASALAZINE

MECHANISM

5-Aminosalicylic acid (ASA) derivative. Decreases inflammatory response in the colon and systemically inhibits prostaglandin synthesis.

USES

An enteric-coated tablet indicated for ulcerative colitis. It can also be used for rheumatoid arthritis.

SIDE EFFECTS

Contraindicated in patients with sulfa allergy. Most patients experience GI intolerance upon initiation of this drug.

ONDANSETRON

MECHANISM

Antiemetic selective serotonin (5-HT$_3$) receptor antagonist. Blocks serotonin on peripheral vagal nerve terminals and in the central chemoreceptor trigger zone.

USES

Prophylaxis for highly emetogenic chemotherapy and for prevention and treatment of postoperative nausea and vomiting.

SIDE EFFECTS

Should be used on a scheduled basis for chemotherapy, not as needed because it is indicated for the prevention of nausea. Side effects include headaches, malaise, and constipation.

ANTACIDS

Antacids are weak bases that decrease gastric acidity by neutralizing gastric acid to form water and a salt. They also affect the action of pepsin, which requires a pH < 4.0. Agents are composed of sodium bicarbonate and aluminum, magnesium, or calcium salts. Aluminum and magnesium salts are most common and promote the healing of duodenal ulcers. Chronic use of antacids, however, may lead to unwanted effects (Table 3-27).

TABLE 3-27.   **Consequences of Antacid Overuse**

Aluminum-containing antacids	Constipation. Binds to tetracycline to form insoluble complex that is not absorbed. Increases absorption of certain drugs such as levodopa. Antacid binds to secreted and ingested phosphate to form insoluble salts; hypophosphatemia may lead to osteomalacia and myopathy.
Sodium-containing antacids	Transient metabolic alkalosis. Fluid retention. Hypernatremia.
Magnesium-containing antacids	Hypermagnesemia, fluid and electrolyte imbalance. Hypophosphatemia. Diarrhea.
Calcium-containing antacids	Milk-alkali syndrome may lead to hypercalcemia, renal stones, and metabolic alkalosis. Constipation.

NOTES

CHAPTER 4

Hematology and Oncology

Embryology

HEMATOPOIESIS

Formation of Blood Cells

The outer layer of the yolk sac, derived from the extraembryonic mesoderm, is the major site for hematopoiesis in the embryo. The hematopoietic stem cells migrate into the yolk sac from **primitive ectoderm** or **epiblast** and leave the yolk sac to start populating the fetal **liver** between the fourth and the fifth weeks of gestation. As the fetus develops, other hematopoietic organs, including the spleen, lymph nodes, thymus, and bone marrow are also involved in the formation of blood cells.

- **Liver:** The major site of hematopoiesis in early embryonic life beginning at week 9.
- **Spleen:** Exclusively hematopoietic organ until 14 weeks of gestation. At around 15–18 weeks, the spleen is populated with T-cell precursors. In the 23rd week, B-cell precursors enter the spleen and form B-cell regions.
- **Thymus:** Populated by lymphocytes derived from the stem cells in the yolk sac, liver, and omentum once it is completely formed.

TYPES OF HEMOGLOBIN

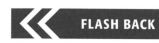

FLASH BACK

Binding of 2,3-BPG causes decreased affinity for O_2. Fetal hemoglobin does not bind with 2,3-BPG, resulting in a greater affinity for O_2.

Hemoglobin is composed of four polypeptide subunits and serves to transport oxygen and carbon dioxide. Hemoglobin is an allosteric molecule whose affinity for oxygen increases as each molecule is bound. This results in a sigmoid oxygen dissociation curve that allows hemoglobin to become saturated with oxygen in the lungs and to effectively unload oxygen in tissues. Elevations in Cl^-, H^+, CO_2, 2,3-bisphosphoglycerate (2,3-BPG), and temperature favor a right shift in the dissociation curve, which facilitates oxygen unloading.

Fetal Hemoglobin (Hb$\alpha_2\gamma_2$)

Contains two α-chains and two γ-chains. It has higher O_2 affinity than adult hemoglobin.

Adult Hemoglobin (Hb$\alpha_2\beta_2$)

The main type of adult hemoglobin contains two α-chains and two β-chains. The transition from fetal to adult hemoglobin concentrations is complete at approximately 6 months of age.

FETAL CIRCULATION

KEY FACT

Prostaglandins are required to keep the patent ductus arteriosus (PDA) open in the fetal period.

Oxygenated blood enters the fetus via the umbilical vein. The oxygenated blood traveling in the umbilical vein (Table 4-1 and see Figure 1-6) is shunted to the inferior vena cava (IVC) via the **ductus venosus,** where it mixes with deoxygenated blood from the trunk and legs. The IVC drains into the right atrium. The **foramen ovale,** a shunt between the right atrium and the left atrium, allows the oxygenated blood from the IVC/right atrium to enter into the left atrium. High resistance in the pulmonary circuit during fetal life secondary to collapsed lungs results in very minimal blood flow in the pulmonary circuit. Hence, a slight amount of deoxygenated blood coming from the unventilated lungs mixes with the oxygenated blood in the left atrium. The

FLASH FORWARD

PDA is seen in congenital rubella syndrome.

TABLE 4-1.   Fetal Circulatory Structures and Adult Remnants

FETAL CIRCULATORY STRUCTURES	ADULT REMNANTS
Umbilical arteries	Medial umbilical ligaments
Left umbilical vein	Ligamentum teres hepatis
Ductus arteriosus	Ligamentum arteriosus
Ductus venosus	Ligamentum venosum
Foramen ovale	Fossa ovale

left ventricle then pumps blood (via the aortic opening) to supply the systemic circulation. At the level of the descending aorta, the **ductus arteriosus** allows for shunting of blood from the pulmonary trunk to the descending aorta. The pulmonary trunk carries deoxygenated blood from the superior vena cava and right ventricle. Finally, deoxygenated blood from the lower limbs and trunk is drained by two umbilical arteries to the placenta for oxygenation.

Changes in Fetal Circulation After Birth

- Opening of the alveoli in the lungs after the first breath causes a sudden drop in pulmonary resistance, which is facilitated by the production of surfactant.
- Increased venous return to the left atrium causes increased pressure in the heart; cessation of the umbilical blood flow causes decreased pressure in the right atrium. This change in pressure results in closure of the foramen ovale.
- Cessation of umbilical blood flow, decreased pulmonary vasculature resistance, and increased venous return to the left atrium and left ventricle result in increased flow of oxygenated blood through the ductus arteriosus. This increase in local O_2 tension causes constriction of the ductus arteriosus.

Anatomy

BLOOD

Blood is a specialized connective tissue containing RBCs, WBCs, and platelets suspended in plasma. See Figure 4-1 for a detailed hematopoietic tree.

Plasma

Plasma is yellow fluid that makes up approximately 55% of the total blood volume.

Cells

There are three major types of blood cells: erythrocytes (RBCs), leukocytes (WBCs), and platelets. Blood cells constitute about 45% of the total blood volume.

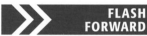

FLASH FORWARD

Indomethacin is a prostaglandin inhibitor that is used to close a PDA in the preterm infant.

FLASH FORWARD

Transposition of the great vessels requires either a PDA or a patent foramen ovale to allow survival of the newborn. This can be achieved by administration of prostaglandins until the condition is surgically corrected.

KEY FACT

Serum = plasma without clotting factors.

KEY FACT

Corticosteroids inhibit polymorphonuclear neutrophil (PMN) migration from the circulation into the periphery, causing benign leukocytosis.

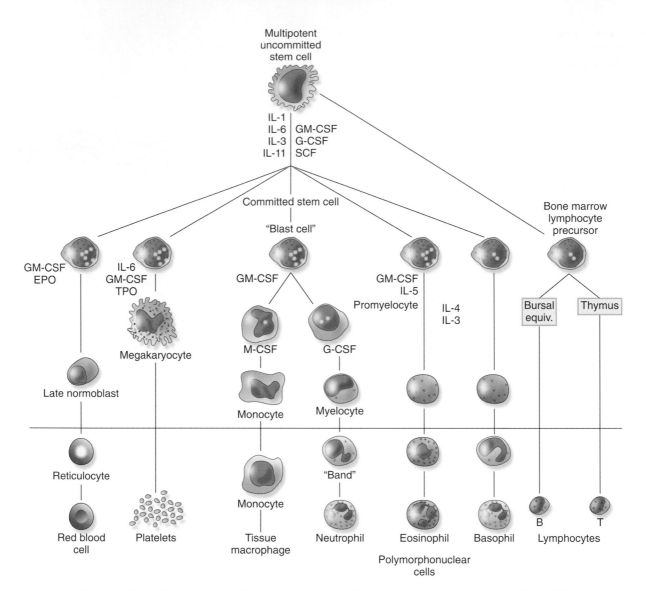

FIGURE 4-1. Hematopoiesis. Development of the formed elements of blood from bone marrow stem cells. Cells below the horizontal line are found in normal peripheral blood. The principal cytokines that stimulate each cell lineage to differentiate are shown. (EPO, erythropoietin; TPO, thrombopoietin; CSF, colony-stimulating factor; G, granulocyte; M, macrophage; IL, interleukin; SCF, stem cell factor.) (Reproduced with permission from Ganong WF. *Review of Medical Physiology*, 22nd ed. McGraw-Hill, 2005.)

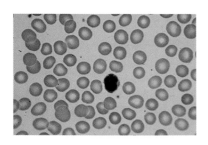

FIGURE 4-2. Anucleated, biconcave red blood cells. (Reproduced with permission from Lichtman MA, Beutler E, Kipps TJ, et al. *Williams Hematology*, 7th ed. New York: McGraw-Hill, 2007: Plate I-1.)

ERYTHROCYTES

The erythrocyte is a biconcave, anucleated cell (Figure 4-2) specialized to carry oxygen. It has a diameter of 7.5–8.7 μm, a volume of 90 fL, and a surface area of 136 μm^2, providing a large surface area:volume ratio. See Table 4.2 for terms used in the evaluation of RBCs.

RBCs exclusively utilize glucose as a source of energy, with 90% anaerobically degraded to lactate and the rest metabolized through the hexose monophosphate (HMP) shunt in the production of NADPH. They survive for an average of 120 days and are destroyed in the spleen by macrophages.

Reticulocytes are immature RBCs that can be identified by specific staining because they contain **polyribosomes**. They account for 0.5–1.5% of RBCs. The reticulocyte count is increased in conditions, such as hemolytic anemia and blood loss, in which RBC production is increased; it is decreased in aplastic anemia.

TABLE 4-2. Key Terms

Hematocrit	Represents the percentage of whole-blood volume composed of erythrocytes.
Mean cell hemoglobin	The average content of hemoglobin per RBC.
MCHC	The average concentration of hemoglobin in a given volume of packed RBCs. The MCHC is low if the RBCs are hypochromic.
MCV	The average volume of an RBC. A normal value is 80–100 fL. More than 100 fL is a macrocytic anemia, whereas < 80 fL is microcytic.
RDW	The coefficient of variation of RBC volume. An increased RDW means that the RBCs vary greatly in size.

MCHC = mean corpuscular hemoglobin concentration; MCV = mean corpuscular volume; RDW = RBC distribution width.

LEUKOCYTES

Leukocytes lead the fight against infection or foreign invasion. The WBC count normally ranges from 4000 to 11,000/µL. WBCs can be divided into five different types of cells: neutrophils, basophils, eosinophils, monocytes, and lymphocytes (Table 4-3 and Figure 4-3).

- **Neutrophils:** Can morphologically be divided into two groups: nonsegmented and hypersegmented.
  - **Nonsegmented** cells are immature neutrophils (also known as bands), which are seen during bacterial infections, leukemias, and other inflammatory conditions.
  - **Hypersegmented** neutrophils (with more than five lobes) are older cells seen in macrocytic anemias associated with vitamin B$_{12}$ and folate deficiencies.

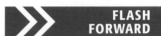

FLASH FORWARD

Chronic granulomatous disease, resulting from a deficiency of reduced nicotinamide adenine dinucleotide phosphate oxidase, results in an increased incidence of infection with catalase-positive organisms.

TABLE 4-3. Leukocytes

LEUKOCYTE	PERCENTAGE	CHARACTERISTICS	FUNCTION
Neutrophil	60–70	Multilobed (3–5), specific and azurophilic granules, lactoferrin	Phagocytic cell, mediator of acute inflammation
Lymphocyte	20–30		
B lymphocyte		Small, round cells, scant cytoplasm, dense nuclei	Humoral immunity
T lymphocyte		Small, round cells, scant cytoplasm, dense nuclei	Cell-mediated immunity
Plasma cell		Eccentric cells, purple nuclei	Produce antibodies
Natural killer cell		Small granules of perforin and proteases	Cell-mediated immunity
Monocyte	2–10	Kidney-shaped nuclei, basophilic and azurophilic granules	Precursor for macrophages and APCs
Eosinophil	1–6	Bilobed nuclei, large eosinophilic granules	Phagocytic cells, defends against parasites and allergic reactions
Basophil	< 0.5	Bilobed nuclei, basophilic granules	Mediates allergic reactions by release of histamine and other vasoactive substances

APCs = antigen-presenting cells.

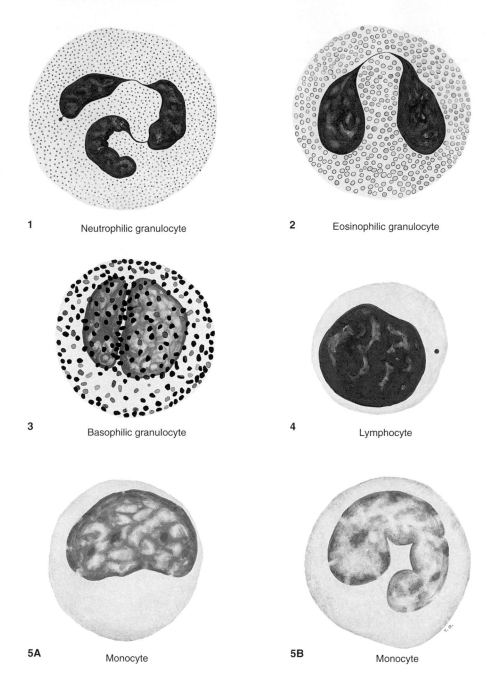

1 Neutrophilic granulocyte

2 Eosinophilic granulocyte

3 Basophilic granulocyte

4 Lymphocyte

5A Monocyte

5B Monocyte

FIGURE 4-3. **The five types of human leukocytes.** (1) Neutrophils, (2) eosinophils, and (3) basophils have granules that stain specifically with certain dyes and are called granulocytes. (4) Lymphocytes and (5A, 5B) monocytes are agranulocytes; they may show azurophilic granules, which are also present in other leukocytes. (Reproduced with permission from Junqueira LC, Carneiro J. *Basic Histology: Text and Atlas*, 11th ed. New York: McGraw-Hill, 2007: 227.)

■ Multilobed (3–5), phagocytic cells with granules in the cytoplasm. They account for 60–70% of all leukocytes and are the prime mediators of acute inflammation. Primarily two groups of granules are present in the cytoplasm: **specific granules** are **peroxidase-negative,** small, and pale-looking, whereas **azurophilic granules** are lysosomes that are **peroxidase-positive,** large, and dense and contain myeloperoxidase enzymes. Neutrophils utilize glucose via the glycolytic pathway and have a life span of 1–4 days in blood. Following phagocytosis, neutrophils consume O_2, producing free radicals that help kill bacteria. Neutrophils also contain **lactoferrin,** which avidly binds with iron, robbing bacteria of this essential nutrient and leading to bacterial death.

- **Lymphocytes:** Small, round cells with scant cytoplasm and densely staining nuclei. There are four different types of lymphocytes:
    - **B lymphocyte:** Matures in **B**one marrow and migrates to peripheral lymphoid tissues (follicles of lymph nodes, white pulp of spleen, and unencapsulated lymphoid tissue). B lymphocytes mediate humoral immunity and express monomeric molecules of **IgM as the receptors for the antigen.** Recognition of the antigen leads to differentiation into plasma cells and production of antibodies (including IgG, IgA, and IgM). They function as memory cells and APCs and express MHC class II.
    - **T lymphocyte:** Matures in **T**hymus. Precursor cells of T lymphocytes originate in the bone marrow. After maturation, T lymphocytes leave the thymus and redistribute in lymphoid tissues. They induce cell-mediated immunity and express **T-cell receptor.** T lymphocytes differentiate into cytotoxic T cells (major histocompatabilty complex I [MHC I] and CD 8), helper T cells (**MHC II, CD 4, and CD 3**), suppressor T cells, and delayed hypersensitivity T cells.
    - **Plasma cell:** Eccentric cells with purple "clock-faced" nuclei. Cytoplasm has abundant blue rough endoplasmic reticulum and well-developed Golgi apparatus. They differentiate from B lymphocytes and produce large amounts of antibodies specific for a particular antigen.
    - **Natural killer (NK) cell:** NK cells are a type of cytotoxic lymphocyte that expresses CD16 and CD56. The cytoplasm contains small granules filled with perforin and proteases that help target and kill cells lacking MHC I, including tumor-derived cells and cells infected with viruses.
- **Monocytes:** Cells with kidney-shaped nuclei. The cytoplasm contains fine azurophilic granules (lysosomes) and appears basophilic with a "frosted-glass" appearance. Monocytes are precursor cells for macrophages and antigen-presenting cells (APCs). They account for 2–10% of all leukocytes.
- **Eosinophils:** Bilobed cells with large eosinophilic granules. Eosinophils comprise 1–6% of all leukocytes. They function as phagocytic cells, release cytokines and chemokines (leukotrienes, platelet-activating factor, prostaglandins E_1 and E_2, thromboxane B_2, histaminase, catalase, and phospholipase D), and defend against parasitic infections. Eosinophils also down-regulate allergic reactions by inactivating basophil-derived histamine.
- **Basophils:** Cells with bilobed nuclei that mediate allergic reactions. Basophils stain with **B**asic stain (**B**lue) and have deeply basophilic granules. Basophils account for < 0.5% of all leukocytes and express **IgE** receptors that, when triggered, release histamine, heparin, prostaglandins, leukotrienes, and other vasoactive amines. They have a causative role in allergic diseases, including asthma and hay fever, and are frequently elevated in myeloproliferative diseases.

MAST CELLS

Granulocytes that are derived from bone marrow precursors and which mature in tissues. They are especially abundant near blood vessels and in tissues exposed to the external environment (eg, skin, respiratory, gastrointestinal, and urogenital systems). Similar to basophils, they express IgE receptors and counter parasitic infections and chronic allergic diseases.

MACROPHAGES

Cells with oval nuclei and blue-gray to pale cytoplasm. Macrophages are derived from monocytes and reside in the tissues. They serve as tissue scav-

MNEMONIC

For prevalence in the blood, greatest to least, remember–

Never Let Monkeys Eat Bananas
Neutrophil
Lymphocyte
Monocyte
Eosinophil
Basophil

MNEMONIC

Causes of eosinophilia–

NAACP
Neoplasia
Asthma
Allergic processes
Collagen vascular diseases
Parasites

FLASH FORWARD

Cromolyn sodium is a mast cell stabilizer used to treat asthma.

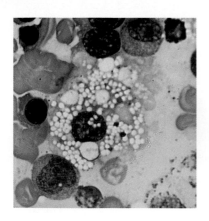

FIGURE 4-4. Active macrophage. (Reproduced with permission from Lichtman MA, Beutler E, Kipps TJ, et al. *Williams Hematology*, 7th ed. New York: McGraw-Hill, 2007: Plate IX-1.)

engers (Figure 4-4) and are phagocytic, consuming bacteria, aged RBCs, and cell debris. Macrophages also serve as APCs and are activated by γ-interferon.

DENDRITIC CELLS

Dendritic cells are sentinels, adjuvants, and controllers of the immune system. They serve as APCs and express MHC II and crystallizable fragment (Fc) receptors on their surface. They are the main inducers of the primary antibody response. Dendritic cells are called Langerhans cells in skin.

Pathology

ANEMIA

Classification and Appearance

An anemia is a reduction in the O_2-transporting capacity of blood. Anemias are classified by mechanism (increased destruction vs. impaired production), RBC size (Table 4-4) and shape (Table 4-5), and hemoglobinization (normochromic vs. hypochromic) (Figure 4-5). Relevant signs and symptoms include weakness, fatigue, pale skin, malaise, dyspnea with exertion, koilonychias (spooning of the nails), cardiac failure, headache, and presyncope/syncope.

Microcytic Anemias

IRON DEFICIENCY ANEMIA

Iron is necessary for the **production of heme**; therefore iron deficiency decreases the O_2-carrying capacity of RBCs. Deficiency can be caused by:

- Increased requirement: **Pregnancy**, infants, and preadolescents.
- Dietary deficiency: Exclusively breast-fed infants after 6 months of age, elderly.
- Chronic blood loss: **Menorrhagia, gastrointestinal bleeding.**

PRESENTATION

Pallor, fatigue, angina pectoris in persons with coronary artery disease (CAD), gastritis, glossitis, koilonychias, pica, can be associated with **Plummer-Vinson syndrome** (upper esophageal web).

> **KEY FACT**
>
> Lab findings in iron deficiency anemia:
> ↑ TIBC
> ↓ Serum iron, ferritin

TABLE 4-4. Morphologic Categorization of Anemias

TYPE	CAUSE	MANIFESTATIONS
Microcytic, hypochromic (MCV < 80 fL)	Iron deficiency, thalassemia target cells, lead poisoning.	Elevated TIBC, decreased ferritin and serum iron.
Macrocytic (MCV > 100 fL)	Megaloblastic folate/vitamin B_{12} deficiency, drugs that block DNA synthesis.	Hypersegmented neutrophils, neurologic abnormalities in vitamin B_{12} deficiency.
Normocytic, normochromic	Acute hemorrhage, G6PD deficiency, HS, bone marrow disorders, hemoglobinopathies, autoimmune hemolysis, anemia of chronic disease.	Decreased TIBC and serum iron, elevated ferritin, decreased serum haptoglobin in hemolysis.

G6PD = glucose-6-phosphate dehydrogenase; HS = hereditary spherocytosis; MCV = mean corpuscular volume; TIBC = total iron-binding capacity.

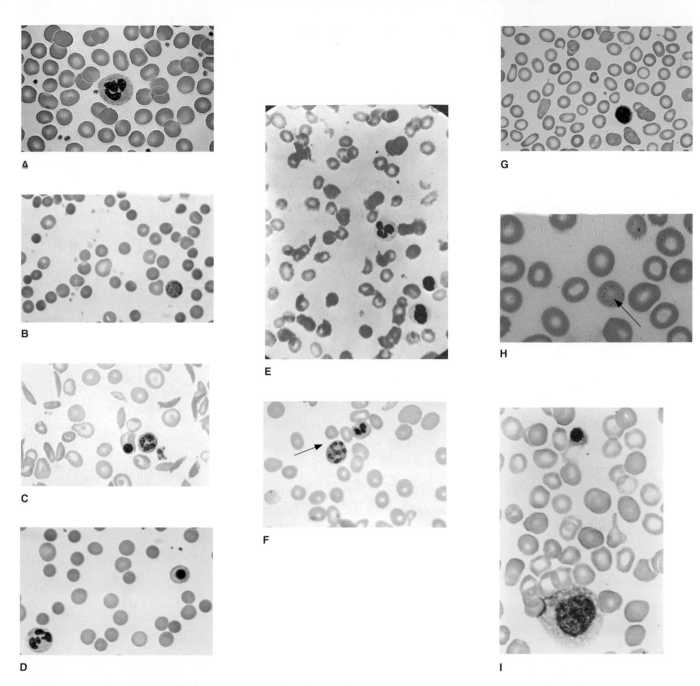

FIGURE 4-5. **Anemias by appearance on peripheral blood smear.** (A) Normal, no anemia: Normochromic, normocytic. (B) Hereditary spherocytosis: Normochromic, normocytic, spherocytosis, reticulocytosis. (C) Sickle cell anemia: Normochromic, normocytic sickle-shaped RBCs, reticulocytosis. (D) Autoimmune hemolytic anemia: Normochromic, normocytic, spherocytosis, reticulocytosis. (E) Microangiopathic anemia or trauma to RBCs: Helmet cells, schistocytes. (F) Megaloblastic anemia: Macro-ovalocyte, macrocytic, hypersegmented neutrophils (*arrow*). (G) Iron deficiency anemia: Microcytic, hypochromic. (H) Lead poisoning: Microcytic, hypochromic, ringed sideroblasts (*arrow*). (I) Myelophthisic anemia: Nucleated RBCs and immature granulocytes. (Parts A–D & F reproduced with permission from Kasper DL, Braunwald E, Fauci AS, eds. *Harrison's Principles of Internal Medicine*, 16th ed. New York: McGraw-Hill, 2005: 331, 609, 596, 613, 400. Parts E & G–I reproduced with permission from Lichtman MA, Beutler E, Kipps TJ, et al. *Williams Hematology*, 7th ed. New York: McGraw-Hill, 2006: 450, Plate I-3, Plate IV-3, 562.)

TABLE 4-5.   Red Blood Cell Forms

RBC SHAPE	ASSOCIATED DISEASE
Spherocytes	HS, autoimmune hemolysis.
Macrocyte	Megaloblastic anemia.
Helmet cell/schistocyte	DIC, traumatic hemolysis.
Sickle cell	Sickle cell anemia.
Teardrop cell	Myelofibrosis.
Acanthocyte	Abetalipoproteinemia, liver disease.
Target cell	Thalassemia, liver disease, hemoglobin C, asplenia.
Poikilocytes	TTP/HUS, microvascular hemolysis, DIC.
Hereditary spherocytosis	TTP/HUS.

DIC = disseminated intravascular coagulation; HS = hereditary spherocytosis; HUS/TTP = hemolytic-uremic syndrome/thrombotic thrombocytopenic purpura.

KEY FACT

Thalassemia is common among African, Indian, Southeast Asian, and Mediterranean populations.

KEY FACT

Thalassemias cause underproduction of *normal* globin proteins. Hemoglobinopathies (eg, sickle cell disease) involve structural abnormalities in globin proteins.

MNEMONIC

β-*ThalaSSemia*—

3 S's
Splenomegaly
Hemo**S**iderosis
Skeletal deformities

DIAGNOSIS

Decreased hemoglobin and hematocrit. Peripheral smear shows **micro-cytic, hypochromic** RBCs. Laboratory studies reveal **decreased serum iron, increased total iron-binding capacity (TIBC)**, and **decreased ferritin.**

TREATMENT

Iron supplementation; management of blood loss, if present.

THALASSEMIA

Genetic syndrome resulting from decreased synthesis of one of the chains in HbA (normally α2β2). Clinical abnormalities are caused by both the low concentration of hemoglobin and the excess of the other chain. There are two types of thalassemias, β- and α-thalassemias, discussed later.

β-THALASSEMIA

Defective β-globin chain. Also known as Mediterranean, or Cooley, anemia. Three forms exist:

- **Minor:** Heterozygote with underproduced β-globin chain.
- **Major:** Homozygote with absent β-globin chain.
- **HbS/β-thalassemia:** Combination of sickle cell and β-thalassemia. Most common form in the United States and in the Mediterranean.

All lead to lack of HbA and **aggregation of α-chains.** Aggregation leads to **decreased RBC life span** and apoptotic death of RBC precursors, resulting in ineffective erythropoiesis. **Fetal hemoglobin is increased** as a compensatory mechanism but is inadequate.

PRESENTATION

Anemia, splenomegaly from extramedullary hematopoiesis, hemosiderosis (from increased iron absorption and repeated transfusion), skeletal deformities (including "crew cut" appearance of skull on X-rays due to thinning of cortical bone and peripheral new bone formation).

DIAGNOSIS

Hemoglobin electrophoresis. Microcytic, hypochromic RBC morphology on peripheral blood smear.

TREATMENT

Blood transfusions.

PROGNOSIS

Complications may include growth retardation, death at an early age, cardiac failure, and other organ damage from hemosiderosis.

α-THALASSEMIA

Decreased production of α-globin due to mutation in one or more of the four α-globin genes. There is no compensatory increase in any other chains, but there is a relative excess of other chains including β, γ, and δ.

- α-Thalassemia is prevalent among **Asian** and **African** populations.
- Hb Bart: Excess γ-globin chains form stable tetramers.

PRESENTATION

Depends on the number of genes mutated or deleted.

- **Silent carrier state:** Only **one** α-globin gene affected; **asymptomatic.**
- **α-Thalassemia trait:** **Two** genes deleted; similar to β-thalassemia minor with **minimal anemia.**
- **Hemoglobin H disease: Three** α-globin genes affected; **HbH** (tetramers of β-globin chains) form; HbH has high O_2 affinity; **anemia disproportionate** to the amount of hemoglobin.
- **Hydrops fetalis:** Deletion of **all four** genes; **Hb Barts** (stable tetramers of γ-globin chains) has extremely high O_2 affinity; severe anemia; leads to **intrauterine death** unless intrauterine transfusion is performed; fetus shows edema, pallor, and hepatosplenomegaly.

DIAGNOSIS

Hemoglobin electrophoresis. Based on **microcytic, hypochromic** cells on blood smear and clinical presentation.

Macrocytic Anemias

MEGALOBLASTIC ANEMIA

Deficiency in vitamin B_{12} or folate (coenzymes in DNA synthesis) leads to **delayed DNA replication,** although cytoplasmic maturation is normal.

Enlargement of erythroid precursors gives rise to large RBCs (macrocytes). The bone marrow is hypercellular.

- **Vitamin B$_{12}$ deficiency** can be caused by:
  - Decreased intake (especially in **vegans**).
  - Impaired absorption (**pernicious anemia,** gastrectomy, malabsorption, **ileal resection,** *Diphyllobothrium latum*/**fish tapeworm** infection, **blind loop syndrome,** broad-spectrum antibiotics).
  - Increased requirement (**pregnancy,** hyperthyroidism).
- **Folic acid deficiency** can be caused by:
  - Decreased intake (**alcoholics**).
  - Impaired absorption (sprue, phenytoin, oral contraceptives).
  - Increased loss (hemodialysis).
  - Increased requirement (**pregnancy,** infancy, increased hematopoiesis).
  - Folic acid antagonist chemotherapy (methotrexate).

PRESENTATION

Anemia; **subacute combined degeneration** of the spinal cord in vitamin B$_{12}$ deficiency.

DIAGNOSIS

Peripheral blood smear may show **pancytopenia, oval macrocytosis,** and **hypersegmented neutrophils** (> 5 lobes); bone marrow shows **megaloblastic hyperplasia.** Methylmalonic acid, homocysteine, vitamin B$_{12}$ and folate levels can be measured.

In pernicious anemia, **anti-intrinsic factor antibodies** are present and the **Schilling test** shows that the absorption of vitamin B$_{12}$ improves with administration of intrinsic factor.

TREATMENT

Requires vitamin B$_{12}$ with/without folate supplementation.

Normocytic Anemias

GLUCOSE-6-PHOSPHATE DEHYDROGENASE DEFICIENCY

Deficiency of G6PD, an enzyme that protects RBCs from oxidants. The enzyme is **abnormally folded** and thus subject to proteolysis in older RBCs, leading to reduced ability to withstand **oxidative stress** (Figure 4-6). The oxidation of sulfhydryl groups causes hemoglobin to precipitate as **Heinz bodies.**

G6PD deficiency is **X-linked** and common in **black and Middle Eastern/ Mediterranean populations.** It is associated with resistance to malarial infection. Women may have both normal and abnormal cells if they are heterozygous. Episodes are **self-limited,** as erythropoiesis leads to the production of reticulocytes with normal enzyme activity. Hemolysis is both **intravascular and extravascular.**

PRESENTATION

Often asymptomatic. History of neonatal jaundice and cholelithiasis. Episodic fatigue, pallor, and other symptoms of anemia may result. Exam may reveal jaundice and splenomegaly. Hemolysis often results from exposure to oxidative stress such as:

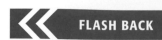

FLASH BACK

Subacute combined degeneration of the spinal cord: Vitamin B$_{12}$ deficiency leads to demyelination of the dorsal and lateral columns of the spinal cord. As a result, patients exhibit ataxia, hyperreflexia, and decreased position and vibration sensation.

KEY FACT

Use the Schilling test to check if vitamin B$_{12}$ deficiency is related to a lack of intrinsic factor.

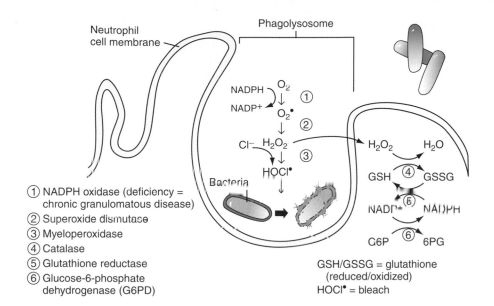

FIGURE 4-6.   Red blood cells and oxidative stress. G6P, glucose-6-phosphate; NADP, nicotinamide adenine dinucleotide phosphate; NADPH, reduced nicotinamide adenine dinucleotide phosphate; 6PG, 6-phosphogluconate.

- **Drugs:** Sulfonamides, primaquine, chloroquine, and nitrofurantoins, among others.
- **Infections:** Viral hepatitis, typhoid fever, pneumonia.
- **Other:** Fava beans.

DIAGNOSIS

Measure **G6PD enzyme activity** (is normal at time of hemolysis due to presence of young cells but is decreased when no hemolysis is present), **indirect bilirubin** ($\uparrow$), and **serum haptoglobin** ($\downarrow$). Complete blood count (CBC) with reticulocyte count reveals **hemoglobinemia** and **decreased hematocrit.** Urinalysis shows hemoglobinuria. Peripheral blood smear shows **Heinz bodies** and **bite cells** (result from splenic removal of Heinz bodies). Abdominal ultrasound may reveal splenomegaly and gallstones. Differential diagnosis includes other anemias (especially hemolytic).

TREATMENT

- Avoid precipitating factors.
- Provide O_2 and rest during episodes.
- Exchange transfusions if severe.
- Phototherapy in infants.

PROGNOSIS

Patients can remain healthy if they avoid precipitating factors, but complications include neonatal jaundice that may lead to kernicterus, a type of brain damage caused by pathologically high levels of bilirubin.

HEREDITARY SPHEROCYTOSIS

Autosomal dominant deficiency of spectrin, ankyrin, or other cytoskeletal protein leads to RBC fragility. The cells are forced into a **spherical shape** because of a **loss of membrane fragments.** Spherical cells are less deformable, become trapped within the spleen, and are then phagocytosed.

FLASH FORWARD

In G6PD-deficient patients, avoid sulfonamides, primaquine, chloroquine, and fava beans.

FLASH FORWARD

Hereditary spherocytosis (HS) results from a defect in the proteins involved in vertical interactions (ankyrin, spectrin, band 3, and protein 4.2), whereas hereditary elliptocytosis results from a defect in the proteins involved in horizontal interactions (spectrin, protein 4.1, and glycophorin). Both groups of proteins work to maintain membrane integrity.

PRESENTATION

Stable course of **anemia, splenomegaly,** and **jaundice.** Some are asymptomatic. Patients may develop **cholelithiasis** as well. There is typically a positive family history, especially in an **autosomal dominant** pattern.

DIAGNOSIS

An **osmotic fragility test** shows lysis of RBCs in hypotonic salt. **Increased MCHC** is seen due to cell dehydration. CBC reveals minimal anemia with reticulocytosis, and a peripheral blood smear shows **spherocytes.** Increased levels of **indirect bilirubin** may be detected. Differential includes anemia, biliary disease, hyperbilirubinemia, and autoimmune hemolytic anemia (which may also have spherocytes).

TREATMENT

- Splenectomy.
- Transfusion if severe.
- Phototherapy in infants.
- Supplemental folic acid and iron for increased RBC turnover.

PROGNOSIS

Possible complications include aplastic crisis triggered by parvovirus infection, infections after splenectomy, cholelithiasis, and hemosiderosis from multiple transfusions.

Immunohemolytic Anemias

Antibodies are produced that lead to destruction of RBCs. Due to the presence of antibodies, these anemias are **Coombs-positive.** Three types of immunohemolytic anemias—warm antibody, cold agglutinin, and erythroblastosis fetalis—are discussed as follows.

WARM ANTIBODY HEMOLYTIC ANEMIA

IgG autoantibodies bind RBCs, leading to spheroidal transformation. Spherocytes are sequestered in spleen (**extravascular** hemolysis).

PRESENTATION

Elevated bilirubin (jaundice, pigment gallstones), reticulocytosis, and splenomegaly. Often associated with **systemic lupus erythematosus (SLE), Hodgkin lymphoma, chronic lymphocytic leukemia (CLL),** or certain drugs (α-methyldopa, penicillin, cephalosporins).

DIAGNOSIS

Spherocytosis, positive direct Coombs test (anti-Ig Ab added to patient's RBCs leads to agglutination if RBCs have IgG attached).

COLD AGGLUTININ IMMUNE HEMOLYTIC ANEMIA

IgM autoantibodies (pathologic cold agglutinins) occur at high titers and react at 28–31°C, and sometimes at 37°C. Some **intravascular hemolysis** is seen, especially in distal body parts. IgM is released when cells warm, leaving **C3b** bound to membrane. Thus, RBCs are also subject to **extravascular hemolysis.**

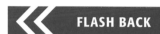

FLASH BACK

Hemoglobin has two forms: T (taut) has a low affinity for O_2, and R (relaxed) has a high affinity.

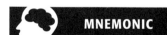

FLASH BACK

O_2 binding is cooperative and is **decreased** by Cl^-, H^+, CO_2, 2-3-diphosphoglycerate (2,3-DPG), and high temperatures.

MNEMONIC

Warm weather is **GGG**reat (IgG).
Cold ice cream ... **MMM** (IgM).

PRESENTATION

Episodic hyperbilirubinemia. May also have hemoglobinemia and hemoglobinuria.

- **Acute:** Often in recovery phase after infectious **mononucleosis** or **mycoplasmal pneumonia.**
- **Chronic:** Associated with **lymphoproliferative neoplasms;** may be associated with **Raynaud phenomenon** (Figure 4-7) due to vascular obstruction.

ERYTHROBLASTOSIS FETALIS

Maternal alloimmunization to **D antigen of Rh blood group** leads to destruction of fetal RBCs. Usually, the mother is D (Rh negative) and the fetus is D (Rh positive). May also occur in setting of **ABO incompatibility;** in these cases, the mother is O and the fetus is A or B.

PRESENTATION

Fetal hemolytic anemia.

DIAGNOSIS

Test maternal and fetal blood for presence of antibodies.

PROGNOSIS

Stillbirth, **hydrops fetalis** (fetal heart failure), **kernicterus** (unconjugated bilirubin damages basal ganglia and other central nervous system [CNS] structures, leading to neurologic damage).

KEY FACT

Erythroblastosis fetalis:
Mom → Rh−
Fetus = Rh+

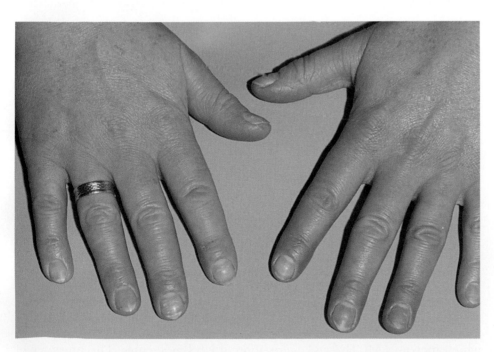

FIGURE 4-7.   Raynaud phenomenon. Note the cyanosis in the distal phalanges of the left hand. (Reproduced with permission from Wolff K, Johnson RA, Surrmon D. *Fitzpatrick's Color Atlas & Synopsis of Clinical Dermatology,* 5th ed. New York: McGraw-Hill, 2005: 403.)

Anemia of Chronic Disease

Usually characterized by marrow hypoproliferation as a result of impaired responsiveness to erythropoietin or impaired iron reutilization. Presents as a normocytic or microcytic anemia. Typical causes include:

- **Chronic infections:** Osteomyelitis and bacterial endocarditis, among others.
- Chronic immune disorders: **Rheumatoid arthritis.**
- **Renal disease.**
- **Neoplasms:** Hodgkin disease and lung carcinoma, among others.

PRESENTATION

Symptoms of the chronic disease along with mild anemia (fatigue, pallor).

DIAGNOSIS

Decreased hemoglobin and hematocrit; peripheral smear may show microcytic, hypochromic RBCs or normocytic, normochromic RBCs; **decreased serum iron, decreased TIBC, increased ferritin,** and **abundant iron stored in marrow macrophages.**

TREATMENT

Anemia may be resolved by administering erythropoietin and treating the underlying condition.

PROGNOSIS

Overall prognosis depends on the underlying condition.

Sickle Cell Disease

Point mutation (substitution of **valine** for glutamic acid at position 6) in the **β-globin chain gene** leads to production of abnormal hemoglobin, **HbS.** Common in populations of **African** heritage.

Adults normally have a large amount of HbA and small amounts of HbA_2 and HbF (fetal hemoglobin). However, those with sickle cell have at least one allele for HbS. Many variants of sickle cell exist including:

- **Sickle cell trait:** Heterozygotes with an HbA and an HbS allele (HbSA); results in resistance against malarial infection.
- **Sickle cell disease:** Homozygotes have two HbS alleles (HbSS).
- **Other:** Heterozygotes with an HbS and an HbC allele (HbSC).
- **Order of severity:** HbSS > HbSC > HbSA.

HbS undergoes aggregation and polymerization when **deoxygenated,** leading to **sickle-shaped** cells, which are subject to **splenic destruction** (Figure 4-8). These cells make the blood **hyperviscous,** which can lead to **microvascular occlusion.** Sickling may occur as a result of **hypoxia or a fall in pH,** which reduces the O_2 affinity of hemoglobin. This is worsened by **dehydration,** which increases MCHC and aggregation of HbS molecules. The presence of HbF prevents polymerization of HbS.

KEY FACT

Lab findings in anemia of chronic disease:
↓ TIBC
↓ Serum iron
↑ Serum ferritin, iron stored in macrophages

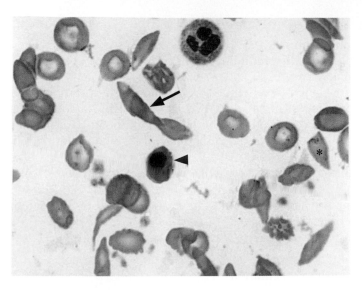

FIGURE 4-8.   Sickle cell peripheral blood smear. Note the sickle cells (*arrow*) as well as anisocytosis, poikilocytosis (*asterisk*), and nucleated red blood cells (*arrowhead*).

PRESENTATION

Because HbF prevents polymerization of HbS, disease may not manifest until newborns are 6 months old.

- Pallor from chronic hemolytic anemia.
- Vaso-occlusion causes strokes, swelling of hands and feet (**hand-foot syndrome**) and pulmonary infiltrate (**acute chest syndrome**).
- **Painful vaso-occlusive crisis** in joints, abdomen, viscera, lungs, liver, and penis.
- Infarctions of lungs and spleen occur, and **autosplenectomy** (Figure 4-9) is complete by age 6 years.
- Increased susceptibility to encapsulated bacteria such as **pneumococcus, N meningitidis** and *Haemophilus influenzae,* as well as to *Salmonella* **osteomyelitis,** secondary to asplenia.
- **Aplastic crises** brought on by **parvovirus** infection.
- Adults may develop chronic leg ulcers.

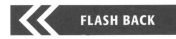

FLASH BACK

Fetal hemoglobin has lower affinity for 2,3-DPG than does adult hemoglobin and, as a result, has higher affinity for O_2.

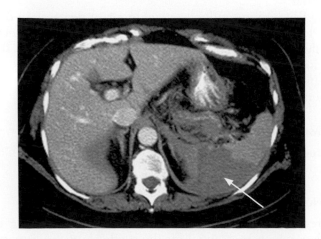

FIGURE 4-9.   Splenic infarction. The splenic artery lacks collateral supply, making the spleen particularly susceptible to ischemic damage. Coagulative necrosis has occurred in a wedge shape along the pattern of vascular supply (*arrow*). Individual sickle cells cause generalized splenic infarcts that result in autospelenctomy.

DIAGNOSIS

- **Hb electrophoresis** reveals high levels of HbS.
- Mixing blood with a **reducing agent** causes sickling; positive in both sickle cell trait and disease.
- CBC shows anemia, reticulocytosis, leukocytosis, thrombocytosis.
- Peripheral smear (Figure 4-8) reveals sickled RBCs, polychromasia, nucleated RBCs, and **Howell-Jolly bodies** (basophilic nuclear remnants).
- Serum bilirubin and fecal/urinary urobilinogen are elevated; haptoglobin levels are low.
- Skull radiograph shows "**crew cut**" pattern due to extramedullary hematopoiesis.
- Differential diagnosis includes other anemias, other hemoglobinopathies, and osteomyelitis.

TREATMENT

- Folic acid supplementation
- Blood transfusion
- Penicillin prophylaxis
- Pneumococcal, *H influenzae*, and meningococcal vaccines
- Pain control
- Bone marrow transplantation
- **Hydroxyurea** (increases concentration of HbF)

Hemolytic Anemias

Result of **premature RBC destruction** causing a build-up of **hemoglobin metabolites** and an increase in **erythropoiesis**. Classified by location of destruction (intravascular vs. extravascular), cause of destruction (extrinsic vs. intrinsic to RBCs), and origin of defect (hereditary vs. acquired), as summarized in Table 4-6.

- **Intravascular:**
  - Due to complement fixation, mechanical injury, or toxins.
  - Look for hemoglobinemia, methemalbuminemia, mild jaundice/elevation in **unconjugated bilirubin,** hemoglobinuria, hemosiderinuria, methemoglobinuria, decreased serum haptoglobin, hemosiderosis of renal tubules, and increased fecal urobilin.
- **Extravascular:**
  - Due to RBC injury, antibody attachment, or decrease in deformability/ability to leave cords of Billroth and enter sinusoids of spleen.
  - Hemolysis usually occurs in mononuclear phagocytic cells in the spleen.
  - Look for jaundice/elevation in unconjugated bilirubin, some decrease in serum haptoglobin, and **splenomegaly.** Minimal hemoglobinemia and hemoglobinuria.

PYRUVATE KINASE DEFICIENCY

Autosomal recessive enzyme dysfunction leading to anemia that is **chronic** rather than episodic.

PAROXYSMAL NOCTURNAL HEMOGLOBINURIA

Rare, **acquired** clonal hematologic disorder that arises from a mutation in the *PIGA* gene, which is essential for the synthesis of the glycosylphosphatidylinositol (GPI) anchors used for surface protein attachment. Many of the GPI-linked proteins inactivate complement, so without them, RBCs are subject to lysis by endogenous complement. Platelets and granulocytes can be affected also.

KEY FACT

Intravascular → hemoglobinemia/hemoglobinuria, decreased serum haptoglobin
Extravascular → splenomegaly

KEY FACT

In G6PD deficiency, RBCs cannot withstand oxidative stress, especially from drugs and infection, leading to hemolysis.

TABLE 4-6.   Hemolytic Anemia

INTRINSIC	EXTRINSIC
Hereditary	**Acquired**
Enzyme deficiencies (IV and EV)	**Antibody mediated (IV)**
HMP shunt: G6PD, glutathione synthetase	Transfusion reactions
	Erythroblastosis fetalis
Glycolytic enzymes: pyruvate kinase, hexokinase	Systemic lupus erythematous
	Malignant neoplasms
Membrane disorders (EV)	Mycoplasmal infection, mononucleosis
Elliptocytosis	Drug-associated
Spherocytosis	Idiopathic
Hemoglobin synthesis derangements (EV)	**Mechanical injury (IV)**
	Microangiopathic hemolytic anemias (TTP, DIC)
Thalassemias	
Sickle cell anemia (can also have IV)	Cardiac traumatic hemolytic anemia
Acquired	**Infection (IV)**
Membrane disorders (EV)	Malaria, babesiosis
Paroxysmal nocturnal hemoglobinuria	**Chemical injury (IV)**
	Lead poisoning
	Excessive destruction by spleen (EV)
	Hypersplenism

DIC = disseminated intravascular coagulation; EV = extravascular; G6PD = glucose-6-phosphate dehydrogenase; IV = intravascular; TTP = thrombotic thrombocytopenic purpura.

PRESENTATION

Hemoglobinuria on awakening; **hemosiderinuria** can lead to iron deficiency.

DIAGNOSIS

Based on clinical presentation. Flow cytometry can detect abnormalities in red cell membranes.

PROGNOSIS

This can evolve into aplastic anemia and acute leukemia.

MICROANGIOPATHIC HEMOLYTIC ANEMIA

Mechanical trauma caused by narrowed vessels leads to **intravascular** hemolysis seen in disseminated intravascular coagulation (DIC), thrombotic thrombocytopenic purpura (TTP), hemolytic-uremic syndrome (HUS), SLE, or malignant hypertension.

PRESENTATION

Related to clinical syndrome causing hemolysis. Hemolysis is usually clinically irrelevant except in TTP and HUS.

DIAGNOSIS

Schistocytes (helmet cells) on peripheral blood smear.

CARDIAC TRAUMATIC HEMOLYTIC ANEMIA

Shear stress due to the turbulent blood flow and abnormal pressures that occur with **prosthetic valves** leads to RBC damage.

Aplastic Anemia

Pancytopenia characterized by severe **anemia, neutropenia,** and **thrombocytopenia.** Failure or destruction of multipotent myeloid stem cells leads to inadequate production or release of differentiated cell lines. Common causes:

- Idiopathic (immune-mediated).
- Radiation.
- Chemicals: Benzene.
- Drugs: Chloramphenicol, sulfonamides, alkylating agents, antimalarial drugs, antimetabolites.
- Viral agents (parvovirus B19, Epstein-Barr virus [EBV], HIV, hepatitis C virus [HCV]).
- Fanconi anemia.

PRESENTATION

Onset usually gradual:

- Anemia → fatigue, malaise, pallor.
- Thrombocytopenia → purpura, mucosal bleeding, petechiae.
- Neutropenia → infection.

DIAGNOSIS

- **CBC:** Decreased RBC, WBC, and platelet count.
- **Marrow biopsy: Hypocellular bone marrow** (Figure 4-10), decreased erythrocytic and granulocytic precursors, decreased megakaryocytes, and **fatty infiltration.**
- **Peripheral smear: Pancytopenia,** normochromic, normocytic, no reticulocytosis, and no splenomegaly.

TREATMENT

- Withdrawal of offending agent.
- Immune therapy: Antithymocyte globulin, cyclosporine.
- Allogenic bone marrow transplantation.
- RBC and platelet transfusion.
- Granulocyte colony-stimulating factor (G-CSF), granulocyte-macrophage colony-stimulating factor (GM-CSF).

PROGNOSIS

- If adverse effect of drug, withdrawal may lead to recovery.
- If idiopathic, poor prognosis.

BLOOD LOSS

Acute Blood Loss

Loss of blood volume leads to a decrease in RBCs; other blood components are also affected.

PRESENTATION

Sudden weakness, fatigue, pale skin, malaise, dyspnea, cardiac failure, headache, presyncope/syncope, and shock. Patients may have history of **trauma** or bleeding. Bleeding may be external or internal.

FLASH BACK

Aplastic anemia is a common adverse effect of chloramphenicol; it may or may not reverse with discontinuation of the drug.

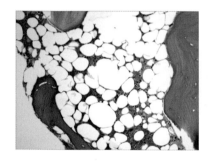

FIGURE 4-10. Bone marrow biopsy specimen of aplastic anemia. Note the hypocellular bone marrow (predominantly fat) with rare hematopoietic precursor cells but no atypical cells. (Reproduced with permission from USMLERx.)

DIAGNOSIS

CBC, peripheral blood smear. Differential includes other anemias (especially hemolytic anemias), hypothyroidism, myelofibrosis, acute porphyria, and SLE. **Hematocrit is initially normal but decreases** as interstitial fluid shifts into the vascular compartment, causing hemodilution. **Reticulocyte count increases** as erythropoiesis peaks at around 1 week. If hemorrhage is external, iron deficiency occurs over time. Peripheral smear is **initially normochromic and normocytic,** but reticulocytes appear later as polychromatophilic macrocytes.

TREATMENT

- Fluids
- Blood transfusion
- Elimination of cause of hemorrhage
- Other measures to prevent shock

Chronic Blood Loss

May lead to anemia when **loss exceeds erythropoiesis** or when **iron stores are diminished.** Presentation, diagnosis, treatment, and complications are similar to those for anemias caused by impaired RBC production. Vitamin B_{12} and folate supplementation is appropriate.

HEME PATHOLOGY

Heme production occurs via the synthetic pathway shown in Figure 4-11. A defect in any of these steps can result in **porphyrias,** a group of diseases that result from the accumulation of heme intermediates.

Acute Intermittent Porphyria (AIP)

Autosomal dominant, leading to a deficiency in porphobilinogen deaminase with subsequent accumulation of upstream metabolites—**porphobilinogen (urinary),** and **δ-aminolevulinic acid (ALA).** These intermediates lead to degeneration of myelin.

PRESENTATION

May be induced by certain medications (sulfa drugs and barbiturates, in addition to *many* others). Symptoms include dark, foul-smelling urine, hallucinations, blurred vision, and gross neurologic manifestations such as foot drop.

> **KEY FACT**
>
> Corrected reticulocyte count (CRC) = actual hematocrit/45 × reticulocyte count. If > 3%, then a good bone marrow response to anemia is present. If < 2%, then erythropoiesis is diminished or a marrow disorder, such as iron deficiency anemia, occurs.

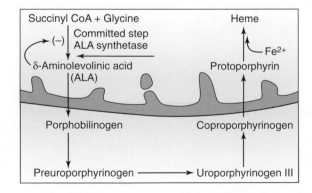

FIGURE 4-11. Heme synthesis. Underproduction of heme results in a microcytic hypochromic anemia. Accumulation of intermediates causes porphyrias.

DIAGNOSIS

Genetic testing; increased urinary secretion of porphobilinogen and porphyrins is pathognomonic. Measuring the activity of porphobilinogen deaminase is of little value, as some patients have normal levels.

TREATMENT

Goal is to decrease heme synthesis, thereby reducing the production of porphyrin precursors. Patients should eat a high-carbohydrate diet during acute attacks. Severe attacks should be treated with hematin.

KEY FACT

AIP differs from other porphyrias because it has no sun-induced lesions.

Porphyria Cutanea Tarda (PCT)

Part of the porphyria spectrum that results from deficient activity of the heme synthetic enzyme uroporphyrinogen decarboxylase (UROD). This leads to elevated porphyrin by-products, including elevated **uroporyphyrin,** iron, and transferrin.

PATHOLOGY

Accumulation of iron leads to siderosis, affecting liver function. Accumulated uroporphyrins lead to bullae and skin lesions that form upon exposure to sunlight.

PRESENTATION

Patients present with cutaneous bullae that form upon exposure to sunlight. Additional organ damage includes liver siderosis and eventual fibrosis. Urine turns dark upon standing. The disease is exacerbated by consumption of alcohol, iron, and estrogens.

DIAGNOSIS

Plasma and urine analysis for elevated uroporphyrin. The activity of the UROD can also be tested in red blood cells.

TREATMENT

- Low-dose antimalarial medications, phlebotomy.
- The porphyria syndromes are summarized in Table 4-7.

TABLE 4-7.   Summary of the Porphyrias

DISEASE	DEFICIT	PRESENTATION	TREATMENT
Acute intermittent porphyria	Porphobilinogen deaminase	Dark, foul-smelling urine (usually following sun exposure or certain medications), and neurologic deficits.	Hematin, high-carbohydrate diet.
Porphyria cutanea tarda	Uroporphyrinogen decarboxylase	Bullae on sun-exposed areas, liver siderosis, dark urine upon standing.	Low-dose antimalarials, phlebotomy. Avoidance of alcohol, sun exposure, estrogens and iron.

PRESENTATION

Usually mild (petechiae, purpura in skin or mucous membranes); occasionally more severe (hemorrhages into joints and muscles, menorrhagia, epistaxis, GI bleeding, hematuria).

DIAGNOSIS

Platelet count, prothrombin time (PT), and partial thromboplastin time (PTT) are usually normal. Bleeding time is occasionally prolonged.

Note: Platelet function assay (PFA)-100 has replaced bleeding time tests in many institutions.

PROGNOSIS

Depends on specific cause.

Platelet Disorders

THROMBOCYTOPENIA

Reduction in number of platelets leads to decreased ability to form clots. Results from decreased production, decreased survival, sequestration, and dilution of platelets. Specific causes include:

- Bone marrow diseases such as **aplastic anemia** and **acute leukemia.**
- Drugs: Alcohol, quinidine, **heparin,** sulfa, **cytotoxic drugs,** and thiazide diuretics.
- Infections such as measles, **HIV,** infectious mononucleosis, cytomegalovirus (CMV), *Haemophilus influenzae* type B.
- **Hypersplenism** leads to sequestration of platelets.
- **Transfusions** result in dilution of platelets and clotting factors; may additionally lead to destruction of platelets.
- SLE.
- DIC: Activation of coagulation cascade leads to **microthrombi** and consumption of platelets and coagulation factors (**especially II, V, VIII, and fibrinogen**); characterized by both thrombosis and hemorrhage; results from the release of tissue thromboplastin or activation of the intrinsic pathway. Common causes include **obstetric** complications (toxemia, amniotic fluid emboli, retained fetus, or abruptio placentae), **gram-negative sepsis,** transfusion, trauma, **malignancy** (especially of the lung, pancreas, prostate, and stomach), acute pancreatitis, nephrotic syndrome.

DIAGNOSIS

Increased PT, PTT, fibrin, fibrin split products (D-dimers), thrombin time, and bleeding time; decreased platelet count. Helmet-shaped cells and schistocytes seen on blood smear occasionally.

PROGNOSIS

Can lead to organ damage and shock; poor prognosis.

TREATMENT

Treat underlying cause and provide supportive therapy.

- **Idiopathic thrombocytopenic purpura:** Thrombocytopenia with normal or increased megakaryocytes. **Antiplatelet antibodies** attach to platelets and lead to removal by splenic macrophages. No splenomegaly. Splenectomy is curative in two-thirds of patients.

FLASH FORWARD

Heparin-induced thrombocytopenia (HIT) results from acquired immunoglobulin G (IgG) antibodies to platelet factor IV/heparin complexes. Antibody binding results in thrombosis despite thrombocytopenia. Cessation of therapy is curative:

- Type I occurs rapidly and is clinically insignificant, resulting from platelet aggregation.
- Type II develops after 5–14 days; life-threatening thrombosis; immune reaction against complex of heparin and platelet factor IV. Can occur earlier if previously exposed to heparin.

- **Children: Acute,** self-limited reaction to viral infection or immunization; treat only if severe.
- **Adults: Chronic,** autoimmune condition; occurs more often in **females;** treat with steroids, Anti-Rh(D) Ig, IVIG, rituximab, and other medications. Ultimately, may need a splenectomy.

■ **Thrombotic microangiopathies:** Result from **hyaline microthrombi** (platelet aggregates surrounded by fibrin) leading to **thrombocytopenia** and microangiopathic anemia (peripheral blood smear shows **schistocytes** and **helmet cells**).

- **TTP:** Associated with a lack of metalloproteinase enzyme, (ADAMTS13) which normally degrades von Willebrand factor (vWF). The resulting multimeric form causes platelet aggregation with the pentad of microangiopathic hemolytic anemia, thrombocytopenia, renal failure, fever, and neurologic deficits. Usually in **adult** females.
- **HUS:** Usually in **children** following *Escherichia coli* O157:H7 infection; Shiga toxin damage of endothelium results in the triad of microangiopathic hemolytic anemia, thrombocytopenia, and renal failure.

KEY FACT

DIC laboratory findings:
↑ PT, PTT, fibrin, fibrin split products, thrombin time, and bleeding time.
↓ Platelet count.

KEY FACT

Laboratory findings in thrombocytopenia:
↓ Platelet count
↑ Bleeding time
No change in PT and PTT.

PRESENTATION

Characterized by bleeding from small vessels, which leads to **petechial, purpural, mucosal, and intracranial hemorrhage** (Figure 4-13). Platelet count below 100,000/mm^3 is considered pathologic, though spontaneous bleeding does not typically occur until the platelet count falls below 20,000/mm^3.

DIAGNOSIS

■ **Decreased platelet count** is the main diagnostic finding.
■ **Prolonged bleeding time** occasionally seen; is often normal and rarely used in diagnosis.
■ Bone marrow aspiration: Megakaryocytes decreased if decreased platelet production, increased if increased platelet destruction; usually not performed.

PROGNOSIS

Varies with underlying cause.

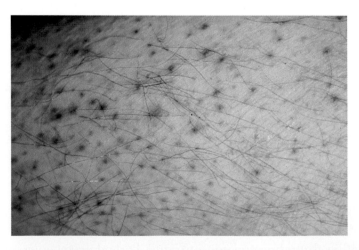

FIGURE 4-13. **Petechiae.** (Reproduced with permission from Lichtman MA, Beutler E, Kipps TJ, et al. *Williams Hematology,* 7th ed. New York: McGraw-Hill, 2006: Figure XXV-32.)

Platelet Function Abnormalities

Qualitative platelet dysfunction that takes place in the setting of normal platelet counts. Caused by:

- Defects in platelet adhesion:
    - **von Willebrand disease:** Most common hereditary bleeding disorder; **autosomal dominant** deficiency of vWF, which normally carries **factor VIII** and mediates adhesion of platelets to endothelium in vascular injury; disease is characterized by normal platelet counts with:
        - Impaired adhesion → prolonged bleeding time.
        - Mild quantitative deficiency of factor VIII → prolonged activated partial thromboplastin time (aPTT).
    - **Bernard-Soulier disease: Autosomal recessive** disorder in which platelets are abnormally large and lack platelet-surface **glycoprotein Ib,** which is needed for platelet adhesion.
- Defects in platelet aggregation:
    - **Aspirin:** Acetylates and irreversibly inactivates cyclooxygenase (COX), an enzyme necessary for the production of **thromboxane A$_2$,** a platelet aggregant.
    - **Glanzmann thrombasthenia:** Hereditary deficiency of platelet-surface **glycoproteins IIb and IIIa,** which are required for forming fibrinogen bridges between platelets.

PRESENTATION

Mucocutaneous bleeding.

DIAGNOSIS

Laboratory tests (PT, PTT, bleeding time, platelet count).

PROGNOSIS

Depends on underlying cause.

Clotting Factor Deficiencies

Lack of clotting factors leads to easy bruising and bleeding. Spontaneous bleeding into joints (hemarthrosis) and other tissues is common. These deficiencies are described in the following sections.

HEMOPHILIA A

X-linked deficiency of factor VIII; also known as classic hemophilia. Prolonged PTT that corrects with mixing studies. Treatment is with infusion of factor VIII.

HEMOPHILIA B

X-linked deficiency of factor IX; also known as Christmas disease. Corrects with normal plasma mixing, but treatment with factor VIII produces no response. Treatment is with factor IX replacement.

VITAMIN K DEFICIENCY

Leads to deficiency of **factors II, VII, IX, X,** and **proteins C and S.** In adults, caused by fat malabsorption due to pancreatic or small-bowel disease. In infants, caused by deficient exogenous vitamin K (not present in breast milk) and incomplete intestinal colonization by bacteria that synthesize vitamin K.

KEY FACT

von Willebrand disease:
↑ Bleeding time
↑ aPTT

FLASH FORWARD

Aspirin: Inhibition of COX-1 and COX-2 prevents the conversion of arachidonic acid to various prostaglandins. It is therefore used to treat fever, inflammation, and prevent adverse consequences of clot formation.

FLASH BACK

PTT: Assesses intrinsic and common pathways; prolongation due to deficiency of **factors V, VIII, IX, X, XI, XII, prothrombin (II), and fibrinogen (I).**

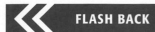

PT: Assesses extrinsic and common pathways; prolonged due to deficiency of **factor V, VII, X, prothrombin (II), or fibrinogen (I).**

Liver Disease

Hepatocellular damage prevents the production of **all coagulation factors except vWF,** as they are exclusively formed in the liver. Liver disease may lead to **hypersplenism** and **overt thrombocytopenia.** As a result, PT, PTT, thrombin time, and bleeding time are prolonged.

PRESENTATION

Macrohemorrhage leads to **hemarthroses** (bleeding into joints), **easy bruising,** and large hematomas rather than petechiae.

DIAGNOSIS

Laboratory test results for PT, aPTT, and thrombin time.

TREATMENT

Vitamin K or fresh frozen plasma.

PROGNOSIS

Depends on severity and type of condition.

WHITE CELL DISORDERS

Leukopenia

Decreased white blood cell count. Can reflect **neutropenia/granulocytopenia** (decreased number of neutrophils) and/or **lymphopenia** (decreased number of lymphocytes).

Neutropenia can result from:

- Decreased production:
  - Aplastic anemia.
  - Certain adverse drug reactions.
  - Inherited conditions.
- Increased destruction:
  - Immunologic disorders.
  - Certain adverse drug reactions.
  - Splenic sequestration.
  - Reduction in numbers due to overwhelming infection.

Lymphopenia may result from:

- HIV
- Steroids
- Cytotoxic drugs
- Viral infections
- Malnutrition

PRESENTATION

- **Neutropenia:** Bacterial or fungal infections; malaise, chills, and fever; other signs of specific infections.
- **Lymphopenia:** Viral infections.

DIAGNOSIS

CBC with WBC count and differential.

PROGNOSIS

Depends on degree of reduction in number of cells and cause.

Reactive Proliferation

LEUKOCYTOSIS

Increased number of white blood cells, usually due to infection or inflammation.

- **Neutrophilic** → bacterial infection.
- **Eosinophilic** → allergies/asthma, parasitic infections, drugs, neoplasms, collagen vascular diseases.

LYMPHADENITIS

Increased number of WBCs in lymph nodes (Figure 4-14), usually due to infection or inflammation. For example: infectious mononucleosis—EBV, especially in young adults, infects B lymphocytes and leads to generalized lymphadenopathy. It is characterized by **atypical lymphocytes**, anti-EBV antibodies, and **heterophile antibodies**. It can be associated with sore throat, fever, and hepatosplenomegaly and is usually self-limited.

Neoplastic Proliferation

Neoplastic proliferation of WBCs can be classified into lymphomas and leukemias. Many are characterized by a specific chromosomal translocation (Table 4-10).

LYMPHOMAS

Lymphomas are proliferations most often in the lymph nodes. These can be divided into **Hodgkin lymphomas**, with characteristic Reed-Sternberg cells, and **non-Hodgkin lymphomas (NHLs)**.

HODGKIN LYMPHOMA

Malignant proliferation of WBCs featuring characteristic **Reed-Sternberg cells** (bi- or multinucleated giant cells with eosinophilic nucleoli or "owl

KEY FACT

Corticosteroids induce a benign neutrophilic leukocytosis.

KEY FACT

Hodgkin	Non-Hodgkin
Reed-Sternberg cells	No Reed-Sternberg cells
Single groups of axial nodes	Multiple groups of peripheral nodes
Contiguous spread	Noncontiguous spread
Constitutional symptoms	Fewer constitutional symptoms
Bimodal (young and old)	Usually seen in those 20–40 years old

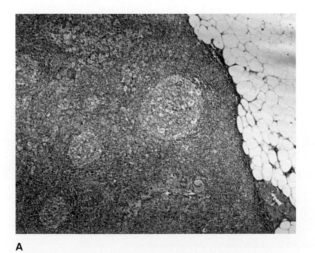

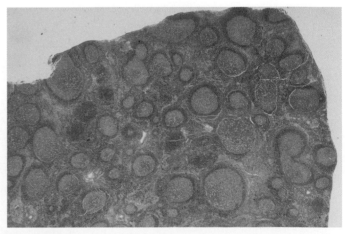

A   **B**

FIGURE 4-14.   Normal (A) and reactive (B) lymph nodes. (Reproduced with permission from Lichtman MA, Beutler E, Kipps TJ, et al. *Williams Hematology*, 7th ed. New York: McGraw-Hill, 2006: Plates XXII-1 and XXII-3.)

TABLE 4-10. Common Chromosomal Translocations

DISEASE	TRANSLOCATION
CML	t(9;22) Ph chromosome
Burkitt lymphoma	t(8;14) c-myc
Follicular lymphoma	t(14;18) bcl-2
AML M3 type	t(15;17) APL: RARA
Ewing sarcoma	t(11;22)
Mantle cell lymphoma	t(11;14)

AML = acute myelogenous leukemia; CML = chronic myelogenous leukemia.

eyes"; of CD30+ and CD15+ B-cell origin) in addition to reactive lymphocytes (Figure 4-15). The majority of cases can be cured. There are four histologic variants: **nodular sclerosing, mixed cellularity, lymphocyte predominant,** and **lymphocyte depleted** (Figure 4-16 and Table 4-11).

PRESENTATION

Constitutional ("B") symptoms: Low-grade fever, night sweats, and weight loss often present. Typically presents with painless mediastinal lymphadenopathy. About half of cases are associated with **EBV infection.** Age distribution is bimodal (young and old). All types affect men more than women except for the nodular sclerosing type, which affects women more. Spread is contiguous.

DIAGNOSIS

Based on biopsy.

TREATMENT

Chemotherapy, radiotherapy.

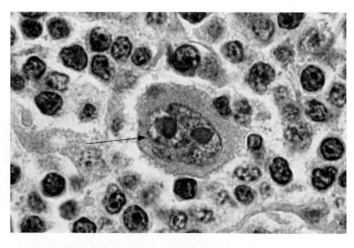

FIGURE 4-15. **Reed-Sternberg cells.** Classic "owl's eye" (*arrow*) appearance. (Reproduced with permission from Lichtman MA, Beutler E, Kipps TJ, et al. *Williams Hematology,* 7th ed. New York: McGraw-Hill, 2006: Plate XXII-32.)

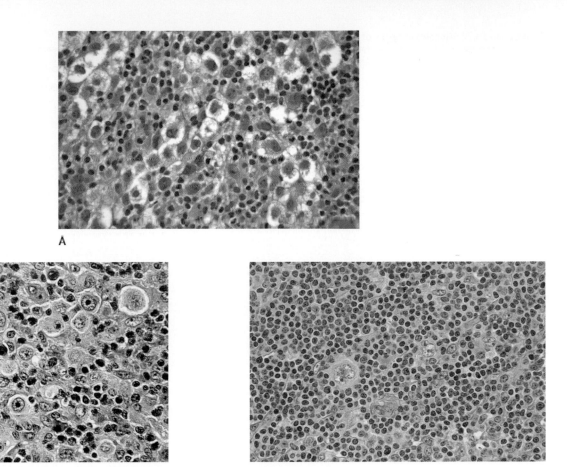

FIGURE 4-16.   Histologic types of Hodgkin lymphoma. (A) Nodular sclerosing; (B) mixed cellularity; (C) lymphocyte-predominant. (Part A reproduced with permission from USMLERx; Figures B and C reproduced with permission from Lichtman MA, Beutler E, Kipps TJ, et al. *Williams Hematology*, 7th ed. New York: McGraw-Hill, 2006: Plates XXII-36, XXII-37.)

PROGNOSIS

Staging, the best predictor of prognosis, is based on the number of lymph node regions involved, involvement of extralymphatic sites, and extent of dissemination. Because of the high rate of cure due to chemotherapy and radiotherapy, survivors often develop secondary cancers.

NON-HODGKIN LYMPHOMA

Malignant lymphoid proliferations of B cells (and occasionally T cells). Often these cases are associated with HIV and immunosuppression. Cells are often located in multiple groups of nodes, and **extranodal** involvement is common. Spread of malignant cells is **noncontiguous.** Can be classified by clinical behavior (low-, intermediate-, or high-grade), by nodular versus diffuse (follicular lymphoma is the only nodular type), and by cytology of small versus large cells.

PRESENTATION

Lymphadenopathy in multiple groups of peripheral nodes. Constitutional symptoms occur less frequently than in Hodgkin lymphomas.

TABLE 4-11. **Histologic Types of Hodgkin Lymphoma and Their Characteristics**

TYPE	PREVALENCE	NO. OF REED-STERNBERG CELLS	NO. OF LYMPHOCYTES	PROGNOSIS
Nodular sclerosing	Most common (70%)	+	+++	Excellent
▪ More common in women than men.				
▪ Cells are grouped into nodules surrounded by **fibrous bands.**				
▪ Usually located in cervical, supraclavicular, or mediastinal nodes.				
▪ **Lacunar cells** (Reed-Sternberg nucleus surrounded by empty space).				
▪ Can be related to EBV infection.				
Mixed cellularity	25%	++++	+++	Intermediate
▪ Typically seen in young men.				
▪ Also often related to EBV infection.				
▪ Complete effacement, multiple nodes.				
▪ Eosinophils, plasma cells, histiocytes, and Reed-Sternberg cells with regions of fibrosis.				
Lymphocyte predominant	6%	+	++++	Excellent
▪ Lymphocytes and histiocytes.				
▪ < 35-year-old men.				
▪ Popcorn cells (Reed-Sternberg cells).				
Lymphocyte depleted	Rare	High relative to lymphocytes	+	Poor
▪ Few lymphocytes with large number of Reed-Sternberg cells and fibrosis.				
▪ Older men with disseminated disease, HIV patients.				

EBV = Epstein-Barr virus.

DIAGNOSIS

Based on clinical presentation and histologic findings on biopsy (Table 4-12 and Figure 4-17 for histologic classifications).

PROGNOSIS

Depends on type. Although average survival is better in low-grade lymphomas, they are rarely cured. Follicular lymphomas have better survival rates than diffuse forms. The prognosis for small-cell lymphomas is better than that for large-cell types.

KEY FACT

Mycosis fungoides is in the skin. Sézary syndrome is in the blood.

CUTANEOUS T-CELL LYMPHOMAS

Neoplastic mature T cells proliferate in the dermis and epidermis in **mycosis fungoides.** In a second, leukemic form of the disease known as **Sézary syndrome,** neoplastic cells circulate as well as concentrate in the skin, resulting in a physical presentation termed **leonine facies.**

TABLE 4-12. Histologic Types of Non-Hodgkin Lymphoma and Their Characteristics

TYPE	EPIDEMIOLOGY	CELL TYPE	GRADE	GENETICS	HISTOLOGY
Small lymphocytic lymphoma ■ Like a focal mass of **chronic lymphocytic leukemia.** ■ **Richter syndrome** or **prolymphocytic transformation** into diffuse B-cell lymphoma occurs in a quarter of cases.	Adults	B	Low		Small, mature-looking lymphocytes; lymph nodes are effaced.
Follicular lymphoma (small cleaved cell) ■ **Common adult** form; indolent and difficult to cure.	Adults	B	Low	**t(14;18),** translocation of *bcl-2* to Ig heavy-chain locus on chromosome 14 leads to overexpression and prevents apoptosis.	Angulated grooved cells typical of those in normal lymphoid follicular center; arranged in nodules.
Diffuse large cell ■ Often presents with extranodal mass. ■ Aggressive, but about half are curable.	Adults: 80%; children: 20%	B: 80%; mature T: 20%	Intermediate		
Mantle cell lymphoma ■ Poor prognosis. ■ Frequent involvement of the GI tract causing lymphomatoid polyposis.	Adults	B		t(11:14)	Resemble cells in the mantle zone of lymph nodes.
Lymphoblastic lymphoma ■ **Most common childhood** form. ■ Very aggressive; 80% cured, but high relapse rate. ■ Often presents with **acute lymphocytic leukemia** and **mediastinal mass.**	Children and adults	Immature T	High		**Cell nuclei appear convoluted; arise from thymic lymphocytes.**
Burkitt lymphoma ■ Associated with **EBV, HIV.** ■ **Very rapidly growing mass.** ■ Jaw involvement common in endemic African form. ■ Pelvic/abdominal involvement often occurs in sporadic form.	Children and adults	B	High	t(8;14), *c-myc* overexpressed once moved next to heavy-chain Ig gene on 14.	**Starry-sky** appearance (sheets of lymphocytes with interspersed nonneoplastic macrophages).

EBV = Epstein-Barr virus.

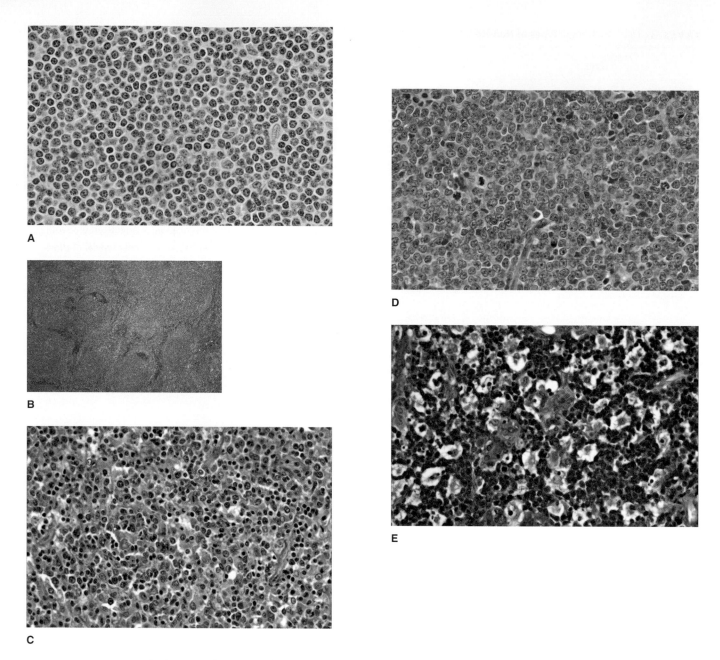

FIGURE 4-17. **Histologic types of non-Hodgkin lymphoma.** (A) Small lymhocytic lymphoma; (B) follicular lymphoma (small cleaved cell); (C) diffuse large cell; (D) lymphoblastic lymphoma; (E) Burkitt lymphoma. (Parts A, D reproduced with permission from Lichtman MA, Beutler E, Kipps TJ, et al. *Williams Hematology*, 7th ed. New York: McGraw-Hill, 2006: Plates XXII-10, XXII-8. Part B, C, E reproduced with permission from USMLERx.)

PRESENTATION

Erythematous lesions develop on the skin in the inflammatory premycotic phase, progress along a typical path to the plaque phase, and finally enter the tumor phase.

DIAGNOSIS

Biopsy reveals CD4+ T cells with characteristic **cerebriform nuclei** proliferating in the dermis. Often there are focal concentrations of neoplastic cells in the epidermis known as **Pautrier microabscesses**.

PROGNOSIS

Indolent, median survival of 8–9 years; can progress to diffuse large-cell lymphoma.

EXTRANODAL MARGINAL ZONE LYMPHOMA (MALT LYMPHOMA)

Low-grade B-cell tumors arising most commonly in **M**ucosal-**A**ssociated **L**ymphatic **T**issue (salivary glands, small and large bowel, and lungs). May occur in the setting of *Helicobacter pylori* infection; in this case, treatment with antibiotics and eradication of the organism leads to tumor regression.

LEUKEMIAS

Leukemias involve the malignant spread of granulocytic or lymphocytic precursors in the bone marrow and the circulation. Cells also frequently infiltrate liver, spleen, and lymph nodes. They can be separated into acute and chronic leukemias. **Acute** forms involve blasts (immature cells), affect children or the elderly, and have a short and drastic course. **Chronic** forms usually involve the proliferation of more mature cells, affect people in mid-life, and have a longer and less devastating course. Leukemias can also be classified by whether they involve **lymphocytic** or **myelogenous** cell types. Often, marrow failure can cause anemia, infections, and hemorrhage by reducing the numbers of RBCs, WBCs, and platelets.

KEY FACT

Leukemia = proliferation in the bone marrow and bloodstream; divided into acute versus chronic and myelogenous versus lymphocytic.

ACUTE LYMPHOBLASTIC LEUKEMIA (ALL)

Neoplasm of lymphoblasts (immature B or T cells).

PRESENTATION

Pre-B-cell leukemias usually affect children. **Pre-T-cell** leukemias often occur with lymphoblastic leukemia; typical clinical picture is an adolescent male with a mediastinal mass. **Onset is sudden,** and patients usually present within days or weeks of symptom onset. **Marrow failure** usually results in fatigue, infection, and bleeding due to anemia, neutropenia, and thrombocytopenia. Bone pain, lymphadenopathy, splenomegaly, hepatomegaly, meningeal spread, and testicular spread are also common. Relapses often occur in the CNS and testis.

DIAGNOSIS

Based on flow cytometry, peripheral smear and bone marrow biopsy. Monomorphic cells with condensed chromatin, **minimal cytoplasm,** and no granules (Figure 4-18). Surface markers are also assessed to differentiate from acute myeloid leukemia.

TREATMENT

Chemotherapy.

PROGNOSIS

Almost all patients go into remission after chemotherapy, and in children about **two-thirds are cured.** This leukemia is the most responsive to therapy. Prognosis is worst for those younger than age 2, those who present in adolescence or later, and those with the Philadelphia translocation, t(9;22). The WBC and platelet counts on admission are also important diagnostic indicators.

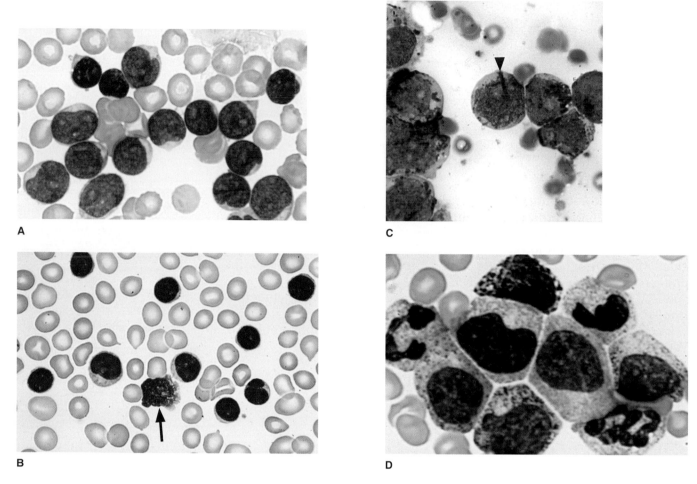

FIGURE 4-18. **Peripheral smears of leukemias.** (A) Acute lymphoblastic leukemia. Lymphoblasts have condensed chromatin with indented nuclei, minimal cytoplasm, and no granules. (B) Chronic lymphocytic leukemia. Small, round lymphocytes are visible in peripheral smears. Smudge cells (*arrow*), the result of the fragility of the neoplastic cells, are frequently seen. (C) Acute myelogenous leukemia. Myeloblasts with delicate chromatin, peroxidase-positive granules, and abundant cytoplasm compared with lymphoblasts. Cells in acute promyelocytic leukemia often contain Auer rods (*arrowhead*) in the cytoplasm. (D) Chronic myelogenous leukemia. Leukocytosis with a mix of neutrophils, metamyelocytes, and myelocytes, and less than 10% myeloblasts. Eosinophilia and basophilia are also common. (Reproduced with permission from Lichtman MA, Beutler E, Kipps TJ, et al. *Williams Hematology*, 7th ed. New York: McGraw-Hill, 2006: Plates XX-11, XX-4, XVI-3, and XIX-2.)

CHRONIC LYMPHOCYTIC LEUKEMIA (CLL)

Neoplastic proliferation of lymphoid cells, usually **CD5+ B cells.** This disease is the same as **small lymphocytic lymphoma (SLL)** except that the majority of the neoplastic cells in CLL are in the circulation and marrow as opposed to nodal or extranodal masses. Cells do not differentiate into antibody-secreting plasma cells.

PRESENTATION

Males are affected twice as often as females, and the average age of presentation is **60 years.** Patients are often asymptomatic or have nonspecific symptoms of weight loss and fatigue. Lymphadenopathy and hepatosplenomegaly are common. Bacterial infections are common as a result of hypogammaglobulinemia. Autoantibodies that develop in reaction to the tumor cells can lead to **warm antibody autoimmune hemolytic anemia** or thrombocytopenia. **Prolymphocytic transformation** into diffuse B-cell lymphoma occurs in one-quarter of cases.

DIAGNOSIS

Small, round lymphocytes are visible in peripheral smears and bone marrow biopsies. **Smudge cells,** the result of the fragility of the neoplastic cells, are frequently seen. Some patients may have a monoclonal Ig "spike."

PROGNOSIS

Survival is typically 4–6 years. If prolymphocytic transformation occurs, survival is less than 1 year.

ACUTE MYELOGENOUS LEUKEMIA

Acquired genetic mutations in stem cells lead to proliferation of undifferentiated myeloid blasts. Also known as acute granulocytic leukemia. Classified as arising from myelodysplasia versus de novo.

One specific type of acute myelogenous leukemia (AML) is **acute promyelocytic leukemia (APL),** which results from a translocation of the retinoic acid receptor-α (**RAR-α**) gene from chromosome 17 to next to the promyelocytic leukemia gene on chromosome 15 [t(15;17)(q22;q12)]. The result is an abnormal receptor that prevents cell differentiation and maturation.

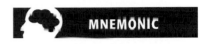

MNEMONIC

Acute promyelocytic leukemia—

A pro's engine **RARs (roars)** at 1715 **myels (miles)** per **Auer (hour).**

PRESENTATION

The de novo form affects **adults** (15–39 years old), but cases arising from myelodysplasia usually affect people in the sixth decade or beyond. Patients have symptoms of fatigue, infection, and bleeding because of anemia, neutropenia, and thrombocytopenia.

DIAGNOSIS

Based on peripheral smear and bone marrow biopsy. Biopsy reveals > 20% myeloid blasts in marrow. On smear, myeloblasts have delicate chromatin, peroxidase-positive granules, and **abundant cytoplasm** compared with lymphoblasts.

Cells often contain **Auer rods** (peroxidase-positive cytoplasmic inclusions) in the cytoplasm, especially in APL. Surface markers can be assessed to differentiate from ALL.

TREATMENT

Chemotherapy (7+3+3 – cytarabine, daunorubicin, etoposide); high-dose **all-*trans*-retinoic acid** can overcome the blockade caused by the abnormal protein in APL with a t(15;17) translocation.

PROGNOSIS

Chemotherapy is successful in producing complete remission in approximately 60% of patients; however, more than half of these people have recurrence of disease within 5 years. Specific genetic alteration influences prognosis. A large portion of patients treated with all-*trans*-retinoic acid also achieve remission, although relapse almost always occurs. Also of note, treatment of APL may release large numbers of Auer rods, which can result in DIC.

CHRONIC MYELOGENOUS LEUKEMIA (CML)

Proliferation of pluripotent cells producing myeloid cells that are capable of terminal differentiation; also known as **chronic myelocytic** or **chronic granulocytic leukemia.** Note that this is both a leukemia and a myeloproliferative disorder. Production of normal cells is prevented because of overcrowding.

Can be associated with the **Philadelphia (Ph) chromosome,** in which the *c-abl* gene is moved from **chromosome 9 to 22,** next to the *bcr* gene. The result is a fusion protein, ***BCR-ABL,*** with tyrosine kinase activity that leads to uncontrolled proliferation.

PRESENTATION

Insidious onset with nonspecific symptoms such as mild anemia and weight loss, typically in middle-aged patients. **Splenomegaly** is common. An **accelerated phase** with increasing anemia and thrombocytopenia often occurs after approximately 3 years. Whether or not there is an accelerated phase, all untreated patients eventually enter a **blast crisis with > 20% blasts on peripheral smear,** a condition similar to acute leukemia.

DIAGNOSIS

Peripheral smear and bone marrow biopsy aid diagnosis, although chromosomal analysis or PCR can be used to definitively detect the ***BCR-ABL* fusion gene.** Leukocytosis with mixed neutrophils, metamyelocytes, myelocytes, and absolute basophilia on smear. The marrow is entirely filled with cells, especially mature granulocytic precursors. Can be differentiated from leukemoid reactions because **leukocyte alkaline phosphatase is not as elevated in CML.**

TREATMENT

- **Gleevec (imatinib mesylate):** Induces apoptosis of leukemic cells; has almost completely replaced other therapies.
- **Low-dose chemotherapy:** Stabilizes early phase, but does not prevent accelerated phase and blast crisis.
- **Allogenic bone marrow transplantation:** Cures up to 75% of cases; most effective in the stable phase.

PROGNOSIS

With or without treatment, initial progression is slow until accelerated phase and blast crisis.

HAIRY CELL LEUKEMIA

Uncommon leukemia distinguished by the presence of leukemic cells that have fine, hair-like cytoplasmic projections. Cells are CD103+ and TRAP+. The hairy cells can usually be seen in the peripheral blood smear.

ADULT T-CELL LEUKEMIA/LYMPHOMA

T-cell neoplasm caused by infection with a retrovirus (human T-cell leukemia virus type 1 [HTLV-1]). Characterized by skin lesions, generalized lymphadenopathy, hepatosplenomegaly, hypercalcemia, and an elevated leukocyte count with multilobed CD4 lymphocytes. May cause progressive demyelinating disease of the CNS.

Plasma Cell Disorders

Include multiple myeloma, Waldenström macroglobulinemia, and monoclonal gammopathy of undetermined significance. These disorders are caused by clonal neoplastic transformation of Ig-secreting, terminally differentiated B cells. Monoclonal Ig is referred to as the **M component.** The balance between light-chain and heavy-chain production is lost, and free light chains, **Bence Jones proteins,** are excreted in the urine.

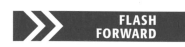

FLASH FORWARD

Gleevec inhibits *BCR-ABL* tyrosine kinase to decrease proliferation and increase apoptosis.

KEY FACT

Tartrate-resistant acid phosphatase (TRAP) is a marker for hairy B-cell leukemia.

MULTIPLE MYELOMA

Neoplastic proliferation of small lymphoid cells leads to clonal expansion of plasma cells. The proliferation and survival of myeloma cells depends on multiple factors, most notably upon interleukin 6 (IL-6).

PRESENTATION

Usually presents in patients **50–60 years old.** Characteristics include:

- **Punched-out bone lesions,** especially in the vertebrae and skull. Fractures of the vertebral column and bone pain are common.
- **Hypercalcemia** from bone destruction.
- **Myeloma kidney,** or renal insufficiency with azotemia, because of excretion of Bence Jones proteins; tubular casts of Bence Jones protein, giant cells, and metastatic calcification may be evident.
- **Marrow failure** leading to anemia and, rarely, leukopenia and thrombocytopenia.
- **Infections,** especially with *Streptococcus pneumoniae*, *Staphylococcus aureus*, and *Escherichia coli*, as a result of clonal Ig, leading to decreased production of normal Ig.
- **Amyloidosis.**
- **Hyperviscosity syndrome** in a minority of cases.

DIAGNOSIS

Hyperglobulinemia may lead to **rouleaux formation** of red cells (an aggregate of erythrocytes stacked like a pile of coins). Electrophoresis usually reveals increased Ig in blood and/or Bence Jones proteins in the urine. **IgG** is the M component in about half of cases; IgA in about one-quarter. Radiography usually reveals **punched-out round skeletal lesions,** but sometimes findings are more consistent with generalized osteoporosis. Cells have a characteristic "**fried-egg**" appearance (Figure 4-19).

PROGNOSIS

Survival varies, with an average of **3–5 years.** Some forms are indolent, but others have a survival of 6–12 months. Death usually occurs from infection or renal insufficiency. Chemotherapy leads to remission in about half of patients. **Bisphosphonates** can inhibit bone resorption. Bone marrow transplantation can improve survival but is not curative.

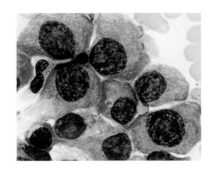

FIGURE 4-19. **Multiple myeloma.** (Reproduced with permission from Lichtman MA, Beutler E, Kipps TJ, et al. *Williams Hematology*, 7th ed. New York: McGraw-Hill, 2006: Plate XXI-4.)

WALDENSTRÖM MACROGLOBULINEMIA

Neoplasm of **plasmacytoid lymphocytes** (cells between B lymphocytes and plasma cells in terms of maturity) with monoclonal **IgM** secretion. Also known as lymphoplasmacytic lymphoma.

PRESENTATION

Typically affects **50+ year-old males.** Nonspecific symptoms of fatigue and weight loss are common, as are lymphadenopathy, hepatomegaly, and splenomegaly. Anemia occurs as a result of marrow failure and sometimes due to IgM **cold antibody autoimmune hemolysis. Hyperviscosity syndrome** often develops and presents with visual impairment such as retinal vascular dilation, neurologic issues, bleeding, and Raynaud phenomenon.

DIAGNOSIS

Electrophoresis of serum reveals a clonal IgM spike, and 10% of cases show Bence Jones proteinuria; no bone lesions.

PROGNOSIS

Incurable and progressive with a median survival of 4 years. Plasmapheresis can treat hyperviscosity and hemolysis. Rarely transforms to large-cell lymphoma.

MONOCLONAL GAMMOPATHY OF UNCERTAIN SIGNIFICANCE

Some healthy, older adults may have benign M proteins with no symptoms or disease. Some, however, may go on to develop multiple myeloma or other plasma cell dyscrasias after 10–15 years. Amyloidosis can also develop.

LANGERHANS CELL HISTIOCYTOSIS

Histiocytosis refers to the proliferation of histiocytes or macrophages. In Langerhans cell histiocytosis there is a clonal proliferation of **dendritic cells** known as Langerhans cells.

PRESENTATION

Typical presentations include:

- **Letterer-Siwe disease:** Acute disseminated histiocytosis; usually before age 2 years; characterized by cutaneous lesions on trunk and scalp; marrow failure, hepatosplenomegaly, and osteolytic lesions develop.
- **Hand-Schüller-Christian disease:** Calvarial lesions, diabetes insipidus, and exophthalmos.
- **Multifocal Langerhans cell histiocytosis:** Affects children; patients develop fever, eruptions on the scalp and in the ear canals, recurrent infections, hepatosplenomegaly, and diabetes insipidus from posterior pituitary involvement.
- **Eosinophilic granuloma:** Unifocal or multifocal expansion of Langerhans cells, usually in marrow space and occasionally in lung; often asymptomatic and benign.

DIAGNOSIS

Electron microscopy reveals **Birbeck granules** in the cytoplasm, which appear like **tennis racquets.** Immunohistochemical techniques aid diagnosis.

PROGNOSIS

Depends on type. The acute disseminated presentation is rapidly fatal if untreated; with chemotherapy, half survive for about 5 years. Unifocal lesions can be excised or irradiated and occasionally heal without treatment. Multifocal histiocytosis can be treated with chemotherapy, although this may also heal without treatment. It has a better prognosis than the acute disseminated form.

MYELOPROLIFERATIVE SYNDROMES

Neoplastic proliferation of myeloid stem cells. Includes CML, polycythemia vera (PCV), and essential thrombocythemia.

Polycythemia Vera

Neoplasm of multipotent myeloid stem cells leading to excessive production of **erythrocytes, granulocytes,** and **megakaryocytes.**

PRESENTATION

Insidious onset at median age of 60. Erythrocytosis causes stagnation of blood flow and cyanosis. Increased risk of **bleeding and thrombosis** leads to deep venous thrombosis, myocardial infarction, ischemic and hemorrhagic stroke, Budd-Chiari syndrome, splenic infarction, and mesenteric infarction. Headache, pruritus, peptic ulceration, and hyperuricemia are common. The **spent phase** of the bone marrow has prominent fibrosis, resulting in extramedullary hematopoiesis. The clinical picture of myelofibrosis with myeloid metaplasia develops. **Splenomegaly** may occur from congestion early on or as a result of extramedullary hematopoiesis.

DIAGNOSIS

Increased hematocrit, decreased EPO, and JAK2 mutations. Bone marrow is hypercellular until the spent phase, when fibrosis is prominent. To differentiate from CML, leukocyte alkaline phosphatase levels are *elevated*, and polymerase chain reaction (PCR) does not reveal the *BCR-ABL* gene.

TREATMENT

Involves frequent **phlebotomy** to maintain normal red cell mass; lengthens survival by approximately 10 years.

PROGNOSIS

Without treatment, death occurs within months.

Myelofibrosis with Myeloid Metaplasia

Neoplastic changes in multipotent stem cells lead to proliferation of cells, including megakaryocytes. The **megakaryocytes** release platelet-derived growth factor and transforming growth factor-β (TGF-β), which encourage growth of non-neoplastic fibroblasts. The fibroblasts produce significant amounts of collagen, and the result is **prominent fibrosis** occurring early in the course of the disease (Figure 4-20). Similar to the spent phase of polycythemia vera (PCV).

PRESENTATION

Usually affects individuals **60+ years of age,** who present with anemia, splenomegaly, nonspecific symptoms, and hyperuricemia (a result of high cell turnover); also infection, bleeding, and thrombosis because of cell abnormalities. Marrow fibrosis necessitates extramedullary hematopoiesis, which results in hepatosplenomegaly.

DIAGNOSIS

Marrow is initially hypercellular but progressively becomes hypocellular and fibrotic. Eventually, the marrow is converted to bone by osteosclerosis. Peripheral smear shows **leukoerythroblastosis,** increased numbers of nucleated erythroid progenitors and early granulocytes, as fibrosis leads to the abnormal release of these cells. **Teardrop erythrocytes,** or **dacrocytes,** are common as well. Lab tests reveal normochromic normocytic anemia and thrombocytopenia as the disease advances.

PROGNOSIS

Survival ranges from 1 to 15 years.

KEY FACT

Polycythemia/erythrocythemia can be:

- Relative: Due to decreased plasma volume (volume contraction) caused by **H₂O deprivation,** prolonged vomiting, diarrhea, or diuretics.
- Absolute: Increased total RBC mass due to polycythemia vera (PCV), increased sensitivity of erythropoietin (EPO) receptor, increased levels of EPO, physiologic changes (lung disease, high altitude, cyanotic heart disease), or EPO secreting tumors.

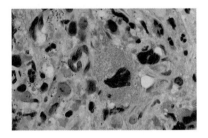

FIGURE 4-20. Myelofibrosis with myeloid metaplasia, bone marrow biopsy specimen. (Reproduced with permission from Lichtman MA, Beutler E, Kipps TJ, et al. *Williams Hematology,* 7th ed. New York: McGraw-Hill, 2006: Plate XIV-11.)

Essential Thrombocythemia

Neoplastic proliferation of myeloid stem cells, which leads to production of megakaryocytes.

PRESENTATION

Indolent course, usually asymptomatic except for episodes of prominent thrombosis and hemorrhage.

DIAGNOSIS

JAK2 mutations. Marrow is moderately hypercellular, and large numbers of normal and **abnormally large megakaryocytes** are seen. No fibrosis develops. Peripheral smear shows extremely large platelets.

PROGNOSIS

Survival is approximately 5–30 years.

SOLID TUMORS

Tumor Nomenclature

Tumors are often first defined by their "aggressiveness" and ability to metastasize (spread to other sites beyond the primary site).

BENIGN

Tumor shows microscopic and gross evidence that it will remain localized and not metastasize. Implies it is amenable to surgical resection.

- **Fibroma:** A benign tumor of fibrous or connective tissue.
- **Chondroma:** A benign tumor of cartilaginous cells.
- **Adenoma:** A benign tumor of glandular cells.
- **Papilloma:** A benign tumor of epithelial tissue that typically has a stalk or pedicle.
- **Polyps:** Similar to a papilloma, any growth, benign or malignant, that has a stalk or pedicle.
- **Cystadenoma:** A tumor of epithelial glandular origin but with production of a substrate, producing cysts within the neoplasm.
- **Hamartoma:** Mass of disorganized tissue elements, not necessarily a neoplasm.

MALIGNANT

Cells that tend to adhere, infiltrate, and destroy surrounding tissue, with characteristics of clonality and abnormal proliferation. Prone to metastasize to distant sites.

- **Sarcoma:** Malignant tumor arising from mesenchymal tissue.
- **Carcinoma:** Malignant tumor of epithelial origin.
- **Teratoma:** Tumor that contains more than one germ cell layer and typically contains immature and mature elements.
- **Leukemias and lymphomas:** See previous section.

Tumor Grading Versus Staging

Grading and staging of tumors guides medical and surgical therapy and provides information on prognosis.

GRADING

Tumors can be graded 1–4 in levels of increasing severity and differentiation based on their microscopic appearance. However, note some grading systems range from 1 to 3. Well-differentiated tumors are grade 1 and tend to be less aggressive. Grade 4 tumors tend to be poorly differentiated and highly aggressive.

STAGING

The extent to which a primary tumor has spread, which helps determine treatment and prognosis. Typically described in the **TNM** staging system, which refers to (**T**) Tumor: the extent of tumor growth; (**N**) Nodes: which and how many lymph nodes are involved; and (**M**) Metastasis: has the tumor metastasized.

Oncogenes

Genes derived from mutations in "proto-oncogenes" to "oncogenes," which promote cell growth in cancer cells. All oncogenes contribute to persistent expression of cellular growth factors (eg, cyclin-dependent kinases).

- **MYC gene:** Oncogene most commonly found in human tumors.
- **Others:** *MYB, JUN, FOS,* and *REL* oncogenes.

Tumor Suppressor Genes

Genes that suppress continued cell growth. Inhibition of these genes makes cells refractory to inhibition of growth.

- **Retinoblastoma (RB):** First tumor suppressor gene to be discovered. Retinoblastoma is a neoplasm of the retina that typically occurs in young children with an abnormal *Rb* gene located on chromosome 13. Findings include leukocoria and loss of red light reflex in infants.
- **Others:** *APC* gene, TGF-β, and *TP53*.
- **Two-hit hypothesis:** In order for a tumor suppressor gene to be rendered inactive both normal alleles must be inactive.

Oncogenic Viruses

Viral infection of cells can lead to unchecked proliferation and tumor development (Table 4-13).

TABLE 4-13.   Oncogenic Viruses

Human T-cell leukemic virus type 1	RNA oncogenic virus. Associated with T-cell leukemia and lymphoma.
Epstein-Barr virus	DNA oncogenic virus. Associated with Burkitt lymphoma, AIDS-related lymphomas, Hodgkin lymphoma, nasopharyngeal carcinoma.
Human papillomavirus	DNA oncogenic virus. Associated with cervical carcinoma.
Human herpesvirus-8	DNA oncogenic virus. Associated with Kaposi sarcoma.
Hepatitis B virus	DNA oncogenic virus. Associated with hepatocellular carcinoma.

TABLE 4-14. **Paraneoplastic Syndromes**

Cushing syndrome	Small-cell cancer of the lung, pancreatic carcinoma.
SIADH	Small-cell cancer of the lung, intracranial neoplasm.
Hypercalcemia	Squamous cell cancer of the lung, breast cancer, renal cell carcinoma.
Myasthenia gravis	Thymoma.
Hypertrophic osteoarthropathy	Lung cancer.
Migratory venous thrombosis (Trousseau syndrome)	Pancreatic carcinoma.
Cancer cachexia	Progressive loss of lean body mass and body fat, weakness, anorexia, and anemia.

SIADH = syndrome of inappropriate secretion of antidiuretic hormone.

Paraneoplastic Syndromes

Complex of symptoms that cannot be explained by the spread of tumor cells. Occur in 10–15% of cancer patients. Certain cancers cause specific paraneoplastic syndromes (Table 4-14).

Pharmacology

CHEMOTHERAPY DRUGS: ALKYLATING AGENTS

These drugs are cell cycle nonspecific. They act by interfering with nucleic acid function in various ways. All are contraindicated in pregnancy and cause myelosuppression and nausea. Antiemetic medications are frequently used in conjunction with chemotherapy. Please refer to Pharmacology section in Chapter 3 (Gastrointestinal).

Cyclophosphamide and Ifosfamide

MECHANISM

Nitrogen mustard alkylating agents that covalently cross-link DNA at guanine N-7. They require activation by the CYP-450 enzyme system in the liver. Cyclophosphamide is also a potent immunosuppressive agent.

USES

Solid tumors and hematologic malignancies.

SIDE EFFECTS

Hemorrhagic cystitis caused by urotoxic metabolite acrolein (seen mainly with Ifosfamide). Prevented by hydration and **coadministration of mesna.**

Nitrosureas (Carmustine, Lomustine, Streptozocin)

MECHANISM

Interfere with DNA and RNA synthesis by alkylation and protein modification. These agents require bioactivation. They are **lipid-soluble** and are able to cross the **blood-brain barrier.**

USES

Used in a variety of malignancies, including CNS tumors (due to its lipophilic properties), hematologic malignancies, adenocarcinomas and hepatomas, and breast and ovarian cancers.

SIDE EFFECTS

CNS toxicity (dizziness and ataxia), myelosuppression and dose-related nephrotoxicity, hepatotoxicity, and pulmonary toxicity (infiltrates or fibrosis).

Cisplatin, Carboplatin, Oxaliplatin

MECHANISM

Cross-link DNA strands, thus inhibiting DNA replication.

USES

Solid tumors and hematologic malignancies.

SIDE EFFECTS

Anaphylactic-like reactions, nephrotoxicity, neurotoxicity, ototoxicity, vomiting.

Busulfan

MECHANISM

Alkylates DNA.

USES

Leukemias/lymphomas.

SIDE EFFECTS

Pulmonary fibrosis, hyperpigmentation, seizures.

ANTIMETABOLITES

These drugs are cell cycle specific (predominantly for the synthesis [S] phase). They structurally resemble purines, pyrimidines, or other endogenous compounds, but are nonfunctional and therefore block nucleic acid synthesis. All are contraindicated in pregnancy and tend to cause myelosuppression.

Methotrexate

MECHANISM

Folic antimetabolite inhibiting dihydrofolate reductase, therefore impairing DNA and protein synthesis.

USES

Leukemias/lymphomas and solid tumors. Also used for abortion, ectopic pregnancy, rheumatoid arthritis, Crohn disease, and psoriasis.

SIDE EFFECTS

Myelosuppression, which is reversible with **leucovorin** (folinic acid). Also causes fatty change in liver (like ethanol and amiodarone). Skin and nephrotoxicity.

Pemetrexed

MECHANISM

A pyrrolopyrimidine antifolate analog with activity in the S phase. It is transported into the cell via the reduced folate carrier and requires activation. Its main mechanism of action is inhibition of thymidylate synthase.

USES

Mesothelioma and other lung cancers.

SIDE EFFECTS

Myelosuppression, skin rash, mucositis, diarrhea, fatigue. Vitamin supplementation with folic acid and vitamin B_{12} appear to reduce these toxicities.

6-Mercaptopurine (6-MP)

MECHANISM

Blocks purine synthesis. Must be activated by hypoxanthine guanine phosphoribosyl transferase (HGPRTase).

USES

Leukemias/lymphomas.

SIDE EFFECTS

6-MP is **metabolized by xanthine oxidase,** so toxicity is increased with coadministration of allopurinol (xanthine oxidase inhibitor). Myelosuppression, hepatotoxicity, nausea and vomiting.

Cytarabine

MECHANISM

Pyrimidine antagonist, terminates chain elongation. Also inhibits DNA polymerase.

USES

Leukemias/lymphomas.

SIDE EFFECTS

Potent myelosuppressive agent: leukopenia, thrombocytopenia, megaloblastic anemia, neurotoxicity.

5-Fluorouracil (5-FU)

MECHANISM

Pyrimidine analog that is bioactivated to 5-fluoro-deoxyuridine monophosphate (5F-dUMP). 5F-dUMP binds folic acid, and this complex **inhibits thymidylate synthase,** thus inhibiting nucleic acid synthesis.

USES

Solid tumors. Used topically for basal cell carcinoma of the skin.

SIDE EFFECTS

"Hand-foot syndrome" (dermopathy after extended use), mucositis, GI toxicity (diarrhea).

TOPOISOMERASE INHIBITORS

Etoposide, Doxorubicin, and Irinotecan

MECHANISM

Inhibit topoisomerases (I or II), thus preventing DNA replication and inducing DNA strand breaks.

USES

Solid tumors and hematologic malignancies.

SIDE EFFECTS

Doxorubicin has cardiac side effects, including myopathy, failure, and arrhythmias. Irinotecan causes severe diarrhea. Etoposide side effects include myelosuppression, mucositis, and is associated with increased risk of leukemia.

DRUGS THAT TARGET TUBULIN

Vinca Alkaloids (Vincristine, Vinblastine)

MECHANISM

Prevent microtubule formation by interfering with tubulin binding. The mitotic spindle cannot form, and the M phase does not proceed.

USES

Leukemias/lymphomas, and solid tumors.

SIDE EFFECTS

VilNcristine causes Neurotoxicity. VinBlastine causes Bone marrow toxicity.

Taxanes (Paclitaxel, Docetaxel)

MECHANISM

Prevents microtubule breakdown by stabilizing tubulin already bound in mitotic spindles. M phase cannot complete.

USES

Solid tumors.

SIDE EFFECTS

Acute hypersensitivity reaction, neurotoxicity.

Ixabepilone, Epothilone

MECHANISM

Microtubule inhibitors active in the M phase of the cell cycle.

USES

Breast cancers.

SIDE EFFECTS

Myelosuppression, hypersensitivity reactions, and neurotoxicity (peripheral sensory neuropathy).

HORMONAL AGENTS

Selective Estrogen Receptor Modulators (SERMs) (Tamoxifen, Raloxifene)

MECHANISM

Estrogen agonist and antagonist properties depending on the individual target organ.

USES

Estrogen-sensitive breast cancers, especially in postmenopausal women. Raloxifene additionally stimulates the bone to increase density, but is used less.

SIDE EFFECTS

Tamoxifen activates estrogen receptors on other types of tissue such as endometrium, increasing endometrial cancer risk. All can cause mild hot flashes and nausea.

Leuprolide and Goserelin

MECHANISM

Agonists of luteinizing hormone-releasing hormone (LHRH). Shuts off LH release when given continuously, thereby inhibiting testosterone or estrogen production.

USES

Prostate cancer, breast cancer in premenopausal women.

SIDE EFFECTS

Hot flashes, decreased bone density, decreased libido.

TARGETED MOLECULAR THERAPEUTICS

Anti-EGRF Antibodies (Cetuximab, Panitumumab)

MECHANISM

Antiangiogenic. The epidermal growth factor receptor (EGFR) is a member of the erb-B family of growth factor receptors. Its signaling pathway is involved in cellular growth and proliferation, invasion and metastasis, and angiogenesis. Cetuximab is an antibody directed against the extracellular domain of the EGFR. Panitumumab is a human monoclonal antibody directed against the EGFR and works through inhibition of the EGFR signaling pathway.

USES

Colorectal cancer and some head and neck cancers.

SIDE EFFECTS

Cetuximab is associated with an acneiform skin rash, hypersensitivity infusion reaction, and hypomagnesemia. Infusion-related reactions are seen only rarely with panitumumab, and its main side effects are acneiform skin rash and hypomagnesemia.

Anti-EGFR Agents (Gefitinib, Erlotinib)

MECHANISM

Antiangiogenic. Inhibitors of the tyrosine kinase domain associated with EGFR.

USES

Non–small-cell lung cancer. Erlotinib has also been approved for use in the treatment regimen of pancreatic cancer.

SIDE EFFECTS

Both drugs have the potential to interact with other drugs metabolized by the liver CYP3A4 system and grapefruit. Acneiform skin rash, diarrhea, and anorexia and fatigue are often seen.

Trastuzumab

MECHANISM

Antibody against erbB2 may facilitate T-cell cytotoxicity against cancer cells with erbB2 expression.

USES

Breast cancers that express erbB2 (~30%).

SIDE EFFECTS

Cardiotoxicity, especially when combined with doxorubicin.

Anti-VEGF Antibodies (Bevacizumab)

MECHANISM

Antiangiogenic. Vascular endothelial growth factor (VEGF) is an important angiogenic growth factor. **Bevacizumab** is a recombinant monoclonal antibody that targets all forms of VEGF-A, binding and preventing interactions with target VEGF receptors.

USES

Colorectal cancer, non–small-lung cancer and breast cancer.

SIDE EFFECTS

Hypertension, increased incidence of arterial thromboembolic events (transient ischemic attack, stroke, angina, and myocardial infarction), wound healing complications and gastrointestinal perforations, and proteinuria.

Anti-VEGF Agents (Sorafenib, Sunitinib)

MECHANISM

Antiangiogenic. Inhibitors of the tyrosine kinase domain associated with VEGF.

USES

Sorafenib is approved for use in renal cell cancer and hepatocellular cancer. **Sunitinib** is used in renal cell cancer and gastrointestinal stromal tumors (GIST).

SIDE EFFECTS

Can have potential interactions with drugs metabolized by the CYP3A4 system, grapefruit, and St. John's wort. Hypertension, bleeding complications, and fatigue are also seen. Skin rash and the hand-foot syndrome is commonly seen with sorafenib use. There is an increased risk of cardiac dysfunction with sunitinib.

Anti-BCR-ABL (Imatinib, Dasatinib, Nilotinib)

MECHANISM

Imatinib inhibits BCR-ABL tyrosine kinase specific to CML by blocking the binding site of ADP substrate. Dasatinib and nilotinib inhibit other tyrosine kinases.

USES

CML with the t(9:22) Philadelphia chromosomal translocation.

SIDE EFFECTS

Mild. Potential interactions exist with other drugs, grapefruit, and St. John's wort, which are also metabolized by the CYP3A4 system.

Anti-CD20 Antibody (Rituximab)

MECHANISM

An antibody against the protein CD20, found on the surface of B cells.

USES

Lymphomas, leukemias, transplant rejection, and some autoimmune diseases.

SIDE EFFECTS

Infusion reactions, tumor lysis syndrome, skin and mouth reactions, infections.

Antiproteasome (Bortezomib)

MECHANISM

Interferes with proteasomes, which normally control the degradation of proteins regulating cell proliferation. Causes apoptosis in tumor cells.

USES

Multiple myeloma, mantle cell lymphoma.

SIDE EFFECTS

Gastrointestinal effects, asthenia, peripheral neuropathy, and myelosuppression.

NATIVE CYTOKINES USED IN CANCER TREATMENT

Interferon-Alfa

MECHANISM

Enhances cell-mediated immunity against some cancers and viruses, possibly by upregulating expression of antigen in tumor cells. May also have direct apoptotic activity.

USES

Melanoma, renal cell carcinoma, CML.

SIDE EFFECTS

Flulike symptoms and aggravation of psychiatric disorders.

Interleukin-2

MECHANISM

Stimulates T-cell survival and activation, enhancing cell-mediated immunity against cancer cells.

USES

Kidney cancers and melanoma.

SIDE EFFECTS

Capillary leak syndrome (hypotension, low vascular resistance, and high cardiac output similar to septic shock).

NOTES

CHAPTER 5

Musculoskeletal and Connective Tissue

Embryology

SKELETAL SYSTEM

Osteogenesis

DEVELOPMENT

Bone develops from two sources: mesenchyme (intramembranous ossification) and cartilage (endochondral ossification).

- **Intramembranous ossification:** Flat bones, such as those that make up the skull, develop directly from mesenchyme in preexisting membranes.
- **Endochondral ossification:** Most bones, including long bones in the appendicular skeleton, develop from mesenchyme that has condensed into cartilage first. The **primary center of ossification** in the cartilaginous model forms the shaft of the bone (diaphysis). The ends of the bone (epiphyses) remain cartilaginous for several years after birth, during which time the **secondary centers of ossification** appear. Bone lengthening occurs in the epiphyseal cartilage plate at the diaphysial-epiphyseal junction until it ossifies by about 20 years of age (Figure 5-1).

CONGENITAL MALFORMATIONS

- **Osteogenesis imperfecta (OI):** Caused by a deficiency in **type I collagen,** usually due to an autosomal dominant gene defect affecting collagen synthesis (Table 5-1). There are eight different types of OI, each differing by the quality and quantity of type I collagen. It is characterized by extremely fragile bones (leading to fracture), blue sclerae, poor wound healing, and hearing loss (in about 50%).
- **Achondroplasia:** This is the most prevalent form of dwarfism (70%). **Autosomal dominant** disorder caused by a mutation in the gene for a fibroblast growth factor (**FGF-3**) receptor on **chromosome 4p.** Constitutive activation of this receptor leads to inhibition of chondrocyte proliferation. Endochondral ossification is impaired, as the epiphyseal growth plate becomes small and disorganized, preventing proper bone growth. This leads to disproportionately short arms and legs and often a disproportionately large head and trunk. In some cases, severe spinal deformity may compress the spinal cord. Homozygotes experience more severe disease that may result in neonatal death. Proportional dwarfism occurs in growth-hormone defi-

MNEMONIC

There is only **1** shaft of the bone (diaphysis); **primary** ossification center is here.

There are **2** ends of the bone (epiphyses); **secondary** ossification centers are here.

KEY FACT

OI is often confused with child abuse, because exuberant healing of fractures creates callus. OI may also mimic osteosarcoma.

KEY FACT

Achondroplasia is a disorder that affects endochondral ossification at the epiphyseal cartilage plates in long bones, resulting in premature closing of the epiphyses and short limbs.

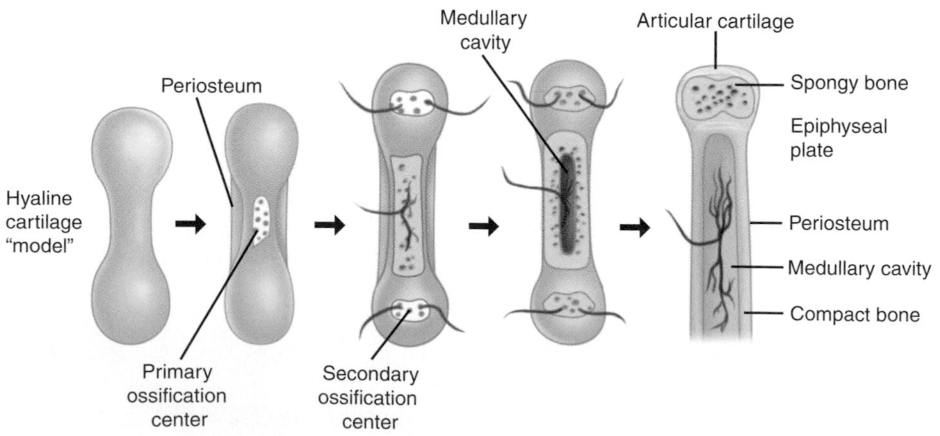

FIGURE 5-1. **Bone growth.** Primary ossification center in the diaphysis; secondary ossification center in the epiphyses.

TABLE 5-1.   Metabolic and Genetic Disease Affecting Bone and Cartilage

DISEASE	ETIOLOGY	CLINICAL PRESENTATION
Dwarfism	Often due to deficiency in growth hormone (GH), but has many other causes (70% of cases are due to achondroplasia); gene mutations, damage to pituitary gland, Turner syndrome, poor nutrition, and stress (psychogenic dwarfism).	Short stature (due to stunted or halted growth), delayed puberty.
Rickets	Due to a deficiency in vitamin D during childhood; causes softening of bones due to defective bone mineralization.	Bone pain, skeletal deformity (bowed legs), muscle weakness, hypocalcemia
Osteomalacia	Due to a deficiency in vitamin D during adulthood; causes softening of bones due to detective bone mineralization.	Weak bones, bone pain, muscle weakness, hypocalcemia, easy fractures.
Hyperparathyroidism	Excess parathyroid hormone causes bone resorption.	Weakness and fatigue, depression, bone pain, kidney stones, muscle soreness (myalgias), decreased appetite. Mnemonic: "Renal Stones, abdominal Groans, painful Bones, and psychiatric Moans."
Osteogenesis imperfecta	Due to a variety of mutations in the *COL1A1* and *COL1A2* genes affecting the synthesis and structure of type 1 collagen; also known as brittle bone disease.	Fragile bones (leading to fractures), blue sclerae, poor wound healing, hearing loss.
Osteoporosis	Commonly postmenopausal or in other cases is more gradual and related to age; a small number of cases are due to mutations in the *COL1A1* and *COL1A2* genes and possibly in the vitamin D receptor gene; bone mineral density (BMD) is reduced leading to disrupted bone architecture.	Fractures (vertebral body, hip, wrist).
Osteoarthritis	Usually develops with age and increasing impact on joints, but a small number are due to mutations in *COL1A* genes.	Articular pain often with movement and in areas of weight bearing; joint swelling with more use throughout day; Heberden and Bouchard nodes are interphalangeal bony enlargements.
Achondroplasia	Due to mutations in the gene encoding FGFR3 (autosomal dominant).	Short limbs, increased spinal curvature, and distorted skull growth.

ciency (ie, pituitary dwarfism). Rarer forms of dwarfism can include hypothyroidism, Turner syndrome, OI, storage disorders, malnutrition. Furthermore, mutations in genes responsible for cartilage and/or bone growth can result in dwarfism.

■ **Marfan syndrome:** An **autosomal dominant** mutation in the gene for the protein **fibrillin** (the fibrillin-1 gene is located on chromosome 15q21.1) causes **abnormal elastin fibers that affect the skeletal, cardiac, and ocular systems.** Skeletal changes include tall stature, long limbs, hyperextendable joints, long and tapering digits, pectus excavatum, and scoliosis (Figure 5-2).

■ **Gigantism and acromegaly: Hyperpituitarism** causes excessive amounts of GH that can result in gigantism in infants (increased height and exces-

KEY FACT

Larson syndrome is another form of dwarfism. It is an **autosomal recessive** disorder in which a **defect in the growth hormone receptor (GHR)** causes a lack of responsiveness to increased levels of GH in the body.

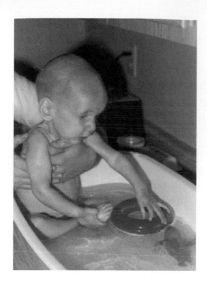

FIGURE 5-2.   Marfan syndrome.
Note bony changes, long limbs, and long, tapering digits. (Courtesy of the Hall family.)

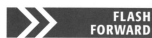
FLASH FORWARD

Ocular findings in Marfan syndrome include **ectopia lentis** (lens dislocation) in 50% of patients. Dislocation is usually upward and toward the temples. This is in contrast to ectopia lentis in homocystinuria, which is usually downward and into the anterior chamber.

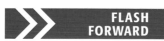
FLASH FORWARD

Marfan syndrome is associated with ascending aortic dissection, mitral valve prolapse, and cerebral berry aneurysms.

sive body proportions) and acromegaly in adults (increased bone growth in the jaw, hands, and feet, as well as increased soft tissue and visceral organ growth). IGF-1 levels are usually elevated secondary to excess GH; this is often seen in adolescence (secondary to puberty), as well as in pathologic conditions. Further diagnostics include the **oral glucose tolerance test (OGTT)**: GH level should decrease after an oral glucose load; if not, it is diagnostic of pituitary GH excess.

■ **Cretinism: A deficiency in fetal thyroid hormone** resulting in **mental retardation, short stature, impaired bone growth,** and neurologic disorders of muscle tone and coordination. There are several possible etiologies:
  ■ Lack of dietary iodine (especially in areas where there is little iodine in the soil and water)
  ■ Mutations in thyroid hormone synthesis
  ■ Agenesis of the thyroid gland

There are over 20 different types of collagen; however, over 90% of the collagen in the body is of type I, II, III, and IV (Table 5-2).

Skull

DEVELOPMENT

Mesenchyme around the fetal brain develops into the skull, which can be divided into two parts:

■ Neurocranium: Includes the flat bones and base of the skull.
■ Viscerocranium: Includes the bones of the face and laryngeal cartilage.

Most of the bones in the neurocranium and viscerocranium are derived from neural crest cells, though there are some exceptions (the base of the

TABLE 5-2.   Collagen Types

COLLAGEN TYPES	REPRESENTATIVE TISSUE
I	Skin, tendon, bone, dentin
II	Cartilage, vitreous body
III	Skin, muscle, blood vessels, frequently together with type I; annulus fibrosus
IV	All basement membranes
V	Fetal tissues, skin, bone, placenta, most interstitial tissues
VI	Most connective tissues
VII	Epithelia
VIII	Endothelium, other tissues
IX	Cartilage, vitreous body
X	Hypertrophic cartilage

(Adapted with permission from Junqueira's *Basic Histology: Text & Atlas,* 12e. New York: McGraw-Hill, 2010. Table 5-3.)

occipital bone comes from the mesoderm of the occipital sclerotomes, and the laryngeal cartilage is derived from the pharyngeal arches 4 and 6).

The flat bones in the skull are separated by five connective tissue **sutures** that allow expansion of the skull while the brain grows:

- Frontal suture
- Sagittal suture
- Lambdoid suture
- Coronal suture
- Squamosal suture

Fontanelles are areas between the flat bones of the skull where the sutures meet. Fontanelles allow room for the brain to finish growing. All fontanelles usually close by about 2 years of age. Exam of the fontanelles can indicate dehydration (sunken fontanelle) or increased intracranial pressure (bulging fontanelle). There are six fontanelles (Figure 5-3; *note*: only the anterior and posterior fontanelles are shown):

- Anterior fontanelle: Closes by the end of the second year and is the last to close.
- Posterior fontanelle.
- Sphenoid fontanelle (one on each side of head).
- Mastoid fontanelles (one on each side of head).

CONGENITAL MALFORMATIONS

- **Microcephaly:** Failure of the brain, and subsequently the skull, to grow. Affected children are severely mentally retarded. The etiology may be an autosomal recessive genetic mutation or in-utero infection.
- **Craniosynostoses:** Premature closure of the sutures may lead to abnormal shapes of the skull.

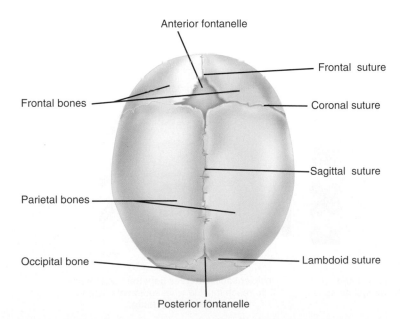

FIGURE 5-3. **Normal skull of a newborn with sutures and fontanelles.**

FLASH BACK

The pharyngeal arches, pouches, grooves, and membranes form much of the head and neck, including arches 4 and 6 that provide part of the structure of the viscerocranium: the laryngeal cartilage.

FLASH BACK

In embryonic development, the neural tube becomes the spinal cord, and the notochord eventually forms the vertebrae.

FLASH BACK

The development of the vertebral column is likely regulated by paired box genes (transcription factors specific for a certain tissue type) and homeobox genes (genes that have "homeobox" sequences containing transcription factors involved in the development of an organism; *Hox* genes are a subset of these involved in development of the body axis).

KEY FACT

The notochord is the embryologic origin of the nucleus pulposus.

Vertebral Column

DEVELOPMENT

At week 4 of embryonic development, the mesenchymal cells from the sclerotomes of the somites begin to surround the notochord, the neural tube, and the body wall. In each of these three areas, significant structures of the vertebral column are formed.

- Around the **notochord:** Each sclerotome consists of a layer of loosely arranged cells cranially and a layer of densely arranged cells caudally. Some of the densely arranged cells move cranially and form the **intervertebral disk.** The rest of the dense cells combine with the loosely arranged cells to form the **centrum,** which will become the body of the vertebra. The notochord degenerates when it is surrounded by the developing vertebral bodies. Between the vertebral bodies, the notochord develops into the **nucleus pulposus** of the intervertebral disk (Figure 5-4). Surrounding the nucleus pulposus is the annulus fibrosus, which develops from sclerotomal cells (Figure 5-5).
- Around the **neural tube:** Mesenchymal cells form the vertebral arch.
- In the **body wall:** Mesenchymal cells form the costal processes that then develop into the ribs.

During week 6 of embryonic development:

- Mesenchyme forms a cartilaginous vertebra.
- **Chondrification centers** appear in the centrum to form a cartilaginous body.
- Chondrification centers in the vertebral arch (originally from the neural tube) fuse with the centrum and each other, giving rise to the spinous and transverse processes.

After puberty, **secondary ossification centers** appear at the tips of the spinous and transverse processes; these centers eventually fuse completely by the age of 25 years.

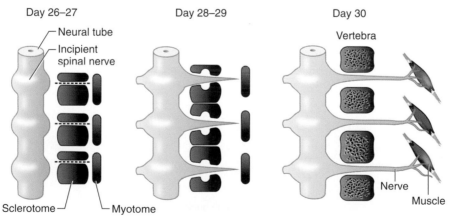

Day 26–27   Day 28–29   Day 30

Neural tube
Incipient spinal nerve
Vertebra
Sclerotome   Myotome
Nerve
Muscle

Segmental sclerotomes split and recombine to form vertebral rudiments.

Incipient spinal nerves penetrate sclerotome to reach muscle while rudiments fuse to become vertebra.

FIGURE 5-4. **Neural tube differentiation and formation of vertebral bodies.** From left to right, the neural tube's incipient spinal nerves penetrate sclerotomes to innervate muscle. In this process, sclerotomes split to fuse with neighboring sclerotomes to form vertebral bodies.

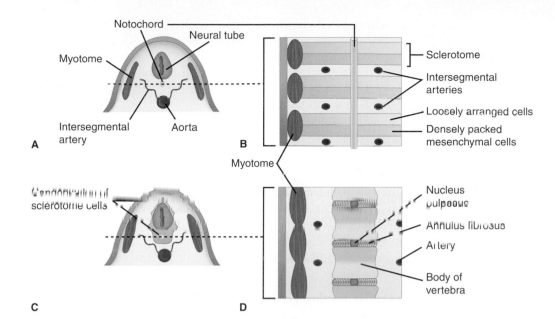

FIGURE 5-5.   **Early vertebral column development.** (A) and (B) show transverse and frontal sections of a 4-week-old embryo, respectively. (C) and (D) show the same sections in a 5-week-old embryo. Note the condensation of sclerotome cells around the neural tube and notochord by week 5. Also note how the loosely arranged cells and densely arranged cells form the body of the vertebra and how the notochord becomes the nucleus pulposus in between the vertebral bodies.

The following vertebrae do not ossify in the previously described manner:

- Atlas (C1): Has no vertebral body.
- Axis (C2): Has a **dens** (odontoid process) that is the developmental remnant of the body of the atlas.
- Sacrum: These five vertebrae fuse together to form a wall of the pelvic cavity.
- Coccyx: Four rudimentary vertebrae fuse into a small triangle at the base of the spine.

The four main spinal areas are associated with four specific curvatures: cervical, thoracic, lumbar, sacral. These curvatures reverse themselves when moving to the next contiguous spinal segment. The cervical and lumbar segments have lordotic curves, but the thoracic and sacral segments are kyphotic.

CONGENITAL MALFORMATIONS

- **Chordoma:** This is a **remnant of the notochord.** One-third of chordomas become slow-growing, malignant tumors that infiltrate surrounding tissues, including bone. They often form at the base of the skull and extend into the nasopharynx; however. Chordomas can occur anywhere along the spine, with **many occurring in the lumbosacral and sacrococcygeal areas as well.** Depending on the location, patients can present with diplopia and headache (if near the skull) or lower back and leg pain (if in the lumbosacral spine). The prognosis is poor, with only half of patients surviving past 5 years.
- **Variations in the number of vertebrae:** The vast majority of people have a total of 33 vertebrae: 7 cervical, 12 thoracic, 5 lumbar, 5 sacral, and 4 fused in the coccyx. Less commonly, people either have one vertebra too many or one too few. It is extremely rare for variations to occur in the cervical region.

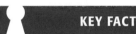

KEY FACT

The annulus fibrosus is made of type III collagen.

- **Klippel-Feil syndrome (brevicollis):** A syndrome of unclear etiology caused by fusion of the cervical vertebrae. Typically involves the following constellation of symptoms:
  - Decreased range of motion in the cervical spine
  - Defects in the thoracic and lumbar spine causing **scoliosis**
  - Renal anomalies
  - Hearing loss
  - Short neck with low hairline

SPINA BIFIDA

FLASH BACK

When a similar bony defect occurs at the base of the skull, a meningocele (protrusion of the meninges and CSF), meningoencephalocele (protrusion of the meninges and brain), or meningohydroencephalocele (protrusion of meninges, brain, and ventricle) may occur.

This spinal defect occurs when the **two halves of the vertebral arch fail to fuse, most commonly in the lumbosacral region** (L5 and/or S1). Because of the defect, the vertebral arch consists of two parts and is hence "bifid." There are many variations of spina bifida, ranging from mild to severe, depending on how much of the spinal cord and/or meninges protrude through the defect (Figure 5-6).

- **Spina bifida occulta:** The mildest version, occurring in 10–25% of the population. The spinal cord and nerves are usually normal, and there are no clinical symptoms other than a small tuft of hair that may grow in the lumbosacral region of the back.
- **Spina bifida with meningocele:** A type of "spina bifida cystica" in which a sac containing meninges and cerebrospinal fluid (CSF) protrudes through the vertebral defect. The spinal cord is not affected.
- **Spina bifida with meningomyelocele:** A more severe type of spina bifida cystica in which the sac protruding through the vertebral defect contains not only meninges and CSF, but the spinal cord and/or nerve roots as well. The patient is more likely to have neurologic symptoms with this disorder.

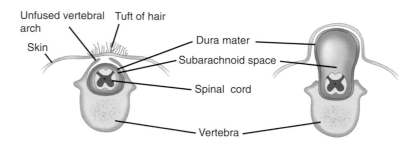

A Spina bifida occulta   **B** Spina bifida with meningocele

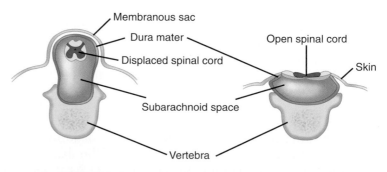

C Spina bifida with meningomyelocele   **D** Spina bifida with rachischisis

FIGURE 5-6. **Spina bifida.** Note the range of spina bifida types, depending on what protrudes through the vertebral arch defect. (A) Spina bifida occulta. (B-D) These defects are all under the umbrella term of "spina bifida cystica" because of their cystlike sac protrusion.

Patients are also more likely to have latex allergies, Arnold-Chiari malformations, and syringomyelia.

- **Spina bifida with rachischisis:** The most severe type of spina bifida cystica in which there is an open neural tube due to the failure of the posterior neuropore to close at the end of week 4 of embryonic development. The spinal cord protrudes through the vertebral defect to the outside of the body. Often fatal.

The maternal **serum level of α-fetoprotein (AFP) is high** in spina bifida. Further evaluation using ultrasound can be done during the first trimester.

Causes of neural tube defects such as spina bifida cystica include **genetic factors, increased alcohol intake during pregnancy, and certain drugs taken during the first trimester,** most notably **valproic acid,** an anticonvulsant. All pregnant women should take folic acid supplements to help prevent neural tube defects.

HEMIVERTEBRA

One of the two chondrification centers in the centrum fails to appear, so only half of the vertebral body is able to form. This produces a lateral curvature and rotation of the spine and is one potential cause of **scoliosis.**

SPONDYLOLYSIS AND SPONDYLOLISTHESIS

The vertebral arch pedicles fail to fuse with the vertebral body (spondylolysis: the connection is "lysed"), which may lead to displacement of a vertebral body relative to the vertebral body below it (spondylolisthesis). The displaced vertebral may move anteriorly (anterolisthesis) or posteriorly (posterolisthesis).

Ribs

DEVELOPMENT

Mesenchymal cells from the sclerotomes of the somites that surround the body wall form the costal processes that develop into ribs. Though costal processes occur at all vertebrae, only the thoracic vertebrae develop ribs. The "true ribs" are the first seven that attach to the sternum. The "false ribs," ribs 8–12, attach to the sternum via other ribs. The last two ribs are "floating ribs" that do not attach to the sternum at all.

CONGENITAL MALFORMATIONS

- **Accessory ribs:** An extra rib can develop from the costal processes of a cervical or lumbar vertebral body. A lumbar rib is more common; however, a cervical rib arising from C7 can cause **thoracic outlet syndrome,** in which the extra rib compresses the neurovascular bundle at the thoracic outlet.
- The lower nerve roots of the brachial plexus (C8 and T1) are affected most commonly, leading to neurologic symptoms such as pain and tingling in the ulnar nerve distribution.
- The upper nerve roots (C5, C6, and C7) can also be compressed, causing similar symptoms in the radial nerve distribution as well as the neck, ear, and torso.
- A compressed subclavian vein can lead to swelling and cyanosis in the upper extremity of the affected side, and a compressed subclavian artery can cause pallor, pulselessness, low blood pressure, coolness, and rare small infarcts in the affected upper extremity.

KEY FACT

The "triple screen" is a blood test done at weeks 16–18 of pregnancy that measures AFP, β-human chorionic gonadotropin, and unconjugated estriol. Elevated **AFP** may indicate **spina bifida** or another congenital disorder such as anencephaly. In contrast, Down syndrome may cause a low ("down") AFP level.

KEY FACT

When testing a patient for thoracic outlet syndrome, look for a positive Adson sign: Have the patient maximally extend the neck and rotate the head toward the side being tested. Look for a decrease in the ipsilateral radial pulse and listen for a subclavian bruit.

FLASH BACK

The **interscalene triangle** is bordered anteriorly by anterior scalene, posteriorly by middle scalene, and inferiorly by medial surface of the first rib. An accessory cervical rib can compress this small area, causing thoracic outlet syndrome.

KEY FACT

The cartilage of the upper limbs develop before that of the lower limbs. The clavicle is the first bone to undergo primary ossification, closely followed by the femurs. The first secondary ossification site is in the knees.

FLASH BACK

Many trisomy syndromes are associated with limb defects.

- Trisomy 21 (Down syndrome): **Clinodactyly** (curving of the fingers).
- Trisomy 18 (Edwards syndrome): Flexed digits (or overlapping) and "rocker-bottom" feet.
- Trisomy 13 (Patau syndrome): **Polydactyly.**

KEY FACT

The critical period of limb development occurs during the third to fifth week. Teratogens ingested early in this period may cause severe defects. In the late 1950s and early 1960s, many mothers took **thalidomide,** a sedative and antiemetic that caused severe teratogenic limb defects including amelia.

FLASH BACK

Today, the only FDA-approved uses for thalidomide are pain relief from erythema nodosum leprosum, the skin manifestation of leprosy, and newly diagnosed multiple myeloma.

Limbs

DEVELOPMENT

Development of the limb bones begins when the early limb buds form at about the fourth week of embryonic development. By the fifth week, mesodermal cells from the lateral plate migrate into the limb buds.

- A thickened region of ectoderm called the **apical ectodermal ridge (AER)** develops at the edge of the limb bud; it produces **FGF** that induces the mesodermal cells to grow outward and form cartilage.
- The **zone of polarizing activity** at the base of the limb bud produces the **sonic hedgehog** protein, which activates **homeobox-containing** (*Hox*) **genes** to direct the patterned organization of the limbs and digits.

The rest of limb development follows this general timeline:

- Week 6: Digital rays develop in the hands and feet; digit formation involves selective **apoptosis** within the AER. By the end of week 6, the cartilaginous models of the limb bones are complete.
- Weeks 7–12: The long bones undergo endochondral ossification as discussed previously, and most of the primary ossification centers develop.
- Before birth: Several secondary ossification centers develop, though many develop after birth as well.
- Adult age: The primary ossification in the diaphysis does not fuse with the secondary ossification in the epiphysis until adult age, allowing for complete bone growth. At this time, the epiphyseal plate between the two finally ossifies, and bone growth ends.

CONGENITAL MALFORMATIONS

Limb anomalies range from issues with limb bud development, resulting in the complete absence of the limb, to problems in the growth or differentiation of limbs, causing shortened or deformed extremities. The limb anomalies listed below may be caused by genetic factors, environmental factors, or both.

- **Amelia:** Complete absence of one or more limbs, often due to maternal ingestion of a teratogen, such as **thalidomide.**
- **Meromelia:** Partial absence of one or more limbs.
- **Cleft hand and foot:** Also known as "lobster-claw deformities." Several of the digital rays fail to develop centrally; the lateral digits fuse, causing a claw-shaped hand or foot.
- **Congenital clubfoot:** A common anomaly occurring about once in every 1000 births, involving any deformity in the ankle bone (talus) of the foot. The most common type of clubfoot is **talipes equinovarus,** in which the foot is inverted and turned in medially. A genetic predisposition seems to be involved. The majority of cases involve abnormal positioning of the feet in the uterus.
- **Polydactyly:** An autosomal dominant trait that causes extra fingers or toes to develop, usually medially or laterally. More common in African Americans. In Caucasians, polydactyly is associated with heart disorders.
- **Syndactyly:** The most common limb anomaly; may be either autosomal recessive or autosomal dominant. Cutaneous syndactyly involves simple webbing of the digits, usually in the toes. A more severe form is osseous syndactyly in which the bones of the digits fuse (as in the lateral digits in clubfoot) when the divisions between the digital rays fail to develop.

- **Brachydactyly:** Hypoplasia of the fingers or toes. It is uncommon, often inherited as an autosomal dominant trait, and usually associated with short stature.
- **Holt-Oram syndrome:** Also known as **heart-hand syndrome.** Due to mutations in the *TBX5* gene on chromosome 12, which is important in both cardiac and upper limb development. Major manifestations include **atrial septal defects** and **abnormalities of the thumbs;** other cardiac abnormalities include ventral septal defects, atrioventricular block, and atrial fibrillation.
- **Congenital hip dislocation:** A very common disorder, affecting about one in every 1000 infants. Predisposing factors include female gender, Native American heritage, first-born status, and breech birth. **Diagnosed by physical exam and/or hip ultrasound.**
    - **Positive Ortolani test:** One hears a low-pitched click when abducting the hip.
    - **Positive Barlow maneuver:** While keeping hips in the adducted position, one hears a click when applying gentle pressure posteriorly.
    - **Positive Galeazzi sign:** One leg appears longer than the other. This may be more reliable for diagnosis in older infants.
    Treatment includes a Pavlik harness; if this fails, then open or closed reduction with spica casting is appropriate (depending on the age and severity of disease).

MUSCULAR SYSTEM

Almost all muscles in the human body develop from mesoderm (the notable exceptions being the dilator pupillae and sphincter of the iris that develop from the neuroectoderm). Cardiac and smooth muscles develop from **splanchnic mesoderm,** whereas most skeletal muscles develop from regions of the somites called **myotomes.** Developmental anomalies can lead to the absence of or variation in muscles, which are generally benign.

KEY FACT

The dilator pupillae and sphincter muscles of the iris originate from neuroectoderm, not mesoderm.

Skeletal Muscle

Mesenchymal cells in the myotome areas of the somites differentiate into **myoblasts** that then elongate and fuse into tubular structures called **myotubes.** Fibroblasts and external laminae that form around the muscle tubules encase the muscle in a fibrous sheath during its development. Myofilaments, myofibrils, and other muscle-specific organelles develop early. Skeletal muscle starts to grow as myotubes fuse together; after the first year, the increase in myofilaments leads to muscle growth.

Different myotomes give rise to different muscles in the body, generally depending on location.

Muscular Development of the Head and Neck

- **Preoptic myotomes** give rise to extraocular muscles.
- **Occipital myotomes** give rise to the tongue muscles.

Muscular Development of the Trunk

Each myotome of each somite in the trunk region divides into two parts: an **epaxial division** on the dorsal side and a **hypaxial division** on the ventral side. Each developing spinal nerve splits to innervate both areas: a **dorsal primary ramus** to the former and a **ventral primary ramus** to the latter.

- **Epaxial myotomes** develop into intrinsic back muscles and extensor muscles of the neck and vertebrae.

- **Hypaxial myotomes** develop into limb, abdominal, and intercostal muscles, as well as the following based on location:
  - Cervical myotomes form the prevertebral, geniohyoid, infrahyoid, and scalene muscles.
  - Thoracic myotomes form the flexor muscles of the vertebrae.
  - Lumbar myotomes form the quadratus lumborum muscle.
  - Sacrococcygeal myotomes form pelvic diaphragm muscles.

Muscular Development of the Limbs

Mesenchyme from the myotomes in the limb buds condense into two areas: posterior and anterior condensations.

The posterior condensations form:

- Extensor and supinator muscles in the upper limbs.
- Extensor and abductor muscles in the lower limbs.

The anterior condensations form:

- Flexor and pronator muscles in the upper limbs.
- Flexor and adductor muscles in the lower limbs.

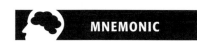

MNEMONIC

Several Parts Build Diaphragm
Septum transversum
Pleuroperitoneal folds
Body wall
Dorsal mesentery of esophagus

Development of the Diaphragm

The diaphragm arises from several different parts of the developing body cavity; its embryonic components include:

- Septum transversum
- Pleuroperitoneal folds
- Body wall
- Dorsal mesentery of the esophagus

At around week 3 of embryonic development, the **septum transversum** develops from the ventral aspect of the body wall, growing dorsally to separate the heart from the liver. It forms the primordium of the **central tendon of the diaphragm,** which is innervated by the phrenic nerves. The septum transversum eventually fuses with the **pleuroperitoneal membranes** and **esophageal mesentery** to complete the primordial diaphragm. The pleuroperitoneal membranes initially make up a large dorsal portion of the primordial diaphragm but contribute very little to the infant's diaphragm. The esophageal mesentery forms the median portion and **crura of the diaphragm.**

Later in embryonic development, between weeks 9 and 12, the internal muscular layer of the lateral body wall fuses with the primordial diaphragm, contributing to its periphery and then forming the costodiaphragmatic recesses (Figure 5-7).

Smooth Muscle

Splanchnic mesenchyme around the primordial gut endoderm develops into the smooth muscle in the GI tract. Somatic mesoderm gives rise to the smooth muscle in the walls of blood and lymphatic vessels.

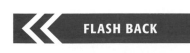

FLASH BACK

Heart muscle (and CNS) can be recognized in the embryo by 4 weeks of gestation.

Cardiac Muscle

Mesenchyme around the heart tube migrates from the lateral splanchnic mesoderm and then develops into cardiac myoblasts. Unlike skeletal muscle, cardiac muscle fibers do not fuse together but rather differentiate and grow as single cells. By week 4 of development, heart muscle can be recognized in the embryo.

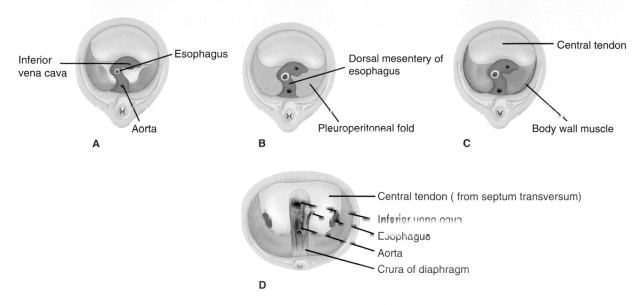

FIGURE 5-7. Development of the diaphragm. The different components making up the diaphragm in an embryo at 5 weeks (A), 6 weeks (B), and 12 weeks (C). The diaphragm of an infant (D). Please note that though the pleuroperitoneal membrane makes up much of the posterior aspect of the diaphragm in the embryo, the muscular ingrowth from the body wall takes over much of that region by the time the infant is born.

CONGENITAL MALFORMATIONS

CONGENITAL DIAPHRAGMATIC HERNIA

Incomplete development of the diaphragm, usually a posterolateral defect on the left, allows abdominal contents to herniate into the thorax. The lungs are not able to expand fully, resulting in pulmonary hypoplasia and possibly pneumothorax. Polyhydramnios is often associated with congenital diaphragmatic hernia. Prenatal diagnosis requires MRI or ultrasound evidence of abdominal organs displaced into the thorax.

PRUNE BELLY SYNDROME

Abdominal musculature is severely underdeveloped or even absent, most likely due to the involvement of myoblasts in the hypaxial myotomes. **Urinary tract defects** are commonly associated, including tortuous and dilated ureters, prostatic hypoplasia, and a thick-walled bladder. Cryptorchidism is extremely common. **Pulmonary hypoplasia is also seen** due to the pressure of the abdominal contents on the thorax. Diagnosis is made with neonatal ultrasound, and treatment includes surgical repair for severe cases.

POLAND SYNDROME

Uncommon anomaly with complete or partial (often just the sternal head) absence of the **pectoralis major** muscle. There may also be partial absence of the ribs and sternum, mammary gland aplasia, nipple hypoplasia, and absence of the serratus anterior and latissimus dorsi muscles. Does not usually cause disability, as the shoulder muscles are able to compensate for the missing muscle.

CONGENITAL TORTICOLLIS

The **sternocleidomastoid (SCM)** muscle is either injured at birth or congenitally shortened, such that the infant's head is rotated and tilted in a fixed position. Contraction of one SCM tilts the head ipsilaterally, but due to the attachment of the SCM to the mastoid process posterior to the fulcrum of the head, **rotation is in the contralateral direction.** So, if the head is turned **right,** the **left** SCM is involved.

ACCESSORY MUSCLES

Generally benign, accessory muscles can occur virtually anywhere in the body. One of the more common (about 6% of the population) and occasionally clinically significant cases is an **accessory soleus muscle,** which can cause pain in the posteromedial area of the ankle after strenuous exercise.

Anatomy

SKELETAL SYSTEM

Two types of connective tissue make up the skeletal system: bone and cartilage. All bones are made up of an outer layer of **compact** bone and an inner mass of **spongy** bone (mainly replaced by a **medullary cavity**), with different bones having different relative amounts of each. Compact bone is primarily for weight bearing, while the medullary cavity and areas around the spongy bone spicules house the formation of blood cells and platelets (Figure 5-8). Cartilage forms in the areas of the skeletal system where movement is required. Unlike bone, cartilage does not have its own blood supply and receives nutrition via diffusion.

There are two main divisions of the skeletal system: the **axial skeleton** (skull, vertebrae, hyoid bone, ribs, and sternum) and the **appendicular skeleton** (limb bones, shoulders, and pelvic girdles).

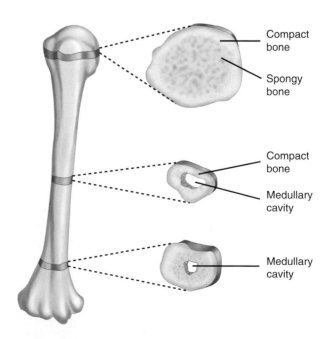

FIGURE 5-8. **Humerus with transverse sections.** Compact bone, spongy bone, and the medullary cavity are shown.

Major Bones

SKULL

The bones of the skull can be divided into two main groups: **neurocranium** and **viscerocranium.**

The **neurocranium** houses the brain and associated blood vessels, cranial nerves, and meninges. It consists of eight mostly flat bones that are connected by sutures:

- Frontal bone
- Parietal bones (2)
- Temporal bones (2)
- Occipital bone
- Sphenoid bone
- Ethmoid bone (along with parts of the temporal and occipital bones, makes up the base of the skull)

The major **sutures** (see Figure 5-3) connecting the bones of the neurocranium are as follows:

- Coronal suture: Connects the frontal bone with the parietal bones.
- Sagittal suture: Connects the two parietal bones.
- Squamosal sutures: Connect the temporal bones with the parietal bones.
- Lambdoid suture: Connects the occipital bone with the parietal and temporal bones.

The **viscerocranium** makes up the "face" of the skull—namely, the orbits, nasal cavities, and jaw. It consists of 14 bones (Figure 5-9):

- Nasal bones (2)
- Lacrimal bones (2)
- Zygomatic bones (2)

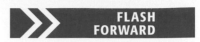

FLASH FORWARD

The **pterion** is the area where four of the bones of the neurocranium meet: frontal, parietal, temporal, and sphenoid. It is at this structurally weak point that the **middle meningeal artery** is easily ruptured in the event of trauma to the side of the head, **causing an epidural hematoma.**

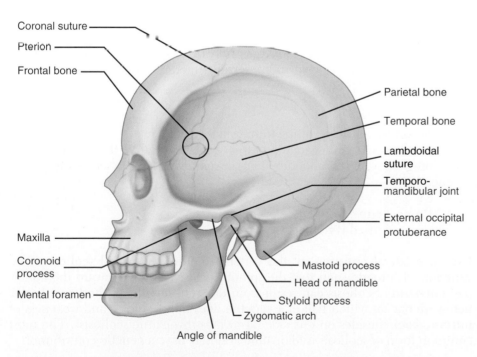

FIGURE 5-9. **Lateral view of the skull.** (Modified with permission from White JS. *USMLE: Road Map: Gross Anatomy,* 2nd ed. New York: McGraw-Hill, 2006: 188.)

MNEMONIC

Structures passing through the superior orbital fissures—

Lazy French Tarts Sit Naked In Anticipation Of Sex

Lacrimal nerve (branch of the ophthalmic nerve, CN V_1)

Frontal nerve (branch of the ophthalmic nerve, CN V_1)

Trochlear nerve (CN IV)

Superior division of the oculomotor nerve (CN III)

Nasociliary (branch of the ophthalmic nerve, CN V_1)

Inferior division of the oculomotor nerve (CN III)

Abducens nerve (CN VI)

Ophthalmic vein

Sympathetic fibers

MNEMONIC

Structures passing through the foramen ovale—

MALE

Mandibular nerve (CN V_3)

Accessory meningeal artery

Lesser petrosal nerve

Emissary veins

FLASH BACK

Spondylolisthesis is a cause of **lordosis.** Due to the failure of the pedicles to form properly, one or more of the lumbar vertebral bodies are free to move anteriorly, causing exaggerated curvature.

- Vomer
- Palatine bones (2)
- Inferior nasal conchae (2)
- Maxillae (2)
- Mandible

The inner surface of the cranial base contains three depressions: the **anterior fossa, middle fossa,** and **posterior fossa.** Through each fossa various nerves and blood vessels are transmitted through holes in the skull called **foramina** (Table 5-3).

VERTEBRAL COLUMN

The vertebral column is made up of 33 vertebrae (Figure 5-10). A typical vertebra has a **vertebral body** anteriorly (to support body weight), a **vertebral arch** posteriorly (made up of pedicles and laminae that serve to protect the spinal cord), and seven processes that serve different functions:

- The **spinous process** projects posteriorly and allows for muscle attachment and movement.
- The two **transverse processes** project posterolaterally and function like the spinous process.
- Four **articular processes** (two superior, two inferior) project from the same place as the transverse processes but serve to guide some movement as well as prevent anterior movement of the superior vertebrae over the inferior vertebrae.

These 33 vertebrae are divided into five areas, each area with a specific curvature:

- Cervical:
  - C1–C7.
  - Secondary curve resulting from the infant lifting its head.
- Thoracic:
  - T1–T12.
  - Primary curve from fetal development.
  - Accentuated **kyphosis**—exaggeration of this (forward) curve—can be due to wedge vertebral compression fractures (from osteoporosis) or disk degeneration.
- Lumbar:
  - L1–L5.
  - Secondary curve resulting from walking.
  - **Lordosis** is an exaggeration of this (backward) curve that can be due to pregnancy, excess abdominal fat, or spondylolisthesis (see below).
- Sacral:
  - S1–S5.
  - Primary curve from fetal development.
- Coccyx = 4 fused vertebrae.

Excessive lateral curvature of the vertebral column is called **scoliosis.** The vertebrae also rotate such that the spinous processes move toward the abnormal curvature. Scoliosis can result from different lengths of the lower limbs, hemivertebra (in which half of a vertebra does not develop), and weakness of intrinsic back muscles on one side (known as myopathic scoliosis). The most common form of scoliosis is idiopathic and may have a genetic contribution.

Between each vertebra (except the C1–C2 space) is an intervertebral disk that serves as a shock absorber and distributes weight. Each disk is made up of

TABLE 5-3.   Structures Transmitted Through Skull Foramina

Foramen	Bone	Fossa	Transmitted Structure(s)
Cribriform plate foramina	Ethmoid	Anterior	Olfactory nerve (CN I).
Optic canals	Sphenoid (lesser wing)	Middle	▪ Optic nerves (CN II). ▪ Ophthalmic arteries.
Superior orbital fissures	Between the lesser and greater wings of the sphenoid	Middle	▪ Ophthalmic veins. ▪ CN III. ▪ CN IV. ▪ CN V$_1$ (ophthalmic). ▪ CN VI. ▪ Sympathetic fibers.
Carotid canal	Between temporal (petrous portion) and sphenoid (greater wing)	Middle	Internal carotid artery.
Foramen rotundum	Sphenoid (greater wing)	Middle	CN V$_2$ (maxillary).
Foramen ovale	Sphenoid (greater wing)	Middle	▪ CN V$_3$ (mandibular). ▪ Accessory meningeal artery. ▪ Lesser petrosal nerve. ▪ Emissary veins.
Foramen spinosum	Sphenoid (greater wing)	Middle	Middle meningeal artery and vein.
Foramen lacerum	Between temporal (petrous portion) and sphenoid	Middle	Nothing transmits through, but the internal carotid artery passes across it.
Internal acoustic meatus	Temporal (petrous part)	Posterior	CNs VII and VIII.
Jugular foramen	Between temporal (petrous portion) and occipital	Posterior	CNs IX, X, and XI, internal jugular vein, sigmoid sinus.
Hypoglossal canal	Occipital	Posterior	CN XII.
Foramen magnum	Occipital	Posterior	Spinal roots of CN XI, vertebral arteries, anterior and posterior spinal arteries, dural veins, medulla, meninges.
Mastoid foramen	Temporal (petrous)	Posterior	Mastoid emissary vein from the sigmoid sinus.

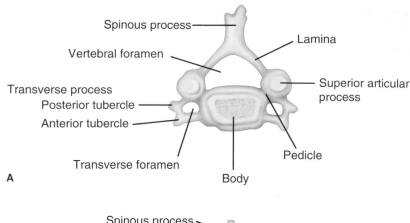

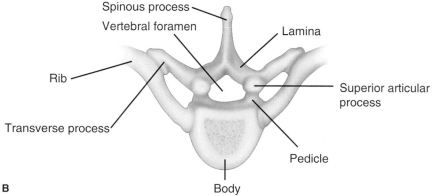

FIGURE 5-10. **A typical cervical and a thoracic vertebra.** (A) Cervical vertebra (B) thoracic vertebra.

an outer fibrous ring known as the **annulus fibrosus** and an inner gelatinous mass known as the **nucleus pulposus.**

PELVIS

The pelvis is made up of two **hip bones** (each consisting of an **ischium, ilium,** and **pubis** that join to form the **acetabulum,** which articulates with the femur), the **sacrum,** and the **coccyx.**

The pelvis is divided into the **greater pelvis** (false pelvis) and **lesser pelvis** (true pelvis) by the pelvic inlet. The **pelvic inlet** is the plane passing through the S1 vertebral body (the **sacral promontory**) and the **terminal lines** (including the pubic crest, iliopectineal line, and arcuate line of the ilium). The **pelvic outlet** is the plane passing through the pubic symphysis anteriorly, the inferior pubic rami and ischial tuberosities laterally, and the coccyx posteriorly.

The greater pelvis is superior to the pelvic inlet and contains abdominal organs such as the ileum and sigmoid colon. It is bound by the abdominal wall anteriorly, the iliac crests laterally, and L5/S1 posteriorly.

The lesser pelvis lies between the pelvic inlet and pelvic outlet. It contains the pelvic viscera (thus making it the "true pelvis") including the urinary bladder, uterus, and ovaries. The pelvic diaphragm lies inferiorly (Figure 5-11).

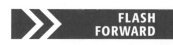
FLASH FORWARD

Dystocia, or abnormal/difficult labor, can be caused by the inability of the infant to pass through the pelvic inlet. The pelvic inlet may be too small (especially in android and platypelloid shaped pelvis) or the baby too large (macrosomia).

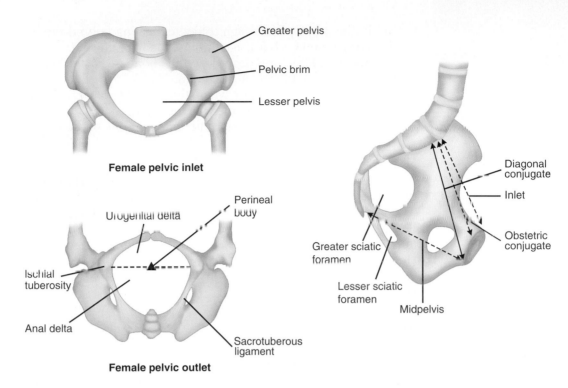

FIGURE 5-11. **Views of the bony pelvis.** (Modified with permission from White JS. *USMLE: Road Map: Gross Anatomy*, 2nd ed. New York: McGraw-Hill, 2006: 105.)

UPPER LIMBS

Each upper limb is made up of four basic skeletal segments:

- Pectoral girdle: Scapula, clavicle
- Arm: Humerus
- Forearm: Ulna (medial), radius (lateral)
- Hand: Carpus, metacarpus, phalanges

The **axillary nerve** runs along the **surgical neck** of the humerus. The **radial nerve** runs in the **radial groove**, as the name suggests. The **median nerve** runs along the **distal humerus**. The **ulnar nerve** runs posterior to the **medial epicondyle** (making this nerve responsible for the "funny bone" sensation).

LOWER LIMBS

Like the upper limbs, each lower limb is made up of four basic segments:

- Pelvic girdle: Hip
- Thigh: Femur
- Leg: Tibia (anteromedial), fibula (posterolateral)
- Foot: Tarsus, metatarsus, phalanges

Common Injuries and Disorders

FRACTURES OF THE SKULL

There are several different types of skull fractures.

- **Linear** skull fractures are the most common and usually result from blunt trauma.
- **Basilar** skull fractures are usually linear and most often involve the temporal bone. Signs of basilar skull fractures are "raccoon eyes" (blood collect-

ing in the orbits), Battle sign (blood collecting behind the ears), blood in the sinuses, and CSF leakage through the nose and ears.

- **Comminuted** fractures occur when the bone is broken into several pieces, some of which can lacerate the brain.
- **Depressed** fractures occur when the bone is depressed inward, putting pressure on and causing damage to the brain.
- A **contrecoup** fracture occurs at the side opposite of the impact.

FRACTURES AND DISLOCATIONS OF THE VERTEBRAE

Fractures and/or dislocations are usually due to **hyperflexion of the neck,** often resulting from car accidents or direct trauma to the back of the head. The most common injury is a crush or compression fracture of the vertebral body. Because the articular surfaces of cervical vertebrae are inclined horizontally, anterior dislocations can occur in this region of the spine without concomitant fractures. On the other hand, in the thoracic and lumbar regions, articular surfaces are arranged vertically, so dislocations are usually seen with fractures.

ATLANTOAXIAL DISLOCATION

The dens of the axis (C2) interlocks with the atlas (C1) through a foramen and is normally held in place by the cruciform, alar, and apical ligaments, as well as the tectorial membrane (a continuation of the posterior longitudinal ligament). When trauma or rheumatoid arthritis causes a tear or degradation in the cruciform ligament, the dens may not move in tandem with the anterior arch of C1, damaging the cervical spinal cord (posterior movement of the dens) and medulla (superior dens movement), often resulting in quadriplegia.

HERNIATION OF THE NUCLEUS PULPOSUS

Also known as a "herniated disk" or "slipped disk," the nucleus pulposus actually pushes into or through the annulus fibrosus. This commonly occurs at the lumbar level but may occur in the cervical region as well. Posterolateral herniation compresses spinal nerve roots, whereas posterior herniation may compress the spinal cord.

KEY FACT

In the lumbar spine, posterolateral disk herniation impinges the spinal nerve numbered for the inferior vertebrae at that disk level (eg, the L5/S1 disk impinges the S1 nerve). Over 90% of clinically evident herniated disks occur at L4/L5 and L5/S1.

- In the elderly, degeneration and wear at the posterior longitudinal ligament and posterior aspect of the annulus fibrosus in the lumbar region may allow the nucleus pulposus to herniate. Nerve root impingement at the L5/S1 intervertebral foramen level can result in radiating low back pain down the back of the thigh into the leg to the foot, called **sciatica.**
- Similar injuries in the cervical spine are also very common. **Hyperflexion** of the neck during head-on traffic collisions may cause rupture of the posterior ligaments and subsequent nucleus pulposus herniation at the C5–C7 levels, resulting in pain in the neck radiating to the shoulders, and arms. Hyperextension of the neck, or **whiplash,** may stretch the anterior ligaments and cause fractures and dislocations of the vertebrae as well.

SPONDYLOLYSIS

Defect or fracture in the **pars interarticularis** (ie, the part of the vertebral arch lamina that connects the inferior and superior articular processes). Though frequently asymptomatic, it can cause lower back pain at the L5 level. Although genetics probably play a role, it is thought that repeated microtrauma to this region may cause stress fractures (occurs in gymnasts). If the defects are bilateral, this condition can progress to **spondylolisthesis,** in which the affected vertebra becomes displaced (Figure 5-12) (males more than females). Spondylolysis on plain radiographs is best demonstrated with oblique views of the spine.

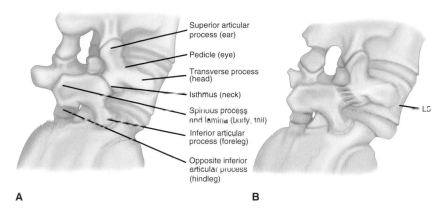

Labels on figure:
- Superior articular process (ear)
- Pedicle (eye)
- Transverse process (head)
- Isthmus (neck)
- Spinous process and lamina (body, tail)
- Inferior articular process (foreleg)
- Opposite inferior articular process (hindleg)
- L5

A   **B**

FIGURE 5-12. A comparison of spondylolysis and spondylolisthesis. (A) Posterior oblique radiographic view mimics shape of Scotty dog. In simple spondylolysis, dog appears to be wearing a collar. (B) In spondylolisthesis, Scotty dog appears decapitated. L5 body and disk are displaced anteriorly. (Modified with permission from White JS. *USMLE: Road Map: Gross Anatomy*, 2nd ed. New York: McGraw-Hill, 2006: 26.)

ANKYLOSING SPONDYLITIS

Chronic, progressive, seronegative arthritis that commonly first affects the lumbar vertebrae and sacroiliac joints. The annulus fibrosus of several vertebrae may become ossified, leading to the formation of syndesmophytes and fusion of vertebrae. Multiple fused vertebrae may appear as a characteristic **"bamboo spine"** seen on plain films. Mainly affects young males and often presents as low back pain that causes awakening from sleep, as well as morning spinal stiffness. Most patients with ankylosing spondylitis are **HLA-B27-positive.** Extraspinal manifestations can include peripheral arthritis (especially in the hips and knees), iritis, and pulmonary involvement.

See Table 5-4 for definitions and common features.

FRACTURES OF THE PELVIS

May occur from anteroposterior compression, lateral compression, and acetabular fractures

- Anteroposterior compression (ie, compression between the steering wheel and seat in automobile accidents) results in fractures of the pubic symphysis and pubic rami.
- Lateral compression can also involve the pubic rami as well as the ala of the ilium.
- Acetabular fractures can result from falls onto the feet with extended legs, causing the head of the femur to push through (protrusio acetabuli). Pelvic organs, vessels, and nerves may also be injured by the femur. Signs of pelvic fracture on exam include pelvic tenderness, palpable instability, and vaginal or urethral bleeding.

TABLE 5-4. Synopsis of Spondylolysis, Spondylolisthesis, and Ankylosing Spondylitis

SPONDYLOLYSIS	SPONDYLOLISTHESIS	ANKYLOSING SPONDYLITIS
Defect/fracture in the pars interarticularis; uncommonly symptomatic	Displacement of a vertebra commonly caused by spondylolysis or degenerative disk disease.	Inflammatory arthritis of spinal joints, causing back stiffness, pain, and limited range of motion; moves cephalad and eventually affects the cervical spine.

FRACTURES OF THE UPPER LIMB

Fractures can occur at many places along the arm, often with concurrent damage to important arteries and nerves.

- **Clavicle:** Most commonly in the middle one-third of the bone. The SCM muscle lifts the proximal piece, and the weight of the arm pulls down the distal piece.
- **Greater tuberosity:** Often associated with separation of the shoulder, as three out of the four rotator cuff muscles attach here (supraspinatus, infraspinatus, teres minor).
- **Surgical neck of the humerus:** May injure the axillary nerve.
- **Distal half of the humerus:** May injure the radial nerve along the radial/spiral groove.
- **Humerus, just superior to the elbow (ie, supracondylar fracture):** May injure the brachial artery and median nerve. Can lead to a Volkmann ischemic contracture, in which ischemia from brachial artery disruption leads to scar tissue formation and hand and forearm muscle flexion contractures.
- **Medial epicondyle:** May injure the ulnar nerve.
- **Distal radius (Colles fracture):** Often includes a fracture of the ulna (styloid process). A common finding is "dinner fork" deformity (dorsal displacement of bone fragments distal to the fracture).
- **Scaphoid:** Very little displacement of the bones with pain in the anatomic snuff box; often missed on X-rays and misdiagnosed as a sprain. X-rays should be repeated in 10 days to confirm a suspected fracture. Whereas a sprain can be treated with rest and ice, fractures usually require casting. Improperly treated fractures may progress to a nonunion, avascular necrosis, and arthritis.

FRACTURES OF THE LOWER LIMB

As in the upper limb, fractures may occur throughout the lower limb.

- **Femoral neck:** Occurs more often in women due to their greater risk of osteoporosis. The blood vessels (medial circumflex femoral artery) that supply the femoral head are frequently ruptured in this fracture, resulting in avascular necrosis. On presentation, the lower limb is usually shortened and laterally rotated.
- **Tibial fractures:** Several types of fractures can occur at the middle of the body of the tibia. A compound fracture can involve both the tibia and fibula, and fragments of the tibia may tear blood vessels and penetrate the skin. Diagonal fractures may occur due to severe torsion of the lower leg. Transverse fractures, or "boot-top" fractures, are comminuted fractures that often occur after a forward fall while skiing, in which the leg is bent over the tops of the rigid boots. Stress fractures are transverse and may occur in normally sedentary people who decide to take a long walk or run.
- **Pott fracture:** The medial (deltoid) ligament is overly stretched during severe foot eversion. The strong medial ligament does not tear, but causes fractures of the medial malleolus (transverse avulsion) and fibula (oblique at the level of the joint).
- **Fracture of the fifth metatarsal:** Occurs during extreme inversion of the foot. This tears the lateral ligament and can fracture the lateral malleolus. This is a common sports injury.

COXA VALGA AND COXA VARA

The angle between the shaft of the femur and the head of the femur varies among people of different ages and genders. When this angle is large, it is termed **coxa valga** and when it is too acute, it is called **coxa vara.** The latter can lead to a shortening of the leg, making it difficult to completely abduct the leg.

LEGG-CALVÉ-PERTHES DISEASE

Idiopathic avascular necrosis of the capital femoral epiphysis of the femoral head (can be bilateral) that causes decreased range of motion and upper leg pain, typically in male children aged 3–12 years. The cause is unknown. It is self-limited because the bone eventually revascularizes, but the prognosis may be complicated by osteoarthritis (OA).

SLIPPED CAPITAL FEMORAL EPIPHYSIS (SCFE)

If an adolescent has a weakened epiphyseal plate due to acute trauma or many microtraumas, the femoral head epiphysis can slowly slip away from the femoral neck, causing a coxa vara. This condition commonly affects obese adolescents during their growth spurt, and the slipped femoral head can present with hip pain **referred to the knee**. Diagnosis is made by X-ray

JOINTS

Types of Joints

Joints are simply defined as those areas where bones meet. There are three main types of joints: **synovial, cartilaginous,** and **fibrous.**

SYNOVIAL JOINTS

The most common in the body; allow for free movement between the two articulating bones. Lubricating fluid known as **synovial fluid** found in the **joint cavity** between the two bones facilitates movement. This cavity is enclosed by two structures: **articular cartilage** at the surface of the bone ends, and a **synovial membrane** that, in conjunction with an outer **fibrous capsule,** makes up the **articular capsule.** The periosteum of the two meeting bones blends together with the articular capsule. These joints are often strengthened by surrounding ligaments, which are especially important when considering common joint injuries.

There are six main types of synovial joints (Table 5-5).

TABLE 5-5. **Types of Synovial Joints**

TYPE OF SYNOVIAL JOINT	EXAMPLES	TYPE OF MOVEMENT
Plane joints	Acromioclavicular joint	Gliding in one axis.
Hinge joints	Elbow joint	Flexion/extension.
Saddle joints	Carpometacarpal joints	Flexion/extension, abduction/adduction, circumduction.
Condyloid joints	Metacarpophalangeal joints	Same as saddle joints, with one axis usually greater than the other.
Ball and socket joints	Hip joint	Flexion/extension, abduction/adduction, circumduction, medial/lateral rotation.
Pivot joints	Atlantoaxial joint	Rotation (pronation/supination as in the radius; rotation of the atlas around the dens in the atlantoaxial joint).

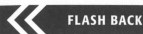

FLASH BACK

The hyaline cartilage in primary cartilaginous joints is made up predominantly of type II collagen.

KEY FACT

Force from the hand to the humerus is transferred from the radius to the ulna through the interosseous ligaments, which are oriented in an inferomedial direction to transfer these pulling forces.

KEY FACT

The Colles fracture involves the distal radius and frequently the styloid process of the ulna as well. Bone fragments are displaced dorsally distal to the fracture, causing what is known as the dinner fork deformity.

CARTILAGINOUS JOINTS

Two types of cartilaginous joints exist in the body throughout development. **Primary cartilaginous joints** are typically temporary articulations of bone made up of **hyaline** cartilage; these are present during development of the long bones and at epiphyseal plates. **Secondary cartilaginous joints** are made up of **fibrocartilage**. An example of this joint type is the intervertebral disks that join the vertebrae together and allow for limited movement of the spine.

FIBROUS JOINTS

The articulating bones are connected by ligaments or fibrous membranes. Movement in these joints may be limited or nonexistent, depending on the fibrous limitations connecting the bones. Examples include the sutures of the skull, the pubic symphysis, and the joint connecting the radius and the ulna.

Major Joints and Common Injuries

VERTEBRA

- **Atlanto-occipital:** Synovial joint between the atlas (C1) and the occipital condyles that allows the head to nod "yes."
- **Atlantoaxial:** Synovial joint between the atlas (C1) and the axis (C2) that allows the head to shake "no."
- **Facet joints:** Synovial joints between the inferior and superior articular facets of the spine.

SHOULDER

- **Acromioclavicular joint:** A plane type of synovial joint between the lateral end of the clavicle and acromion of the scapula. Despite the strong ligaments keeping it in place, this joint may become separated following a fall onto the shoulder or outstretched arm.
- **Glenohumeral:** Ball-and-socket type of synovial joint between the humeral head and glenoid fossa. Because this fossa is shallow, the humeral head may be dislocated anteriorly or posteriorly. Anterior dislocation may result in damage to the axillary nerve. More rare posterior dislocations are caused by electrocution injuries.

ELBOW

This hinge-type synovial joint is actually made up of three different joints:

- **Ulnohumeral:** Reinforced by the medial collateral ligament.
- **Radiohumeral:** Reinforced by the lateral collateral ligament.
- **Radioulnar:** Reinforced by the **annular ligament. A pulled elbow,** or nursemaid's elbow, may occur when a child is lifted forcibly by the arms while the forearm is pronated. This tears the annular ligament and causes subluxation of the radial head. Pain results from pinching of the annular ligament in the elbow joint, and pronation/supination becomes very limited. The elbow is reduced by supinating the forearm while the elbow is flexed.

WRIST

Radiocarpal joint. A condyloid type of synovial joint between the radius and carpal bones. The most common type of fracture at this site is from a **FOOSH** (Fall On OutStretched Hand), which leads to a **Colles fracture** ("dinner fork" deformity).

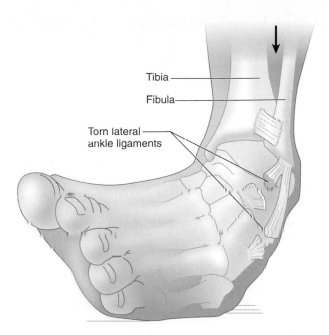

FIGURE 5-13. **Ligament injury of ankle.** With typical inversion ankle injury, the antero-talofibular ligament is sprained or torn.

HIP

A ball-and-socket joint between the femoral head and acetabulum. Fractures involving this area have been discussed previously.

KNEE

A hinge-type synovial joint between the tibia, femur, and patella, with multiple associated ligaments.

- **Medially:** The fibrocartilaginous **medial meniscus** is firmly attached to the **medial (tibial) collateral ligament.** Trauma to the lateral side of the knee causing excessive valgus deformity will often result in injury to both of these structures.
- **Laterally:** The **lateral meniscus** is fibrocartilage that is **not** firmly attached to the **lateral (fibular) collateral ligament.** Trauma to the medial side of the knee causing excessive varus deformity may result in injury to the lateral ligament. Tears of the lateral meniscus are less common since it has fewer points of attachment.
- **Anteriorly:** The **anterior cruciate ligament** starts at the anterior tibia and extends posterolaterally to the lateral condyle of the femur. This ligament prevents excessive anterior movement of the tibia when the knee is flexed. A tear of this ligament can be demonstrated with a positive **anterior drawer sign,** in which the examiner flexes the knee and pulls on the tibia, causing abnormal anterior displacement.
- **Posteriorly:** The **posterior cruciate ligament** starts at the posterior tibia and extends anteromedially to the medial condyle of the femur; it prevents excessive posterior movement of the tibia when the knee is flexed. A tear can be demonstrated with a positive **posterior drawer sign,** in which the examiner flexes the knee and pushes on the tibia, causing abnormal posterior displacement.

A common soccer injury, called the **"unhappy triad,"** occurs when an athlete is hit from the lateral side and twists the flexed knee. The **tibial ligament** tears first, followed closely by the **medial meniscus,** and finally the **anterior cruciate ligament.** In this case, one would see abnormal passive abduction (valgus deviation) and a positive anterior drawer sign.

ANKLE

Talocrural joint. A hinge-type synovial joint between the ends of the tibia/fibula and the talus. **Inversion** (foot rolls in) results in sprain (tearing) of the **lateral ligament (anterotalofibular ligament,** ie, ATFL) (Figure 5-13). Extreme **eversion** (foot rolls out) places stress on the **medial ligament (deltoid)** and may result in a **Pott fracture** of the fibula and medial malleolus, as discussed previously.

MUSCULAR SYSTEM

Types of Muscle

There are three basic types of muscle fibers that allow the human body to move, as well as provide form and heat: **skeletal, smooth,** and **cardiac.**

SKELETAL MUSCLE

Skeletal muscle is composed of large, elongated, multinucleated fibers that show strong, quick, voluntary contractions.

Most skeletal muscles produce movements of the skeleton and are attached to bone or cartilage either directly or via tendons. There are many exceptions to this, however, such as eye muscles, superficial facial muscles, and the diaphragm. Nerve impulses in the somatic nervous system innervate muscle fibers to cause contraction. This is often under voluntary control, though some skeletal muscles, such as the diaphragm, are under involuntary control.

Though new muscle cells can be formed to a limited degree, the primary growth response (ie, to exercise) is through hypertrophy (increase in size, not number).

Skeletal muscle fibers of humans are classified into three types based on their physiologic, biochemical, and histochemical characteristics:

- **Type I** or slow, red oxidative fibers contain many mitochondria and abundant myoglobin, a protein with iron groups that bind O_2 and produce a dark red color. Red fibers derive energy primarily from aerobic oxidative phosphorylation of fatty acids and are adapted for slow, continuous contractions over prolonged periods, as required, for example, in the postural muscles of the back.
- **Type IIa** or fast, intermediate oxidative-glycolytic fibers have many mitochondria and much myoglobin, but also have considerable glycogen. They utilize both oxidative metabolism and anaerobic glycolysis and are intermediate between the other fiber types both in color and in energy metabolism. They are adapted for rapid contractions and short bursts of activity, such as those required for athletics.
- **Type IIb** or fast, white glycolytic fibers have fewer mitochondria and less myoglobin, but abundant glycogen, making them very pale in color. They depend largely on glycolysis for energy and are adapted for rapid contractions, but fatigue quickly. They are typically small muscles with a relatively large number of neuromuscular junctions, such as the muscles that move the eyes and digits.

SMOOTH MUSCLE

Smooth muscle is composed of grouped, mononucleated fusiform cells with weak, involuntary contractions.

Smooth muscle lacks the striations of skeletal and cardiac muscles and is found mainly within the walls of visceral organs and the tunica media of blood vessels.

- Unlike skeletal muscle, their contractions are slow and rhythmic, helping to move food (**peristalsis**) and regulate the flow of blood (**vasoconstriction**), in addition to other functions (**sphincteric activity**).
- Like cardiac muscle, the autonomic nervous system innervates smooth muscle, and contraction is involuntary.

Smooth muscle cells can undergo hypertrophy (increase in size) and hyperplasia (increase in number).

KEY FACT

Smooth muscle is also found at the base of hair follicles (erector pili muscles) and in the iris and ciliary body of the eye.

CARDIAC MUSCLE

Cardiac muscle is composed of irregular branched cells bound together longitudinally by intercalated disks and shows strong, involuntary contractions.

The muscle of the heart (ie, myocardium) is composed of cardiac muscle. The cells are striated and contain a single (sometimes two) central nuclei. Actions of these cells are involuntary but are also under the control of specialized intrinsic pacemaker cells (in the SA and AV nodes) that are influenced by the autonomic nervous system.

Unlike skeletal or smooth muscles, cardiac muscle cannot regenerate, though hypertrophy can result from increased demand on the heart (ie, hypertension).

Important Muscles

HEAD AND NECK MUSCLES

MASTICATION MUSCLES

There are four main muscles that move the mandible for chewing, all of which are innervated by various branches of CN V_3 (the mandibular branch of the trigeminal nerve):

- **Temporalis:** Elevates and retracts the mandible (closes the jaw).
- **Masseter:** Elevates and protrudes the mandible (closes the jaw).
- **Medial pterygoid:** Elevates and helps (slightly) to protrude the mandible (closing and grinding the jaw).
- **Lateral pterygoid:** Depresses (slightly) and protrudes the mandible as well as moves it from side to side (opening and grinding the jaw).

The main force that opens the jaw is gravity, though the lateral pterygoid as well as suprahyoid and infrahyoid muscles assist.

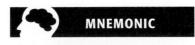

MNEMONIC

Three muscles CLOSE the jaw (the **M**s **M**unch): **M**asseter, **M**edial pterygoid, and te**M**poralis.
One muscle OPENS the jaw (the **L** **L**owers): **L**ateral pterygoid.

MUSCLES WITH "GLOSSUS" AND "PALAT"

As a general rule, all of the muscles that end in "glossus" are innervated by CN XII (hypoglossal nerve), and all of the muscles that have "palat" in them are innervated by CN X (vagus nerve). The following muscles follow these rules:

- **Genioglossus:** CN XII; depresses and protrudes the tongue.
- **Hyoglossus:** CN XII; depresses and retracts the tongue.

MNEMONIC

All muscles that end with **GLOSSUS** (except the palatoglossus—"palat" is first!) are innervated by the hypo**GLOSSAL** nerve.
All muscles with **PALAT** are innervated by the **VAGUS** (except the tensor veli palatini, which is too **TENSE** to be with the rest).

FLASH BACK

The second through fourth branchial clefts usually merge and involute; when the second branchial cleft persists, a fistula can be formed between the pharynx and skin. This fistula is usually located along the anterior border of the upper third of the SCM.

- **Styloglossus:** CN XII; retracts and elevates the tongue for swallowing.
- **Levator veli palatini:** CN X; elevates the soft palate for swallowing/yawning.
- **Palatopharyngeus:** CN X; tenses the soft palate and moves the pharynx for swallowing.

There is one exception to each rule: The **palatoglossus** muscle, which elevates the posterior tongue *and* brings the soft palate to the tongue, follows the "palat" rule ("palat" is first in palatoglossus) and is innervated by the vagus nerve. The **tensor veli palatini**, which tenses the soft palate and opens the auditory tube during swallowing/yawning, does **not** follow the "palat" rule, but instead is innervated by a branch of CN V$_3$ (mandibular branch of the trigeminal nerve).

STERNOCLEIDOMASTOID (SCM)

Attaches superiorly to the mastoid and divides inferiorly into two heads that form attachments to the sternum and clavicle. Contraction of one SCM tilts the head to the ipsilateral side, while flexing and rotating the head to the contralateral side. The SCM is important for both anatomic and clinical reasons:

- It divides the neck anatomically into anterior and posterior triangles.
- It is an important landmark for branchial anomalies that may occur during embryologic development.
- Congenital torticollis occurs when the SCM is congenitally shortened or injured at birth, causing a fixed tilted, rotated, and flexed position.
- Spasmodic torticollis (a.k.a. "cervical dystonia" or "wry neck") occurs with abnormally increased tone in the SCM. It is often associated with spasms of intense neck pain.

LARYNX

Muscles are divided first into extrinsic and intrinsic groups. The **extrinsic muscles** function to **move the hyoid bone and larynx superiorly or inferiorly,** while the **intrinsic muscles** make fine adjustments to the **vocal folds** and **rima glottidis** to aid in speaking, whispering, and respiration.

The extrinsic laryngeal muscles are further divided into **suprahyoid** and **infrahyoid** muscles (Table 5-6). The suprahyoid muscles and **stylopharyngeus** elevate the hyoid and larynx, while the infrahyoid muscles depress these structures.

The intrinsic laryngeal muscles work together to alter the shape and tension of the vocal folds in order to change the size and shape of the space between

TABLE 5-6. **Extrinsic Muscles of the Larynx**

SUPRAHYOID MUSCLES	INFRAHYOID MUSCLES
Mylohyoid	Sternohyoid
Geniohyoid	Omohyoid
Stylohyoid	Sternothyroid
Digastric	Thyrohyoid

the folds, called the rima glottidis. Dividing them into functional groups is helpful:

- Adductors (close the rima glottidis for phonation):
  - Lateral cricoarytenoid muscles: Main adductors.
  - Transverse and oblique arytenoid muscles: Adductors and sphincters to protect during swallowing.
  - Aryepiglottic muscles: Sphincters.
- Abductor (open the rima glottidis for breathing): Posterior cricoarytenoid muscles: The **only abductors** of the intrinsic muscles of the larynx (without these muscles, we would be unable to breathe!).
- Tensors (raise the pitch of the voice): Cricothyroid muscles.
- Relaxers (decrease the pitch of the voice, and used for singing):
  - Thyroarytenoid muscles
  - Vocalis muscles (for fine adjustments).

Almost all motor innervation of the inner laryngeal muscles comes from **below** via the **recurrent laryngeal nerve** (a branch of the **inferior** laryngeal nerve). Damage to the recurrent laryngeal nerve therefore causes hoarseness (if unilateral), and possible breathing difficulties and aphonia (if bilateral). Damage may occur following surgery, including thyroidectomy or compression from laryngeal cancer.

All sensory innervation comes from **above** via the **internal laryngeal nerve** (a branch of the **superior** laryngeal nerve). Damage to the superior laryngeal nerve therefore causes anesthesia of the laryngeal mucosa. This is dangerous as foreign bodies are more likely to pass, but this nerve is often temporarily blocked in order to pass an endotracheal tube. Laryngeal elevation is the primary mechanism for preventing aspiration during swallowing.

UPPER LIMB MUSCLES

ROTATOR CUFF MUSCLES

Four muscles collectively known as the rotator cuff muscles help to stabilize the humeral head in the glenohumeral joint while the shoulder moves. Subscapularis inserts onto lesser tuberosity; remaining muscles insert on greater tuberosity.

- **Supraspinatus:** Innervated by the suprascapular nerve; also helps the deltoid muscle to abduct the arm for the first 15°.
- **Infraspinatus:** Innervated by the suprascapular nerve; externally rotates the arm.
- **Teres minor:** Innervated by the axillary nerve; externally rotates the arm.
- **Subscapularis:** Innervated by subscapular nerves; internally rotates the arm.

ARM/FOREARM MUSCLES

The muscles of the arm and forearm are divided into anterior and posterior compartments. Knowing the innervation and actions of these muscles enables clinicians to predict how patients will present following different types of trauma.

The **anterior compartment of the arm** contains three flexor muscles, all innervated by the musculocutaneous nerve:

- **Biceps brachii:** Flexes and supinates the forearm.
- **Brachialis:** Flexes the forearm.
- **Coracobrachialis:** Flexes and adducts the arm.

KEY FACT

In rheumatoid arthritis hoarseness can be the product of synovitis involving the cricoarytenoid joints, in the absence of nerve damage, as these joints are always used in the production of the voice.

KEY FACT

The cricothyroid muscle is the one exception to this rule. **Both** its motor and sensory innervation comes from **above** via branches of the superior laryngeal nerve: the external branch for motor and the internal branch for sensory.

MNEMONIC

Rotator cuff muscles—

SItS
Supraspinatus, **I**nfraspinatus, **t**eres minor, **S**ubscapularis (small "t" for teres **minor;** also the only rotator cuff muscle not innervated by a scapular nerve).

FLASH BACK

It may be helpful to review the brachial plexus (in Chapter 6) at this time.

MNEMONIC

THenar muscles for the THumb.

KEY FACT

The adductor pollicis has different innervation than the rest of the thenar muscles (the ulnar nerve instead of the recurrent median nerve).

MNEMONIC

For the actual order of the muscles, remember—

A OF A OF A
Thenar, lateral to medial:
Abductor pollicis brevis
Opponens pollicis
Flexor pollicis brevis
Adductor pollicis
Hypothenar, lateral to medial:
Opponens digiti minimi
Flexor digiti minimi
Abductor digiti minimi

KEY FACT

In 12% of people, the sciatic nerve splits, and one branch pierces the piriformis. Compression leads to symptoms of sciatica termed **piriformis syndrome,** which is common in mountain climbers who develop hypertrophic piriformis muscles.

The **posterior compartment of the arm** contains only one extensor muscle, innervated by the radial nerve: the **triceps brachii**—extends the forearm.

The **anterior compartment of the forearm** contains **pronators** of the forearm and **flexors** of the forearm, hand, and fingers. All are innervated by the **median nerve,** except the flexor carpi ulnaris and the medial part of the flexor digitorum profundus, which are innervated by the **ulnar nerve.**

The **posterior compartment of the forearm** contains **extensors** and **supinators** (with the exception of the brachioradialis, which flexes the forearm). All are innervated by the **radial nerve.**

Upper nerve damage is discussed in Table 5-7.

THENAR/HYPOTHENAR

Thenar muscles control actions of the thumb and are innervated by the recurrent branch of the median nerve (**except** the adductor pollicis, which is innervated by the ulnar nerve):

- Abductor pollicis brevis: Abduction
- Opponens pollicis: Opposition
- Flexor pollicis brevis: Flexion
- Adductor pollicis

Hypothenar muscles control actions of the fifth digit and are innervated by the ulnar nerve:

- Opponens digiti minimi: Opposition
- Flexor digiti minimi: Flexion
- Abductor digiti minimi: Abduction

LOWER LIMB MUSCLES

GLUTEAL MUSCLES

This region of the body contains two main groups of muscles.

The glutei mainly extend and abduct the thigh and are innervated by the gluteal nerves:

- Gluteus maximus: Inferior gluteal nerve; extends thigh.
- Gluteus medius and minimus: Superior gluteal nerve; abducts and medially rotates the thigh.

The smaller muscles of the gluteal region are covered by the gluteus maximus and help to **laterally rotate** the thigh:

- **Piriformis:** Ventral rami of S1 and S2.
- **Obturator internus:** Nerve to obturator internus (L5, S1).
- **Gemelli superior and inferior:** L5 and S1.
- **Quadratus femoris:** Nerve to quadratus femoris (L5, S1).

THIGH/LEG MUSCLES

Like the arm/forearm muscles, the thigh and leg muscles are organized into compartments. The thigh muscles are organized into three compartments: Anterior, medial, and posterior; the leg muscles are organized into anterior, lateral, and posterior compartments.

TABLE 5-7.   Upper Limb Nerve Damage

INJURY	NERVE AFFECTED	CLINICAL FINDING	ETIOLOGIES
Fracture of the surgical neck of the humerus	Axillary n.	Impaired shoulder abduction (deltoid) and lateral rotation (teres minor)	Trauma
Shoulder dislocation	Axillary n.	Impaired shoulder abduction (deltoid) and lateral rotation (teres minor)	Occurs during sports (overhead reaching) and electrocutions
Midhumerus fracture	Radial n.	Wrist drop (triceps is spared because innervation by radial n. is above this area of injury)	Trauma
Radial head dislocation	Radial n.	Wrist drop (triceps is spared because innervation by radial n. is above this area of injury)	Falling on outstretched arm or pulling on child's arm
Bullet shot to anterior biceps	Musculocutaneous n.	Impaired elbow flexion and forearm supination	Trauma
Supracondylar fracture (elbow)	Median n.	Impaired wrist flexion, flexion of digits 1–3, and pronation of the forearm → deficits make "hand of benediction"; can cause interruption of brachial artery and subsequent Volkmann ischemic contracture of the forearm/arm	Fall on outstretched arm
Fracture of lateral epicondyle of humerus	Median n.	Impaired wrist flexion, flexion of digits 1–3, and pronation of the forearm → deficits make "hand of benediction"	
Carpal tunnel	Median n. (superficial branch spared)	Sensory/muscular deficits in digits 1–3, impaired thenar muscles, palm sensation intact	Wrist overuse, obesity, pregnancy, volume overload, synovitis
Fracture of medial epicondyle of humerus	Ulnar n.	Impaired interossei muscles, impaired digit 4–5 flexors and lumbricals, impaired hypothenar; impaired wrist flexion on ulnar side, leading to a claw-hand deformity	
Fracture of hook of hamate	Ulnar n.	Impaired interossei muscles, impaired digit 4–5 flexors and lumbricals, impaired hypothenar	Fall onto hand

The **anterior compartment of the thigh** contains **flexors of the hip** and **extensors of the knee.** Most of them are innervated by the **femoral nerve,** though there are exceptions noted below. The **femoral artery** courses in this compartment as well.

- Muscles:
  - Sartorius: Flexes, abducts, and laterally rotates the thigh, and flexes the knee.
  - Quadriceps (rectus femoris, vastus lateralis/medialis/intermedius): Flexes hip and extends knee.

KEY FACT

The sciatic nerve innervates the entire leg except the inner medial calf. As such, sciatica and piriformis syndrome spares the part of the leg innervated by the saphenous nerve, the termination of the femoral nerve (L2, 3, 4).

KEY FACT

The anterior tibial artery becomes the dorsalis pedis (DP), which courses over the anteromedial aspect of the dorsal foot between the first and second ray. This is where the DP pulse is palpated.

MNEMONIC

What courses behind the medial malleolus? (*Note:* The great saphenous vein runs anterior to the medial malleolus.)
"**T**om, **D**ick, **AN**d **H**arry:
1. "**T**om": **T**ibialis posterior muscle
2. "**D**ick": Flexor **D**igitorum longus muscle
3. **AN**d: Posterior tibial **A**rtery (PT pulse) tibial **N**erve
4. "**H**arry": flexor **H**allucis longus muscle

- Iliopsoas: Innervated by ventral rami of lumbar nerves (psoas) along with the femoral nerve (iliacus); flexes the hip.
- Pectineus: Flexes, adducts, and helps to medially rotate the thigh.
- Tensor fascia lata: Innervated by the superior gluteal nerve; flexes, abducts, and medially (internally) rotates the thigh, and keeps the knee extended. Becomes the iliotibial (IT) band.
- Artery: Femoral artery.
- Nerve: Femoral nerve, superior gluteal nerve (tensor fascia lata).

The **medial compartment of the thigh** contains the **adductors:**

- Muscles: Adductor longus/brevis/magnus, gracilis, obturator externus (laterally rotates thigh).
- Artery: Obturator artery.
- Nerve: Obturator nerve.

The **posterior compartment of the thigh** contains the **hamstrings,** which are extensors of the thigh and flexors of the leg. From medial to lateral:

- Muscles: Semitendinosus, semimembranosus, biceps femoris (long and short head).
- Artery: Profunda femoral artery, inferior gluteal artery, and the perforating arteries.
- Nerve: Sciatic nerve, common peroneal/fibular (short head of biceps femoris).

The anterior compartment of the leg contains dorsiflexors of the ankle and extensors of the toes:

- Muscles: Tibialis anterior, extensor hallucis longus, extensor digitorum longus, peroneus tertius.
- Artery: Anterior tibial vessels.
- Nerve: Deep peroneal/fibular nerve.

The lateral compartment of the leg contains the ankle evertors:

- Muscles: Peroneus longus and brevis
- Nerve: Superficial peroneal/fibular nerve

The posterior compartment of the leg (superficial and deep posterior) contains the plantar flexors of the ankle and flexors of the toes (exceptions noted below):

- Superficial posterior:
  - Muscles: Gastrocnemius, soleus, plantaris.
  - Artery/Vein: Posterior tibial artery, small (short) and great (long) saphenous vein.
  - Nerve: Sural nerve.
- Deep posterior:
  - Muscles: Flexor hallucis longus, flexor digitorum longus, tibialis posterior, popliteus.
  - Artery: Peroneal and posterior tibial artery.
  - Nerve: Tibial nerve.

NERVE DAMAGE AFFECTING THE MUSCLES OF THE LOWER LIMB

- **Piriformis syndrome:** The sciatic nerve enters the greater sciatic foramen very closely related to the piriformis muscle (usually the nerve is inferior to the muscle, though it can occasionally pierce the muscle or run superiorly). Some people who use the muscles in the gluteal region extensively (eg, skaters, mountain climbers, and cyclists) can overdevelop their piriformis muscle, resulting in pinched-nerve, sciatica-like symptoms. Women are more susceptible.

- The **Trendelenburg sign** occurs following damage to the **superior gluteal nerve** (affecting the gluteus medius and minimus). To test for this, observe the patient's back while the patient raises each foot off the ground. If the right pelvis falls when the right foot is lifted, the **left** superior gluteal nerve is damaged; if the left pelvis falls when the left foot is lifted, the **right** superior gluteal nerve is damaged. This sign can also occur in patients with a hip dislocation or fracture of the neck of the femur.
- Trauma in the femoral triangle region may damage the **femoral nerve**, causing weakened ability to flex the thigh (weak iliacus and sartorius), as well as loss of extension of the thigh (quadriceps femoris muscle).
- Injury to the **tibial nerve** is uncommon in the popliteal region because it runs deep (though deep knife wounds can injure it). Symptoms include loss of flexion of the leg, loss of plantar flexion of the ankle, and loss of flexion of the toes and inversion of the foot. There may also be loss of sensation on the sole of the foot.
- The **common fibular (peroneal) nerve** is the most commonly injured nerve in the lower leg because of its superficial course around the fibular neck, a common fracture site. Damage results in loss of function of all muscles in the anterior and lateral compartments, resulting in inability to dorsiflex the foot, evert the foot, and extend the toes. This is known as a **footdrop,** and the patient will develop a high-stepping gait to compensate.

OTHER ANATOMIC LANDMARKS OF THE LOWER EXTREMITY

DIAPHRAGM

The diaphragm separates the thoracic and abdominal cavities and is the most important muscle for inspiration. Important structures pass through the diaphragm at various levels.

- T8: The IVC passes through.
- T10: Esophagus and vagus nerve.
- T12: The aorta, thoracic duct, and azygos vein.

Cervical nerves C3, C4, and C5 make up the somatic **phrenic nerve.** Irritation of the diaphragmatic pleura or peritoneum causes pain that is referred to the shoulder. There are many etiologies including intra-abdominal abscess, fluid (secondary to perforated organ or abdominal trauma), or air (secondary to perforated organ) near the diaphragm.

Physiology

MUSCLE TYPES

Skeletal Muscle

OVERVIEW

Each skeletal muscle fiber receives neural input from a motor neuron via the **neuromuscular junction.** A single motor neuron and the muscle fiber it innervates are known as a **motor unit.** Large motor units in large muscle groups execute coarse movements (eg, the quadriceps muscles), and small motor units control fine movements (eg, extraocular muscles).

MNEMONIC

What muscles insert on the medial tibia via the pes anserinus?
"**S**er**G**ean**T** pes": **S**artorius muscle, **G**racilis muscle, semi**T**endinosus muscle

KEY FACT

What courses behind the lateral malleolus?
Peroneus longus and brevis muscles, small saphenous vein

MNEMONIC

I 8 (ate) 10 EGGs AT 12
IVC at T**8.**
T**10: E**spha**G**us and va**G**us.
Aorta/**A**zygos and **T**horacic duct at T**12.**

MNEMONIC

C3, 4, 5 keeps the diaphragm alive!

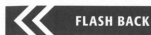

FLASH BACK

Acetylcholinesterase is a common target for pharmacologic paralysis in neuromuscular blockade.

KEY FACT

Skeletal muscle is a structurally complex organ, containing several levels of organization. They are listed below, from smallest to largest:
- Myofilament
- Sarcomere
- Myofibril
- Muscle cells
- Muscle fiber
- Muscle fasciculus
- Whole muscle

In the synaptic cleft, the action potential (AP) that has propagated along the neuron is transferred to the **myocyte,** or muscle cell. The neurotransmitter **acetylcholine (ACh)** is released from the axonal bouton (Figure 5-14). The myocyte's postsynaptic membrane, known as the **motor end plate,** contains specialized **nicotinic ACh receptors.** These receptors are transmembrane cation channels (Na^+ and K^+) that open when bound to ACh. Activation of these ligand-gated channels results in increased local cation flux, leading to membrane depolarization that is propagated to the nearby **transverse tubule (T-tubule)** system (Figure 5-15). Excess ACh is hydrolyzed by the enzyme **acetylcholinesterase,** which resides on the postsynaptic or postjunctional membrane, into acetate and choline. Choline is reabsorbed by the presynaptic neuron, via Na^+-coupled transport, for production of more ACh.

EXCITATION-CONTRACTION COUPLING

Myofibrils are the functional components of contraction. The T-tubules, a system of plasma membrane invaginations (see Figure 5-15), allow the AP to propagate deep into the cytoplasm, facilitating Ca^{2+} release from the sarcoplasmic reticulum. This increase in intracellular calcium triggers **excitation-contraction coupling** among longitudinally arranged intracellular contractile

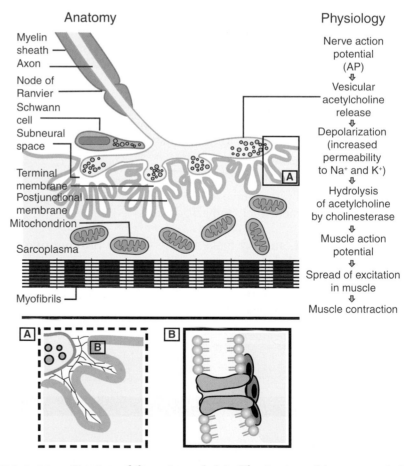

FIGURE 5-14. Structure of the motor end plate. The structure of the motor end plate is shown above on the left, and the sequence of events from liberation of ACh by the nerve AP to contraction of the muscle fiber are indicated by the right column. The insets are enlargements of the indicated structures. The highest magnification depicts the receptor in the bilayer of the postsynaptic membrane. (Modified with permission from Brunton LL, Parker KL, Buxton I, Blumenthal DK. *Goodman & Gilman's The Pharmacological Basis of Therapeutics*, 11th ed. New York: McGraw-Hill, 2006: 225.)

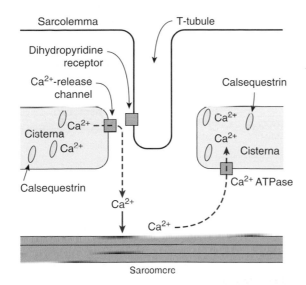

FIGURE 5-15. **Schematic of transverse tubule system.** Diagram of the relationships among the sarcolemma (plasma membrane), a T-tubule, and two cisternae of the sarcoplasmic reticulum of skeletal muscle (not to scale). The T-tubule extends inward from the sarcolemma. A wave of depolarization, initiated by ACh binding, is transmitted from the sarcolemma down the T-tubule. It is then conveyed to the Ca^{2+} release channel (ryanodine receptor), perhaps by interaction between it and the dihydropyridine receptor, which are shown in close proximity. Release of Ca^{2+} from the Ca^{2+}-release channel into the cytosol initiates contraction. Subsequently, Ca^{2+} is pumped back into the cisternae of the sarcoplasmic reticulum by the Ca^{2+} ATPase (Ca^{2+} pump) and stored there, in part bound to calsequestrin. (Modified with permission from Murray RK, Granner DK, Rodwell VW. *Harper's Biochemistry*, 27th ed. New York: McGraw-Hill, 2006: 572.)

proteins in the **sarcomere.** Repeating units of sarcomeres comprise **myofibrils** within a single multinucleate myocyte (Figure 5-16).

Each myofibril contains interdigitating **thick** and **thin myofilaments.**

- Thick filaments contain a large-molecular-weight protein, **myosin,** which itself is made of heavy and light chains. The light chains contain **actin-binding sites** and an **ATP** cleavage site.
- Thin filaments have three components:
  - **Actin:** Bound by myosin, it contributes to **cross-bridge** formation that allows for movement of myosin filaments and change in myofibril length.
  - **Tropomyosin:** At rest, this protein occupies potential **myosin-binding sites** on the actin protein, preventing contraction.
  - **Troponin:** Ca^{2+} released from the sarcoplasmic reticulum binds troponin, inducing a conformational change that consequently moves tropomyosin, freeing actin's myosin-binding sites for contraction.

Once tropomyosin uncovers actin's myosin-binding sites, actin binds myosin light chains, creating **cross-bridges.** The myosin light chains pivot, and the myosin heavy chain slides along the actin filament. This event is known as a **twitch** and develops the tension that exerts force (proportional to the number of cross-bridges) during muscle contraction. Returning the pivoted or flexed myosin light chains to their original state requires the cleavage of ATP to ADP + P_i. Once regenerated, the myosin light chain binds a new molecule of ATP for future cross-bridge coupling (see Figure 5-16).

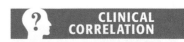

CLINICAL CORRELATION

A lack of ATP can keep the muscle in "twitch," leading to cramps and rigor mortis.

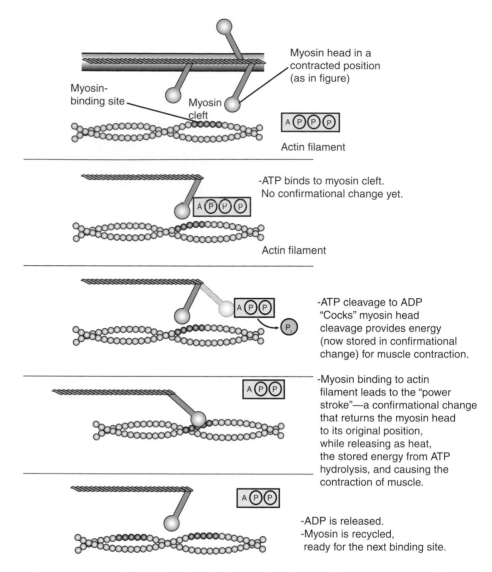

Myosin head in a contracted position (as in figure)

Myosin-binding site

Myosin cleft

Actin filament

-ATP binds to myosin cleft. No confirmational change yet.

Actin filament

-ATP cleavage to ADP "Cocks" myosin head cleavage provides energy (now stored in confirmational change) for muscle contraction.

-Myosin binding to actin filament leads to the "power stroke"—a confirmational change that returns the myosin head to its original position, while releasing as heat, the stored energy from ATP hydrolysis, and causing the contraction of muscle.

-ADP is released.
-Myosin is recycled, ready for the next binding site.

FIGURE 5-16. **Myofibrils and excitation-contraction coupling.** Arrangement of thick and thin filaments in the sarcomere. (Modified with permission from Murray RK, Granner DK, Rodwell VW. *Harper's Biochemistry*, 27th ed. New York: McGraw-Hill, 2006: 567.)

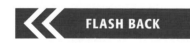
FLASH BACK

Clostridium tetani induces tetanus via an exotoxin that maintains high intracellular Ca^{2+}.

This process continues as long as the cytoplasmic Ca^{2+} concentration remains high. The Ca^{2+}-ATPase functions to ensure Ca^{2+} reuptake into the sarcoplasmic reticulum, thus reducing the cytoplasmic Ca^{2+} concentration. When the calcium concentration has returned to low levels, troponin returns to its original state and tropomyosin again blocks the myosin-binding sites on actin. If a muscle fiber is stimulated repeatedly without allowing sufficient time for Ca^{2+} to reaccumulate in the sarcoplasmic reticulum, the sustained high cytoplasmic Ca^{2+} concentration leads to sustained muscle contraction, or **tetanus**.

The sarcomere is the most basic contractile unit. Under light microscopy, it appears as a series of bands and lines (Figures 5-17 and 5-18), spanning the space between **Z lines**.

Within a given muscle, the maximum force or tension that can be produced is dependent upon the length of the muscle. The tension a muscle is able to produce is proportional to both the number of cross-bridges formed and the number that *could* be formed. At the extremes of myofibril length (very long

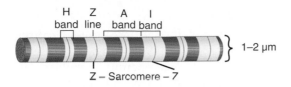

FIGURE 5-17. Myofibril.

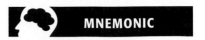

MNEMONIC

Contraction results in HIZ shrinkage:
H, I, and **Z** bands shorten during muscle contraction, while the A band's length remains constant.

and very short) either the number of existing cross-bridges or the number of available new cross-bridges is limited, thus reducing the tension the muscle fiber can produce.

Smooth Muscle

OVERVIEW

Smooth muscle differs from skeletal muscle in at least three important ways. First, the myofilaments are not organized into sarcomeres and thus do not appear striated. Second, innervation is primarily via the autonomic nervous system, not the somatic nervous system. And third, the excitation-contraction cascade within smooth muscle differs from that of skeletal muscle. These differences allow smooth muscle to perform its functions more efficiently than skeletal muscle could.

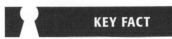

KEY FACT

Smooth muscle locations:
Vasculature (larger than capillaries)
Airways (larger than terminal bronchioles)
GI tract
Urinary bladder and ureters
Uterus
Muscles within the eye

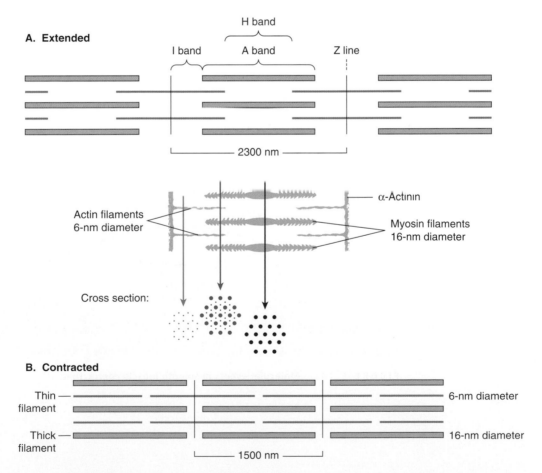

FIGURE 5-18. Arrangement of thick and thin filaments in the sarcomere. (Modified with permission from Murray RK, Granner DK, Rodwell VW. *Harper's Biochemistry*, 27th ed. New York: McGraw-Hill, 2006: 567.)

EXCITATION-CONTRACTION COUPLING

Smooth muscle lacks troponin. Instead, the protein **calmodulin** acts as the cross-bridging gatekeeper (Figure 5-19). Similar to skeletal muscle, the cascade begins with an AP. This leads to opening of voltage-gated Ca^{2+} channels and an increase in the intracellular Ca^{2+} concentration. Calmodulin then binds Ca^{2+} and activates **myosin light-chain kinase (MLCK),** which in turn phosphorylates myosin. Activated myosin is able to bind and release actin, repeatedly forming and breaking cross-bridges. Like skeletal muscle, each cycle consumes one molecule of ATP.

However, when the Ca^{2+} concentration decreases (again due to a Ca^{2+}-ATPase), and myosin is dephosphorylated via **myosin light-chain phosphatase,** the dephosphorylated form of myosin can still interact with actin via **latch-bridges.** These are residual attachments that allow for the maintenance of tonic tension within smooth muscle without consuming energy. In this way, (unlike skeletal muscle) smooth muscle can maintain tonic contraction without continually cleaving ATP. When combined with **gap junctions,** these capabilities allow smooth muscle to produce the coordinated tonic contractions necessary for aiding digestion, maintaining BP, voiding urine, and accomplishing labor and delivery.

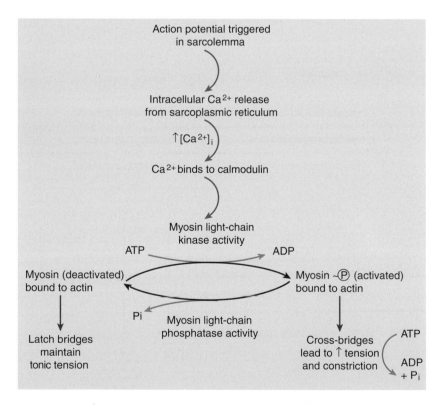

FIGURE 5-19.   **Molecular events in smooth muscle contraction.**

METABOLISM

Cross-bridging of skeletal muscles requires a constant supply of ATP. At rest, muscles may be responsible for 30% of the body's O_2 consumption, while during exercise this number tops off at around 90%. The major energy source that fuels muscle contraction is **carbohydrate metabolism**. Secondary sources of energy include **fatty acid** and **amino acid metabolism.**

Glucose

In the well-fed state, glucose is readily available to supply the energy needs of muscle. Therefore, simple glycolysis, coupled with the Krebs cycle, can meet the needs of muscles. Following a carbohydrate-rich meal, an increase in the intracellular transport of glucose occurs via insulin signaling. Each glucose molecule is immediately phosphorylated (to glucose-6-phosphate) upon entering the cell and then shuttled into glycolysis.

Glycogen

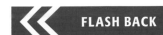
FLASH BACK

The structure of glycogen and the regulation of hepatic glycogen metabolism were introduced in the biochemistry section.

As the major storage form of glucose, glycogen is essential to **anaerobic glycolysis** in active muscle. The main storage sites of glycogen are the liver and skeletal muscles. Hepatic glycogen sustains the blood glucose level while muscle glycogen provides a readily available source of glucose during muscle contraction.

Regulation of glycogen metabolism occurs on two levels:

- Allosteric enzymatic regulation.
- Hormonal regulation by insulin.

ALLOSTERIC REGULATION

Glycogen synthase, the enzyme responsible for intramuscular glycogen production, is allosterically favored by increased levels of the substrates of glycogen synthesis, such as glucose-1-phosphate. Simultaneously, **glycogen phosphorylase,** responsible for glycogen catabolism, is inhibited by glucose-6-phosphate and ATP, products of glycolysis and successful glycogen degradation.

In contrast, glycogen degradation occurs in the presence of molecules and messengers of muscle activity. Specifically, increased intracellular Ca^{2+} and **AMP** (a product of ATP hydrolysis) lead to enhanced glycogen phosphorylase activity. Once the muscle relaxes and Ca^{2+} returns to the sarcoplasmic reticulum or AMP is consumed to produce ATP, these effects are lost. The end result is that active muscle sends signals that increase the breakdown of glycogen into glucose, thus increasing available energy substrates.

INSULIN REGULATION

In the fed state, the body increases serum insulin levels. Specifically, in the liver, insulin depresses gluconeogenesis and increases glycogen production. Within skeletal muscle, insulin increases glucose transport into cells, where it is phosphorylated and enters metabolic pathways ending in ATP production.

The absence of insulin exerts opposite effects. In this state, the liver mobilizes glycogen and adipose tissues mobilize fatty acids in order to maintain systemic glucose levels. Within muscles, a decrease in insulin-mediated glucose transport leads to glycogenolysis. More information on insulin's actions can be found in the endocrine physiology section in Chapter 2.

Lipid and Protein Metabolism

In a state of starvation, muscle is able to use fatty acids and ketones for energy. By the third week of starvation, muscle is able to operate almost entirely on mobilized fatty acids.

At the onset of a state of starvation, rapid muscle protein turnover occurs, resulting in the release of amino acids to the liver for gluconeogenesis. As the brain begins to use alternative sources of energy, thus reducing its need for glucose, protein breakdown decreases.

Exercise

During strenuous activity, skeletal muscle's metabolic needs are the greatest. Depending on the intensity of the activity, potential energy sources (glucose, glycogen, fatty acids, and protein) are utilized in different proportions. When energy demands are greatest (ie, during sprinting), anaerobic metabolism predominates. Intracellular glucose and glycogen are the primary fuels for rapid energy requirements. In fact, anaerobic metabolism can begin sustaining ATP stores before O_2 delivery to muscle increases. When energy needs are low, however (ie, during walking), oxidation of circulating glucose and fatty acids is favored. This form of metabolism extracts far more energy from fuel (~38 ATP molecules per glucose molecule) and therefore can sustain muscle activity much longer than inefficient substitutes like anaerobic metabolism.

At the onset of aerobic exercise, hepatic glycogenolysis supplies ~40% of the increased energy needed by muscles. In these early stages, there is an exercise-induced translocation of GLUT 4 glucose transporters to the muscle plasma membrane. This insulin-independent response is thought to be mediated by AMP kinase. As time progresses, hepatic gluconeogenesis becomes more important in the maintenance of circulating glucose. Alanine and lactate, produced in peripheral anaerobic metabolism, become important substrates. In fact, resting muscle can transform glycogen stores into lactate for systemic release, leading to hepatic conversion to glucose and redistribution to active muscle.

At later stages of lengthy exercise, glucose use within skeletal muscle decreases and fatty acid oxidation increases from its original ~60% share to provide nearly all of the necessary substrates for aerobic exercise metabolism.

Nutritional Deficiency

SCURVY

Vitamin C deficiency leading to bone disease in growing children and to hemorrhages and healing defects in both children and adults.

RICKETS (CHILDREN)/OSTEOMALACIA (ADULTS)

Vitamin D deficiency leading to hypocalcemia and activation of parathyroid hormone (PTH). This causes loss of bone mass in adults (osteopenia) and bowing of the legs in children.

IMPORTANT LABORATORY VALUES

TABLE 5-8. Laboratory Values Pertinent to Musculoskeletal and Connective Tissue Disorders

LAB TEST	ABBREVIATION	MARKER FOR . . .
Erythrocyte sedimentation rate	ESR	Systemic inflammation.
Creatine kinase	CK	Muscle injury.
CK isoenzyme (myocardial bound)	CK-MB	Cardiac injury or regenerating muscle.
Antineutrophil cytoplasmic antibody (ANCA)	c-ANCA (cytoplasmic)	Wegener granulomatosis.
	p-ANCA (perinuclear)	Microscopic polyangiitis, Churg-Strauss vasculitis **or** focal necrotizing and crescentic glomerulonephritis.
C-reactive protein	CRP	Direct marker for systemic inflammation.
Antinuclear antibody	ANA	Nonspecific; numerous autoimmune diseases and falsely positive in 5–10%.
Rheumatoid factor	RF	Rheumatoid arthritis and other autoimmune and chronic inflammatory diseases; falsely positive in 5–10%.
Anticyclic citrullinated peptide	Anti-CCP	Rheumatoid arthritis.
Alkaline phosphatase	Alkaline phosphatase	Bone turnover.
Serum calcium	Ca^{2+}	Disordered calcium homeostasis.
Parathyroid hormone	PTH	Parathyroid gland function.
Parathyroid hormone-related peptide	PTHrP	Protein secreted by neoplastic cells, mimics PTH; its activity may lead to disordered calcium and/or phosphate homeostasis.

MNEMONIC

Primary tumors that metastasize to bone—

BLTT with a Cool Kosher Pickle
Breast
Lung
Thyroid
Testes
Colon
Kidney
Prostate

KEY FACT

The three most common bony sites for metastases (in descending order):
- Vertebrae
- Proximal femur
- Pelvis

Pathology

SKELETAL ONCOLOGY

The most common tumor found in bone is a metastasis from another organ system. Prostate, breast, and lung carcinomas account for 80% of bony metastases. The majority of these metastases spread hematogenously; rarely, however, these cancers can invade through local infiltration. Once in the bone, tumors may lead to osteolysis, osteogenesis, or both. Osteolysis can be elicited either through **parathyroid hormone-related peptide (PTHrP)** or through cytokines like interleukin-1 (IL-1) and tumor necrosis factor-alpha (TNF-α), which increase osteoclast differentiation and activation. Conversely, osteogenesis occurs in response to lesions that stimulate osteoblastic differentiation.

PRESENTATION

Although they are often **asymptomatic,** bony metastases may present with pain, swelling, nerve compression, or pathologic fracture. Marrow infiltration by lymphomas can present with symptoms of bone marrow suppression known as **myelophthisis.** Pain usually develops gradually over several weeks and is most intense at night, often waking the patient. If neurologic symptoms such as numbness, weakness, or radiculopathy accompany back pain, an emergent spinal cord evaluation is indicated.

DIAGNOSIS

All patients should be screened with plain films and serum calcium levels. Osteolytic lesions > 1 cm in size, common with metastatic renal cancer, can regularly be detected with plain radiographs and often cause **hypercalcemia.** Osteoblastic lesions, commonly seen in breast and prostatic metastases, are best detected with radionucleotide bone scans, which will show increased uptake. In these instances, plain films may reveal focal sclerosis. These patients often have increased serum **alkaline phosphatase** levels and, if disease is widespread, hypocalcemia.

TREATMENT

The therapeutic approach depends on the source of the underlying malignancy and symptomatology. Bisphosphonates, agents that inhibit osteoclast function, are adjuvant medications used to preserve bone health and relieve pain. Severe bone pain in the terminal stages of cancer is very common, and adequate attention to pain symptoms may require relatively high doses of narcotic analgesics to maintain patient quality of life. Pain from bone cancer is one of the most difficult types of pain to treat and should never be neglected.

PROGNOSIS

Overall survival varies greatly, depending on the primary diagnosis.

Primary Cancers

BENIGN

There are five important primary benign tumors of bone (Table 5-9):

- **Giant-cell tumor:** Benign tumor composed of spindle-shaped cells with multinucleated giant cells (osteoclasts). It is most commonly found at epiphyseal ends of long bones, such as the distal femur or proximal tibia. The peak incidence is in females between the ages of 20 and 40 years. It car-

TABLE 5-9.   Common Bone Tumors

TYPE	EPIDEMIOLOGY	LOCATION	DESCRIPTION
Benign			
Enchondroma	No special incidence.	Small distal bones of hands and feet.	Risk for chondrosarcoma. Can have multiple tumors.
Giant-cell tumor	Females 20–40 years of age.	Epiphysis of distal femur and proximal tibia.	Locally aggressive; multinucleated giant-cell tumor. "Soap-bubble" appearance on radiograph
Osteoblastoma	Males < 25 years of age.	Vertebral column	Similar to osteoid osteoma except for location.
Osteochondroma	Most common benign tumor. Males < 25 years of age.	Long bones; especially metaphysis of the distal femur.	Outgrowth of mature bone capped by benign cartilage.
Osteoid osteoma	Males < 25 years of age.	Proximal femur.	Interlacing trabeculae of woven bone.
Osteoma	Males of any age.	Facial bones and skull.	Associated with Gardner syndrome (FAP). Mature bone continues growing on itself.
Malignant			
Chondrosarcoma	Men 30–60 years of age.	Pelvis, proximal femur.	Malignant cartilage tumor. May be primary or from osteochondroma. Metastasize to lungs.
Ewing sarcoma	Males 10–20 years of age.	Pelvis and long bones.	Anaplastic small blue-cell tumor. "Onion-skin" appearance of bone on plain film. Associated with 11;22 translocation.
Osteogenic sarcoma (osteosarcoma)	Most common primary bone tumor. Males 10–25 years of age. Risk factors: Paget disease, familial retinoblastoma, irradiation.	Metaphysis of distal femur and proximal tibia.	Malignant osteoid formation. "Sunburst" appearance on radiograph from elevation of periosteum.

FAP = familial adenomatous polyposis.

ries a distinct histologic appearance (Figure 5-20) and has a characteristic "double-bubble," or "soap-bubble" radiographic appearance.

- **Enchondroma:** Benign cartilage cyst found within the bone marrow, often affecting the smaller bones of the hands and feet. This is one of the few tumors that can be in multiple locations. On plain film, this tumor appears as a lytic area in the bone marrow with stippled calcification. On MRI, this tumor has a popcorn appearance.
- **Osteochondroma:** The most common benign bone tumor, usually occurring in males younger than age 25 years. It often arises from the long metaphysis of the distal femur. On plain film, the tumor appears as a cartilage-capped bony outgrowth. Malignant transformation to chondrosarcoma is rare.

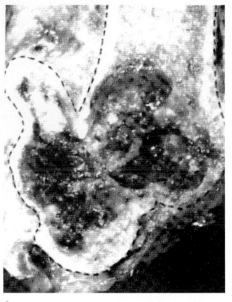
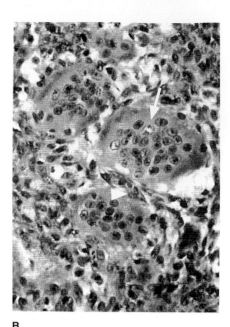

A   **B**

FIGURE 5-20. **Giant-cell tumor pathology.** (A) Giant-cell tumor of the distal end of the femur, showing expansion of the bone end by a well-circumscribed mass composed of fleshy tumor that has replaced the bone. A thin rim of bone is present around the mass. The outline of the bone is indicated by the dotted lines. (B) Histology of giant-cell tumor of bone, showing numerous osteoclast-like giant cells (*arrow*) and intervening small spindle cells (*arrowhead*). (Reproduced with permission from Chandrasoma P, Taylor CR. *Concise Lange Pathology*, 3rd ed. Stamford, CT: Appleton & Lange, 1998. Copyright © 2006 McGraw-Hill.)

- **Osteoid osteoma:** A benign bone-forming tumor seen in adolescent males. It typically presents with night pain that improves with nonsteroidal anti-inflammatory drug (NSAID) use.
- **Osteoma:** Benign tumor found in the facial bones of males. There is a strong association with Gardner polyposis syndrome.

MALIGNANT

There are three important malignant primary bone tumors (see Table 5-9):

- Chondrosarcoma
- Ewing sarcoma
- Osteosarcoma

CHONDROSARCOMA

One-quarter of all bone sarcomas are chondrosarcomas, with a peak incidence in the fourth to sixth decades. Primarily arising in flat bones like the shoulder and pelvic girdle, these tumors typically develop de novo by sporadic mutation. Rarely, they deviate from this pattern and appear in the diaphyses of long bones or arise by malignant transformation of enchondromas or osteochondromas.

PRESENTATION

Like other bone sarcomas, pain and swelling are the principal symptoms. New-onset pain, inflammation, and/or a gradually growing mass, especially in the scapula or pelvis, are commonly associated with this tumor.

DIAGNOSIS

Radiography reveals a lobular mass with mottled, punctate, or annular calcifications of the cartilaginous matrix.

TREATMENT

Surgical resection is the mainstay of therapy, as nearly all chondrosarcomas are resistant to chemotherapy.

PROGNOSIS

Chondrosarcomas follow an indolent course, eventually metastasizing to the lungs if not treated.

EWING SARCOMA

Comprising only 10–15% of bone sarcomas, this anaplastic blue cell tumor has its peak incidence in adolescents. The underlying genetic abnormality is overexpression of the **MIC2 gene,** whose product is a cell-surface marker, and a simultaneous **t(11;22) translocation.** These genetic abnormalities are common in those with primitive neuroectodermal tumors (PNETs), the family of tumors to which Ewing sarcoma belongs.

PRESENTATION

Most often found in diaphyses of long bones, pelvis, scapula, or ribs. Patients can complain of fever and anemia.

DIAGNOSIS

Radiography reveals a characteristic **"onion-peel"** periosteal reaction with a soft tissue mass (Figure 5-21). Pathologic examination uncovers sheets of small, round, undifferentiated blue cells that can be confused with lymphoma or small-cell carcinomas.

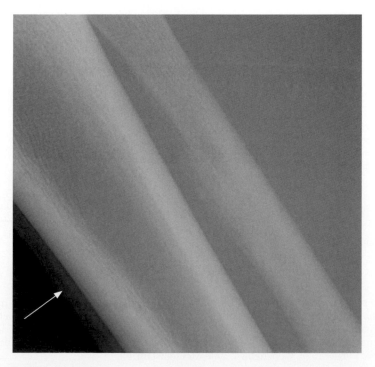

FIGURE 5-21. **Radiograph of Ewing sarcoma.** Lower leg demonstrating subtle cortical irregularity of the proximal fibular diaphysis with raised periosteal reaction (*arrow*). (Reproduced with permission from USMLERx.com.)

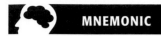

MNEMONIC

Going out for E**wing**'s and **onion** rings. (E**wing** sarcoma results in an **onion**-peel periosteal reaction.)

TREATMENT

The foundation of treatment is systemic chemotherapy to shrink the size of the tumor, followed by surgery.

PROGNOSIS

This condition is very aggressive and is treated as a systemic disease due to the high probability of early metastases. Common sites of metastasis include the lungs and other bones. Patients with disease of the distal extremities have a 5-year survival rate of 80%.

OSTEOSARCOMA

The most common primary bone malignancy (45%), this cancer results in the production of unmineralized bone (**osteoid**) and is therefore also known as **osteogenic carcinoma** (Figure 5-22). The majority of cases occur in male children and adolescents. Those that occur late in life (~10%) are often secondary to predisposing risk factors such as radiation exposure, familial retinoblastoma, benign transformation (as in Paget disease), or bone irradiation. These tumors often metastasize to the lungs.

PRESENTATION

Osteosarcoma has an affinity for the metaphysis of long bones, specifically the distal femur, proximal tibia, and proximal humerus. Patients usually complain of pain and swelling of the affected region.

DIAGNOSIS

A plain film reveals osteolysis with a "moth-eaten" appearance and a periosteal "sunburst" reaction. New bone formation at the margin of the soft tissue mass leads to elevation of the periosteum known as the characteristic **Codman triangle**. Chest radiography and CT are employed to rule out lung metastases, whereas a bone scan can uncover bony metastases.

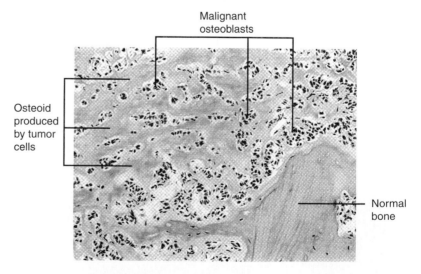

FIGURE 5-22. **Histology of malignant osteosarcoma.** Histology showing small malignant osteoblastic cells surrounded by osteoid, which appears as a homogeneous material between the malignant cells. Contrast this with the residual normal bone spicule. (Reproduced with permission from Chandrasoma P, Taylor CR. *Concise Lange Pathology*, 3rd ed. Stamford, CT: Appleton & Lange, 1998. Copyright © 2006 McGraw-Hill.)

TREATMENT

Preoperative chemotherapy, limb-sparing surgery, and postoperative chemotherapy is the usual regimen.

PROGNOSIS

The most important prognostic indicator is response to chemotherapy. Long-term survival in extremity sarcoma lies in the range of 60–80%.

NONONCOLOGIC MUSCULOSKELETAL DISEASE

Osteoarthritis

Arising from "cartilage failure" of the diarthrodial (movable, synovium-lined) joints, osteoarthritis (OA) is the most common form of joint disease. Although age is the strongest risk factor, other systemic factors (genetics, nutritional and metabolic factors) and biomechanical factors (obesity, malalignment, joint injury or overuse, muscle weakness) contribute to the risk for degradation of articular cartilage. Cartilage loss occurs when the limited reparative capacity of hyaline cartilage is overcome by degradative processes. Loss of cartilage may be accompanied by new bone formation in and around the joint. Joint pathology may include some or all of the following changes:

- **Loss of articular cartilage:** As the cartilage degrades, it is unable to sufficiently repair itself, leading to changes in joint stress and architecture. Progressive cartilage loss may ultimately expose subchondral bone.
- **Sclerosis:** Increased mechanical stress transmitted to bone beneath degrading articular cartilage produces increased subchondral bone density, detected on radiographs as subchondral sclerosis (eburnation).
- **Osteophytes:** Increased stress causes bone to remodel; producing bone spurs at the edges of articular surfaces.
- **Bone cysts:** Microfractures beneath the cortex form due to increased stress. The bone gets reabsorbed, and the cyst fills with fluid and fibrous tissue.

Soft tissue pathology may also include synovitis with mild hypertrophy and thickening of the joint capsule. Synovitis when detected arthroscopically is localized to near the site of cartilage injury. Cellular and inflammatory mediators from the synovitis serve to perpetuate cartilage degeneration.

PRESENTATION

Patients complain of a deep aching pain in weight-bearing diarthrodial joints after prolonged use. This pain often **improves with rest, and stiffness in the morning usually resolves within 15 minutes of awakening.** On physical examination of the hands, pain and bony swelling are most pronounced in the distal and proximal interphalangeal (DIP and PIP) joints. Swelling and bony crepitus may be evident in affected joints (Figure 5-23). Advanced disease may result in gross deformity, noticeable bony hypertrophy, partial dislocation (known as **subluxation**), and loss of joint motion. There are **no associated systemic symptoms.**

DIAGNOSIS

Based on clinical and radiographic findings, joint space narrowing occurs early in disease progression. Subchondral bone may contain cysts or sclerosis. Sclerotic regions have an ivory-like appearance radiographically, representing a phenomenon called **eburnation.** An altered joint contour or subluxation can also be seen. Despite this list of possible changes, however, radiographic

MNEMONIC

Osteoarthritis leads to SMASHED joints:
Subchondral cysts
Mechanical damage to
Articular cartilage
Synovial
Hypertrophy
Eburnation
DIP joints = Heberden nodes

KEY FACT

Osteophytes at DIP joints are known as **Heberden nodes,** and those at PIP joints are known as **Bouchard nodes.**

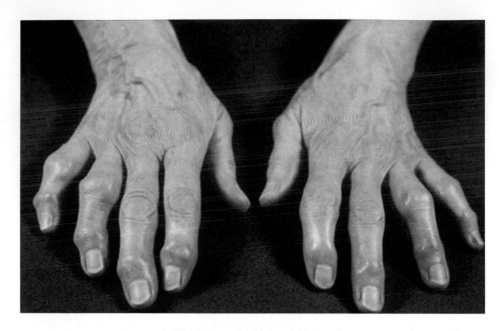

FIGURE 5-23. **Osteoarthritic changes in the hand.** Notice that anatomic changes—bony enlargement of the distal (DIP) and proximal interphalangeal (PIP) joints—do not affect the wrists. (Reproduced with permission from Fauci AS, et al, eds. *Harrison's Principles of Internal Medicine*, 17th ed. New York: McGraw-Hill, 2008.)

appearance often does not correlate with symptom severity. Laboratory tests are usually normal in primary OA, though synovial fluid analysis may be helpful if OA is secondary to another cause (eg, a crystalline or septic arthritis). Common characteristics of OA as compared with RA are shown in Table 5-10.

TREATMENT

Treatment goals include reducing pain, maintaining mobility, and preventing disability. Reducing joint loading through improved posture, reducing malalignment, exercise, and weight loss are often the first steps in mild OA. Although many patients avoid exercise for fear of pain, moderate to vigorous exercise does not seem to exacerbate it. In fact, patients who are physically active tend to report a decrease in their pain and an increased quality of life. NSAIDs and acetaminophen are palliative pain relievers but do not prevent disease progression. Other short-term interventions include glucocorticoid or hyaluronic acid injections. Generally used in patients who fail conservative therapy or are not surgical candidates, injections provide only limited-duration relief.

PROGNOSIS

The natural history of OA is progressive joint degeneration and decreasing range of motion that worsens with age, use, and wear. End-stage OA can be relieved with total joint arthroplasty, most commonly done for hips and knees.

Rheumatoid Arthritis

Rheumatoid arthritis (RA) is characterized by a chronic autoimmune process resulting in inflammatory synovitis of diarthrodial joints. It is more common in women and has a strong genetic association with **HLA-DR4** haplotypes. Smoking is a recently described risk factor. Chronic inflammation leads to encroachment of synovial hypertrophy, referred to as **pannus,** over bone and cartilage leading to erosion within the affected joint.

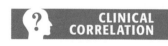

CLINICAL CORRELATION

Watch out for GI complications (peptic ulcer disease and/or hemorrhage), renal insufficiency, and aggravation of hypertension in patients regularly taking NSAIDs!

TABLE 5-10. Differences Between Osteoarthritis and Rheumatoid Arthritis

	OSTEOARTHRITIS	RHEUMATOID ARTHRITIS
Epidemiology	Men = Women. People > 40 years of age. ~10% prevalence.	Women > Men. Usually people 20–60 years of age but can occur anytime. ~1–2% prevalence.
Mechanism of injury	Biomechanical: Cartilage failure (degradation exceeds repair).	Autoimmune: Immune system attacking the synovium and other intra-articular structures.
Symptoms and signs	Joint pain, bony enlargement, crepitus. Morning stiffness lasting < 30 min.	Joint pain, synovitis, and systemic symptoms. Morning stiffness > 1 hour.
Joint distribution (Figure 5-24)	PIPs, DIPs, first CMCs. C/L/S spine. Hips, knees, midfoot, 1st MTP.	Wrists, MCPs, PIPs. C-spine but spares T/L spine. Ankles, MTPs.
Radiology	Joint space narrowing. Osteophytes usually present.	Marginal erosions and subluxations. Osteophytes usually absent.
Treatment	NSAIDs, acetaminophen, joint replacement.	DMARDs, NSAIDs.

CMC, carpometacarpal; DIP, distal interphalangeal; DMARD, disease-modifying antirheumatic drug; NSAID, nonsteroidal anti-inflammatory drug; PIP, proximal interphalangeal.

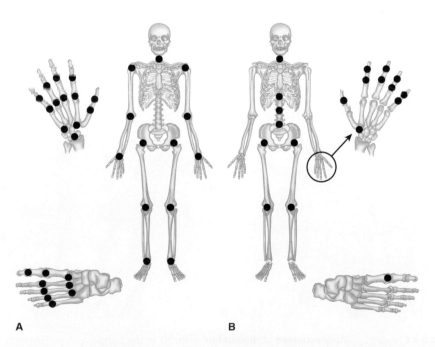

A   B

FIGURE 5-24. Distribution of rheumatoid and osteoarthritis. The joint distribution of the two most common types of arthritis are compared: Rheumatoid arthritis (RA) (A) and Osteoarthritis (OA) (B). RA involves almost all synovial joints in the body. OA has a much more limited distribution. Importantly, RA rarely, if ever, involves the distal interphalangeal joints, but OA commonly does. (Modified with permission from Imboden J, Hellmann DB, Stone JH. *Current Rheumatology Diagnosis & Treatment*, New York: McGraw-Hill, 2004: 162.)

The inciting cause of RA is unknown. The initiation and propagation of synovitis is complex, involving T and B cells, synovial fibroblasts, and a network of cytokines, chemokines, and degradative enzymes. Synovitis includes B-cell production of **rheumatoid factor (RF)**. RF complexes are IgM RF-autoantibodies directed against the F_c portion of an IgG. RF immune complexes participate in the pathogenesis of RA through activation of complement and attraction of neutrophils, leading to acute inflammation. Proliferation of chronically inflamed synovial tissue results in pannus formation. If not treated, the end result is reactive fibrosis in the affected joints leading to deformity and loss of function.

PRESENTATION

Characteristically affecting small to medium joints at onset (proximal interphalangeal [PIP], metacarpophalangeal [MCP], wrist joints, ankles, and metatarsophalangeal [MTP] joints), RA is marked by morning stiffness lasting > 1 hour but **improving with use.** Joint involvement is symmetrical and may be associated with systemic complaints: fever, fatigue, and/or anorexia. Affected joints become swollen, tender, and warm, with a reduced range of motion.

As the disease progresses, joint laxity, subluxation, and cartilage degradation develop. In late stages, joint fibrosis and soft tissue contractures may predominate. Specifically, MCP joint subluxation with ulnar deviation of the fingers is common, as are finger deformities. Hyperextension of the PIP joint with DIP joint flexions is referred to as a "swan-neck" deformity, whereas hyperextension of the DIP joint with PIP joint flexions known as a **"boutonnière" deformity** (Figure 5-25). Knee involvement can result in inflamed synovium within the popliteal fossa, creating the characteristic **Baker cyst.**

Patients often suffer from a variety of extra-articular symptoms. Muscle weakness and atrophy are common adjacent to affected joints. Twenty percent of patients may develop **rheumatoid nodules:** centralized zones of necrotic tissue surrounded by macrophages and granulation tissue, appearing in areas of mechanical pressure. Although the prevalence of rheumatoid vasculitis has declined due to aggressive RA management, pleuritis and pericarditis can be seen with active disease.

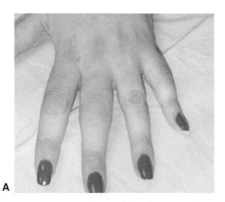 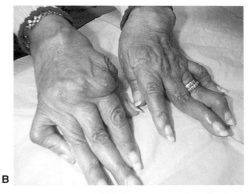

A   B

FIGURE 5-25. Manifestations of rheumatoid arthritis in the hand. (A) A patient with early rheumatoid arthritis (RA); there are no joint deformities, but the soft tissue synovial swelling around the third and fifth proximal interphalangeal (PIP) joints is easily seen. (B) A patient with advanced RA; severe joint deformities including dorsal wrist swelling, subluxation at the metacarpohalangeal joints, and "swan-neck" deformities (hyperextension at the PIP joints), are prominent. (Reproduced with permission from Imboden J, Hellmann DB, Stone JH. *Current Rheumatology Diagnosis & Treatment*, New York: McGraw-Hill, 2004: 163.)

DIAGNOSIS

RA is primarily a clinical diagnosis, although laboratory evaluation may reveal an elevated erythrocyte sedimentation rate (ESR) and C-reactive protein (CRP), a positive RF test (in up to 80% of RA patients) and/or anti-CCP antibody. Patients also often exhibit an anemia of chronic disease (normochromic, normocytic) with reactive thrombocytosis. Joint aspiration yields opaque watery (inflammatory) fluid with a WBC count of > 2000.

Radiography, though not necessary for establishing the diagnosis, may show osteopenia, adjacent to the joint, and bone erosion typically at the margins of the joint (Figure 5-26).

TREATMENT

Therapeutic goals include (1) pain relief, (2) reduction of inflammation, (3) anatomic preservation, (4) functional maintenance, and (5) systemic control. Physical therapy and rest are effective for pain relief, and orthotics can be used to support weakened joints.

Medical management includes five modalities:

- **Aspirin and NSAIDs:** Alleviate pain of inflammation but do not stop disease progression.
- **Low-dose oral or intra-articular glucocorticoids:** Reduce inflammation and bone erosion but may cause many systemic side effects.
- **Disease-modifying antirheumatic drugs (DMARDs):** These include methotrexate, leflunomide antimalarials, and sulfasalazine. They slow disease progression by decreasing inflammatory mediators. DMARDs may inhibit or reduce the progression of bony erosions.
- **Biologic agents:** Proteins (antibodies, fusion proteins) engineered to target proinflammatory cytokines (TNF-α, IL-1, IL-6), T-cell activation (CD28), or pre-plasma cell B-cells (CD-20). Best in combination with DMARD therapy.
- **Immunosuppressive and cytotoxic agents:** Azathioprine, cyclosporine, and cyclophosphamide can be used but are often reserved for more resistant cases.

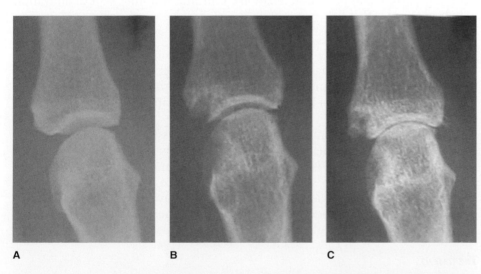

A   B   C

FIGURE 5-26. **Progressive destruction of a metacarpophalangeal joint by rheumatoid arthritis.** Shown are sequential radiographs of the same second metacarpophalangeal joint. (A) The joint is normal 1 year prior to the development of rheumatoid arthritis. (B) Six months following the onset of rheumatoid arthritis, there is a bony erosion adjacent to the joint and joint space narrowing. (C) After 3 years of disease, diffuse loss of articular cartilage has led to marked joint space narrowing. (Reproduced with permission from Imboden J, Hellmann DB, Stone JH. *Current Rheumatology Diagnosis & Treatment*, New York: McGraw-Hill, 2004: Figure 15-3.)

RA varies greatly in prognosis, ranging from mild disease with minimal joint injury to progressive polyarthritis and significant disability. Often, the common clinical characteristics develop within 1–2 years of disease onset. Although not practically considered to be curable, disease can be put into remission, particularly with early, aggressive management.

Osteomyelitis

Whether acute or chronic, osteomyelitis begins as a phagocytic response to a bacterial infection of the bone, leading to ostcolysis. Causes include direct inoculation of bacteria into the bone during trauma, spread from nearby skin infection, and hematogenous spread. In adults, the majority of cases are caused by the hematogenous spread of *Staphylococcus aureus* into the bone; however, *Pseudomonas aeruginosa* and *Serratia* species are common in IV drug users as causative pathogens. Acute osteomyelitis is most commonly seen in the vertebral bodies, especially when caused by tuberculosis or brucellosis (Figure 5-27). Diabetes, hemodialysis, and IV drug use all increase the risk of vertebral infection. In contrast, sickle cell patients are known for their susceptibility to *Salmonella* species and *S aureus* infections within long bones.

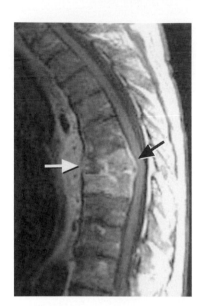

FIGURE 5-27. MRI of vertebral osteomyelitis. Osteomyelitis of the thoracic spine demonstrated on a sagittal, fat-suppressed T1-weighted MRI after the administration of IV gadolinium. At T8–T9, there is involvement of the adjacent vertebral bodies and intervening disk. Abnormally enhancing inflamed tissue extends from the disk space anteriorly (*white arrow*) as well as posteriorly into the epidural space, compressing the thecal sac (*black arrow*). (Reproduced with permission from Kasper DL, Braunwald E, Fauci A, et al. *Harrison's Principles of Internal Medicine*, 16th ed. New York: McGraw-Hill, 2005: 747.)

PRESENTATION

In children, acute osteomyelitis is predominantly hematogenous in origin, often accompanied by a history of blunt trauma. When the infection breaks through the periosteum, cutaneous erythema and swelling may be present.

In adults, vertebral infection often presents with neck or back pain, although it may present with abnormal pain in the extremities due to nerve root irritation. Bony pain at night, awakening the patient from sleep, is a clue not to be dismissed. Symptoms are accompanied by **low-grade fever** and dull pain that slowly increases over 2 or 3 months. Vertebral percussion elicits tenderness, accompanied by paraspinal muscle spasm. Chronic osteomyelitis is marked by fluctuating activity with periodic exacerbations. Sinus tracts between bone and skin often drain purulent fluid and necrotic bone fragments. Increased pain and ESR accompany exacerbations. Chronic immune system activation may lead to a positive RF.

DIAGNOSIS

In addition to these clinical findings, most patients have a normal or only mildly elevated white count. Elevated ESRs (> 100 mm/h) and CRPs are also common. Only 20–30% of blood cultures return positive.

Radiographically, early plain films may show soft tissue swelling. At 10 days, a periosteal reaction appears. Lytic changes appear after 2–6 weeks, once 50–75% of bone density is lost. Within the vertebrae, irregular erosions of adjacent vertebral bodies suggest infection because tumors do not usually extend to adjacent vertebrae. MRI is the best modality for detecting early bony changes and epidural abscesses, the latter a complication of vertebral osteomyelitis, and should be performed in all suspected cases.

TREATMENT

Early diagnosis and high-dose antibiotic therapy are essential for preventing bone necrosis. ESR and CRP levels can be monitored to assess response to treatment.

In children with acute hematogenous infections, oral antibiotics follow 5–10 days of IV antibiotics. In adults, IV treatment for 4–6 weeks should prove effective in both acute hematogenous and vertebral infections. Chronic osteomyelitis can be treated with surgical debridement and long-term antibiotic therapy; however, the risks (including potential limb amputation) can outweigh the benefits. Intermittent antibiotic therapy is effective for suppressing exacerbations.

Osteoporosis

The primary pathology of osteoporosis is a reduction of bone mass in spite of normal bone mineralization. Osteoporosis is defined by the World Health Organization as a reduction in bone mass of ≥ 2.5 standard deviations below the mean for young, healthy, gender- and race-matched controls. This measure, also known as a **T-score**, is clinically useful because it correlates with fracture risk as a sequela of reduced bone density. Risk factors for osteoporosis include increasing age, female gender, history of fractures, low body mass index, family history, poor calcium intake, steroid use, and smoking.

KEY FACT

T-score classifications:
≤ 2.5 = Osteoporosis
< 1.0 = Low bone density (osteopenia), with an increased risk for osteoporosis

Bone density maintenance is a balance between bone deposition (osteoblastic activity) and resorption (osteoclastic activity). These two opposing components of **bone remodeling** serve to repair microfractures, maintain skeletal strength, and regulate serum calcium levels. However, any factor favoring resorption over deposition leads to an overall loss in bone mass.

Several key hormones influence the remodeling process:

- **Estrogens:** Deficiency results in increased osteoclast differentiation and activity, leading to increased rates of resorption.
- **Vitamin D:** The active form, 1,25-dihydroxyvitamin D, is produced by coordinated chemical modifications in the skin, liver, and kidney. It increases GI absorption of dietary calcium.
- **PTH:** PTH increases bone resorption and reduces renal calcium excretion in order to raise serum calcium levels. PTH also causes increased phosphate excretion in the urine.
- **Thyroid hormone:** Hyperthyroidism is associated with increased bone loss.
- **Locally produced growth factors:** These include insulin-like growth factors (IGFs), ILs, transforming growth factor beta (TGF-β), and PTHrP.

PRESENTATION

Reduced bone density does not produce specific symptoms; therefore, osteoporosis is often undetected until the patient fractures an affected bone. For this reason, the physician's index of suspicion must be elevated, especially in elderly women. According to the National Osteoporosis Foundation, **bone mineral density (BMD)** should be determined in all postmenopausal women with risk factors or all women aged **65 and older**. In addition to age and female gender, the intrinsic and extrinsic modifiers of bone remodeling mentioned earlier should all be considered risk factors. Furthermore, any risk for falls (impaired strength, coordination, or mentation), the most common precipitant of fracture, should be cause for initiation of an osteoporosis workup.

Older patients who present with sudden-onset back pain may have suffered a vertebral compression fracture (Figure 5-28). These patients may also show loss of height and kyphosis. Hip fractures typically fit a history of a recent fall with pain and weakness in the affected hip and the inability to bear weight. Distal radius (Colles) fractures are also common.

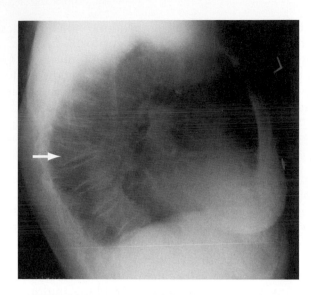

FIGURE 5-28. **Vertebral compression fracture.** Lateral spine radiograph showing severe osteopenia and a severe wedge-type deformity (severe anterior compression, *arrow*). (Reproduced with permission from Kasper DL, Braunwald E, Fauci A, et al. *Harrison's Principles of Internal Medicine*, 16th ed. New York: McGraw-Hill, 2005: 2269.)

DIAGNOSIS

Dual-energy X-ray absorptiometry (DEXA) scans have become the most popular method of measuring bone density, although quantitative CT provides helpful information regarding vertebral trabecular bone. Typically, DEXA scans of the hip and lumbar spine define clinical BMD measures. If BMD is reduced, modifiable risk factors should be sought and treated appropriately.

TREATMENT

When osteoporosis is discovered, a variety of therapies are available. First, calcium and vitamin D deficiencies should be corrected and, if possible, moderate weight-bearing exercise should be incorporated into the patient's lifestyle.

Bisphosphonates (alendronate, ibandronate, risedronate, and zoledronic acid) are chemical analogs of pyrophosphate and act to reduce osteoclast number and function, allowing the balance between bone deposition and resorption to be restored. Bisphosphonates are available in orally and intravenously dosing regimens and lead to fracture risk reduction of 40–50%. **Calcitonin** and the recombinant human PTH-analog **teriparatide** both have anabolic effects on bone, thus preventing vertebral fractures. Though teriparatide reduces vertebral fractures by 65% and nonvertebral fractures by 45%, it is reserved for patients at very high risk for fracture or who have failed treatment with a bisphosphonate. Animal studies have demonstrated a risk of osteosarcoma with supratherapeutic doses.

For postmenopausal women, estrogen replacement therapies can be effective. However, they carry increased risks for cardiovascular disease, stroke, deep vein thrombosis, and breast cancer, and these possible risks must be weighed against the benefits for each individual patient. Alternatively, **selective estrogen receptor modulators (SERMs)** are available. These medications (**tamoxifen** and **raloxifene**) activate estrogen receptors on bone but act as partial agonist or antagonists on other estrogen tissues, somewhat reducing the risks associated with hormone replacement therapy.

PROGNOSIS

Disease progression depends greatly on severity at diagnosis and intensity of intervention. Most patients can do well, though risk increases with age.

Osteopetrosis

Marble bone disease (also known as Albers-Schönberg disease) actually refers to a class of disorders sharing the common feature of defective osteoclastic bone resorption leading to "too much bone." The infantile (congenital or malignant) form is more severe, arising from an autosomal recessive mutation in the osteoclast cell-surface proton pump. The less severe adult forms (types I and II), also referred to as benign osteopetrosis, are autosomal dominant with varying levels of penetrance. Type II is caused by a mutation in the chloride channel that allows for bicarbonate exchange and continued proton production.

PRESENTATION

The infantile form occurs in 1 in 200,000 to 1 in 500,000 live births. The failure in bone remodeling can lead to cranial nerve paralysis due to foraminal narrowing. Inadequate marrow space can lead to extramedullary and splenic hematopoiesis. The adult forms are typically discovered incidentally by radiography while evaluating a fracture. The prevalence is between 1 in 100,000 and 1 in 500,000. Though referred to as "benign," the adult forms can present with complications such as deafness, psychomotor deficits, and osteomyelitis.

DIAGNOSIS

Radiographic changes indicative of increased thickness of both cortical and trabecular bone include:

- Thickened cranium and hearing loss.
- Decreased size of paranasal and mastoid sinus cavities.
- Widened diaphyses and metaphyses of long bones.
- Alternating bands of lucency and sclerosis in the iliac crest.

TREATMENT

The infantile form is best treated with HLA-matched bone marrow transplantation to repopulate functional osteoclast progenitors (of the monocyte lineage). Success rates are highest when performed before the age of 4 years. If left untreated, the infantile form is fatal by the age of 5 years. The adult form, if mild, requires no specific therapy.

Osteomalacia

Calcium and vitamin D deficiencies result in hypocalcemia and hypophosphatemia, leading to impaired bone mineralization. Alternatively, chronic hypophosphatemia due to renal phosphate wasting can trigger osteomalacia. The key feature is a poorly mineralized bone matrix that is mechanically inferior to normal bone. This can result in bowed extremities, fractures, and proximal myopathy.

PRESENTATION

As mentioned earlier, these patients suffer from bone pain, increased fractures, and bowed long bones. Due to the importance of vitamin D in maintaining muscle function, patients may present with decreased muscle tone, weakness, and abnormal gait.

DIAGNOSIS

A serum 25(OH)-vitamin D level < 15 ng/mL is associated with hypocalcemia and increased serum PTH. The elevated PTH causes increased bone resorption and serum alkaline phosphatase levels.

Radiologically, thinned cortical bone and widespread lucency are apparent. In addition, pseudofractures—radiolucent lines having the appearance of a fracture but lacking any clinical signs—are common in the scapula, pelvis, and femoral neck.

TREATMENT

Vitamin supplementation with vitamin D and calcium is integral, though therapy should certainly address the underlying disorder (eg, poor dietary intake, poor vitamin D absorption due to celiac sprue). If renal vitamin D activation is impaired, active forms of vitamin D must be given. If the patient is taking medications that increase vitamin D metabolism or lead to resistance, pharmacologic rescue doses (> 5000 IU for 3–12 weeks) may be required.

Osteitis Fibrosa Cystica

A result of primary hyperparathyroidism, osteitis fibrosa cystica (also known as von Recklinghausen disease of bone) is marked by cystic spaces within the bone, lined by active osteoclasts. These sites of bone resorption often contain disorganized osteoid stroma and old blood, earning them the name "brown tumors." Physiologically, elevated serum PTH levels increase bone turnover and act on the kidneys to increase total serum calcium and decrease total serum phosphate. PTH also increases vitamin D activation within the kidney.

PRESENTATION

Patients may experience bone pain or tenderness, bowing of bones, and pathologic fractures.

DIAGNOSIS

Serum levels of calcium and alkaline phosphatase are elevated, whereas phosphorus is decreased. Radiographic examination reveals a "ground-glass" appearance of cranial bones.

TREATMENT

The best therapy is to correct the underlying hyperparathyroidism via surgical resection of the parathyroid glands.

Fibrous Dysplasia

Fibrous dysplasia is a sporadic genetic disorder in which expanding lesions composed of mesenchymal cells arise within medullary bone, leading to skeletal abnormalities. In addition, patients may suffer from disordered pigmentation (café-au-lait spots) and endocrine excess (precocious puberty). Together, this triad is known as **McCune-Albright syndrome.** The specific genetic mutation leads to constitutive activation of the $G_s\alpha$ G-protein subunit. This causes autonomous activation of several cellular processes, including bone resorption, pigmentation, thyroid hormone production, and ovarian hormone release.

PRESENTATION

Whereas fibrous dysplasia occurs equally across both genders, the McCune-Albright triad predominates in women (10:1). More frequently, patients suffer

KEY FACT

Fibrous dysplasia + café-au-lait spots + precocious puberty = McCune-Albright syndrome only a single skeletal lesion (mono-ostotic form) arising in the third decade. However, patients with multiple lesions (polyostotic form) typically present at < 10 years of age. Early onset generally correlates with greater severity. The polyostotic form afflicts the bones of the face, ribs, proximal femur, and tibia (Figure 5-29). Expansion of lesions, often exacerbated during pregnancy or hormonal therapy, leads to pain, deformity, fracture, and possible nerve entrapment.

Diagnosis

Patients presenting with bone pain and café-au-lait spots with rough borders should have plain films taken. Skeletal lesions appear as radiolucent regions with a ground-glass appearance and a thin cortex. Patients may also display symptoms of other endocrinopathies, such as thyrotoxicosis, acromegaly, hyperprolactinemia, hyperparathyroidism, or Cushing syndrome. Typically, serum **alkaline phosphatase** may be elevated, but calcium, PTH, and 25(OH)-vitamin D levels are normal.

Treatment

There is no definitive therapy. Surgical intervention is employed to prevent fractures, maintain threatened joints, or decompress nerves.

Gout

Most commonly affecting middle-aged men and postmenopausal women, intra-articular **monosodium urate** crystal deposition can result in significant arthropathy. Several metabolic abnormalities may underlie this pathology, leading either to increased production or to decreased excretion of uric acid. Dietary excess, physical stressors (eg, trauma, surgery, or myocardial infarction), excess alcohol ingestion, diuretics, and adrenocorticotropic hormone (ACTH) or glucocorticoid withdrawal can all precipitate an acute attack. Eventually, periodic episodes of acute gout give way to a chronic symmetrical synovitis.

Presentation

Acute monarticular arthritis, often of the first metatarsophalangeal (MTP) joint of the great toe, is the most common presentation. Classically, acute episodes occur at night, waking patients from sleep to find a warm, red, tender, swollen toe (**podagra**). Early attacks resemble cellulitis, but resolve after 3–10 days. Chronic tissue deposition of excess urate may present clinically as subcutaneous foci (**tophi**), for example in the Achilles tendon, at the olecranon, or on the external ear.

Diagnosis

Diagnosis must be confirmed by joint aspiration and examination of the fluid for **negatively birefringent needle-shaped crystals** (Figure 5-30). Synovial white counts are also elevated (~60,000 cells/μL). Synovial fluid cultures should be performed if there is clinical suspicion of simultaneous septic arthritis. A 24-hour urinary uric acid level may help delineate an underlying metabolic cause.

Treatment

Anti-inflammatory medications (**colchicine**, NSAIDs, and intra-articular or systemic glucocorticoid injections) are employed during acute episodes for pain relief. Notably, colchicine and NSAIDs can be toxic to elderly patients and those with renal insufficiency or GI disorders. Once acute attacks have

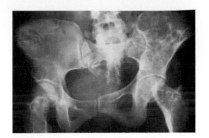

FIGURE 5-29. Radiograph of polyostotic fibrous dysplasia of the pelvis. (Reproduced with permission from Skinner HB. Current Diagnosis & Treatment in Orthopedics, 4th ed. New York: McGraw-Hill, 2006: 320.)

KEY FACT

Conditions predisposing patients to gouty arthritis:
Lesch-Nyhan syndrome
Phosphoribosyl pyrophosphate (PRPP) synthetase excess
Decreased uric acid excretion (ie, renal failure or diuretic use)
Glucose-6-phosphatase deficiency

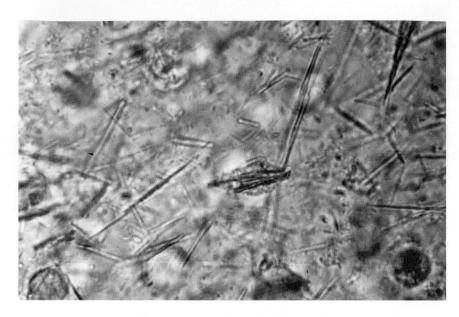

FIGURE 5-30. **Monosodium urate (MSU) crystals.** Extracellular and intracellular MSU crystals, as seen in a fresh preparation of synovial fluid, illustrate needle- and rod-shaped strongly negative birefringent crystals (compensated polarized light microscopy; 400 × magnification). (Reproduced with permission from Kasper DL, Braunwald E, Fauci A, et al. *Harrison's Principles of Internal Medicine*, 16th ed. New York: McGraw-Hill, 2005: 2047.)

KEY FACT

Treatment for gouty attacks:
Acute—**C**olchicine
Chronic—**A**llopurinol

subsided, urate-lowering therapies are used to prevent recurrence. **Probenecid** increases uric acid excretion and is especially useful in patients with poor uric acid excretion and preservation of renal function. **Allopurinol** is best for uric acid overproduction, underexcretion from renal failure, or when a uricosuric is either contraindicated or not tolerated by the patient.

Pseudogout

Calcium pyrophosphate dihydrate deposition disease (CPPD), also known as pseudogout, results in the precipitation of crystals in the joint space through an unknown mechanism. Neutrophil phagocytosis of crystals leads to chemotactic recruitment of more inflammatory cells, as in true gout, perpetuating tissue injury. Very few CPPD patients have concurrent metabolic abnormalities or a heritable genetic basis.

Pseudogout occurring in patients < 50 years old should prompt a search for a metabolic basis. Possible culprits include the "four **H**s":

- Hyperparathyroidism
- Hemochromatosis
- Hypophosphatasia (low activity of alkaline phosphatase)
- Hypomagnesemia

It is speculated that hyperparathyroidism and hemochromatosis lead to elevated serum calcium and iron, respectively, which inhibit local pyrophosphatases, resulting in increased pyrophosphate crystal precipitation.

PRESENTATION

Though often asymptomatic, many individuals with CPPD suffer from acute and chronic arthritis resembling true gout. However, chronic CPPD can lead to a **symmetrical** proliferative synovitis (more common in familial forms) resembling RA ("pseudo-RA"), or intervertebral disk calcification that mimics ankylosing spondylitis. In spite of these peculiar traits, the most common presentation is knee pain ("pseudo-OA"), although the wrist, shoulder, elbow, and ankle can also be affected (unlike in classic OA). Pseudogout attacks may be accompanied by low- to high-grade fevers.

DIAGNOSIS

Just as with true gout, joint aspiration is necessary for definitive diagnosis. Phagocytosed **basophilic, rhomboid crystals with weak positive birefringence** are present. Radiographically, radiodense CPPD crystal deposits in menisci or hyaline cartilage is termed **chondrocalcinosis** and may be present in asymptomatic joints. Is presumptive evidence of CPPD disease.

TREATMENT

Colchicine, joint aspiration, NSAIDs, and intra-articular glucocorticoid injections are the mainstays of therapy during acute attacks, sometimes shortening episodes from 1 month to 10 days in duration. Low-dose colchicine prophylaxis may aid those suffering from frequent attacks. Severe polyarticular attacks are best treated with steroids, but progressive large-joint destructive disease may necessitate surgical treatment.

CONNECTIVE TISSUE DISORDERS

Polymyositis and Dermatomyositis

Inflammatory muscle disorders are the most common cause of acquired skeletal muscle weakness, affecting 1 in 100,000 persons. Though polymyositis (PM) is primarily in adults, dermatomyositis (DM) can affect both children and adults, and women more often than men. The most dramatic clinical distinction between these two disorders is the **prominent rash that occurs in DM,** though they also differ in their underlying pathophysiology. Humoral autoimmunity leads to microangiopathy and muscle fiber ischemia through antibody-mediated damage in DM. In contrast, cytotoxic T-cell-mediated damage is associated with PM, leading to muscle necrosis.

PM is an autoimmune disorder, often mimicked by other myopathies and is considered a diagnosis of exclusion, occurring in the **absence** of the following symptoms: rash, extraocular or facial muscle weakness, family history of neuromuscular disease, myotoxic drug exposure, muscular dystrophy, neurogenic disorders, endocrinopathy, muscle enzyme deficiencies, and viral or bacterial infections.

The photosensitive rash of DM, clinically distinguishes it from PM. Most commonly, it appears as puffy, purple eyelids (**heliotrope rash**), but it can also be seen as a macular red rash on the face and trunk, or as a purple papular eruption on the knuckles (**Gottron rash**) (Figure 5-31).

PRESENTATION

Most commonly, the myopathies present with **subacute, symmetrical, proximal, and girdle muscle weakness** that progresses over weeks and months. It is significant enough to inhibit daily activities (rising from a chair, combing one's hair, lifting objects, and climbing stairs). Fine motor movements are affected only late in disease progression, and extraocular and facial muscles are spared completely in both syndromes. **Myalgia is uncommon.**

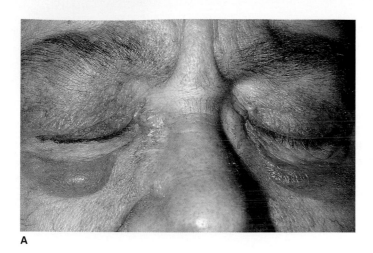

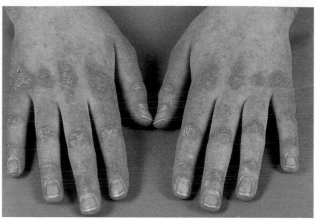

A

B

FIGURE 5-31. **Rashes of dermatomyositis.** (A) Heliotrope erythema of upper eyelids and edema of the lower lids. (B) Gottron papules on the dorsa of the hands and fingers, especially over the metacarpophalangeal and interphalangeal joints. (Reproduced with permission from Wolff K, Johnson RA, Suurmond D. *Fitzpatrick's Color Atlas and Synopsis of Clinical Dermatology*, 5th ed. New York: McGraw-Hill, 2005: 373, 375.)

DIAGNOSIS

Serum muscle enzyme levels aid in diagnosis. Increases in **creatine kinase (CK)** usually indicate increased disease activity. In addition, electromyography **(EMG)** may help rule out neurogenic disorders.

Ultimately, muscle biopsy is definitive. PM is a primary inflammatory condition in which T-cell infiltrates are found among healthy muscle fibers, eventually leading to necrosis and phagocytosis. The underlying CD8/major histocompatability complex (MHC) lesion is definitive. In DM, endomysial inflammation occurs in the immediate vicinity of the small vessels. The resulting angiopathy leads to perifascicular ischemic injuries within the muscle and peripheral perifascicular atrophy.

Myositis-specific autoantibodies may be helpful to define disease subsets. Patients who have the antisynthetase syndrome (eg, anti-Jo-1 antibody positive), the most prevalent subset (~20%) have a higher prevalence of interstitial lung disease, arthritis, and "mechanics hands."

TREATMENT

Immunosuppressive therapy is employed to improve muscle strength and relieve extramuscular symptoms. Plasma CK levels can be followed as evidence of response to treatment, but improvement in muscle strength is the primary end point. Patients usually begin on high-dose (1 mg/kg) oral prednisone, tapering over months. Azathioprine, methotrexate, and cyclophosphamide are common second-line agents if treatment with glucocorticoids fails or the patient cannot tolerate the side effects.

PROGNOSIS

Most patients improve with therapy and achieve meaningful functional recovery through maintenance therapy. PM morbidity usually results from interstitial lung disease, respiratory muscle involvement, or cardiac complications. DM can be indicative of an underlying malignancy, and a symptom-based investigation into a possible source should be undertaken.

Seronegative Spondyloarthropathies

These diseases are characterized by RF-negative inflammatory arthritis of the spine and/or extremities (asymmetrical, oligoarticular distribution). They occur more commonly in males and are strongly associated with **HLA-B27**, which is a gene that encodes for **HLA MHC I.**

ANKYLOSING SPONDYLITIS

Ankylosing spondylitis (AS) is a seronegative spondyloarthropathy that targets the bilateral sacroiliac joints in young men. Ninety percent of patients with AS are HLA-B27 positive.

The underlying cause of AS is unknown, inflamed sacroiliac joints have CD4 and CD8 infiltrates with high levels of TNF-α. Inflammation at this site leads to adjacent marrow edema, bony erosions, fibrous progression, and eventual ossification.

PRESENTATION

Symptomatic disease onset occurs in early adulthood, beginning with insidious dull lumbar or gluteal pain. Morning stiffness that improves with movement but returns at night and disrupts sleep is also typical. Bony pain may predominate at sites of enthesitis, including the major bony prominences of the trunk, girdle, and pelvis.

Several extra-articular symptoms can accompany AS. **Acute unilateral anterior uveitis** occurs in 30% of patients and may precede ankylosis. Up to 60% of patients suffer symptoms of bowel inflammation. **Aortitis, leading to aortic insufficiency** and sometimes precipitating congestive heart failure, is a rare but serious extra-articular manifestation of severe and prolonged disease. Interstitial lung disease may occur in upper lung fields.

At later stages, decreased lumbar range of motion leads to loss of lordosis and decreased flexion and extension of the torso. Restriction of chest expansion becomes significant, leading to a restrictive pulmonary defect. End-stage spinal involvement may result in fracture of brittle, osteoporotic vertebrae, leading to spinal cord injury.

DIAGNOSIS

Definitive diagnosis is established by radiographic evidence of sacroiliitis in addition to one of the three following criteria:

- History of inflammatory back pain.
- Limitation of lumbar range of motion (frontal and sagittal planes).
- Limited chest expansion.

Patients may have an asymmetrical, oligoarticular (medium to large joint) arthritis.

Radiographically, sacroiliitis is revealed by blurred cortical margins, bony erosions, and sclerosis. "Pseudo-widening" of the joint space, due to erosive disease, may be seen before joint obliteration by fusion occurs. Osteitis of vertebral corners leads to "squaring" on plain films and eventual fusion of vertebrae thru syndesmophyte formation, resulting in the pathognomonic **"bamboo" spine** seen on radiography (Figure 5-32). Early changes (bone marrow edema and enthesitis) are best seen on CT or MRI.

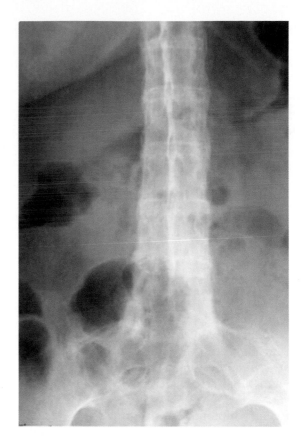

FIGURE 5-32. **Radiograph of ankylosing spondylitis.** Radiograph demonstrating "bamboo spine" deformity due to fusion of the vertebral bodies and posterior elements. (Reproduced with permission from Chen MYM, Pope TL, Jr., Ott DJ. *Basic Radiology.* New York: McGraw-Hill, 2004: Figure 7-38.)

No specific laboratory test is diagnostic of AS; however, many nonspecific tests are positive, including elevated ESR and CRP as markers of inflammation and a low RBC count from anemia of chronic disease.

TREATMENT

Immunomodulation with anti-TNF-α therapies has revolutionized AS therapy. Traditional therapy has included NSAIDs and physical therapy, although these show little effect on disease progression. Traditional DMARDs, such as methotrexate, may improve extremity joint disease but have little to no effect on spinal involvement. Uveitis, specifically, is treated with local glucocorticoids. Surgery, in the form of total hip arthroplasty, is reserved for patients with severe hip arthritis, and often results in immediate resolution of pain.

PROGNOSIS

End-stage AS is a chronic progressive disease, significantly reducing patient quality of life. Most patients suffer increasing pain, stiffness, and disability despite traditional therapy as they age and the disease progresses.

REACTIVE ARTHRITIS

The **reactive arthritides (ReAs)** are a group of seronegative inflammatory arthritides in which up to 85% of sufferers share the **HLA-B27** antigen. It is thought that patients with this haplotype have a genetic susceptibility to arthritis if infected with certain enteric and genital pathogens. In addition, HIV-positive individuals are susceptible to these infections and subsequent ReAs. Several pathogens have been implicated, including:

- *Shigella*
- *Salmonella*
- *Yersinia*
- *Campylobacter*
- *Chlamydia trachomatis*

Most commonly affecting 18- to 40-year-old males, the pathogenesis is unknown, although many theories have been proposed. Each of the inciting pathogens produces **lipopolysaccharide (LPS)** and can invade host cells, surviving intracellularly. In addition to similarities in causative pathogens, patients with the B27 haplotype have been found to share a conserved T-cell receptor, which may contribute to the T_H2 mediated inflammation found in ReAs.

PRESENTATION

Reiter syndrome was the term used for the symptom triad of **arthritis, urethritis,** and **conjunctivitis.** Usually, patients report an antecedent GI or GU infection less than 1 month prior to the onset of an asymmetrical progressive arthritis. Lower extremities (knees, ankles, and feet) are more commonly involved, though wrists and hands may also be affected. Joint effusions, dactylitis, tendinitis, and fasciitis are all common. Associated pathology may include ocular disease, which ranges from conjunctivitis to uveitis, as well as mucosal and urethral ulcers and sores of the palms and soles.

DIAGNOSIS

As a clinical diagnosis, reactive arthritis should be considered in patients suffering from inflammatory back pain and/or an oligoarticular, usually asymmetrical extremity joint arthritis occurring in close temporal proximity to an episode of dysuria or diarrhea.

TREATMENT

Acute arthritic symptoms are alleviated to varying degrees by NSAIDs, although chronic resistant disease may require immunomodulators such as sulfasalazine and methotrexate. Prompt treatment of concomitant GU infection may prevent the development of subsequent ReA in susceptible individuals.

SYSTEMIC LUPUS ERYTHEMATOSUS

Systemic lupus erythematosus (SLE) is an autoimmune connective tissue disease mediated by autoantibodies and immune complexes, causing inflammation and injury primarily to joints, skin, blood, and internal organs. Lupus is characterized by simultaneous and sequential interactions involving:

- T cells, B cells, and antigen-presenting cells
- Cytokines
- (Auto)antibodies
- (Auto)antigens
- Immune complexes
- Complement

The prototype immune complexes of antibodies directed against double-stranded DNA may circulate and deposit in tissues or form in situ. Tissue injury occurs thru immune complex activation of complement, and complement- and Fc-

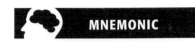

MNEMONIC

Can't **see** (uveitis/conjunctivitis).
Can't **pee** (urethritis).
Can't climb a **tree** (arthritis).

KEY FACT

In a young female with fever, fatigue, rash, and joint pain, always think of SLE.

receptor-mediated recruitment and activation of inflammatory cells. SLE is a disease driven by T_H2 cytokines, particularly interferon-alpha (IFN-α).

Ninety percent of SLE patients are women between the ages of 14 and 45. This disease is three times more common in African American than Caucasians. Those at risk for increased mortality include younger age at onset, non-Caucasian ancestry, and male gender. Infection is the leading cause of death.

PRESENTATION

Definitive classification of a patient as having SLE requires the documentation of 4 of 11 criteria over the course of the patients' medical history (specificity and sensitivity: ~95% and 75%, respectively) (Table 5-11). In addition, **antinuclear antibodies** (ANAs) are positive in > 95% of patients; thus, repeated negative results make the diagnosis less likely. The most common symptoms over time include constitutional symptoms, rash, arthritis, and serositis (pleuritis and/or pericarditis). Less clinically prevalent symptoms include glomerulonephritis, nonbacterial verrucous endocarditis, and Raynaud phenomenon.

With the potential to affect nearly every organ system, SLE sequelae are quite diverse. Descriptions of high-yield major organ system manifestations are shown in Table 5-12.

TABLE 5-11. Classification Criteria for the Diagnosis of Systemic Lupus Erythematosus

A patient must have 4 of the following 11 criteria at any time during disease history in order to be diagnosed with SLE.	
Immunologic disorder	**Anti-ds-DNA**, anti-Sm, and/or aPLs.
Malar rash	Rash on cheeks, flat or raised.
Discoid rash	Erythematous circular raised patches on skin; may result in scarring.
Antinuclear antibody	An abnormal ANA titer (in the absence of drugs known to induce ANAs).
Mucositis (oral ulcers)	Oral and nasopharyngeal ulcers.
Neurologic disorder	Seizures or psychosis.
Serositis	Pleuritis or pericarditis.
Hematologic disorder	Hemolytic anemia or leukopenia, lymphopenia, or thrombocytopenia in the absence of offending drugs.
Arthritis	Nonerosive arthritis of ≥ 2 peripheral joints (tenderness, swelling, and/or effusion).
Renal disorder	Proteinuria (> 0.5 g/d or 3+) and/or cellular casts.
Photosensitivity	Rash resulting from exposure to ultraviolet light.

ANAs = antinuclear antibodies; aPL = antiphospholipid (antibodies).

TABLE 5-12.   Organ System Manifestations of Systemic Lupus Erythematosus

ORGAN SYSTEM	MANIFESTATION	NOTES
Cutaneous	Lupus dermatitis	Most commonly a photosensitive, red, scaly **malar rash** over the cheeks and nose sparing the nasolabial folds.
Musculoskeletal	Polyarthritis and synovitis	Symmetrical, small and medium extremity joint swelling and tenderness without bony erosions.
	Myalgias and weakness	Must be distinguished from steroid side effect, metabolic causes, and pain syndromes.
Renal	Lupus nephritis	Morbid SLE complication; elevated creatinine with hematuria and proteinuria that may progress to ESRD.
Nervous	Cognitive dysfunction	Decreased memory and reasoning.
	Headaches	Intensify with SLE flares; may simulate meningitis.
	CNS vasculitis	May lead to stroke.
	Psychosis	Must be distinguished from steroid side effect.
Pulmonary	Pleuritis	With or without pleural effusion.
	Interstitial inflammation	Dyspnea, with reduced DLco on pulmonary function testing.
Cardiovascular	Accelerated atherosclerosis	Inflammatory state and thrombotic and embolic disease lead to increased MI and stroke risks.
	Myocarditis	Can result in arrhythmias.
	Libman-Sacks endocarditis (subacute endocarditis)	Leads to valvular insufficiency and embolic CVAs.
Hematologic	Anemia of chronic disease	Normochromic, normocytic.
	Hemolytic anemia	Low haptoglobin, high LDH, Coombs-positive.
	Thrombocytopenia	Immune mediated.
	Leukopenia	Primarily lymphocytopenia.
Gastrointestinal	Vasculitis	Leads to perforations, ischemia, and bleeding.
	Lupus pancreatitis	Disease-related vs drug-induced.
Ocular	Sicca syndrome	a.k.a. secondary Sjögren syndrome.
	Retinal vasculitis	May be vision threatening; treated with aggressive steroid therapy.
	Optic neuritis	

DLco = diffusion capacity of the lung for carbon monoxide; CVA = cardiovascular accident; ESRD = end-stage renal disease; MI = myocardial infarction; SLE = systemic lupus erythematosus.

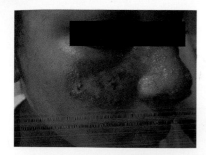

FIGURE 5-33. Cutaneous manifestation of systemic lupus erythematosus. Erythematous sharply demarcated plaques with scale in a butterfly pattern on the face of a 14-year-old girl with arthritis, chest pain, and facial rash. (Reproduced with permission from USMLERx.com.)

■ **Cutaneous: Lupus dermatitis** (Figure 5-33) can be discoid, systemic, or subacute. Most commonly, this occurs as the photosensitive and erythematous **malar rash** over the cheeks and nose (sparing the nasolabial fold). The rash can also spread to the ears, chin, neck, and back, and is mediated by immune complex deposition at the dermal-epidermal junction.

■ **Musculoskeletal:** Most patients experience intermittent polyarthritis, synovitis, and swelling or tenderness in the feet, ankles, knees, hands, and wrists. Bony erosions are rare; if seen, consider RA as an alternative diagnosis. Persistent pain in any one joint should increase clinical suspicion for **ischemic necrosis**, especially in those patients receiving systemic glucocorticoid therapy.

■ **Renal: Lupus nephritis** is a common cause of morbidity in SLE. Every SLE patient should be regularly screened for asymptomatic nephritis with a urinalysis, urine microalbumin, and serum blood urea nitrogen/creatinine (BUN/Cr) level. African Americans are more likely than Caucasians to progress to end-stage renal disease (ESRD).

■ **Cardiovascular:** Vascular occlusive diseases are increased in lupus, especially in those patients with **antiphospholipid antibodies (aPL)**. These aPLs may lead to false-positive results on syphilis rapid plasma reagin/Venereal Disease Research Laboratory (RPR/VDRL) tests. Accelerated atherosclerosis leads to significantly increased risk of stroke and myocardial infarction. SLE, like RA, should be considered a cardiac risk factor. Long-term anticoagulation may be indicated in hypercoagulable patients. In addition to vascular manifestations, inflammatory pericarditis is frequently seen. More worrisome, however, is the development of lupus myocarditis, or **Libman-Sacks** endocarditis. Valvular disease from endocarditis may lead to mitral and aortic valve insufficiency and an increase in stroke risk secondary to emboli arising from the damaged valves.

■ **Gastrointestinal:** Nausea, vomiting, and diarrhea can be manifestations of SLE, typically resulting from vascular disease within the abdomen. Vasculitis involving the intestine is an uncommon yet very serious complication and may result in perforation, ischemia, GI bleeds, diffuse abdominal peritonitis and, potentially, sepsis.

DIAGNOSIS

The most important laboratory test is the antinuclear antibody (**ANA**), which is positive in > 95% of patients with SLE. ANA is very sensitive, but it is not specific for SLE and can also be elevated in RA, and other connective tissue diseases, other chronic inflammatory states including chronic infections, and from certain medications. High anti-double-stranded DNA (**anti-ds-DNA**) and anti-Smith (**anti-Sm**) titers are both specific for lupus and, when present, make it very likely the patient has SLE. Antiphospholipid antibodies, although not specific for SLE, fulfill 1 of 11 classification criteria for diagnosis and thus should be tested for, particularly in women with recurrent spontaneous abortions. Women of childbearing age should receive a screen for anti-Ro antibodies because of a correlation with increased risk of fetal congenital heart block.

Antihistone antibodies are found in drug-induced lupus and are helpful in distinguishing this from SLE.

TREATMENT

NSAIDs are the front-line therapy for patients with arthritis and myalgias. Dermatitis, arthritis, and fatigue are addressed with antimalarials. In the case of life-threatening lupus nephritis, glucocorticoids and cytotoxic agents are the mainstays of pharmacologic intervention. **High-dose systemic steroids to**

KEY FACT

Many medications can cause drug-induced lupus, including:
- Chlorpromazine
- Hydralazine
- Isoniazid
- Methyldopa
- Penicillamine
- Procainamide
- Quinidine
- Sulfasalazine

Distinguish this from SLE using **antihistone antibodies.**

control acute symptoms are recommended for short periods of time only so as to reduce the incidence of steroid side effects. Some patients may require long-term low-dose therapy with glucocorticoids, azathioprine, mycophenolate, or other immunosuppressive agents.

PROGNOSIS

Most patients experience a disease course with relatively quiescent stretches punctuated by acute exacerbations, but complete regression is rare. Most patients are affected chronically by varying degrees of skin and joint disease. ESRD is also common.

SARCOIDOSIS

A chronic disorder of waxing and waning course, sarcoidosis affects men and women from age 20 to 40 years. In the United States most commonly found in African American females, it is characterized by immune-mediated **noncaseating granulomas** and elevated serum angiotensin-converting enzyme (ACE) levels. Arising from disordered immune responses of unknown etiology, T_H1 lymphocytes accumulate within organs due to one of two possible inciting events:

- The presence of persistent antigens (or self-antigens).
- Decreased efficacy of T-suppressor cells.

Mononuclear phagocytes then infiltrate tissues in response to released IL-2. In the tissue, the phagocytes differentiate and fuse to produce the multinucleated giant cells that reside in the center of noncaseating granulomas (Figure 5-34). Local tissue inflammation, fibrosis, and functional deficits lead to patient symptomatology.

Pathology includes epithelial granulomas containing microscopic **Schaumann bodies** (calcium + protein) and **multinucleated giant cells.** These epithelioid giant cells are believed to produce elevated levels of 1,25-dihydroxyvitamin D, leading to enhanced calcium absorption in the gut and hypercalciuria, with or without hypercalcemia.

PRESENTATION

Although sarcoidosis is a systemic disease, the lungs are most commonly and severely affected. Patients may present in the asymptomatic state when a chest radiograph is performed for other reasons. Acute or subacute cases develop over short time courses (weeks) and present with constitutional symptoms of fatigue, low-grade fever, night sweats, malaise, anorexia, and weight loss. Pulmonary symptoms include cough, dyspnea, retrosternal chest discomfort, and hemoptysis. More insidious disease progression may develop over months and causes respiratory symptoms in the absence of constitutional symptoms.

Within the lung, sarcoidosis is primarily an interstitial restrictive lung disease that affects alveoli, terminal bronchi, and vasculature. Auscultation reveals dry rales. Nontender lymphadenopathy is very common, often occurring in the cervical, axillary, tracheal, thoracic, mediastinal/hilar, and inguinal distributions.

About 25% of patients experience skin manifestations, such as **erythema nodosum**—tender deep-seated nodules or plaques on the lower extremities. Other cutaneous manifestations include infiltrated papules about the

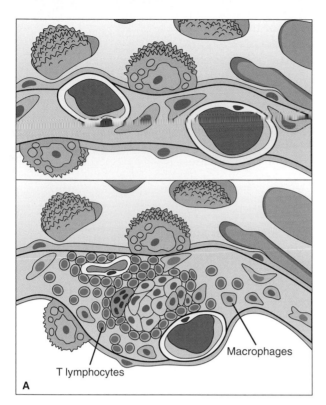

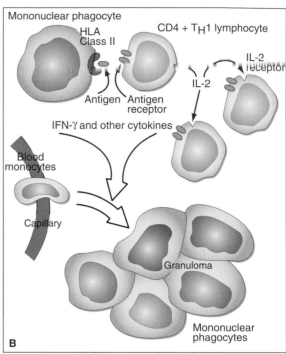

FIGURE 5-34. **Pathogenesis of sarcoidosis.** (A) Histologic abnormalities. Normal alveoli (*top*) and alveoli in active sarcoidosis (*bottom*). The latter are distorted by the accumulated CD4+ T$_H$1 lymphocytes, alveolar macrophages, and macrophages aggregated into granulomas. There is mild damage to alveolar epithelial and endothelial cells. (B) The exaggerated processes of T$_H$1 lymphocytes in affected organs result in the accumulation of these cells along with macrophages and macrophages aggregated into granulomas. The trigger for the T$_H$1 lymphocytes is unknown. The immune response is exaggerated and skewed to produce activated T$_H$1 lymphocytes that release interleukin 2 (IL-2), which drives the accumulation of more T lymphocytes. The activated T$_H$1 lymphocytes also release interferon-γ (IFN-γ). Together with cytokines such as IL-12, macrophage inflammatory protein 1α, and granulocyte-macrophage colony-stimulating factor released in the local milieu, there is recruitment and activation of blood monocytes and subsequent granuloma formation. (Modified with permission from Kasper DL, Braunwald E, Fauci A, et al. *Harrison's Principles of Internal Medicine*, 16th ed. New York: McGraw-Hill, 2005: 2018.)

nose and erythematous or violaceous papules on the upper extremities (Figure 5-35). The combination of erythema nodosum, hilar lymphadenopathy, and arthritis/periarthritis (typically in and around the ankle) is called **Lofgren syndrome.** Another 25% suffer eye involvement that can lead to blindness. Posterior uveitis is most common, presenting with blurred vision, lacrimation, and photophobia. Retinal vasculitis and conjunctival involvement may occur. Lacrimal gland inflammation leads to sicca syndrome.

Several other organs outside of the lungs can be involved.

DIAGNOSIS

Sarcoidosis should be considered in any patient between the ages of 20 and 40 who has respiratory complaints, blurry vision, erythema nodosum, and hilar lymphadenopathy. Hilar or mediastinal lymph nodes are known as "potato nodes." Laboratory tests for lymphocytopenia, eosinophilia, increased ESR, hyperglobulinemia, and elevated **ACE** levels all can support the diagnosis. Definite diagnosis requires biopsy evidence of the typical pathologic changes. Chest films can be used to screen the patient for lymphadenopathy, but chest CT scanning is often required to document alveolitis and interstitial disease. Pulmonary function tests may reveal a restrictive pattern with decreased lung volumes and diffusing capacities.

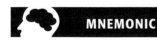

MNEMONIC

GRAIN
Gammaglobulinemia
Rheumatoid factor
ACE increase
Interstitial fibrosis
Noncaseating granulomas

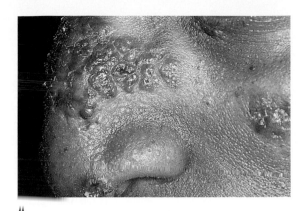
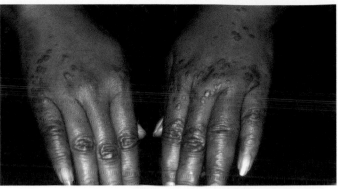

A

B

FIGURE 5-35. **Cutaneous manifestations of sarcoidosis.** (A) Brownish-to purple papules coalescing to irregular plaques, occurring on the face of this man who also had massive pulmonary involvement. (B) Papular brownish to violaceous lesions on the dorsa of a 10-year-old woman who also had pulmonary involvement. Note swelling of the fourth digit of the left hand and of the fifth digit of the right hand. (Reproduced with permission from Wolff K, Johnson RA, Suurmond D. *Fitzpatrick's Color Atlas & Synopsis of Clinical Dermatology*, 5th ed. New York: McGraw-Hill, 2005: 430, 431.)

TREATMENT

The therapy of choice is a high-dose glucocorticoid taper. Methotrexate, antimalarials, TNF-α inhibitors, and immunosuppressants have all been used in refractory cases.

PROGNOSIS

Most patients suffering from acute disease achieve remission with no significant long-term sequelae. Half of all patients experience mild permanent organ damage that rarely progresses; 20% are left with intermittent recurring disease, and only 10% succumb to direct sequelae of sarcoidosis.

Systemic Sclerosis

Systemic sclerosis (SSc) is a systemic disease primarily characterized by excessive production of collagen primarily in the skin that results in sclerosis, thickening, and tightening. Also known as scleroderma, it is a heterogeneous disorder in terms of both the involvement of internal organs and joints and of the pace and severity of its clinical course. SSc is most commonly seen in women (female-to-male ratio of 3:1) between the ages of 35 and 64 years. It is slightly more common in African Americans.

PRESENTATION

In **localized scleroderma** (eg, morphea, linear scleroderma), cutaneous changes consistent with dermal fibrosis are seen without organ involvement. **Systemic sclerosis** is classified as either diffuse or limited based on the extent of skin disease, but patients in both forms are at risk for internal organ involvement. **Diffuse systemic sclerosis** includes extensive fibrotic skin changes with early internal organ involvement including pulmonary, renal, and cardiac systems. **Limited SSc** presents a slowly progressive course over years with fibrotic skin limited to the hands, forearms, feet, neck, and face (Figure 5-36). Patients usually present with Raynaud phenomenon and over time may develop telangiectasias, GI involvement, skin calcifications, and late pulmonary hypertension.

 KEY FACT

CREST syndrome was the older terminology for limited SSc, and stood for **C**alcinosis, **R**aynaud phenomenon, **E**sophageal dysmotility, **S**clerodactyly, and **T**elangiectasias.

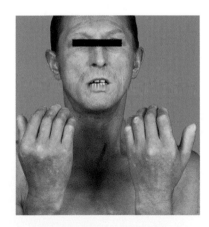

FIGURE 5-36. **Scleroderma.** Localized cutaneous systemic sclerosis showing involvement of the face that has a mask-like appearance, with inability of opening the mouth, sclerodactyly, and digital ulcerations. (Reproduced with permission from Wolff K, Goldsmith LA, Katz SI, et al. *Fitzpatrick's Dermatology in General Medicine*, 7th ed. New York: McGraw-Hill, 2008: Figure 158-4.)

DIAGNOSIS

Diagnosis is based on clinical symptoms and confirmed with laboratory tests. A positive ANA is seen in over 90%. **Anticentromere antibody** is present and very specific in patients with limited SSc, whereas patients with diffuse systemic sclerosis are characterized by **antitopoisomerase I** (or antiscleroderma 70) antibody.

Complications can be detected using pulmonary function testing (for restrictive lung disease) and barium swallow to look for esophageal dysmotility. Echocardiogram can indirectly screen for the presence of pulmonary hypertension.

TREATMENT

Treatment is primarily symptomatic as no therapy has been definitively successful in reversing the course of disease. Calcium channel blockers are useful in treating Raynaud phenomenon. Pulmonary hypertension may be treated with calcium channel blockers and anticoagulants. Unfortunately, no effective therapy currently exists for skin involvement. The only medication known to reduce the mortality of patients with scleroderma are ACE inhibitors, used for patients with renal crisis.

PROGNOSIS

The major cause of mortality and morbidity is involvement of internal organ systems; specifically, renal failure and pulmonary hypertension. Though the average survival time following diagnosis is 12 years, this prognosis is strongly affected by the disease subtype. The limited cutaneous form has a much better prognosis than the diffuse cutaneous type.

Mixed Connective Tissue Disease

Mixed connective tissue disease (MCTD) is an autoimmune disorder wherein the patient may show clinical and lab features of more than one connective tissue disease, including SLE, RA, myositis, and progressive SSc. The exact pathophysiologic mechanism of MCTD remains unknown. It is 15 times more common in women than in men.

PRESENTATION

Patients generally present with arthralgias or arthritis, commonly associated with skin changes. Raynaud phenomenon is seen in 90% of patients, and myositis is present in 75% of patients early in the course of disease. Involvement of the lungs is common in MCTD, although most patients do not initially present with pulmonary symptoms.

DIAGNOSIS

Major clinical findings include Raynaud phenomenon, swelling over the dorsum of the hands, arthritis, esophageal dysmotility, myositis, and pulmonary hypertension, with or without SSc. Most importantly, a high level of anti-U1 ribonucleoprotein autoantibodies (**anti-RNP Ab**) in the absence of the anti-Smith autoantibody (**no anti-Sm Ab**) is required for diagnosis.

TREATMENT

Generally, SLE-like features, arthritis, and pleuritis are treated with **NSAIDs,** antimalarials (**hydroxychloroquine**), low-dose **corticosteroids,** and methotrexate. Raynaud phenomenon is treated symptomatically with **calcium channel blockers.**

PROGNOSIS

The major cause of mortality is progressive pulmonary hypertension and its cardiac sequelae. MCTD rarely affects the kidneys and is generally considered to have a better prognosis than SLE.

Sjögren Syndrome

A systemic disease most frequently manifested by dry mouth (**xerostomia**), dry eyes (**xerophthalmia**), and, in one-third of patients, **enlargement of the parotid glands** (Figure 5-37), resulting from lymphocytic infiltration of exocrine glands. It affects predominantly middle-aged women, with a 9:1 female-to-male ratio. Patients are at a 44-fold greater risk of developing **non-Hodgkin B-cell lymphomas** than are age-matched controls.

PRESENTATION

In addition to **sicca** (dryness)—of the eyes, mouth, upper respiratory tract, and vagina—patients may present with constitutional symptoms.

DIAGNOSIS

Primary Sjögren syndrome is diagnosed in a patient with dry eyes, dry mouth, and lymphocytic infiltration of the salivary glands seen on histology. Secondary Sjögren syndrome presents with the same symptoms but is diagnosed when the patient already has another connective tissue disease.

Abnormal serologies include positive RF, positive ANA, and/or positive anti-SSA (anti-Ro) or anti-SS-B (anti-La). Lab abnormalities may include cytopenias, cryoglobulinemia, distal renal tubular acidosis, and a polyclonal hypergammaglobulinemia.

TREATMENT

Treatment is mainly symptomatic. Artificial tears and saliva preparations can be used to relieve dryness. Cholinergic drugs (ie, pilocarpine) can increase exocrine secretion. The complications of xerostomia and xerophthalmia are best prevented by good dental and ophthalmologic care, respectively. Severe extraglandular disease may require high-dose systemic corticosteroids. Yearly lab testing to screen for transition to a lymphoproliferative disorder includes serum and urine protein electrophoresis, cryoglobulins, and complement. In patients with secondary Sjögren, treatment of the underlying connective tissue disease is often key.

PROGNOSIS

Typically, patients have a normal life expectancy. In patients who have associated disorders, the prognosis generally depends on those diseases.

DERMATOLOGY

Terminology

Many specific terms are used to describe skin lesions (Table 5-13).

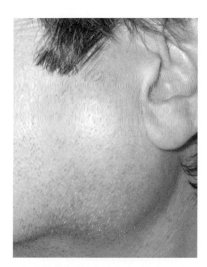

FIGURE 5-37. Sjögren syndrome. Clinical appearance of parotid gland enlargement in Sjögren's syndrome. (Reproduced with permission from Imboden JB, Hellmann DB, Stone JH. *Current Rheumatology Diagnosis & Treatment*, 2nd ed. New York: McGraw-Hill, 2007: Figure 27-3.)

TABLE 5-13. **Key Terms in Dermatology**

Lesion Name	Description
Bulla	Fluid-filled raised lesion > 5 mm across.
Excoriation	Traumatic lesion characterized by breakage of the epidermis, causing a raw linear area (ie, a deep scratch); often self-induced.
Macule	Circumscribed lesion ≤ 5 mm in diameter characterized by flatness and usually distinguished from surrounding skin by its coloration.
Nodule	Elevated lesion with spherical contour > 5 mm across.
Papule	Elevated dome-shaped or flat-topped lesion ≤ 5 mm across.
Patch	Flat lesion (like a macule) > 5 mm.
Plaque	Elevated flat-topped lesion usually > 5 mm across (may be caused by coalescent papules).
Pustule	Discrete, pus-filled, raised lesion.
Scale	Dry, horny, platelike excrescence; usually the result of imperfect cornification.
Vesicle	Fluid-filled raised lesion ≤ 5 mm across.

Skin Disorders and Dermatitis

COMMON

ALLERGIC CONTACT DERMATITIS

Delayed-type hypersensitivity (type IV) reaction to a topical irritant (often poison ivy, cosmetics, or jewelry). The rash appears in a linear distribution mirroring the site of contact with the irritant.

ATOPIC DERMATITIS (ECZEMA)

Immune-mediated skin disease (type I hypersensitivity) causing scaly and vesicular eruptions, which rupture and crust over on flexor surfaces. The rash is pruritic. It is often associated with other allergic conditions.

NEVOCELLULAR NEVUS

A fancy term for the benign common mole.

PSORIASIS

Caused by unregulated proliferation of keratinocytes, psoriasis is identified by well-demarcated papules and plaques with silvery scale. These areas are usually nonpruritic. Biopsy often shows parakeratosis, which is characterized by stratum corneum that has retained nuclei. Approximately 10% of patients have associated psoriatic arthritis.

KEY FACT

Atopic triad: allergic rhinitis, asthma, and eczema.

ROSACEA

An inflammatory condition predominantly affecting the central face, leading to telangiectasias, central redness, and superficial pustules. This is a chronic condition predominantly affecting women and may begin with facial flushing in response to certain stimuli (ie, alcohol, embarrassment, heat).

SEBORRHEIC KERATOSIS

A common benign epidermal tumor that arises spontaneously (mainly on the trunk) and is clinically described as round, flat, coinlike plaques that look "pasted on." The lesions are tan to dark brown (due to melanin pigmentation of basaloid cells) and show a velvety to granular surface. It is usually seen in the elderly and is easily treated by excision.

URTICARIA

More commonly known as hives, this is an intensely pruritic skin elevation that can occur anywhere on the body. It is described as a "wheal-and-flare reaction" in which mast cell release of histamine causes edema (the wheal) with surrounding erythema (flare) (Figure 5-38). Urticaria can also be due to IgE-mediated reactions following exposure to certain foods, insect bites, and drugs. An individual urticarial lesion should last no longer than 24 hours. Individual lesions lasting greater than 24 hours would support the possibility of urticarial vasculitis. Treatment of urticaria includes antihistamines and removal of the causative agent. **Hereditary angioneurotic edema** is an inherited deficiency of C1 esterase inhibitor that results in uncontrolled activation of the early components of the complement cascade and is similar in presentation to hives.

PIGMENTED LESIONS

ALBINISM

Patients with albinism have a normal melanocyte count, but these melanocytes have decreased melanin production secondary to a deficiency of tyrosinase. Clinically, patients may present with silvery white hair and lightly pigmented or nonpigmented skin. Albinism is a risk factor for future skin cancer development, and patients should be closely monitored.

MELASMA

Hyperpigmentation of the skin around the face or on the abdomen that is associated with increased estrogen exposure. Thus, it is commonly seen in women who are pregnant or using oral contraceptive pills.

VITILIGO

Autoimmune destruction of melanocytes, leading to patchy areas of complete depigmentation.

INFECTIOUS

CELLULITIS

An infection of the dermis and subcutaneous tissue, cellulitis is usually caused by gram-positive organisms, especially *Streptococcus pyogenes* or *Staphylococcus aureus*. Patients usually present with an acute and extremely painful erythematous region of skin that demonstrates progressive spread. Treatment is with antibiotics.

FIGURE 5-38. **Urticaria.** (Reproduced with permission from Bondi EE, Jegasothy BV, Lazarus GS, ed. *Dermatology: Diagnosis & Treatment*. Orginally published by Appleton & Lange. Copyright © 1991 McGraw-Hill.)

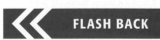

FLASH BACK

Vitiligo is often associated with thyroid disease, diabetes, and Addison disease.

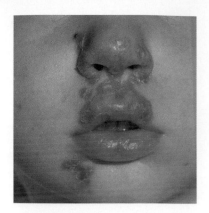

FIGURE 5-39. Impetigo. Crusted erythematous erosions becoming confluent on the nose, cheek, lips, and chin in a child with nasal carriage of *S aureus* and mild facial eczema. (Reproduced with permission from Wolff K, Johnson RA. *Fitzpatrick's Color Atlas & Synopsis of Clinical Dermatology*, 6th ed. New York: McGraw-Hill, 2009: Figure 24-11.)

IMPETIGO

Impetigo is a highly contagious, superficial skin infection that is most often caused by *S aureus* or *S pyogenes*. It usually begins on the face and is characterized by vesicles and pustules that rupture and form a honey-colored crust (Figure 5-39). Treatment is with antibiotics.

NECROTIZING FASCIITIS

Unlike cellulitis, necrotizing fasciitis involves the deeper layers of tissue down to the deep fascia. Usually caused by anaerobic bacteria or group A streptococci, it often manifests with fever and an area of erythema. If not treated, the tissue begins to turn gray/black, and crepitus can be elicited due to CO_2 and methane production during tissue destruction. Amputation, shock, and death can result. Treatment includes surgical exploration and debridement and IV antibiotics.

STAPHYLOCOCCAL SCALDED SKIN SYNDROME

S aureus releases certain exfoliative toxins that bind to a cell adhesion molecule (desmoglein 1) and cleave it, leading to a loss of cell-to-cell adhesion. Desmoglein 1 is only found in the upper part of the epidermis, thus the epidermolysis occurs between the stratum spinosum and stratum granulosum. Staphylococcal scalded skin syndrome is usually seen in newborns or children. It begins with fever and generalized rash, followed by sloughing of the upper layers of the dermis.

VERRUCAE

More commonly known as warts, verrucae are caused by human papillomavirus (a DNA virus). Epidermal hyperplasia leads to cauliflower-like lesions that are more commonly found on children's hands and feet. No extensive diagnostic testing is required, and treatment involves cryotherapy, salicylic acid, or cantharidin.

CONDITIONS WITH BLISTERS

BULLOUS PEMPHIGOID

A type II hypersensitivity reaction caused by autoantibodies targeting hemidesmosomes at the basement membrane. The bullae are below the epidermis and do not tend to rupture when touched. They can be found throughout the body but usually spare the oral mucosa (Figure 5-40). Bullous pemphigoid shows linear immunofluorescence but only at the basement membrane.

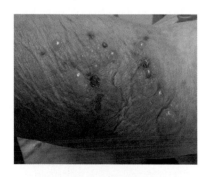

FIGURE 5-40. Bullous pemphigoid. Tense bullae and urticarial plaques. (Reproduced with permission from USMLERx.)

KEY FACT

Treatment for dermatitis herpetiformis is a gluten-free diet.

DERMATITIS HERPETIFORMIS

Rare disorder characterized by extremely pruritic urticaria and grouped vesicles that are mainly along the extensor surfaces. This disease is associated with celiac disease and responds to a gluten-free diet. The IgA antibodies developed against gluten cross-react with reticulin (a component of the anchoring fibrils that tether the epidermal basement membrane to the superficial dermis).

ERYTHEMA MULTIFORME

An uncommon, self-limited disorder that appears to be a hypersensitivity response to certain infections and drugs. It is probably caused by cytotoxic T-cells targeting cross-reactive antigens in, or near, the basal cell layer of the skin and mucosa. It is distinguishable by its target lesions—red papules that have a pale central area.

- **Stevens-Johnson syndrome:** A febrile version of erythema multiforme that is marked by erosions and crusting of the mucosal surfaces of the lips, conjunctivae, oral cavity, urethra, and anogenital region along with bulla formation. Less than 10% of the body surface area must be covered in order to make the diagnosis. It is commonly associated with drug reactions and carries a high mortality rate.
- **Toxic epidermal necrolysis:** Results in diffuse necrosis and sloughing of cutaneous and mucosal epithelial surfaces, producing a clinical situation analogous to an extensive burn. This is the most severe version, affecting > 30% of the body surface area. Prognosis is poor, with a high mortality rate.

PEMPHIGUS VULGARIS

Pemphigus vulgaris is a rare autoimmune blistering disorder affecting the mucosa and skin (scalp, face, groin, and trunk) that, like bullous pemphigoid, is a type II hypersensitivity reaction. Early lesions appear as superficial vesicles and bullae that are suprabasal and easily rupture when touched (Figure 5-41). It is caused by a loss of integrity of normal intercellular attachments within the epidermis and mucosal epithelium.

Acantholysis is the term for dissolution, or lysis, of the intercellular adhesion sites within a squamous epithelial surface. This is common to all forms of pemphigus.

MISCELLANEOUS

ACANTHOSIS NIGRICANS

Caused by hyperplasia of the stratum spinosum. Patients present with a velvety, light-brown patch often in the axilla or on the back of the neck. It is almost always associated with insulin resistance or underlying malignancy. Treatment involves eliciting the underlying cause and treating appropriately.

LICHEN PLANUS

Pruritic, purple, polygonal papules are the presenting signs of this disorder of skin and mucous membranes. Resolving spontaneously in 1–2 years, it often leaves zones of postinflammatory hyperpigmentation. Typically, there are multiple lesions on the extremities, wrists, elbows, or even the glans penis. In 70% of cases, oral lesions are present. Histologically, a lymphocytic infiltrate along the dermoepidermal junction gives the junction a zigzag contour known as a "saw-tooth" appearance.

Skin Cancer

ACTINIC KERATOSIS

Premalignant (dysplastic) lesions that result from chronic sun exposure and are associated with a build-up of excess keratin. Lesions are < 1 cm in size and skin-colored with a sandpaper consistency. If too much keratin is deposited, "cutaneous horns" can develop.

SQUAMOUS CELL CARCINOMA (SCC)

This is the most important tumor arising on chronically sun-exposed sites generally in older people. Exposure to UV light with subsequent unrepaired DNA damage is the most frequent cause, although others exist. Prior to breaking through the basement membrane, SCC appears as a sharply defined, red, scaling plaque. It can become invasive or nodular, may develop hyperkerato-

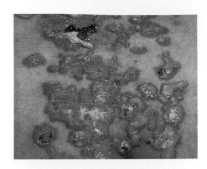

FIGURE 5-41. Pemphigus vulgaris. Widespread confluent flaccid blisters on the lower back of a 40-year-old male who had a generalized eruption including scalp and mucous membranes. The eroded lesions are extremely painful. (Reproduced with permission from Wolff K, Johnson RA. *Fitzpatrick's Color Atlas & Synopsis of Clinical Dermatology*, 6th ed. New York: McGraw-Hill, 2009: Figure 6-10.)

 KEY FACT

A positive Nikolsky sign (rubbing of the skin results in complete separation of the outermost layer) is associated with pemphigus vulgaris and erythema multiforme. This sign is absent in bullous pemphigoid.

 FLASH BACK

Patients with xeroderma pigmentosum cannot repair damaged DNA and are at increased risk for developing SCC.

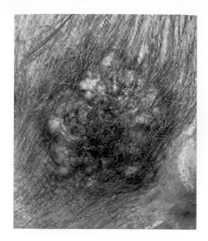

FIGURE 5-42. Squamous cell carcinoma. This nodule with central ulceration slowly developed over 1 year. (Reproduced with permission from Knoop KJ, Stack LB, Storrow AB, Thurman RJ. *The Atlas of Emergency Medicine*, 3rd ed. New York: McGraw-Hill, 2010: Figure 13-73.)

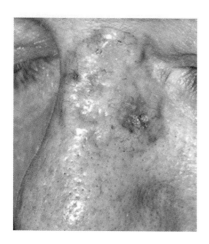

FIGURE 5-43. Basal cell carcinoma (BCC). Aggressive BCC. Note the very subtle clinical features with an indurated plaque, pearly texture with telangiectasia present. (Reproduced with permission from Halter JB, Ouslander JG, Tinetti ME, et al. *Hazzard's Geriatric Medicine and Gerontology*, 6th ed. New York: McGraw-Hill, 2009: Figure 100-3.)

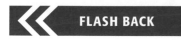

FLASH BACK

Goodpasture syndrome is an example of a type II hypersensitivity reaction.

sis, and may ulcerate (Figure 5-42). Histologically, atypia is present in all layers of the epidermis, and keratin "pearls" can be seen. Only 5% metastasize.

Basal Cell Carcinoma (BCC)

These common, slow-growing tumors also arise from chronic sun exposure (Figure 5-43). Clinically, they present as pearly papules, often containing prominent, dilated subepidermal blood vessels (telangiectasias). The cells forming the periphery of the tumor cell islands tend to be arranged radially with their long axes in approximately parallel alignment (palisading nuclei).

Malignant Melanoma

In contrast to nevi, melanomas exhibit striking variations in pigmentation, appearing in shades of black, brown, red, dark blue, and gray. The borders of melanomas are irregular and notched. Clinical warning signs include a mole that has enlarged, begins itching, or becomes painful; development of newly pigmented lesions in adults; irregular borders; and variegation of color within a pigmented lesion. The most important clinical sign is a change in color or size of a pigmented lesion. The depth of the tumor correlates directly with the risk of metastasis. Dysplastic nevi are precursors to malignant melanoma.

VASCULITIDES

Goodpasture Syndrome

Goodpasture syndrome is an autoimmune disorder of unknown origin, characterized by a triad of diffuse **pulmonary hemorrhage, glomerulonephritis, and antiglomerular basement membrane (anti-GBM) antibodies.** Anti-GBM antibodies are specifically targeted against type IV collagen, which makes up most of the basement membrane. The disease is associated with **HLA-DR2;** there is a male predominance.

PRESENTATION

Most patients present with hemoptysis, cough, and dyspnea. Fever, chills, nausea, and vomiting can often accompany the pulmonary symptoms. Renal symptoms may rapidly progress to include azotemia and volume overload. Generally, the disease represents a medical emergency in young men and elderly women.

DIAGNOSIS

A diagnosis is made by demonstrating circulating anti-GBM antibodies based on suspicion raised by the clinical picture. A lung or renal biopsy may be needed to demonstrate the presence of anti-GBM antibodies in the tissues.

TREATMENT

Aggressive treatment for Goodpasture syndrome includes corticosteroids, cyclophosphamide, and plasmapheresis in order to remove the circulating anti-GBM antibodies. Patients in acute renal failure may require dialysis.

PROGNOSIS

Goodpasture syndrome is a medical emergency, and prognosis depends on the progression of the disease at diagnosis. Currently, the 5-year survival rates are about 80%. However, most patients who survive develop ESRD, with approximately 30% requiring long-term dialysis.

Giant-Cell Arteritis (Temporal Arteritis)

Giant-cell arteritis (GCA) is primarily a large-vessel vasculitis, characterized by granulomatous inflammation of the internal elastic lamina. It typically affects the temporal artery but can involve any of the large branches of the carotids or arteries originating from the aorta. Clinically, GCA is manifested by temporal headache and tenderness, jaw claudication, and occasional visual changes. Approximately 50% of patients have symptoms of polymyalgia rheumatica (neck and proximal upper and lower extremity myalgias).

PRESENTATION

Patients usually complain of headaches, typically with scalp tenderness, vision disturbances, jaw claudication, and constitutional symptoms. The disease affects older individuals (rarely < 50 years of age). With increasing age, the incidence of GCA increases; it is almost 10 times more common among patients in their 80s than those in their 50s. It is predominantly reported in white women (female-to-male ratio of 2:1) of Northern European descent.

DIAGNOSIS

The vast majority of patients present with an ESR > 50 mm/h, making this the most useful laboratory test, although it has low specificity. The diagnosis is usually suspected based on the clinical syndrome, but definitive diagnosis requires positive findings on temporal artery biopsy, including fragmentation of the intima with mononuclear and giant-cell infiltrates. However, the arteritis may have segmental involvement, so a negative biopsy does not exclude the diagnosis.

TREATMENT

High-dose prednisone remains the cornerstone of therapy and is begun based on high clinical suspicion rather than awaiting the results of biopsy. Treatment with slowly tapering doses of steroids usually continues for 12–18 months. Some patients are chronically maintained on very low dose (< 5 mg/day) prednisone or may require steroid-sparing medication (eg, methotrexate). Long-term steroid therapy requires prophylaxis against steroid-induced osteoporosis.

PROGNOSIS

The most dreaded complication, and a major source of morbidity, is loss of vision. This occurs in up to 15% of patients and is due to ischemic optic neuritis.

The risk of death from temporal arteritis appears to be increased within the first 4 months of starting therapy; this is mainly due to vascular complications such as stroke or myocardial infarction.

Polyarteritis Nodosa

Polyarteritis nodosa (PAN) is characterized by inflammation of small and medium-sized arteries and typically affects the vessels of skin, peripheral nerves, kidneys, joints, and the GI tract. Histologically, the findings involve a transmural necrotizing inflammation of small- and medium-sized arteries, which can lead to arterial wall weakening, luminal obstruction, and aneurysm formation with resultant downstream ischemic damage.

PRESENTATION

PAN is a rare disorder that primarily affects individuals 40–60 years of age. It is more common in **males,** with a male-to-female ratio of 2:1. Key clinical features suggestive of PAN include skin lesions (palpable purpura, tender nodular lesions, livedo reticularis, and infarcts of the fingertips), peripheral neuropathy, hypertension with renal sediment abnormalities, orchitis in males (swelling of the testicles), and constitutional symptoms. GI involvement due to mesenteric arteritis is seen in 30% of the patients.

DIAGNOSIS

Elevated ESR, normocytic anemia, and decreased complement are usually present but findings are nonspecific. Hepatitis B surface antigen is present in 10–50% of the cases. By definition, antineutrophil cytoplasmic antibodies (ANCA) are absent in PAN. Definitive diagnosis requires obtaining a biopsy specimen from accessible involved tissue (eg, skin, muscle, nerve) or imaging (ie, angiography). The pathologic feature defining classic PAN is a focal segmental necrotizing vasculitis of medium-sized and small arteries (Figure 5-44).

TREATMENT

High-dose corticosteroids remain the standard of care. Cytotoxic medications, such as cyclophosphamide, are added to corticosteroids in patients with major organ involvement.

PROGNOSIS

Outcome depends on the presence and extent of visceral and central nervous system (CNS) involvement. Most deaths occur within the first year, usually as a result of uncontrolled vasculitis, delay in diagnosis, or complications of treatment. Left untreated, PAN has a 3-month mortality rate approaching 50%. However, corticosteroid therapy drastically improves prognosis, raising

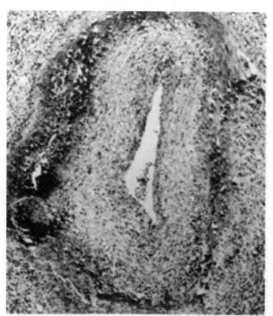 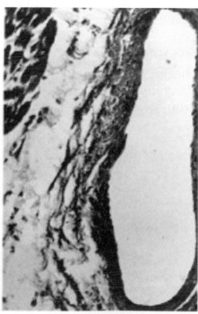

FIGURE 5-44. **Polyarteritis nodosa (PAN).** Histologic appearance (heamatoxylin and eosin stain) of a typical acute lesion of PAN in a medium-sized artery (*left*) compared with a normal artery (*right*). (Reproduced with permission from Fuster V, O'Rourke RA, Walsh RA, Poole-Wilson P, et al, eds. *Hurst's The Heart*, 12th ed. New York: McGraw-Hill, 2008: Figure 55-37.)

the 5-year survival rate to about 50% with a single agent and 70% with multiple agents.

Buerger Disease

Buerger disease, also known as thromboangiitis obliterans (TAO), is a vasculopathy of small- and medium-sized arteries. Characterized by segmental vascular inflammation and the absence of atheromas, it is most notable for a strong association with **heavy tobacco smoking.** Most people affected are 20–45 years of age and generally male. However, this gender discrepancy is thought to be due to the higher prevalence of smoking among males

PRESENTATION

Usually presenting in younger patients who smoke, Buerger disease is characterized by distal extremity ischemia, claudication, and pain at rest (Figure 5-45). Persistent ischemic ulcers or gangrene of the digits and Raynaud phenomenon are also commonly present.

DIAGNOSIS

No specific laboratory tests or definitive histologic findings are helpful in establishing the diagnosis, which is based on clinical (including angiographic) findings. TAO is a diagnosis of exclusion, as many conditions, including atherosclerosis, emboli, autoimmune disease, hypercoagulable states, and diabetes, can mimic the symptoms.

TREATMENT

The only proven treatment for Buerger disease is the **complete discontinuation of tobacco use,** which has been shown to stop disease progression. Treatment of local ischemic ulceration can be attempted with a trial of calcium channel blockers. Limb amputation is sometimes necessary if the degree of damage is severe.

PROGNOSIS

There is a stark difference in prognosis for those patients who completely discontinue tobacco use and those who do not. More than 94% of patients who quit smoking avoid amputation, whereas among those who do not, 8-year amputation rates approach 43%. Of note, even when amputations are

 KEY FACT

Treat Buerger disease with smoking cessation!

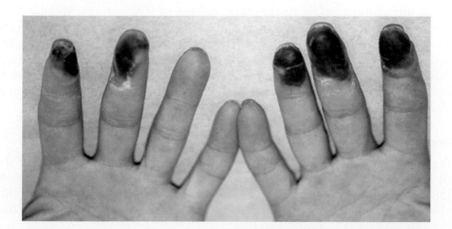

FIGURE 5-45. **Buerger disease.** Clinical appearance of the hands in a patient with Buerger disease, displaying digital ischemia and gangrene. (Reproduced with permission from Imboden JB, Hellmann DB, Stone JH. *Current Rheumatology Diagnosis & Treatment*, 2nd ed. New York: McGraw-Hill, 2007: Figure 42-1.)

not required, claudication and Raynaud phenomenon often persist in those unwilling to abstain from tobacco use.

Takayasu Arteritis

Takayasu arteritis (TA), or **pulseless disease,** is a granulomatous inflammatory vasculitis of large arteries, including the aorta and its branches. Its mortality and morbidity arise from inflammation leading to aneurysm formation, stenosis, and thrombosis of large arteries. Inflammation may also eventually cause ischemic changes such as stroke, transient ischemic attacks, visual disturbances, and chest and abdominal pain.

PRESENTATION

Patients are typically young women, ranging in age from teens to thirties. The disease is particularly common in Asian populations. The presenting symptoms are usually constitutional (malaise, fever, and weight loss), and diagnosis is often delayed. Not uncommonly, the diagnosis is made when a mediastinal mass suspected to be a tumor turns out to be an aortic aneurysm. Up to 10% present without symptoms—the incidental finding of unequal pulses, unequal blood pressures, bruits, or hypertension prompts further evaluation.

DIAGNOSIS

There are no specific markers for TA. An important diagnostic clinical sign is a blood pressure that differs by more than 30 mm Hg between the two arms. Additionally, asymmetrical pulses, abdominal bruits, and retinal hemorrhages can be seen. Arteriography and magnetic resonance angiography (MRA) are imaging modalities commonly used for diagnosing TA. The lesions are most often long-segment stenoses or arterial occlusions of the aorta and visceral vessels at their aortic origin. Due to the involvement of large arteries, biopsies are not performed.

TREATMENT

The main treatment for TA is high-dose systemic steroid therapy. Methotrexate and cyclophosphamide are used in patients who do not respond or in those patients in whom the minimally effective steroid dose is inappropriately too high for chronic use.

PROGNOSIS

Given the chronic relapsing-remitting nature of TA, patients require long periods of steroid treatment, which carries significant risks and side effects. Although the overall 15-year survival rate is reported to be as high as 90%, the morbidity and mortality depend on the degree of vascular and organ damage. This damage can include aneurysm formation, aortic insufficiency, hypertension, and vision changes. Sudden death may occur as a result of myocardial infarction, stroke, or aneurysm rupture.

Wegener Granulomatosis

Wegener granulomatosis (WG) is a small-vessel necrotizing vasculitis of the upper and lower respiratory tracts, extravascular granulomatous inflammation, glomerulonephritis, and variable involvement of other organ systems (Table 5-14). Renal involvement is usually asymptomatic until advanced uremia develops—a very poor prognostic sign.

TABLE 5-14. Comparison of Wegener Granulomatosis and Goodpasture Syndrome

	WEGENER GRANULOMATOSIS	GOODPASTURE SYNDROME
Pathogenesis	Autoimmune destruction of medium- and small-sized blood vessels.	Antibodies against the basement membrane.
Systems affected	Upper respiratory, lung, and renal involvement.	Lung and renal involvement.
Diagnosis	(+) c-ANCA.	(+) Anti-GBM. Linear staining on Immunofluorescence

c-ANCA = cytoplasmic antineutrophilic antibody; GBM = glomerular basement membrane.

PRESENTATION

WG affects patients of all ages, both sexes, and all races, although it is more commonly seen in whites. Patients usually present with constitutional symptoms, chronic sinusitis, epistaxis, mucosal ulcerations, oral ulcers, and occasionally chronic otitis media. Care must be taken in diagnosis, as the initial presentation is often misinterpreted as allergic or infectious in origin.

Pulmonary manifestations range from a complete lack of symptoms to chronic cough, alveolar hemorrhage, and pneumonitis. Renal disease is present in approximately 15% of patients initially and ultimately affects 50%.

DIAGNOSIS

In addition to clinical findings, diagnosis of WG is suspected by demonstrating the presence of cytoplasmic antineutrophilic antibody (**c-ANCA**) and anti-proteinase 3 antibodies (98% specificity). Diagnostic, biopsy results include small-vessel vasculitis, focal necrosis, and granulomatous changes.

TREATMENT

The mainstay of treatment is initially with high-dose systemic steroids and an additional immunosuppressive. Additional treatments include methotrexate for disease limited to the upper respiratory tract and cyclophosphamide for more aggressive disease involvement. Trimethoprim-sulfamethoxazole (TMP-SMX) is used for maintenance therapy and while on cyclophosphamide to prevent *Pneumocystis jiroveci* pneumonia (PCP). IV immunoglobulins and plasmapheresis have been used in cases refractory to immunosuppressive therapy and in those with rapidly progressive glomerulonephritis.

PROGNOSIS

When left untreated, WG is a rapidly fatal disease. Mortality is usually caused by renal failure and pulmonary complications within 5 months of diagnosis. However, aggressive immunosuppressive therapy leads to improvement in more than 90% of patients, with about 75% achieving remission. Unfortunately, due to its relapsing nature, WG still carries an associated 20% mortality rate.

Churg-Strauss Vasculitis

Churg-Strauss syndrome is a necrotizing vasculitis affecting both medium and small vessels. It is often characterized by constitutional symptoms, prominent involvement of the respiratory tract with asthma-like symptoms, and skin lesions, including palpable purpura and subcutaneous nodules.

PRESENTATION

Patients usually present with new-onset allergies and asthma or sudden worsening of preexisting allergic conditions. If severe, they may also have skin, kidney, heart, or liver involvement.

DIAGNOSIS

As the symptoms can often be confused with WG, laboratory studies are helpful to distinguish between the two. Unlike WG, patients with Churg-Strauss have a positive perinuclear antineutrophilic antibody (p-ANCA). They also often have marked peripheral eosinophilia. Definitive diagnosis is made by biopsy of involved tissue showing a prominence of eosinophils.

TREATMENT

Treatment consists of high-dose steroids and immunosuppressives, as with many of the other vasculitides.

PROGNOSIS

Unfortunately, even with steroids, prognosis is poor. The 5-year survival rate is only 50%, with death occurring primarily due to cardiac and pulmonary complications.

Kawasaki Disease

Kawasaki disease (KD) is a febrile vasculitis of childhood characterized by fever, rash, conjunctivitis, (usually unilateral) cervical adenopathy, mucocutaneous symptoms, and coronary artery aneurysms. Although its cause remains unknown, it is likely due to a combination of infectious and autoimmune causes. Currently, KD is the leading cause of acquired cardiac disease in young children.

PRESENTATION

Diagnosis of KD is challenging due to its nonspecific and general presentation. It is a disease of young children with a peak incidence at 9–12 months of age. Children < 2 years of age typically present with fever that is unresponsive to antibiotics, and they are often found to be disproportionately irritable. Presenting signs also include erythema, desquamation and edema of the extremities, conjunctivitis, rash, lymphadenopathy, strawberry tongue, and swollen/fissured lips (Figure 5-46). KD is more common in the Japanese population and slightly more prevalent in males but can occur in any race and both genders.

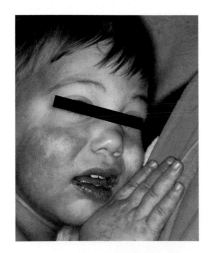

FIGURE 5-46. Kawasaki disease. Young patient presenting with cherry-red lips with hemorrhagic fissures, as well as erythema and edema of the fingertips. (Reproduced with permission from Wolff K, Johnson RA, Suurmond D. *Fitzpatrick's Color Atlas & Synopsis of Clinical Dermatology*, 5th ed. New York: McGraw-Hill, 2005: 425.)

DIAGNOSIS

Criteria for the diagnosis of KD include:

- Prolonged high-grade fever > 5 days.
- Conjunctivitis.
- Cracking and fissuring of lips with inflammation of mucosal membranes (strawberry tongue).
- Unilateral cervical lymphadenopathy.

- Rash involving the trunk and extremities.
- Erythema and edema of the hands and feet, progressing to desquamation.

To meet the diagnosis, four of the above criteria plus prolonged fever must be present.

TREATMENT

Treatment of KD is aimed at the prevention of coronary artery aneurysm formation and the resultant cardiac sequelae. IV immunoglobulins and high-dose aspirin are used as anti-inflammatory agents. Anticoagulation with dipyridamole is also considered. For those patients who do develop coronary artery complications, surgical stenting, bypass, and even heart transplantation may be necessary.

PROGNOSIS

Acute KD is self-limiting; however, the main source of long-term morbidity and mortality is the development of cardiac complications. These include myocarditis, pericarditis, congestive heart failure, and aortic insufficiency. Twenty percent of all patients develop **coronary artery aneurysms,** with a peak incidence in the first 1–2 weeks of illness.

Henoch-Schönlein Purpura

This small-vessel vasculitis is characterized clinically by palpable purpura, colicky abdominal pain, arthritis, and hematuria. Although its exact cause is unknown, histologically it is caused by IgA, C3, and immune complex deposition in arterioles, venules, and capillaries. Henoch-Schönlein purpura (HSP) is a multisystem disease and tends to involve skin, connective tissues, joints, kidneys, the GI tract, and the scrotum. Importantly, HSP and IgA nephropathy are related disorders, with the key difference being that IgA nephropathy generally only involves the kidneys and affects young adults almost exclusively, whereas HSP has other organ involvement and predominantly affects younger children.

PRESENTATION

Patients with HSP typically present in the spring, fall, or winter. The median age at presentation is 4 years, and the male-to-female ratio is about 1.5:1. Close to 50% have a history of preceding upper respiratory tract infection. Even when not evident on presentation, almost all patients develop rash and palpable purpura, predominantly on the lower extremities, at some time during their illness. Palpable purpura refers to large areas of raised bruising stemming from extravasation of RBCs from vessels secondary to low or nonfunctional platelets. Renal involvement is usually mild. Testicular swelling and a history of bloody stools may also be elicited.

DIAGNOSIS

HSP is a clinical diagnosis, as most laboratory values tend to be within normal ranges. Renal tests and urinalysis may be abnormal if the kidneys are involved.

TREATMENT

Treatment is mainly conservative and symptomatic. NSAIDs are used to relieve joint pain. Even though NSAIDs do not seem to result in further platelet inhibition or increased purpura, caution must still be taken in patients with affected kidney function. Although no data exist to support their effectiveness, corticosteroids are occasionally used.

TABLE 5-15. **Common Symptoms and Findings in High-Yield Vasculitides**

DISORDER	VASCULITIS	EPIDEMIOLOGY/ETIOLOGY	CLINICAL/LAB FINDINGS
Large artery			
Takayasu arteritis ("pulseless disease")	Granulomatous thickening of aortic arch and associated vessels.	Asian women < 40 years old.	Absent/weak upper extremity pulses, ocular disturbances, fever, arthritis, stroke.
Medium artery			
Giant-cell (temporal) arteritis	Most common vasculitis affecting medium and large arteries. Granulomatous vasculitis commonly involving the superficial temporal artery.	Elderly women > 50 years of age.	Unilateral temporal headache, jaw claudication and impaired vision from ophthalmic artery occlusion. Associated with polymyalgia rheumatica and ↑ ESR.
Polyarteritis nodosa	Necrotizing immune complex inflammation of medium arteries (typically renal and visceral vessels).	Middle-aged men. Associated with hepatitis B in 30% of patients.	Vessels at all stages of inflammation. Organ infarctions in kidneys, heart, bowels, and skin lead to renal failure, acute MI, bloody diarrhea, ischemic ulcers.
Kawasaki disease	Necrotizing vasculitis involving coronary arteries.	Self-limiting disease in children < 4 years of age.	Fever, congested conjunctiva, desquamating rash, swelling of hands and feet, cervical adenopathy. Abnormal ECG.
Thromboangiitis obliterans (Buerger disease)	Idiopathic, segmental, thrombosing vasculitis.	Seen in heavy smokers.	Intermittent claudication, Raynaud phenomenon, may lead to gangrene.
Small artery			
Wegener granulomatosis	Focal necrotizing vasculitis and granulomas in the upper airways, lungs, and kidneys.	Children and adults.	Perforation of nasal septum, sinusitis, otitis media, cough, hemoptysis, hematuria. c-ANCA (+)/anti-PR3 (+).
Microscopic polyangiitis	Similar to Wegener granulomatosis but lacking granulomas.	Children and adults.	Vessels at same stage of inflammation. p-ANCA (+).
Churg-Strauss syndrome	Granulomatous vasculitis with eosinophilia.	Often seen in atopic patients.	Allergic rhinitis, asthma, and eosinophilia. p-ANCA (+).
Henoch-Schönlein purpura	Involves skin, GI tract, renal vessels.	Most common form of childhood vasculitis.	Palpable purpura of buttocks and lower extremities, polyarthritis, glomerulonephritis, and GI bleeding.

c-ANCA = cytoplasmic antineutrophilic antibody; ECG = electrocardiogram; ESR = erythrocyte sedimentation rate; MI = myocardial infarction; p-ANCA = perinuclear antineutrophilic antibody.

PROGNOSIS

Most (97%) children have a self-limited course lasting 1–2 weeks. However, approximately 20% have a recurrence during the first year. A small percentage of patients have persistent purpura, with or without renal involvement. Less than 1% of all cases progress to ESRD.

See Table 5-15 for high-yield features of each of the previously discussed vasculitides.

Pharmacology

DRUGS USED TO TREAT DISORDERS OF BONE

Bisphosphonates (Risedronate, Alendronate, Clodronate, Etidronate, Ibandronate, Pamidronate, Tiludronate, Zoledronate)

MECHANISM

Bind to bone, inhibit osteoclast-mediated bone resorption, and indirectly stimulate osteoblast activity.

USES

Osteoporosis, Paget disease, hypercalcemia, metastatic bone disease.

SIDE EFFECTS

GI disturbances (dyspepsia, reflux esophagitis, peptic ulcers), and bone pain.

Calcitonin

MECHANISM

Inhibits bone resorption, leading to decreased blood calcium and phosphate. Calcitonin binds to receptors on osteoclasts and inhibits their action. In the kidney, calcitonin decreases the resorption of both calcium and phosphate in the proximal tubules.

USES

Hypercalcemia, neoplasia, Paget disease, postmenopausal osteoporosis, corticosteroid-induced osteoporosis.

SIDE EFFECTS

Nausea, vomiting, tingling sensation in the hands, unpleasant taste in the mouth.

Teriparatide (Recombinant Parathyroid Hormone [Forteo])

MECHANISM

Stimulates Ca^{2+} absorption in the renal distal convoluted tubules and the release of calcium from bone through a G protein-coupled receptor.

USES

Osteoporosis.

MNEMONIC

Calci**ton**in **tones** down serum calcium levels by inhibiting osteoclast action and calcium phosphate resorption.

SIDE EFFECTS

Nausea, headache, dizziness, hypercalcemia, leg cramps.

Selective Estrogen Receptor Modulators (SERMs) (Raloxifene, Tamoxifen)

MECHANISM

Activates estrogen receptors in bone and the cardiovascular system but has antagonist activity on estrogen receptors in mammary tissue or the uterus. SERMs also inhibit cytokines, recruit osteoclasts, and block PTH's bone-resorbing, calcium-mobilizing action.

USES

Osteoporosis prevention, breast cancer.

SIDE EFFECTS

Hot flashes, postmenopausal vasomotor symptoms, flushing, and increased risk of deep vein thrombosis and pulmonary embolism—tamoxifen is contraindicated in patients with a history of either. Tamoxifen may increase the risk of endometrial carcinoma via partial agonist effects.

TNF-α Antagonists (Adalimumab, Certolizumab, Etanercept, Golimumab, Infliximab)

MECHANISM

Block inflammatory cytokine TNF-α.

USES

RA, psoriasis, psoriatic arthritis, ankylosing spondylitis.

SIDE EFFECTS

Hypersensitivity, infection, exacerbation of heart failure, neuropathy, and risk of malignancy (skin cancer, possibly development of lymphoproliferative diseases).

DRUGS USED TO TREAT GOUT

Colchicine

MECHANISM

Prevents neutrophil and leukocyte migration into the joint by binding to tubulin, depolymerizing microtubules, and interfering with motility and degranulation.

USES

Prophylaxis or relief of **acute** gout attack.

SIDE EFFECTS

GI disturbances, nausea, vomiting, abdominal pain, hepatic toxicity, and rarely neuromyotoxicity. Severe diarrhea and GI hemorrhage may be a problem with large doses or standard doses in the setting of renal insufficiency. Since NSAIDs and steroids are potentially less toxic, they are more commonly used in acute attacks.

Xanthine Oxidase Inhibitors (Allopurinol, Febuxostat)

MECHANISM

Reduces the synthesis of uric acid by inhibiting the enzyme xanthine oxidase (Figure 5-47). For chronic use to prevent gout by lowering serum urate levels, but ineffective, and may aggravate acute gout.

USES

Both agents used in the long-term prevention of gout. Allopurinol is additionally used for prevention of urate nephrolithiasis and tumor lysis syndrome.

SIDE EFFECTS

- Allopurinol: GI disturbances, liver function test abnormalities, and allergic skin reactions.
- Febuxostat: GI disturbances, liver function test abnormalities.

Probenecid

MECHANISM

Inhibits the absorption of uric acid in the proximal convoluted tubule, thus increasing uric acid excretion (see Figure 5-47). Be careful prescribing penicillins for patients on probenecid, as coadministration can lead to increased penicillin levels. Must have adequate renal function and is contraindicated if the patient has a history of nephrolithiasis.

USES

Chronic gout.

SIDE EFFECTS

Dyspepsia and peptic ulceration. Hypersensitivity reactions occur occasionally as skin rashes. Drug-induced nephritic syndrome has been reported.

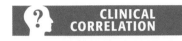

Allopurinol is also used in lymphoma and leukemia to prevent tumor lysis syndrome and is associated with urate neuropathy

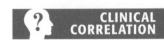

Probenecid promotes plasma penicillin levels.

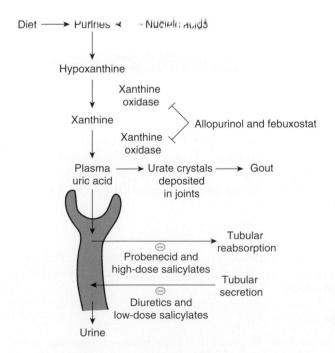

FIGURE 5-47. **Pharmacologic interventions in gout.**

DRUGS USED TO TREAT CONNECTIVE TISSUE DISEASES

Corticosteroids

MECHANISM

By complexing with cytosolic receptors, corticosteroids can enter the nucleus and alter gene expression through tissue-specific nuclear response elements. This leads to inhibition of inflammatory cytokine production and relief of mucosal inflammation. Corticosteroids also reduce bronchial reactivity, increase airway caliber, and reduce the frequency of asthma exacerbations.

USES

Reduction of disease flare-ups, acute inflammation, and asthma.

SIDE EFFECTS

With short-term use, these can include sleeping difficulties, dyspepsia, increased appetite, tremulousness, and anxiety/psychosis. Long-term use can lead to Cushing syndrome, obesity, diabetes, osteoporosis, and immune suppression.

Cyclophosphamide

MECHANISM

The liver metabolizes cyclophosphamide into its active form, phosphoramide mustard. This form cross-links DNA and inhibits T- and B-cell function.

USES

Severe disease in patients with SLE, RA, vasculitis syndromes, and certain cancers (breast, ovarian and non-Hodgkin lymphoma).

SIDE EFFECTS

Ovarian failure, infertility, bone marrow suppression, **hemorrhagic cystitis,** increased risk for malignancy.

DRUGS USED TO TREAT PAIN

Opioids

MECHANISM

Opiates facilitate the opening of potassium channels, causing hyperpolarization that inhibits calcium channel opening and transmitter release. There are three different types of opioid receptors: μ (morphine), δ (enkephalin), and κ (dynorphin). All opioid receptors are linked through G proteins and inhibition of adenylate cyclase.

USES

Pain relief, cough suppression (dextromethorphan), diarrhea (loperamide and diphenoxylate), acute pulmonary edema, and as maintenance for opioid addicts (methadone).

SIDE EFFECTS

Sedation, respiratory depression, constipation, nausea, miosis (pinpoint pupils), and additive CNS depression with other drugs. Opioid antagonists such as naloxone and naltrexone can be given for overdose, as these drugs occupy the opioid receptors without exerting any effect. Supplemental O_2 is contraindicated in morphine overdose in the patient with COPD, as it might further suppress the patient's respiratory drive and contribute to respiratory failure.

Aspirin

MECHANISM

Acetylates and **irreversibly** inhibits cyclooxygenase (both COX-1 and COX-2) to prevent conversion of arachidonic acid to prostaglandins. Aspirin may increase bleeding but has no effect on PT or PTT.

USES

Antipyretic, analgesic, anti-inflammatory, antiplatelet activity, Kawasaki disease, OA, and inflammatory arthritides.

SIDE EFFECTS

Gastric ulceration, bleeding, hyperventilation, Reye syndrome, tinnitus.

Nonsteroidal Anti-inflammatory Drugs (Ibuprofen, Naproxen, Indomethacin, Ketorolac, and Others)

MECHANISM

Reversibly inhibit arachidonic acid and cyclooxygenase (COX-1 and COX-2), thus inhibiting production of prostaglandins and thromboxanes (Figure 5-48). COX-1 is a constitutive enzyme expressed in most tissues, including platelets. COX-2 is induced in inflammatory cells upon activation. NSAIDs increase bleeding time but have no effect on prothrombin time (PT) or partial thromboplastin time (PTT).

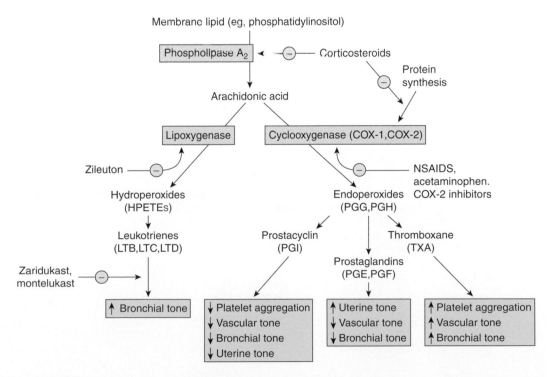

FIGURE 5-48. **Mediators derived from arachidonic acid.** Summary of mediators derived from arachidonic acid and their actions, and sites of action for anti-inflammatory drugs. (Adapted with permission from Katzung BG, Trevor AJ. *Pharmacology: Examination and Board Review,* 5th ed. Stamford, CT: Appleton & Lange, 1998: 150. Copyright © McGraw-Hill.)

USES

Anti-inflammatory, analgesic, antipyretic, and antiplatelet effects. Indomethacin is used to close a patent ductus arteriosus.

SIDE EFFECTS

Renal damage, aplastic anemia, GI distress, ulcers, fluid retention, and hypertension.

Cyclooxygenase-2 Inhibitors (Celecoxib)

MECHANISM

Selectively inhibit cyclooxygenase-2 (COX-2) found in inflammatory cells. Unlike nonspecific NSAIDs, COX-2 inhibitors spare the gastric mucosa from the corrosive effects of COX-1 inhibition.

USES

Analgesic effects for headache, dysmenorrhea, backache, and bony metastases. COX-2 inhibitors are also used for anti-inflammatory effects in chronic or acute inflammatory conditions such as RA, related connective tissue disorders, gout, muscle strains, and soft tissue diseases.

SIDE EFFECTS

Side effects are similar to those of other NSAIDs but with less GI mucosa toxicity (ie, lower incidence of ulcers and bleeding). There is a small, but potentially clinically relevant, increased risk of cardiovascular events with COX-2 inhibitors when compared with nonselective NSAIDs although even selective NSAIDs may increase risk.

Acetaminophen

MECHANISM

Reversibly and weakly inhibits cyclooxygenase and is peripherally inactivated. Most of the effects are centered in the CNS.

USES

Antipyretic and analgesic but no effect on inflammation.

SIDE EFFECTS

Significant hepatic necrosis can occur with high doses, as hepatic metabolism of acetaminophen depletes glutathione supplies needed for their antioxidant properties. Liver damage can be prevented if N-acetylcysteine or methionine are given, as they regenerate glutathione.

CHAPTER 6

Neurology

Embryology

NERVOUS SYSTEM DEVELOPMENT

KEY FACT

By week 3, there are three layers of embryonic tissue: the ectoderm, the mesoderm, and the endoderm.

The nervous system is one of the first systems to develop. In the third gestational week, following gastrulation, the neural tube forms, and neural crest cells emerge and migrate, beginning the precisely controlled development of the central and peripheral nervous systems, respectively.

Gastrulation

During week 3 of embryogenesis, the three layers of embryonic tissue form through a process known as gastrulation (Figure 6-1):

- Ectodermal cells detach from the epiblast, the surface layer of the embryo, invaginate inward into a groove known as the **primitive streak,** and form the mesoderm and endoderm.
- Mesodermal cells in the primitive streak then migrate toward the head until blocked by the fused buccopharyngeal membrane at the primitive node (the most rostral part of primitive streak).
- In parallel, prenotochordal cells also invaginate and move rostrally, forming a line known as the **notochord** from the primitive node to the prechordal plate.

KEY FACT

Remnants of the **primitive streak** can become *sacrococcygeal teratomas.*

Neurulation

The primitive streak regresses and disappears, dragging the notochord toward the buccopharyngeal membrane.

The steps of neurulation are summarized in Figure 6-2.

- The notochord induces the overlying region of the ectoderm to form the **neural plate.**
- The neural plate begins to invaginate along the longitudinal axis and forms the **neural groove.**
- The neural groove continues to invaginate until the surrounding neural folds meet to form an open **neural tube,** the precursor to the central nervous system (CNS).
- The open neural tube then closes, starting in the center (at the middle of the future body) and progressing caudally and rostrally.

KEY FACT

The **notochord** becomes the nucleus pulposus, which lies within the vertebral column in the adult. Herniation of the nucleus pulposus through the annulus fibrosus may result in spinal root impingement and pain.

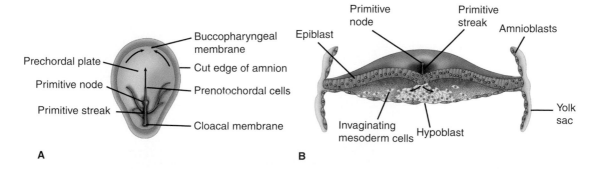

FIGURE 6-1. **Gastrulation.** (A) Topographical view of migrating cells during gastrulation. Invaginating mesoderm cells (prenotochordal cells) detach from the epiblast and migrate along the longitudinal axis to form the notochord. (B) Cross-sectional view of mesodermal cells detaching from the epiblast.

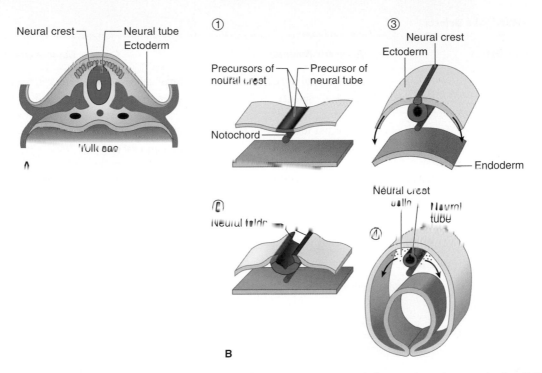

FIGURE 6-2. **Neurulation (in cross-section).** (A) The neural groove invaginates and closes to form the neural tube. (B1) The notochord initiates neural tube development by inducing formation of neuroepithelium. (B2) The neural tube precursors begin to fold and (B3) form the neural tube. (B4) Neural crest cells then initiate migration.

NEURAL TUBE DEFECTS

Failure of the neural tube to close at either end leads to birth defects.

- Failure of rostral neuropore closure leads to anencephaly, a condition characterized by the absence of the scalp, skull, and large portions of the cortex.
- Failure of caudal neuropore closure leads to spina bifida (Figure 6-3)

VARIATIONS OF SPINA BIFIDA

The clinical manifestations and severity of spina bifida vary depending on the degree of closure of the caudal/rostral neuropore as well as the location of the fusion defect (Table 6-1). Elevated α-fetoprotein in maternal serum or amniotic fluid is often suggestive of fetal neural tube defects.

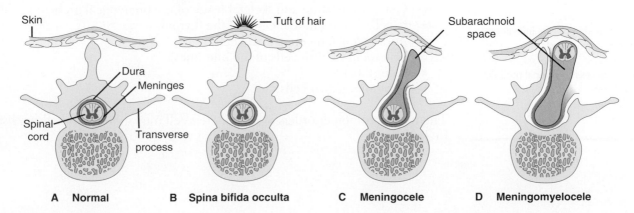

FIGURE 6-3. **Types of spina bifida.** (A–D) The severity of spina bifida correlates with the degree of herniation of the contents: (B) none, (C) meninges, and (D) meninges and spinal cord.

TABLE 6-1. Neural Tube Defects

NEURAL TUBE DEFECT	ABERRANT ANATOMY	CLINICAL MANIFESTATION
Spina bifida occulta	Failure of vertebral arches to close without herniation of intraspinal contents.	Small tuft of hair overlying the defect without any visible herniated contents.
Meningocele	Failure of vertebral arches to close with herniation of meninges but not spinal cord.	Protrusion of the dura and arachnoid, forming a lumbosacral cyst.
Meningomyelocele (*myelo* = neurons/cord)	Failure of vertebral arches to close with herniation of both meninges and spinal cord.	Herniated lumbosacral sac and, depending on the location, paralysis and loss of deep tendon reflexes and sensation in the lower extremities as well as incontinence. Associated with type II Arnold-Chiari syndrome.
Meningoencephalocele (*encephalo* = brain)	Herniation of meninges and brain.	Mental retardation.
Meningohydroencephalocele (*hydro* = CSF)	Herniation of meninges, brain, and CSF-containing ventricles.	Mental retardation.

CSF = cerebrospinal fluid.

CROSS-SECTION OF THE NEURAL TUBE

- The **neural tube** gives rise to the CNS, including the brain, brain stem, and spinal cord. In the brain stem and spinal cord, the dorsal alar plate, the ventral basal plate, and the intervening sulcus limitans develop within the central canal of the neural tube.
  - **Alar plate:** Gives rise to sensory neurons (lateral).
  - **Basal plate:** Gives rise to motor neurons (medial).
  - **Sulcus limitans:** Separates the two plates.
- **Neural crest cells** are derived from ectodermal cells. Ectoderm at the edges of the neural folds is induced by the neural tube to form neuroepithelia. These neural crest cells then migrate and give rise to multiple adult derivatives (see Figures 6-2 and 6-4), including:
  - Peripheral nervous system (PNS) ganglia and neurons.
  - Schwann cells.
  - Chromaffin cells of the adrenal medulla.
  - Melanocytes in the skin.
  - Connective tissue and skeletal tissue of the pharyngeal arches.
  - C cells (parafollicular cells) of the thyroid.
  - Aortic arch and conotruncal cells.
  - Enterochromaffin cells of the intestines.
  - Odontoblasts.
  - Leptomeningeal cells.

The most common disorders of neural crest cell migration include those listed in Table 6-2.

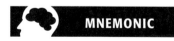 **MNEMONIC**

Neural Crest Derivatives—

ACE PreSCHOOL
Aortic arch
Connective/skeletal tissue of pharyngeal arches
Enterochromaffin cells of intestines
Peripheral nervous system
Schwann cells
CHromaffin cells of adrenal medulla
Odontoblasts
Melan**O**cytes
Leptomeninges

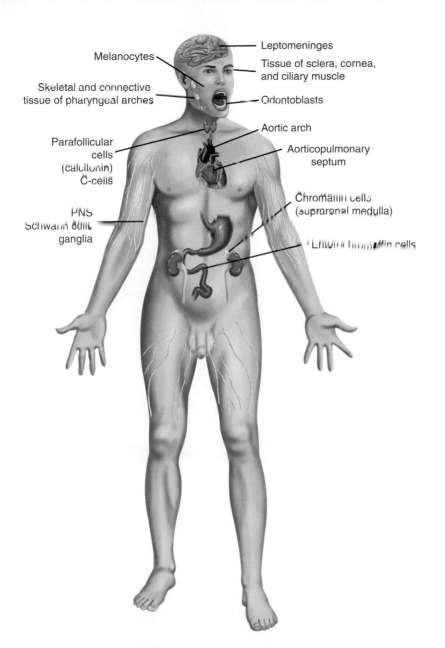

FIGURE 6-4.   Neural crest derivatives. The neural crest cells migrate peripherally from the neural tube to develop into the peripheral nervous system and other important structures.

TABLE 6-2.   Neural Crest Derivatives and Their Corresponding Defects

NEURAL CREST DERIVATIVE	DEFECT
Aortic arch/aorticopulmonary septum.	Great-vessel deformities.
Pharyngeal pouches 3 and 4.	DiGeorge syndrome.
Enterochromaffin cells.	Hirschsprung disease, achalasia.
Melanocytes.	Albinism.

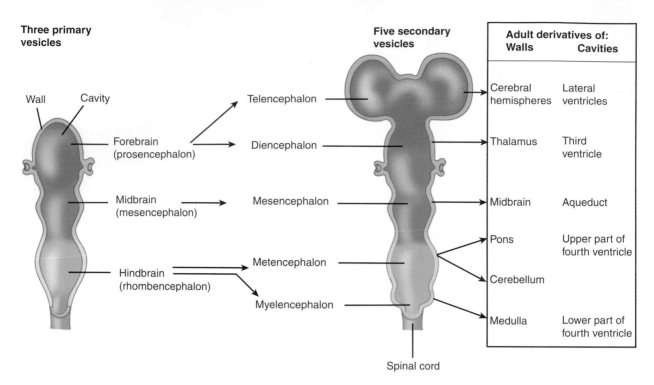

F I G U R E 6 - 5 .   **Development of brain vesicles.**

BRAIN DEVELOPMENT

Formation of Brain Vesicles

From week 6 onward, the neural tube forms three primary brain vesicles that give rise to five secondary vesicles. These secondary vesicles develop into various structures in the adult brain and associated CSF-filled cavities (Figure 6-5).

The three primary vesicles are:

- Forebrain (prosencephalon).
- Midbrain (mesencephalon).
- Hindbrain (rhombencephalon).

The five secondary vesicles are:

- Telencephalon (derived from the prosencephalon).
- Diencephalon (derived from the prosencephalon).
- Mesencephalon.
- Metencephalon (derived from the rhombencephalon).
- Myelencephalon (derived from the rhombencephalon).

Congenital Malformations

ARNOLD-CHIARI

Arnold-Chiari syndrome involves congenital herniation of the cerebellum through the foramen magnum (Figure 6-6).

- Occurs in 1 in 1000 live births.
- Type I: Herniation of cerebellar tonsils only.

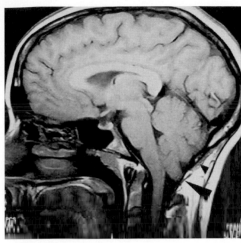
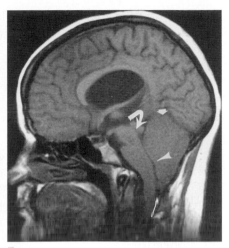

A   B

FIGURE 6-6. **Arnold-Chiari syndrome types I and II.** (A) The cerebellar tonsils (*large arrowhead*) herniate anterior to the posterior arch of the foramen magnum (*small arrowhead*). (B) A small posterior fossa is present, resulting in cerebellar tonsillar ectopia (*long arrow*), towering of the cerebellum (*short arrow*), breaking of the tectum (*curved arrow*), and compression of the fourth ventricle (*arrowhead*) with resulting hydrocephalus. Partial agenesis of the rostrum and splenium of the corpus callosum is noted. (Part A reproduced with permission from Brunicardi F. *Schwartz's Manual of Surgery*. New York: McGraw-Hill, 2006: 1651. Part B reproduced with permission from Chen M. *Basic Radiology*. McGraw-Hill, 2006: 334.)

- Type II: Breaking of the tectal plate, aqueductal stenosis, herniation and unrolling of the vermis into the vertebral canal, and stretching of cranial nerves (CN) IX, X, and XI. May also present with syringomyelia in C8–T1 and lumbar meningomyelocele.

PRESENTATION

- Type I may not show neurologic symptoms until adolescence or adult life and may include cerebellar ataxia, obstructive hydrocephalus, brain stem compression, and syringomyelia.
- Type II may manifest with:
  - Difficulty swallowing (due to compression of the nucleus ambiguus).
  - Loss of pain/temperature sensation along the back of the neck and shoulders secondary to syringomyelia, which interrupts the ascending afferent sensory fibers in the spinothalamic tract.
  - Mental retardation secondary to coincident meningomyelocele, a visible cyst containing spinal cord matter protruding from the dorsum of the spine.
  - Hydrocephalus due to occlusion of cerebrospinal fluid (CSF) flow through the foramen magnum.

PROGNOSIS

Depends on the degree of severity.

- Type I: Normal life span.
- Type II: Fifteen percent die within 1 year of birth. Death is usually due to cranial nerve and brain stem dysfunction resulting in respiratory failure.

DANDY-WALKER SYNDROME

Dandy-Walker syndrome occurs in 1 in 25,000 births, far less common than Arnold-Chiari syndrome. It is characterized by cerebellar vermis hypoplasia

> **KEY FACT**
>
> Syringomyelia = fluid-filled cavity (cyst) within the spinal cord that often manifests with a "capelike" distribution of sensory loss.

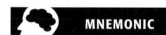

CLINICAL CORRELATION

Arnold-Chiari syndrome:

Features:

- Aqueductal stenosis
- Herniation and unrolling of vermis into vertebral canal

Type 1:

- May not show neurologic symptoms until adolescence or adulthood
- More common (1:1000)
- Only tonsils herniate

Type 2:

- Small posterior fossa
- True herniation of brain stem
- Psychomotor retardation and developmental delays are frequently observed
- Cervical syringomyelia and lumbar meningomyelocele often associated

Dandy-Walker syndrome:

Features:

- Cerebellar vermis hypoplasia
- Dilation of the fourth ventricle

MNEMONIC

Dandy-**Walker** has trouble with **walking.**

and failure of the foramina of Luschka and Magendie to open, resulting in dilation of the fourth ventricle (Figure 6-7).

PRESENTATION

Hydrocephalus, ataxia, and mental retardation.

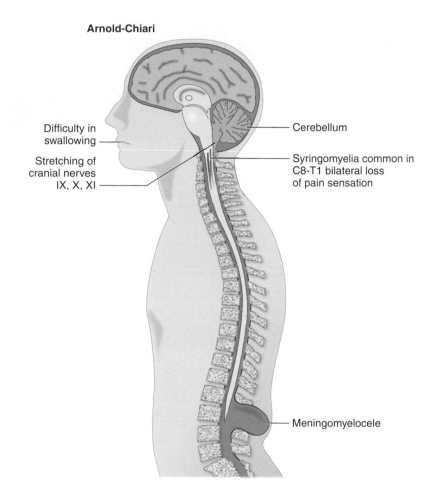

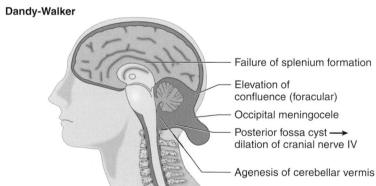

FIGURE 6-7. Comparison of Arnold-Chiari syndrome types I and II and Dandy-Walker syndrome. Arnold-Chiari syndrome is much more common and involves a "falling through" of the cerebellum. Dandy-Walker syndrome is an agenesis of the cerebellum and a expansion of the posterior fossa.

PROGNOSIS

Varies dramatically. Some patients may lead completely normal lives, and others die soon after birth. Overall, it carries a 12–50% mortality rate.

HYDROCEPHALUS

Hydrocephalus is defined as an abnormal accumulation of CSF in the ventricles, which in turn may lead to an increased intracranial pressure (ICP). The most common congenital cause is aqueductal stenosis, a consequence of maternal infection (eg, cytomegalovirus [CMV] or toxoplasmosis).

PRESENTATION

Enlarged cranium with thinning of the bones of the skull and cerebral cortex. Cranial sutures (fissures between plates of bones that make up the skull) do not close until many years after birth. The increased intracranial pressure pushes the bones apart, enlarging the skull and head circumference.

TREATMENT

Placement of an extraventricular shunt (eg, from the ventricle to the peritoneum), endoscopic third ventriculostomy (surgically reopening the blockage), or cauterization of ependymal cells to reduce CSF production.

PROGNOSIS

Depends on the degree of increased pressure. In severe cases, brain tissue is compressed and cannot form properly, resulting in mental retardation.

MICROCEPHALY

Microcephaly is characterized by small brain size. Growth of the skull depends on growth of the brain, so the head circumference is decreased secondary to the underlying defect in brain development. This may be due to genetic causes, prenatal infection, or exposure to teratogens (eg, toxoplasmosis, alcohol, radiation).

PRESENTATION

Small head size; 50% of patients have some degree of mental retardation.

PROGNOSIS

Depends on the severity and degree of mental retardation.

HOLOPROSENCEPHALY

Failure of midline cleavage of the forebrain. This can be seen in severe fetal alcohol syndrome and Patau syndrome (trisomy 13). The forebrain may lack midline features, including the corpus callosum, resulting in a single ventricle in the middle of the brain rather than bilateral ventricles (Figure 6-8).

PRESENTATION

Clinical symptoms can range from mild to severe. Extremely mild cases may only be identified via a single incisor. Severe cases, however, can present with cycloplegia, a lack of central midline structures, and a single ventricle. The degree of mental retardation depends on the extent to which structures are affected.

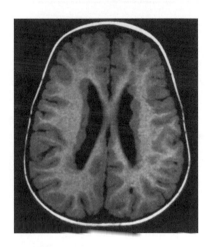

FIGURE 6-8. Holoprosencephaly. Note the lack of brain matter dividing the two hemispheres. (Reproduced with permission from Chen M. *Basic Radiology*. New York: McGraw-Hill, 2006: 332.)

 KEY FACT

Fetal alcohol syndrome is the most common cause of mental retardation. It is characterized by microcephaly, congenital heart disease, abnormal facies, and, in severe cases, holoprosencephaly.

KEY FACT

Patau syndrome (trisomy 13) is characterized by holoprosencephaly, microcephaly, polydactyly, cleft palate, narrow fingernails, and apneic spells. It is the rarest form of the viable trisomies (21, 18, and 13). Death occurs within 1 year.

MNEMONIC

The meninges PAD the brain from inside out:
Pia mater
Arachnoid
Dura mater

CLINICAL CORRELATION

Epidural hematoma:
- Lucid interval in 50% ("talk and die" syndrome).
- Middle meningeal artery is most commonly ruptured.

Subdural hematoma:
- More common than epidural.
- Cortical atrophy in elderly puts tension on bridging veins.
- May be associated with contusion, subarachnoid, and other hemorrhages.

Subarachnoid hemorrhage:
- Ruptured berry aneurysm.
- High intensity: "Worst headache of my life."
- Sudden onset: "thunderclap headache."
- Marfan, Ehlers-Danlos type 4.
- Autosomal dominant polycystic kidney disease, hypertension, smoking, blacks, ↑ age.

Intracerebral/parenchymal hemorrhage:
- Trauma, infarct, amyloid angiopathy, diabetes, hypertension (Charcot-Bouchard aneurysm).
- Many localize to basal ganglia or thalamus.

PROGNOSIS

Depends on severity. In mild cases, individuals may lead a normal life; in more severe cases, the condition may result in mental retardation and early death.

Key Terms

- Gyrus (pl. *gyri*) = outpouching fold of the brain.
- Sulcus = groove between gyri.
- Cortex = layers of gray matter that overlie the deeper white matter of the brain.
- Sylvian fissure = oblique groove that divides the temporal lobe from the parietal and frontal lobes.
- Central sulcus = major sulcus that runs coronally, dividing the frontal lobe from the parietal lobe.
- Nuclei = collection of neuron cell bodies (as opposed to axons) in the CNS, usually sharing a common function.

Meninges

Connective tissue that surrounds the CNS, including the brain and spinal cord. The meninges consist of **three** membranes:

- **Pia mater:** Delicate and highly *vascular;* closely adheres to the surface of the brain and spinal cord.
- **Arachnoid:** Delicate, *nonvascular* layer with **granulations** that absorb CSF.
- **Dura mater:** Dense, tough exterior layer.

The membranes form several potential and real spaces:

- **Subarachnoid space:** Lies between the pia and the arachnoid and contains CSF. It is a relatively narrow space over the surface of the cerebral hemispheres, but it becomes much wider at the base of the brain. It terminates at the S2 vertebrae.
- **Subdural space:** Lies between the arachnoid and the dura and is traversed by **bridging veins** in the brain.
- **Epidural space:** Potential space outside the dura that contains meningeal arteries. In the spinal cord, it contains fatty areolar tissue, lymphatics, and venous plexuses.

PATHOLOGY OF THE MENINGES

Meningeal tissues can be involved in several pathologic processes, including congenital malformation, bleeding, infection, and cancer. Bleeding in the meningeal spaces manifests differently depending on the source and location of the bleed.

EPIDURAL HEMORRHAGE

Usually due to blunt head trauma resulting in rupture of the middle meningeal artery. Imaging shows a biconvex collection of blood bordered by suture lines with lens-shaped enhancement and smooth borders.

SUBDURAL HEMORRHAGE

Usually due to deceleration injury resulting in rupture of the bridging veins. Venous bleeding accumulates slowly. Often accompanied by intracranial bleeds or contusions and presents as decline in mental status over days to weeks. Imaging shows enhancement of a crescent-shaped area that does *not* cross the midline but does cross dural attachments (suture lines), unlike **epidural hemorrhage.** Subdural hemorrhage is seen most often in the elderly as cortical atrophy puts increasing tension on bridging veins but can also be seen in alcoholics and shaken babies.

SUBARACHNOID HEMORRHAGE (SAH)

Usually due to a ruptured berry aneurysm in the circle of Willis. Presents as the sudden onset of the "worst headache of my life." Imaging may show enhancement in the area of the hemorrhage. Risk factors include hypertension, smoking, autosomal dominant polycystic kidney disease (ADPKD), and older age.

MENINGITIS

Inflammation of the meninges is often caused by bacterial, viral, or fungal infections.

- Bacterial meningitis: High fever, headache, nuchal rigidity, Kernig and Brudzinski signs present. The organism involved depends on the age of the patient.
- Viral meningitis (aseptic meningitis): Similar to bacterial, but less acute in onset with less severe symptoms.
- Fungal meningitis: Seen in immunocompromised patients, often due to *Cryptococcus.*
- Diagnosis made by lumbar puncture (Figure 6-9 and Table 6-3).

MENINGIOMA

Benign, well-circumscribed, slow-growing tumors. These occur more commonly in females than males. The patient often presents with headache or sudden paralysis and can be treated by resection or, rarely, radiation. These tumors are slow-growing and carry a favorable prognosis.

CARCINOMATOUS MENINGITIS

The meningeal space is a common site for metastatic spread from cancer outside the CNS. This condition is life threatening and may manifest with mental status changes and headaches. Cranial nerve deficits may be found on clinical exam. Treatment consists of chemotherapy delivered to the CSF (intrathecal).

Ventricles

Ventricles are interconnected spaces in the skull that contain CSF. CSF buffers the brain from impact, transports hormones, and removes waste products. CSF is produced by the **choroid plexus,** a tissue rich in blood vessels and covered with ciliated ependymal cells. It projects into the lateral, third, and

TABLE 6-3. Cerebrospinal Fluid Characteristics of the Different Types of Meningitis

	BACTERIAL	**FUNGAL**	**VIRAL**
Cell Type	PMN predominant	Lymphocyte predominant	Lymphocyte predominant
Glucose	Decreased	Decreased	Normal
Protein	Elevated	Slightly elevated	Slightly elevated

PMN = polymorphonuclear neutrophil.

KEY FACT

Meningismal signs manifest when the inflamed meninges are stretched.
- **Kernig sign:** Pain elicited while straightening knee with hip flexed at 90 degrees.
- **Brudzinski sign:** Patient flexes knees in response to passive flexion of the neck.

KEY FACT

In a lumbar puncture, the needle encounters the following layers:
- Skin
- Subcutaneous tissue
- Supraspinous/interspinous ligaments
- Ligamentum flavum
- Epidural fat
- Epidural space
- Dura mater
- Arachnoid mater
- Subarachnoid space

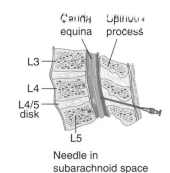

FIGURE 6-9. Lumbar puncture. The correct position may be located by finding the space between the spinous processes at the level of the iliac spine.

fourth ventricles, and contributes to the **blood-brain barrier (BBB),** a tight barrier that separates circulating blood from the CSF. Other components of the BBB combine to form a functional "neurovascular unit":

- Tight junctions between capillary endothelial cells.
- Basement membrane.
- Astrocyte processes.

The permeability of the BBB is characterized by:

- Increased permeability to nonpolar/lipid-soluble substances versus polar/water-soluble substances.
- Permeability to glucose and amino acids via carrier-mediated transport.
- Specialized circumventricular organs have an incomplete BBB and therefore can directly sense the concentrations of many compounds in the bloodstream without the need for specialized transport systems (eg, **area postrema, basal hypothalamus**).

VENTRICULAR SYSTEM

- Two lateral ventricles communicate with the third ventricle through the foramen of Monro (Figure 6-10).
- The third ventricle communicates with the fourth ventricle through the cerebral aqueduct (of Sylvius).
- The **fourth ventricle** communicates with the subarachnoid space via three outlet foramina: two **foramina of Luschka** and one **foramen of Magendie.** The foramina of Luschka drain laterally, and the foramen of Magendie drains medially (see Figure 6-10).

KEY FACT

The aqueduct is the most common site of stenosis.

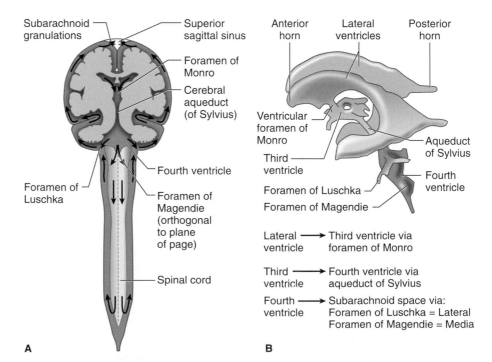

FIGURE 6-10. **Ventricular system.** (A) Note the flow of CSF from the lateral ventricles through the foramen of Monro to the third ventricle, through the aqueduct to the fourth ventricle, into the subarachnoid space through the foramina of Luschka and Magendie, and back into the dural venous sinuses via arachnoid granulations. (B) The same structures shown in sagittal view. (Part A adapted with permission from Morgan GE, Mikhail MS, Murray MJ. *Clinical Anesthesiology*, 4th ed. New York: McGraw-Hill, 2006: Figure 25-4.)

Hydrocephalus develops as a result of an excess accumulation of CSF in the ventricles, which in turn causes ventricular dilation. There are several forms:

- **Noncommunicating hydrocephalus:** Ventricles *do not* communicate with subarachnoid space, but CSF production remains constant. Obstruction between or within the ventricles (eg, congenital aqueductal stenosis).
- **Communicating hydrocephalus:** Ventricles *do* communicate with subarachnoid space. Can arise from three causes: (1) CSF oversecretion (eg, choroid papilloma); (2) CSF circulation blockage (eg, tumor in the subarachnoid space); and (3) poor CSF absorption through arachnoid granulations (eg, meningitis, postmeningitis adhesions, dural venous sinus thrombosis).
- **Normal pressure hydrocephalus:** Chronic form of communicating hydrocephalus with equilibration of CSF formation and absorption, often preceded by a high-pressure phase. Classic triad of symptoms includes urinary incontinence, dementia, and gait disturbance ("wet, wacky, and wobbly").
- **Hydrocephalus ex vacuo:** Expansion of ventricular volume secondary to loss of brain tissue, as seen in neurodegenerative conditions such as Alzheimer disease.
- **Pseudotumor cerebri** (benign intracranial hypertension): Increased resistance to CSF outflow. Seen in young obese women who present with headache, visual changes, and, less frequently, menstrual abnormalities or a history of oral contraceptive use. Exam reveals papilledema, increased ICP (detected by lumbar puncture), and slitlike ventricles on neuroimaging.

The site of ventricular dilation can indicate the site of mechanical obstruction in CSF flow:

- Obstruction in the **foramen of Monro** leads to dilated **lateral** ventricles.
- Obstruction in the **aqueduct of Sylvius** leads to a dilated **third** ventricle and **lateral** ventricles.
- Obstruction in the **fourth ventricle** leads to a dilated **aqueduct, third ventricle, and lateral ventricles.**

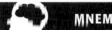

MNEMONIC

Mnemonic for normal pressure hydrocephalus: **wacky, wobbly, wet**
1. Progressive dementia **(wacky)**
2. Ataxic gait **(wobbly)**
3. Urinary incontinence **(wet)**

MNEMONIC

Pseudotumor cerebri can be caused by **A LOT A Stuff:**
Amiodarone
Lupus
Oral contraceptives
Tetracycline/venous **T**hrombosis
Vitamin **A** in high doses
Steroids

Blood Supply

CIRCLE OF WILLIS

The circle of Willis is a network of arteries that sits at the base of the brain in the area encircling the optic chiasm and pituitary gland. It is fed by two major arterial systems: the internal carotids (anterior circulation) and the vertebrobasilar system (posterior circulation; Figure 6-11).

The internal carotid artery gives rise to several branches before joining the circle of Willis:

- Ophthalmic artery: The first branch of the ophthalmic artery gives rise to the **central artery of the retina.** Its occlusion leads to sudden-onset blindness (amaurosis fugax).
- Anterior choroidal artery: Supplies the lateral geniculate nucleus (thalamic relay nucleus for vision), globus pallidus, and internal capsule.

Major components of the circle of Willis:

- Anterior cerebral artery (ACA): Supplies the medial aspect of the frontal lobes, including the lower extremity regions of the motor and sensory cortices.
- Anterior communicating artery: Most common site of **aneurysm** in the circle of Willis, giving rise to **bitemporal hemianopia.**

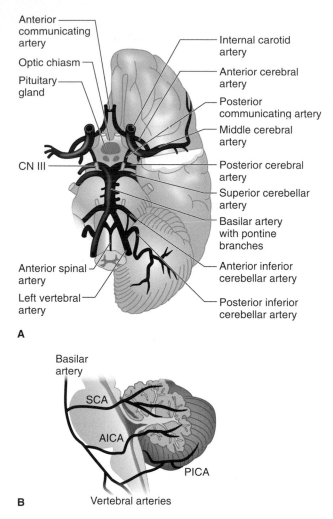

FIGURE 6-11. An inferior view of the Circle of Willis and a sagittal view of cerebellar blood supply. (A) At the center are the optic chiasm and the pituitary gland. Note how the basilar artery sprawls over the pons and how CN III emerges between the posterior cerebral artery (PCA) and the superior cerebellar artery (SCA). The location of CN III predisposes it to compression by PCA aneurysms. (B) Note the three regions of the cerebellum supplied by the SCA, anterior inferior cerebellar artery (AICA), and posterior inferior cerebellar artery (PICA).

- Middle cerebral artery (MCA): Supplies the lateral aspect of the hemispheres, including the trunk–face–upper extremity area of the motor and sensory cortices, as well as Broca and Wernicke speech areas. It is the most commonly involved artery in embolic stroke.
- The lateral striate branches of the MCA, which supply the internal capsule and basal ganglia, can be involved in nonembolic lacunar infarctions and commonly lead to pure motor hemiparesis, pure sensory hemiparesis, or mixed sensorimotor hemiparesis (Table 6-4).
- Posterior cerebral artery (PCA): Supplies the occipital lobe; hypoperfusion may lead to contralateral homonymous hemianopia with macular sparing. Aneurysms may be associated with CN III palsy.
- Posterior communicating artery: Another common site of aneurysms, which may be associated with CN III palsy.

Vertebrobasilar system:

- Anterior spinal artery: Supplies the ventral portion of the spinal cord; hypoperfusion manifests with weakness, loss of pain and temperature sensation, but sparing of position and vibratory sensation.

TABLE 6-4. **Neurologic Deficits Associated with Common Strokes**

RELEVANT CEREBRAL ARTERY	ASSOCIATED NEUROLOGIC DEFICIT
ACA	Contralateral lower extremity hemiplegia and/or sensory deficits.
MCA	Upper branch: face and arm hemiparesis, hemisensory loss, and nonfluent (Broca) aphasia. Lower branch: Fluent (Wernicke) aphasia.
PCA	Contralateral homonymous hemianopia.
PICA	Lateral medullary (Wallenberg) syndrome: ipsilateral facial and contralateral body pain/temperature sensory loss, nystagmus, ipsilateral vocal cord paralysis, and Horner syndrome.

ACA = anterior cerebral artery; MCA = middle cerebral artery; PCA = posterior cerebral artery; PICA = posterior inferior cerebellar artery

- Posterior inferior cerebellar artery (PICA): Supplies the medulla and the posterior inferior cerebellum; hypoperfusion manifests with lateral medullary (Wallenberg) syndrome.
- Anterior inferior cerebellar artery (AICA): Supplies the pons, CN VII, and the anterior inferior surface of the cerebellum; hypoperfusion manifests with lateral pontine syndrome.
- Pontine arteries (from basilar artery): Supply the base of the pons, including the corticospinal fibers and CN VI; hypoperfusion presents with "locked-in" syndrome in which the patient is aware but suffers from paralysis of all muscles except for those controlling extraocular movements.
- Superior cerebellar artery (SCA): Supplies the pons, the superior surface of the cerebellum, and CN VII and VIII; an aneurysm of the SCA can lead to compression of CN III, which manifests as a dilated pupil on the affected side.

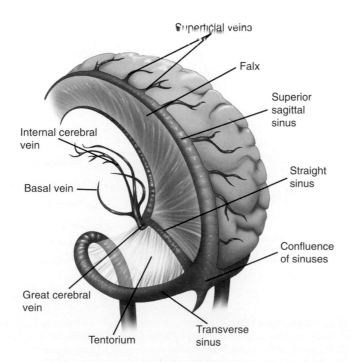

FIGURE 6-12. **Venous sinuses of the brain.** (Reproduced with permission from Waxman SG. *Clinical Neuroanatomy*, 26th ed. New York: McGraw-Hill, 2009.)

KEY FACT

The dural venous sinuses provide pathogens and neoplastic cells with a valveless path from the face/ sinuses through bridging veins to the brain.

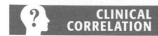
CLINICAL CORRELATION

Cavernous sinus syndrome results from increased pressure in the cavernous sinus and leads to **ophthalmoplegia and facial sensory loss.**

DURAL VEINS AND SINUSES

Superior cerebral ("bridging") veins drain into the superior sagittal sinus to the confluence of sinuses. Meanwhile, the **great cerebral vein of Galen** drains deep cerebral veins into the **straight sinus,** and then the confluence of sinuses (Figure 6-12). The superior sagittal sinus, great cerebral vein, and occipital sinus all drain into the confluence of sinuses, which in turn empties into the transverse sinus, the sigmoid sinus, the internal jugular vein, and finally into the superior vena cava. The cavernous sinuses drain into the superior and inferior petrosal sinuses, which drain into the transverse sinuses and sigmoid sinuses, respectively.

The **cavernous sinus** is a collection of venous sinuses surrounding the pituitary gland. It drains blood from the eye and superficial cortex and feeds into the jugular vein (Figure 6-13).

The cavernous sinus contains several structures.

- CN III, IV, V_1, V_2, VI, and postganglionic sympathetic fibers that supply the orbit.
- CN III, IV, V_1, and V_2 are attached to the wall of the sinus; CN VI is free floating and is most susceptible to impingement by an enlarging pituitary tumor.
- The internal carotid arteries pass through both sides of the sinus.
- Venous drainage from the face drains to the cavernous sinus, providing a route through which skin infections can reach the brain.

Cerebral Cortex

The cortex is composed of specialized regions that are responsible for specific functions. Thus, injury and lesions in different areas of the brain produce deficits appropriate to the function of that area (Figure 6-14). Brodmann labeled different areas of the brain by number; some of these areas are still referred to by these numbers (Figure 6-15).

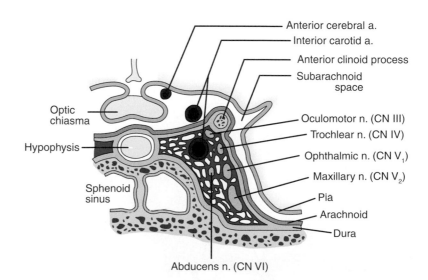

FIGURE 6-13. **Cavernous sinus.** Coronal cut through the cavernous sinus showing passage of cranial nerves and internal carotid through the sinus. Note that the relatively medial position of CN VI makes it the cranial nerve most susceptible to impingement by an expanding pituitary tumor. (Adapted with permission from Kasper DL, Braunwald E, Fauci AS, et al. *Harrison's Principles of Internal Medicine,* 16th ed. New York: McGraw-Hill, 2005: 2438.)

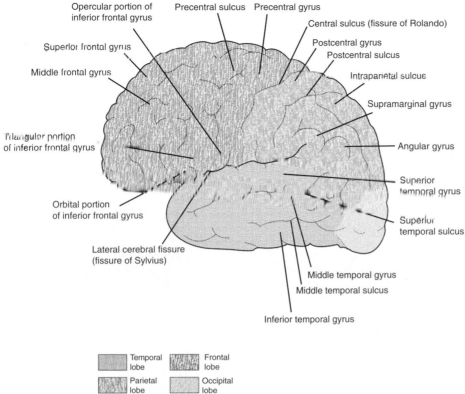

A

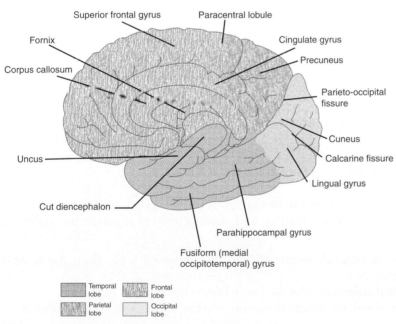

B

FIGURE 6-14.   Basic surface anatomy of the cerebrum. (A and B) Major structures of note are the four major lobes, precentral sulcus/gyrus, central sulcus, Sylvian fissure, cingulate gyrus, corpus callosum, uncus, and hippocampal gyrus.

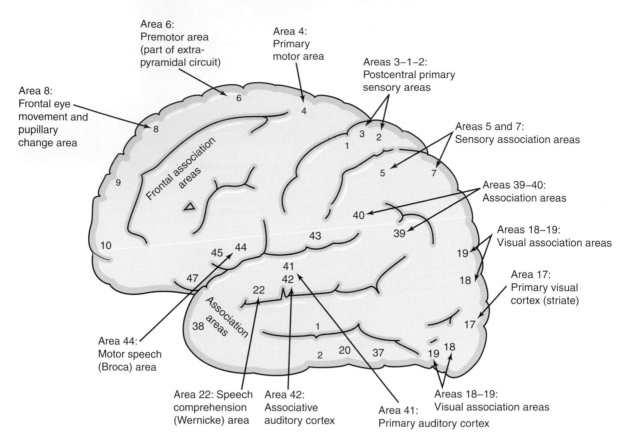

FIGURE 6-15. **Brodmann areas of the brain.** Areas of note include areas 3–1–2 = primary sensory cortex; area 4 = primary motor cortex; area 8 = frontal eye fields; area 44 = Broca area; area 22 = Wernicke area; and area 17 = primary visual cortex. (Reproduced with permission from Waxman SG. *Neuroanatomy with Clinical Correlations*, 26th ed. New York: McGraw-Hill, 2004.)

ORGANIZATION

The cerebral cortex is composed of six layers of cells; the relative size of each layer varies among regions of the brain. Each layer consists of different types of cells and is specialized to send and receive input to and from different areas of the brain. Layer 5 in the primary motor cortex is known for the large motor neurons of the corticospinal tracts known as **Betz cells.**

The cortex is divided into the frontal, parietal, temporal, and occipital lobes (see Figure 6-14). Major fissures and sulci (grooves) separate the different lobes.

- The **Sylvian (lateral) fissure** divides the temporal lobes from the frontal and parietal lobes.
- The **central sulcus** divides the frontal from the parietal lobe.
- The **sagittal sulcus** divides the brain into the left and right hemispheres.

Frontal Lobe

LOCATION

Anterior to the central sulcus.

MAJOR AREAS

Prefrontal cortex, premotor cortex, primary motor cortex, frontal eye fields, Broca area.

FUNCTIONS

- **Movement (primary motor and premotor cortex):** Areas in charge of movement include the primary motor cortex and premotor cortex, located anterior to the central gyrus. The primary motor cortex is closest to the central sulcus, and the premotor cortex is located more anteriorly. The **premotor cortex** plans movements in response to external cues and is particularly active when sequential movements follow visual cues. The **primary motor cortex** executes the planned movement via the descending motor neurons of the corticospinal tract. Areas of the motor cortex correspond geographically to the body parts they control, as mapped out by the motor homunculus (Figure 6-16).

- Lesion of a motor strip causes spastic paralysis of the contralateral region corresponding to the region depicted on the motor homunculus (see Figure 6-16A).

- **Eye movements (frontal eye fields):** The frontal eye fields (also known as area 8) control eye movements. Lesions of the frontal eye fields:
  - Ischemic lesion (ie, stroke): Eyes drift toward the side that is injured.
  - Hyperactivity (ie, seizure): Eyes drift away from the side of hyperactivity.

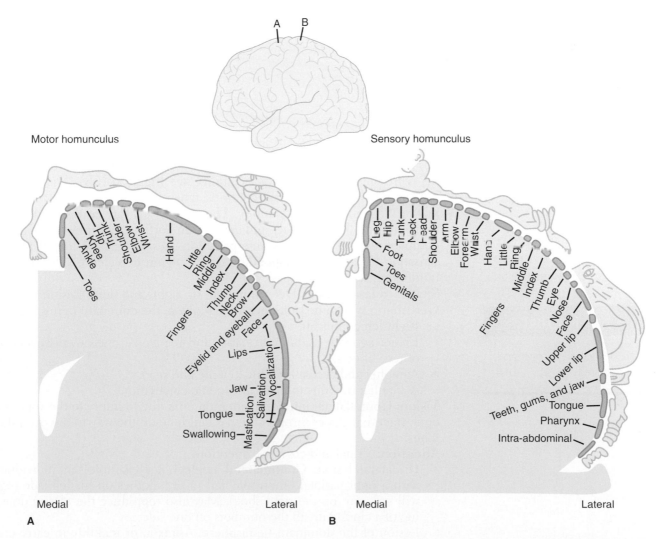

FIGURE 6-16. **Motor (A) and sensory (B) homunculi.** (Part A modified with permission from Ropper AH, Brown RH. *Adams and Victor's Neurology*, 8th ed. New York: McGraw-Hill, 2005. Part B modified with permission from Kandel ER, Schwartz JH, Jessel TM. *Principles of Neural Science*, 4th ed. New York: McGraw-Hill, 2000.)

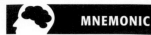

MNEMONIC

The eyes look toward a stroke and away from a seizure.

- **Social judgment (prefrontal cortex):** The frontal lobe is responsible for inhibiting impulsive thoughts to tailor behavior to fit social norms. Lesion of the prefrontal cortex may result in disinhibition. For example, Phineas Gage, a formerly mild-mannered man who survived severe frontal lobe damage, became rude, obnoxious, and defiant of social norms.
- **Language production (Broca area):** Broca area, or area 44 (Figure 6-15), is involved in language production. Lesion in Broca area results in an inability to produce coherent speech. Patients appear to have difficulty forming words and speak very slowly and laboriously. Comprehension is intact, however.
- **Executive functions:** Concentration, orientation, abstraction, judgment, mood, and inhibition of primitive reflexes. Lesion can lead to unmasking of primitive reflexes such as suckling, grasp, and rooting reflexes.

BLOOD SUPPLY

ACA and MCA.

Parietal Lobe

LOCATION

The parietal lobes are located lateral to the sagittal sulcus and posterior to the central sulcus.

MAJOR AREAS

Primary sensory cortex.

FUNCTIONS

- **Sensation (primary sensory cortex):** The primary sensory cortex is just posterior to the central sulcus. Like the motor cortex, a sensory homunculus represents the anatomic correlations (see Figure 6-16B). The ascending spinothalamic and dorsal columns synapse in the thalamus and project to the primary sensory cortex. The primary sensory cortex then sends projections to the secondary and association cortices that integrate sensory components into a cohesive interpretation. Lesion leads to loss of tactile sensation in regions corresponding to the region depicted on the sensory homunculus.
- **Spatial relationships:** Determination of right and left. Lesion causes **Gerstmann syndrome** (inferior parietal lobe of the dominant hemisphere).
    - Right-left confusion.
    - Finger agnosia: Inability to name and recognize one's own fingers or others' fingers.
    - Agraphia and alexia: Inability to write and read.
    - Acalculia: Inability to make arithmetic calculations.
- **Vision:** Contralateral inferior quadrantanopia due to injury to the superior optic tract that passes through the parietal lobe on the way to the occipital lobe.
- **Attention:** Visual and cognitive attention.
    - Unilateral lesion: **Contralateral neglect,** for example, an individual with a right parietal lesion may fail to put clothes on his left side (eg, will only put on the right shoe). May also reproduce the classic drawing of a clock with all the numbers on one side.
    - Lesion of the dominant hemisphere: **Apraxia,** or inability to carry out learned movements (combing hair, brushing teeth). Patients often are

KEY FACT

Clarification: **Dys**lexia is congenital; **A**lexia is **A**cquired.

unable to perform an action when commanded to, but are able to imitate or perform the action in response to other triggering stimuli.

- Bilateral lesions: **Balint syndrome,** a form of visual agnosia, in which patients are unable to scan visual space and to grasp an object in space.

BLOOD SUPPLY

ACA and MCA.

Occipital Lobe

LOCATION

Most posterior region of the brain.

MAJOR AREAS

Primary visual cortex, association visual cortex.

FUNCTIONS

- **Vision (primary and association visual cortices):**
  - Visual pathway: Retina → fibers cross at the optic chiasm → synapse at the lateral geniculate nucleus (LGN) → primary visual cortex within the occipital lobe.
  - Visual signals are processed through inputs from the primary visual cortex to the visual association cortex in the occipital lobe.
- **Visual recognition (association cortices):**
  - Lesion results in visual agnosia, the inability to recognize objects one sees.
  - Lesion causes alexia without agraphia, the acquired inability to read while retaining the ability to write.

BLOOD SUPPLY

PCA.

Temporal Lobes

The temporal lobes contain structures vital for hearing, memory, and emotion.

LOCATION

Inferolateral to the Sylvian fissure.

MAJOR AREAS

Primary auditory cortex, hippocampus, amygdala, Wernicke area.

FUNCTIONS

- **Hearing (primary auditory cortex):** Located within the superior temporal gyrus and transverse temporal gyrus (Heschl gyrus).
- **Auditory pathway:** Cochlea → CN VIII → medullary cochlear nuclei → fibers cross just prior to the superior olivary nuclei, travel along the lateral lemniscus tract → synapse in the medial geniculate nucleus (MGN) → primary auditory cortex.
  - Lesion proximal to the CN VIII decussation and superior olivary nuclei leads to unilateral hearing loss with potential deafness.
  - Lesion distal to the CN VIII decussation and medullary cochlear nuclei causes bilateral diminished hearing without deafness.

KEY FACT

Types of memory loss include anterograde and retrograde.
Anterograde: Inability to create new memories after the injury.
Retrograde: Inability to recall memories prior to the injury.

■ **Memory (hippocampus):** The hippocampus is responsible for learning and consolidation of short-term memory, before memories are later integrated diffusely throughout the cortex. The hippocampus is part of the Papez circuit, an important pathway in the limbic system, which contains structures presumed to play a role in memory and emotion (Figure 6-17). Hippocampal lesion results in anterograde memory loss (inability to form new memories).

■ **Emotion:** The temporal lobe is part of the limbic system. Memory and emotion are intimately related, both structurally and functionally.

■ Fear: Emotional responses, such as the fear response, are mediated by the amygdala.

■ Lesion leads to ablation of the fear response, or **Klüver-Bucy syndrome:**

■ Psychic blindness (visual agnosia)

■ Personality changes (abnormal docility)

■ Hyperorality (puts everything in one's mouth)

■ Hypersexuality and loss of sexual preference (mounts anything in sight).

■ **Seizure activity** is commonly associated with vivid hallucinations. The temporal lobe is one of the common foci for epilepsy.

■ **Language comprehension (Wernicke area):** Wernicke area, or area 22, is responsible for comprehension of language. It is also critical for production of *coherent* language.

■ Lesion in Wernicke area: Patients are unable to understand what is spoken to them. They produce speech fluently that consists of either real

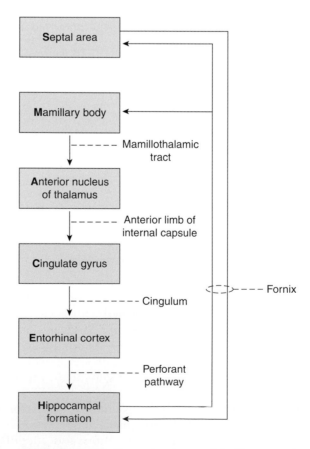

FIGURE 6-17. **Papez circuit.** The Papez circuit was originally proposed as a circuit for memory and emotional processing. Although it is not a true circuit, structures of the "circuit" contribute to memory and emotional processing and constitute the limbic system.

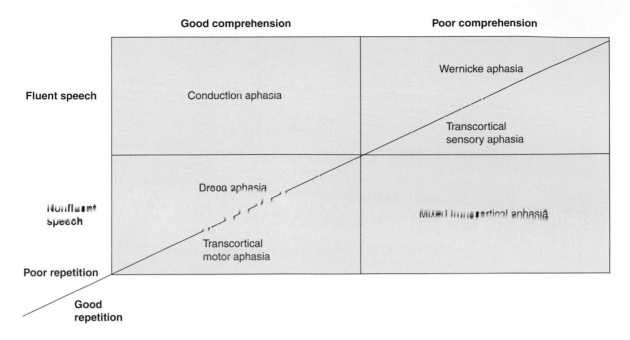

FIGURE 6-18. **Aphasia square.** The six most commonly tested aphasias.

or made-up words (neologisms) and phrases, but it does not make any sense.

- The aphasia square (Figure 6-18) summarizes the various forms of aphasia.
  - Broca aphasia: Inability to produce speech or repeat sentences. Also has trouble with written expression. Comprehension is intact.
  - Wernicke aphasia: Inability to comprehend both verbal and written language, produce coherent speech, or repeat sentences.
  - Conduction aphasia: Inability to repeat after hearing a sentence.
  - Mixed transcortical aphasia: Inability to spontaneously produce words or coherent speech, however, repetition is intact.
  - Global aphasia: All language function is impaired.

DEEP BRAIN STRUCTURES

Basal Ganglia

LOCATION

Lateral to the internal capsule bilaterally.

STRUCTURES

Striatum (caudate + putamen), globus pallidus internus and externus, and the substantia nigra (Figure 6-19).

FUNCTIONS

- Initiation of purposeful movement (Figure 6-20) via the direct and indirect pathways.
  - Dopamine (DA) is released into the caudate/putamen from neurons that originate in the substantia nigra pars compacta.
  - Direct pathway (promotes movement):
    - Cortex → caudate/putamen → globus pallidus internus → thalamus → spinal cord.
    - DA activates this pathway via D_1 receptors, promoting movement.

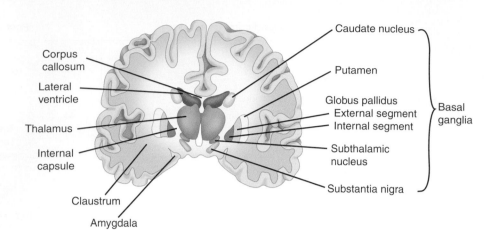

FIGURE 6-19. **Major structures of the basal ganglia.**

- Indirect pathway (inhibits movement):
  - Cortex → caudate/putamen → **globus pallidus externus → subthalamic nucleus** → globus pallidus internus → thalamus → spinal cord.
  - DA inhibits this pathway via D_2 receptors, promoting movement.

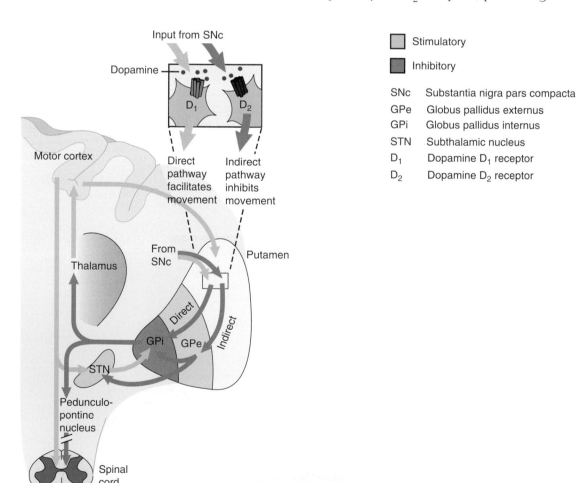

FIGURE 6-20. **Basal ganglia direct and indirect pathways.** (Modified with permission from Kandel ER, Schwartz JH, Jessel TM. *Principles of Neural Science*, 4th ed. New York: McGraw-Hill, 2000.)

- Lesions and corresponding deficits:
  - Substantia nigra DA neurons: lesion results in **Parkinson disease.**
  - Small and medium spiny GABAergic neurons of the caudate and putamen: lesion associated with **Huntington disease.**
  - Subthalamic nucleus: lesion results in **hemiballismus.**

Thalamus

LOCATION

Surrounding the third ventricle, just above the midbrain.

STRUCTURES

Nine nuclei (Table 6-5 and Figure 6-7.)

FUNCTIONS

- **Sensory relay station:**
  - The thalamus receives sensory input of all sensory modalities.
  - Sensory input is "filtered."
  - The thalamus sends processed signals to other areas of the cortex.
- **Emotion and memory:** The thalamus is part of the Papez circuit, which is involved in emotion and memory.
- **Motor relay station:** The thalamus receives input from the motor cortex and basal ganglia and sends signals to the descending motor tracts.
- **Lesion associated with motor and sensory deficits:** Involving multiple areas of the body, and **thalamic pain syndrome,** which is pain perceived without an appropriate stimulus.

TABLE 6-5. Nuclei and Functions of the Thalamus

NUCLEUS	FUNCTION	INPUTS	OUTPUTS
Ventral posterior-lateral	Relay somatic sensory information from the trunk and limbs.	Spinothalamic tract, dorsal columns	Primary sensory cortex
Ventral posterior-medial	Relay somatic sensory information from the head.	Trigeminal tract	Primary sensory cortex
Ventrolateral	Relay motor information.	Cerebellum, globus pallidus	Primary motor cortex and supplementary motor area
Ventroanterior	Relay motor planning information.	Cerebellum, globus pallidus	Prefrontal cortex
Anterior nuclei	Relay emotion/memory information; part of Papez circuit.	Mamillary bodies	Cingulate gyrus
Medial dorsal	Relay cognitive/ memory information.	Prefrontal cortex, olfactory, and limbic systems	Prefrontal association cortex

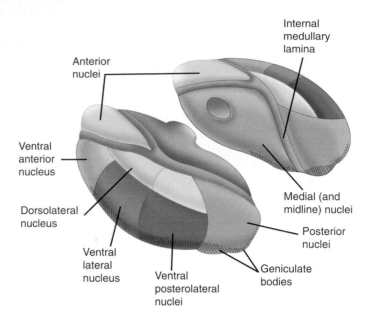

FIGURE 6-21. **Thalamic nuclei.** The thalamus has two lobes, one on each side of the third ventricle. The geniculate bodies include the medial and lateral geniculate bodies/nuclei that relay auditory and visual sensory information, respectively. (Modified with permission from Waxman SG. *Clinical Neuroanatomy,* 25th ed. New York: McGraw-Hill, 2003.)

 KEY FACT

Lesions of the **internal capsule** are more likely to affect multiple areas of the body than are lesions of the motor or sensory cortex. Cortical lesions generally involve isolated parts of the body, depending on the affected segment of the homunculus.

BLOOD SUPPLY

Posterior communicating artery, anterior choroidal artery (a branch of the internal carotid artery; see Figure 6-11).

Internal Capsule

The internal capsule is the site of convergence of all ascending and descending white matter tracts to and from the cortex.

LOCATION

White matter lateral to the thalamus and caudate, and medial to the lenticular nucleus (globus pallidus and putamen) as illustrated in Figure 6-22.

DIVISIONS

Anterior limb, posterior limb, genu (the bend between the anterior and posterior limbs), retrolenticular limb, and sublenticular limb.

- Anterior limb: Frontopontine fibers (between frontal cortex and pons), thalamocortical fibers (between medial/anterior nuclei of thalamus and frontal lobes).
- Posterior limb: Descending corticospinal tract, ascending sensory fibers (medial lemniscus, anterolateral/spinothalamic tract).
- Genu (the bend or "elbow"): Descending corticobulbar tract (between cortex and brain stem).
- Retrolenticular limb: Optic radiation (between lateral geniculate nucleus and primary visual cortex).
- Sublenticular limb: Auditory radiation (between medial geniculate nucleus and primary auditory cortex).

Lesion causes motor (genu, posterior limb) and sensory (posterior limb) deficits involving multiple areas of the body.

 KEY FACT

The **lateral striate arteries** are the penetrating arteries of the MCA and are called the "arteries of stroke" because they are most often affected in **nonembolic lacunar infarctions** and in **Charcot-Bouchard microaneurysms.** Charcot-Bouchard microaneurysms occur in the walls of small penetrating vessels weakened from chronic hypertension.

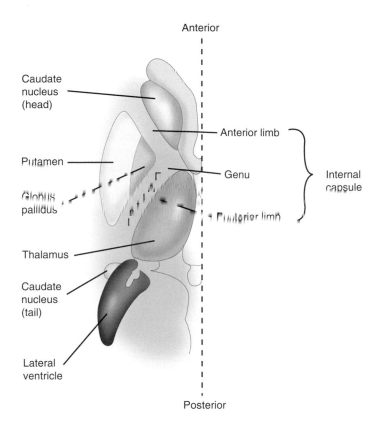

FIGURE 6-22. **Axial cut of the brain through the internal capsule.** Notice that descending motor fibers for the face, arm, and leg (F, A, and L) run anterior to the ascending sensory fibers (f, a, and l) in the posterior limb of the internal capsule.

BLOOD SUPPLY

Medial striate branches from the ACA and lenticulostriate branches from the MCA.

Hypothalamus

The hypothalamus is involved in homeostasis and instinctive actions, such as eating, drinking, sleeping, and sex. Like the thalamus, it is divided into several nuclei controlling various functions (Figure 6-23 and Table 6-6).

DISEASES OF THE HYPOTHALAMUS

- **Central diabetes insipidus:**
  - Lesion of the antidiuretic hormone (ADH) pathways to the posterior lobe of the pituitary gland leads to inappropriately low ADH secretion.
  - Polyuria and polydipsia with hypernatremia.
- **Syndrome of inappropriate ADH (SIADH):**
  - May be due to direct injury to the hypothalamus.
  - Can also be due to lung tumors that secrete ADH-like hormone (small-cell lung carcinoma) or drugs that increase ADH secretion (carbamazepine, chlorpromazine).
  - Manifests as fluid retention with hyponatremia.
- **Craniopharyngioma:**
  - Congenital tumor originating from remnants of the Rathke pouch (oral ectoderm).
  - Often calcified, resembling tooth enamel.
  - Most common supratentorial tumor and cause of hypopituitarism in children.

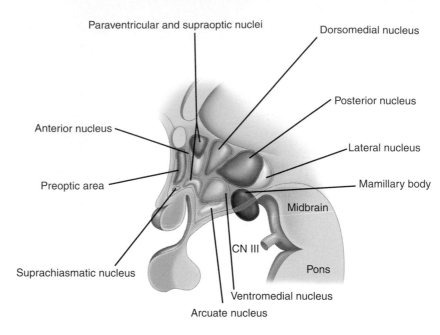

FIGURE 6-23. **Hypothalamic nuclei.**

TABLE 6-6. **Hypothalamic Nuclei and Major Functions**

NUCLEUS	FUNCTION
Supraoptic and paraventricular nuclei	Synthesizes ADH, oxytocin, CRH. Neurophysins serve as carrier peptides for ADH and oxytocin transport to the posterior pituitary for release. Regulates water balance via ADH. Lesion → **diabetes insipidus.**
Anterior nucleus	Temperature regulation (heat dissipation). Lesion → **hyperthermia.** Stimulates parasympathetic nervous system.
Preoptic	Releases gonadotropic hormones. Sexual dimorphic nucleus. Lesion → arrested sexual development, impotence, amenorrhea.
Suprachiasmatic nucleus	Regulates circadian rhythms (eg, cyclic release of CRH, melatonin). Input from retina, output to pineal gland.
Dorsomedial nucleus	Stimulation → obesity, disinhibition.
Posterior nucleus	Temperature regulation (heat conservation). Lesion → **poikilothermia** (poor thermoregulation). Stimulates sympathetic nervous system.
Lateral nucleus	Feeding center: Stimulation → increased eating (lateral nucleus causes you to grow laterally). Lesion → starvation.
Mamillary body	Damaged in Wernicke encephalopathy/Korsakoff psychosis (confabulation, amnesia, and ataxia). Hippocampus → fornix → mamillary body → anterior nucleus of thalamus (part of Papez circuit).
Ventromedial nucleus	Satiety center: Stimulation → decreased eating (ventromedial nucleus causes you to shrink medially), lesion → obesity, hyperphagia, "savage" behavior.
Arcuate nucleus	Produces hypothalamic releasing and inhibiting factors that act on the anterior pituitary. Inhibits prolactin release via dopamine (prolactin-inhibiting factor).

ADH = antidiuretic hormone; CRH = corticotropin-releasing hormone.

- Pressure on the optic chiasm results in **bitemporal hemianopia;** pressure on CN VI within the cavernous sinus can lead to abducens nerve palsy (see Figure 6-13).
- Pressure on the hypothalamus results in hypothalamic syndrome (loss of function of the hypothalamus).
- **Pituitary adenomas:**
  - Although not officially part of the hypothalamus, the pituitary is closely related both spatially and functionally.
  - Location of 15% of clinically symptomatic intracranial tumors.
  - Rarely seen in children (unlike craniopharyngiomas).
  - Produce symptoms similar to those of craniopharyngioma (bitemporal hemianopia and hypothalamic syndrome).
  - If endocrine-active, produce endocrine abnormalities (eg, amenorrhea, galactorrhea from prolactin-secreting tumor or acromegaly/gigantism from a growth hormone-secreting tumor).

KEY FACT

The pituitary gland, or adenohypophysis, is formed from an outpouching of the ectodermal diverticulum of the primitive mouth cavity, the **Rathke pouch.** The pouch ascends until it is adjacent to the neurohypophysis, forming the adenohypophysis/ neurohypophysis complex that rests in the **sella turcica.** Remnants of the Rathke pouch may give rise to a **craniopharyngioma.**

CEREBELLUM

The cerebellum extends dorsally from the level of the pons at the base of the brain. Important structures include the tuber **vermis,** situated medially, and the hemispheres on either side. It is divided into three lobes: the **anterior, posterior,** and **flocculonodular** (Figure 6-24). Major functions include coordination of movement and posture. The hemispheres primarily control purposeful limb movements, and the vermis primarily controls axial posture. Lesions of the cerebellum can result in dysdiadochokinesia (inability to alternate contraction between antagonistic muscle groups), action tremor, dysmetria, nystagmus, scanning speech, and ataxia.

Anatomy

- **Peduncles** (see Figure 6-26):
  - **Superior cerebellar peduncle (SCP):** Contains major output from the cerebellum, including the dentatorubrothalamic tract, and an afferent pathway, the ventral spinocerebellar tract.
  - **Middle cerebellar peduncle (MCP):** Contains incoming pontocerebellar fibers.
  - **Inferior cerebellar peduncle (ICP):** Contains three major afferent tracts: the dorsal spinocerebellar tract, the cuneocerebellar tract, and the olivocerebellar tract from the contralateral inferior olivary nucleus.
- **Layers** (Figure 6-25):
  - **Molecular layer:** Outer layer containing stellate cells, basket cells, the dendritic arbor of Purkinje cells, and parallel fibers of granule cells.
  - **Purkinje cell layer:** Contains cell bodies of Purkinje cells.
  - **Granule layer:** Innermost layer containing granule cell bodies, Golgi cells, and cerebellar glomeruli.
  - **Cerebellar glomeruli:** Consists of a mossy fiber rosette, granule cell dendrites, and a Golgi cell axon.
- **Neurons and fibers** (Table 6-7).
- **Deep nuclei:** The deep cerebellar nuclei process input from the cerebellar hemispheres and transmit output signals through the superior cerebellar peduncle (Figure 6-26).
  - **Dentate nucleus:** Receives input from Purkinje cells in the lateral cerebellar hemispheres and transmits output through the dentatorubrothalamic tract.

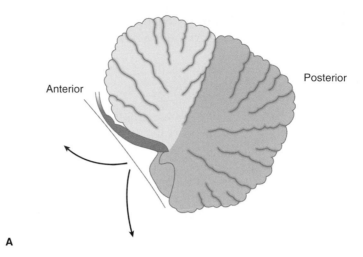

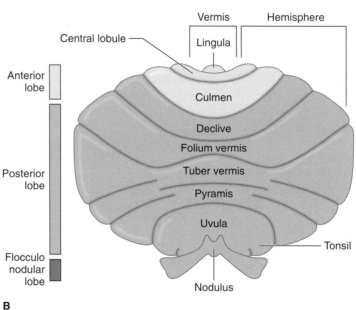

FIGURE 6-24. Regional anatomy of the cerebellum. The cerebellum is divided into anterior and posterior segments in the sagittal plane (A) and into the midline vermis and lateral hemispheres in the axial plane (B). (Modified with permission from McPhee SJ, Hammer GD. *Pathophysiology of Disease: An Introduction to Clinical Medicine*, 6th ed. New York: McGraw-Hill, 2010.)

- **Emboliform and globose nuclei:** Transmits cerebellar output relating to the upper and lower limbs after a movement has been initiated.
- **Fastigial nucleus:** Transmits cerebellar output relating to axial stability, especially during standing or walking.

Major Pathways

- Climbing fibers arising from the inferior olivary nucleus project via the olivocerebellar tract through the inferior peduncle to the cerebellar cortex and synapse on Purkinje cells.

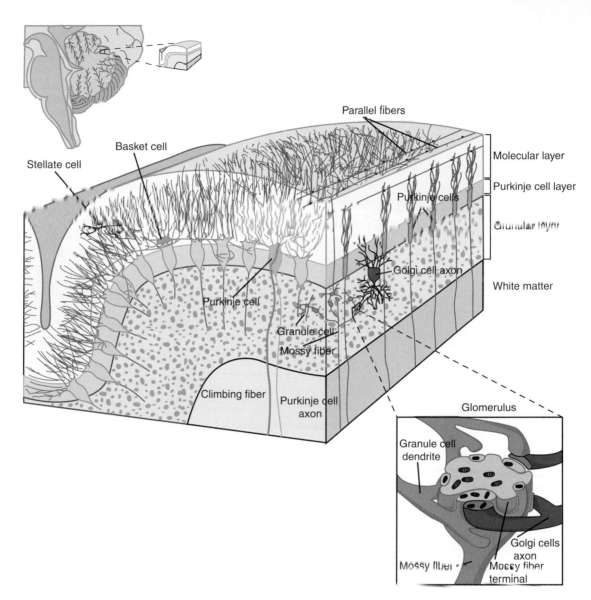

FIGURE 6-25. **Histologic organization of the cerebellum.** Purkinje cells have trees of dendrites that spread along a plane perpendicular to the parallel fibers, forming a matrix for information processing. (Modified with permission from Kandel ER, Schwartz JH, Jessel TM. *Principles of Neural Science*, 4th ed. New York: McGraw-Hill, 2000.)

- Purkinje cells of the cerebellar cortex project to the deep cerebellar nuclei, especially the dentate nucleus, and form the only inhibitory (GABA-ergic) synapses in the cerebellar circuitry.
- Dentate nucleus cells project via the dentatorubrothalamic tract to the red nucleus and the ventral lateral motor nucleus of the thalamus (see Figure 6-26).
- Thalamic neurons project to the primary motor cortex.
- The motor cortex projects to the pontine nuclei via the corticopontine tract.
- Pontine nuclei project via the pontocerebellar tract (MCP) to the contralateral cerebellar cortex (mossy fibers), completing the cerebrocerebellar circuit.

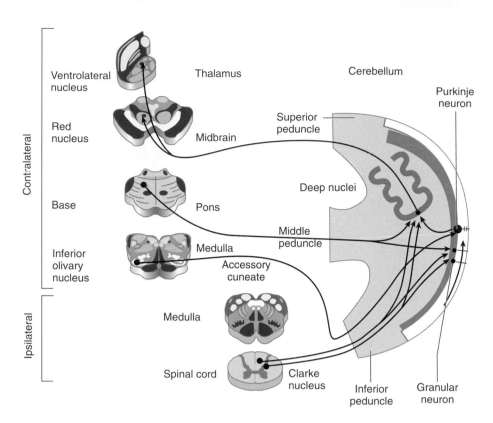

FIGURE 6-26. **Cerebellar pathways.** Major cerebellar pathways traversing the three peduncles.

TABLE 6-7. **Neurons and Fibers of the Cerebellum**

CELL/FIBER	LOCATION	PATHWAY	NEUROTRANSMITTER
Purkinje cells	Cell body in Purkinje cell layer; dendritic tree in molecular layer.	Only output from cerebellar cortex. Receives input from parallel fibers (granule cells) and climbing fibers (inferior olivary nucleus). Project to deep cerebellar nuclei.	GABA
Granule cells	Cell body in granule cell layer; axons (parallel fibers) in molecular layer.	Receive input from Golgi cells and mossy fibers from spinal cord, medulla, and pons. Project to Purkinje, basket, stellate, and Golgi cells through parallel fibers.	Glutamate
Parallel fibers	Molecular layer.	Axons of granule cells.	Glutamate
Mossy fibers	Cell bodies in spinal cord, pons, and vestibular nuclei; terminate in granule cell layer.	Originate in spinocerebellar, pontocerebellar, and vestibulocerebellar tracts. Terminate as mossy fibers on granule cell dendrites.	Glutamate
Climbing fibers	Cell bodies in inferior olivary nucleus; terminate on Purkinje cell dendrites.	Carry information from olivocerebellar tract to cerebellar nuclei and Purkinje cells.	Aspartate

GABA = γ-amino butyric acid.

Cerebellar Dysfunction and Syndromes

■ Signs of cerebellar dysfunction frequently include:
  ■ **Disequilibrium** (loss of balance, truncal and gait ataxia).
  ■ **Dyssynergia** (loss of coordination) includes dysmetria, intention tremor, dysdiadochokinesia, and coarse nystagmus more prominent when gazing toward the side of the lesion.
  ■ **Hypotonia.**
■ Lesions of the hemispheres usually cause *ipsilateral* cerebellar signs with ataxia of the extremities.
■ Lesions of the vermis usually cause gait or truncal ataxia. The classic cerebellar gait is wide-based.

BRAIN STEM

The brain stem lies between the thalamus and the spinal cord. It consists of three main components, in descending order: midbrain, pons, and medulla (Figure 6-27). It develops from the mesencephalon (midbrain), the metencephalon (pons), and the myelencephalon (medulla).

Midbrain

The midbrain is the most superior aspect of the brain stem. Strokes or lesions in the midbrain give rise to several well-known syndromes (see Figures 6-27 and 6-28 and Tables 6-8 through 6-10).

■ Blood supply: PCA, SCA, branches of the basilar artery (BA).
■ Consists of a dorsal tectum (roof), an intermediate tegmentum (floor), and a base.

> **KEY FACT**
>
> Brain stem lesions produce a **Brown-Séquard like syndrome:** Ipsilateral loss of some functions and contralateral loss of other functions. Many of the tracts that travel to and from the brain and spinal cord synapse and cross the midline within the brain stem.

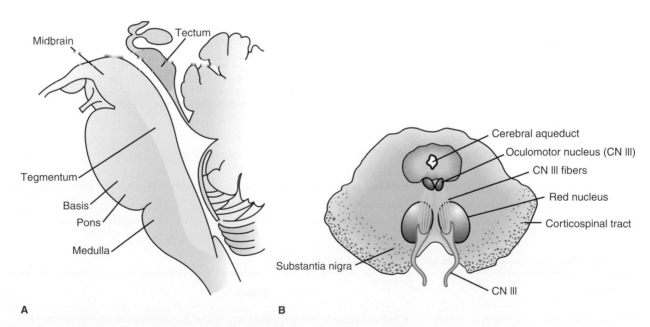

FIGURE 6-27.   Brain stem and cross-section of the midbrain. (A) Basic parts of the brain stem include the midbrain, pons, and medulla. Tegmentum = "floor"; tectum = "roof." (B) The tectum is above the aqueduct, the tegmentum below. (Part A modified with permission from Waxman SG. *Clinical Neuroanatomy*, 25th ed. New York: McGraw-Hill, 2003.)

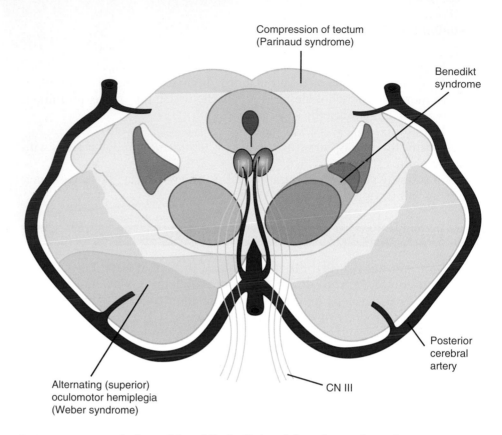

Compression of tectum
(Parinaud syndrome)

Benedikt
syndrome

Posterior
cerebral
artery

CN III

Alternating (superior)
oculomotor hemiplegia
(Weber syndrome)

FIGURE 6-28. Lesions of the midbrain. Parinaud (loss of upward gaze due to compression of superior colliculus frequently by a pineal gland tumor), Benedikt (paramedian midbrain syndrome that can be caused by occlusion of the posterior cerebral artery), and Weber syndromes (CN III palsy with contralateral hemiparesis).

TABLE 6-8. Parinaud Syndrome: Lesion of the Dorsal Tectum of the Midbrain

STRUCTURE	DEFICIT
Superior colliculus and pretectal area	Paralysis of upward (less frequently downward) gaze, pupillary disturbances, absence of convergence.
Cerebral aqueduct	Obstruction leads to noncommunicating hydrocephalus (bilateral papilledema).
Pineal gland	If the underlying cause of **Parinaud syndrome** is a pineal tumor, inadequate *melatonin* production may result in insomnia. Pineal cysts are often asymptomatic.

TABLE 6-9. Benedikt Syndrome: Lesion of the Tegmentum of the Midbrain

STRUCTURE	DEFICIT
CN III nucleus/root	Ptosis (paralysis of the levator palpebrae muscle), fixed and dilated ipsilateral pupil, complete ipsilateral oculomotor paralysis, causing the eye to be "down and out" due to unopposed actions of the lateral rectus (CN VI) and superior oblique (CN IV) muscles.
Dentatothalamic fibers	Contralateral cerebellar ataxia with intention tremor.
Medial lemniscus	Contralateral loss of light touch and position sensation from the extremities.

TABLE 6-10. **Weber Syndrome: Lesion of the Base of Midbrain**

STRUCTURE	DEFICIT
CN III nucleus/root	See Table 6-9.
Corticospinal tracts	Contralateral spastic paralysis of extremities.
Corticobulbar fibers	Contralateral weakness of the lower face (CN VII), tongue (CN XII), and palate (CN X); the uvula points away from the lesion, but the protruded tongue points toward the lesion

Pons

The pons is the region of the brain stem shown in Figure 6-29.

- Blood supply: Paramedian branches of the basilar artery and AICA.
- Contents and lesions (Tables 6-11 and 6-12).

The pons contains an important structure for conjugate gaze, known as the **medial longitudinal fasciculus (MLF).** The MLF connects the CN VI nucleus with the contralateral CN III nucleus to achieve lateral conjugate gaze. A lesion of the MLF produces **MLF syndrome (internuclear ophthalmoplegia):**

- Medial rectus palsy on attempted lateral conjugate gaze and nystagmus in the abducting eye.
- Often seen in **multiple sclerosis** (MS).

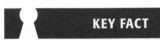

KEY FACT

Charcot triad of MS includes:
1. Scanning speech
2. Intention tremor
3. Nystagmus (MLF syndrome/ internuclear ophthalmoplegia; see discussion)

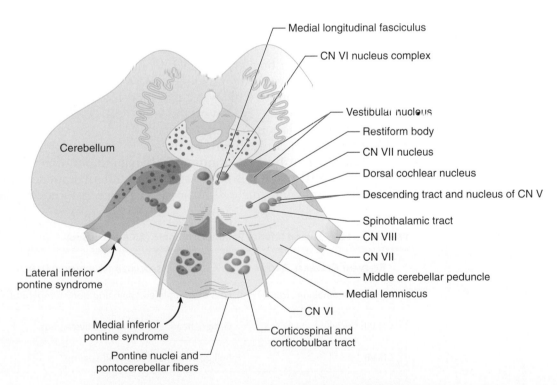

FIGURE 6-29. **Cross-section through the pons.** Note the regions of the lateral inferior pontine syndrome and medial inferior pontine syndrome due to occlusions of the anterior inferior cerebellar artery and the paramedian branches of the basilar artery, respectively. (Modified with permission from Ropper AH, Brown RH. *Adams and Victor's Neurology*, 8th ed. New York: McGraw-Hill, 2005: 683.)

TABLE 6-11.   **Contents and Lesions of the Medial Pons (Result from Occlusion of Paramedian Branches of the Basilar Artery)**

STRUCTURE	DEFICIT
Medial longitudinal fasciculus (MLF)	MLF syndrome (internuclear ophthalmoplegia, see previous discussion).
Abducens nucleus (CN VI)	Lateral rectus palsy.
CN VII (lower motor neuron)	Ipsilateral Bell palsy without forehead sparing.
Medial lemniscus	Loss of contralateral light touch and proprioceptive sensation.
Corticospinal tract	Contralateral hemiparesis.

MNEMONIC

Remember the direction of nystagmus with **COWS:**
Cold–**O**pposite
Warm–**S**ame

MNEMONIC

The cerebellopontine angle is the angle formed by the cerebellum, pons, and medulla. Five brain tumors are often found here **(SAMEE):**

Schwannoma (75%)
Arachnoid cyst (1%)
Meningioma (10%)
Ependymoma (1%)
Epidermoid (5%)

Caloric nystagmus is used to test brain stem function. Nystagmus has two phases: a slow phase in one direction (tracking movement), followed by a fast phase (resetting movement) in the opposite direction. The direction of nystagmus is determined by the direction of the fast phase (Figure 6-30).

- Conscious:
  - Cold water irrigation of the external auditory meatus → reduction of signaling through ipsilateral vestibular afferents (simulating contralateral head turn) → ipsilateral gaze deviation with nystagmus toward contralateral side (ie, cold water in left ear causes left gaze deviation with right beating nystagmus).
  - Warm water irrigation of the external auditory meatus → increased signaling through ipsilateral vestibular afferents (simulating ipsilateral head turn) → contralateral gaze deviation with nystagmus toward the ipsilateral side (ie, warm water in left ear causes right gaze deviation with left beating nystagmus).
- Unconscious with brain stem intact: Cold water irrigation leads to deviation of the eyes toward the ipsilateral side.
- Bilateral MLF lesion: Cold water irrigation leads to deviation of only the ipsilateral (abducting) eye toward the same side.
- Low brain stem lesion: No response.
- Other important clinical correlations:
  - **Acoustic neuroma (schwannoma):** Benign tumor of the Schwann cells of CN VIII that arises in the area of the internal auditory meatus and cerebellopontine angle. If bilateral, frequently associated with **neurofi-**

TABLE 6-12.   **Lateral Inferior Pontine Syndrome (AICA Occlusion)**

RELEVANT CEREBRAL ARTERY	ASSOCIATED NEUROLOGIC DEFICIT
Lateral spinothalamic tract	Loss of contralateral pain and body temperature sensation.
CN VIII nuclei	Vertigo, hearing loss, tinnitus, nystagmus.
CN VII	Bell palsy without forehead sparing.
Middle cerebellar peduncle	Ipsilateral ataxia.
Spinal trigeminal nucleus/tract	Ipsilateral pain/temperature sensation loss (face).
Descending sympathetics	Ipsilateral Horner syndrome.

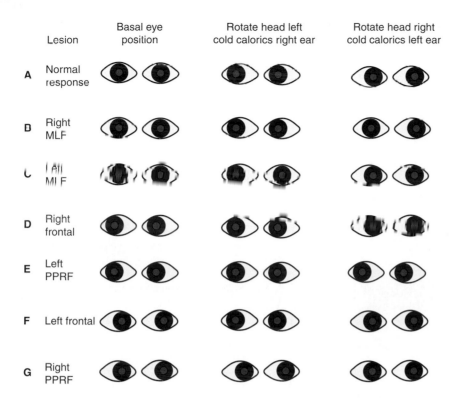

	Lesion	Basal eye position	Rotate head left cold calorics right ear	Rotate head right cold calorics left ear
A	Normal response			
B	Right MLF			
C	Left MLF			
D	Right frontal			
E	Left PPRF			
F	Left frontal			
G	Right PPRF			

FIGURE 6-30. **Responses to cold caloric testing in brain stem injury.** (A) Normally, cold calorics in the right ear simulates a left head turn and induces a right lateral gaze. Calorics in the left ear induces a left lateral gaze. (B) In right MLF syndrome, the right medial rectus does not contract on left lateral gaze, and the right eye remains fixed in midline. (C) In left MLF syndrome, the left medial rectus does not contract on right lateral gaze, and the left eye remains fixed in midline. (D) A right frontal eye field lesion leads to fixed right lateral gaze at rest but does not inhibit left lateral gaze in response to calorics. (E) A left PPRF lesion leaves the eyes fixed in right lateral gaze. (F) A left frontal eye field lesion leads to fixed left lateral gaze at rest but does not inhibit right lateral gaze in response to calorics. (G) A right PPRF lesion leaves the eyes fixed in left lateral gaze. MLF, medial longitudinal fasciculus; PPRF, paramedian pontine reticular formation.

bromatosis II (NF II). May impinge on several cranial nerves that pass near the cerebellopontine angle:
- CN VIII leads to tinnitus, unilateral sensorineural deafness, vertigo, nystagmus, nausea, vomiting, unsteady gait.
- CN VII results in ipsilateral facial weakness and loss of corneal reflex (efferent limb).
- CN V is associated with paresthesias, anesthesia of the ipsilateral face, loss of corneal reflex (afferent limb).
- **"Locked-in" syndrome:** Lesion of the base of the pons from infarction, trauma, tumor, or demyelination.
    - Affects bilateral corticospinal and corticobulbar tracts, and is associated with complete paralysis from head to toe.
    - Spares the oculomotor and trochlear nerves; the patient is only able to communicate with eye movements.
    - Patient is awake and aware.
- **Central pontine myelinolysis:** Demyelination of the base of the pons, associated with alcoholism or rapid correction of hyponatremia. Affects the corticospinal and corticobulbar tracts and results in spastic quadriparesis, pseudobulbar palsy, mental changes; may progress to "locked-in" syndrome.

KEY FACT

Neurofibromatosis II is often associated with **bilateral** acoustic neuromas.

KEY FACT

The medulla is the level at which the corticospinal tract crosses the midline (decussates). The crossing fibers of the corticospinal tract constitute the **pyramidal decussation.**

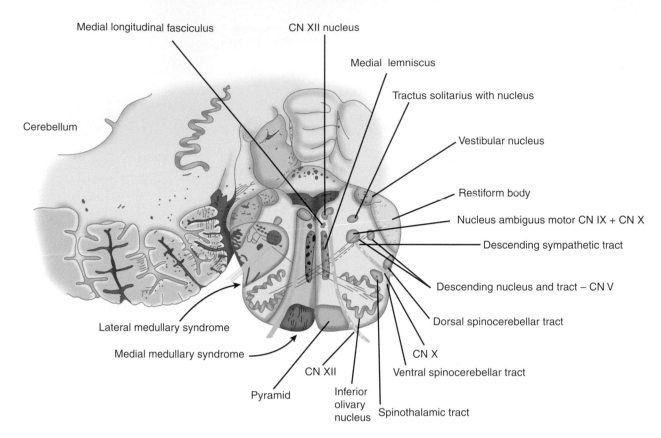

FIGURE 6-31. **Cross-section through the medulla.** Note the regions involved in the lateral medullary (Wallenberg) syndrome and medial medullary syndrome due to occlusion of the posterior inferior cerebellar artery and anterior spinal artery, respectively. (Modified with permission from Ropper AH, Brown RH. *Adams and Victor's Neurology*, 8th ed. New York: McGraw-Hill, 2005: 678.)

 KEY FACT

Horner syndrome:
- Ptosis
- Miosis
- Hemianhidrosis (lack of sweating)
- Apparent enophthalmos (sunken eyeball)

 FLASH FORWARD

Causes of Horner syndrome include Pancoast tumor, carotid artery dissection, and upper brachial plexus injury.

Medulla

- Blood supply: Vertebral artery (VA), anterior spinal artery (ASpA), PICA.
- Contents are shown in Figure 6-31.
- Lesions result in important clinical syndromes (Tables 6-13 and 6-14). **Wallenberg syndrome** is particularly common as a result of occlusion in PICA.

Other functions of the medulla include:

- **Vomiting center (chemoreceptor trigger zone):** Neurons at the base of the fourth ventricle (**area postrema**) sample CSF and send inputs to the nucleus of the solitary tract and other autonomic control centers in the brain stem.

TABLE 6-13. **Medial Medullary Syndrome (VA or BA occlusion)**

STRUCTURE	DEFICIT
Corticospinal tract	Contralateral spastic hemiparesis.
Medial lemniscus	Contralateral loss of tactile, vibrational, and proprioceptive sense from trunk and extremities.
CN XII nucleus/fibers	Ipsilateral flaccid hemiparalysis of the tongue (tongue points to side of lesion).

TABLE 6-14. Lateral Medullary/Wallenberg/Posterior Inferior Cerebellar Artery Syndrome

STRUCTURE	DEFICIT
Vestibular nuclei	Nystagmus, vertigo.
Inferior cerebellar peduncle	Ipsilateral cerebellar signs.
Nucleus ambiguus	Dysarthria, hoarseness, dysphagia, loss of gag reflex.
Spinothalamic tracts/spinal trigeminal nucleus and tract	Contralateral loss of pain and temperature sensation from trunk and extremities, with *ipsilateral* loss of pain and temperature sensation in the face.
Descending sympathetic tract	Ipsilateral Horner syndrome.

- **Respiratory regulation:** At low blood pH, receptors in the medulla activate the **reticular formation** (a diffuse group of neurons controlling vital functions) within the medulla. The phrenic nerve is then activated via CN IX and X, stimulating contraction of the diaphragm and inspiration. Lesion causes respiratory depression, decreased response to hypercapnia.
- **Consciousness:** Disruption of the reticular formation secondary to lesions or alterations in neurotransmitters may lead to changes in consciousness (eg, coma) and even death. Injuries to the reticular formation may result from neck trauma, tumor, and cerebellar herniation through the foramen magnum due to increased ICP.
- **Blood pressure regulation:** Receptors in the medulla, the carotid bodies, and the aorta sense stretching of the vessel and send signals to the medulla to increase or decrease BP as needed. Lesion results in hypotension, orthopnea.

NEUROTRANSMITTERS

Several neurotransmitters have important diffuse functions in the brain. They are present in high concentrations within certain groups of cells that control their release (Table 6-15).

SPINAL CORD

The spinal cord continues caudally from the brain stem as a long cordlike structure that gives off branches along the length of the spine.

Blood Supply

Anterior and posterior spinal arteries.

Function

The spinal cord carries information from the brain and brain stem to different parts of the body.

Levels of the Spinal Cord

Cervical spinal nerves C1–C7 share the same number as the vertebral segment **below** it. Spinal nerve C8 exits below the C7 vertebrae, and all spinal

TABLE 6-15.   Major Diffuse Neurotransmitters of the Nervous System

NEUROTRANSMITTER:	ACETYLCHOLINE	DOPAMINE	NOREPINEPHRINE	SEROTONIN
Functions	Peripheral nervous system.	Movement.	Excess in anxiety, panic attacks.	Low in depression.
	Neuromuscular junction.	Reward pathway.	Low in mood disorders.	Mediates pain during migraines.
	Parasympathetic nervous system.	Inhibits release of prolactin.		
	Preganglionic sympathetic fibers.			
	Postganglionic sympathetic fibers of sweat glands and blood vessels.			
Major sites in the brain	Nucleus basalis of Meynert (degenerates in Alzheimer disease).	Substantia nigra of midbrain (degenerates in Parkinson disease).	Locus ceruleus of pons and midbrain.	Pontine raphe nuclei.
	Caudate and putamen.	Arcuate nucleus of hypothalamus.		

nerves below C8 share the same number as the spinal segment **above** it. Each spinal segment receives sensory input from dermatomal regions of the body and sends motor output to myotomal regions (Figure 6-32).

- Cervical (C1–C8)
- Thoracic (T1–T12)
- Lumbar (L1–L5)
- Sacral (S1–S5)
- Coccygeal

KEY FACT

During growth, the spinal column elongates much more than the spinal cord within it. Thus, the spinal cord terminates at a more cranial level in adults than in newborns.

Unique Structures

- **Conus medullaris:** Terminal end of the spinal cord at L3 in newborns and at the lower border of L1 in adults (Figure 6-33).
- **Cauda equina ("tail of the horse"):** At its caudal end (conus medullaris), the spinal cord splits into multiple separate motor and sensory roots, which exit the vertebral canal through the lumbar intervertebral and sacral foramina.

Myotatic Reflex

The myotatic reflexes are monosynaptic, ipsilateral **muscle stretch reflexes,** also known as deep tendon reflexes. Interruption of either the afferent or efferent limb results in **areflexia.** The pathway of the myotatic reflex is as follows (Figure 6-34):

- Afferent limb: Muscle spindle (receptor) → Ia fiber → dorsal root ganglion neuron.
- Efferent limb: Ventral horn motor neuron → striated muscle (effector).

Reflexes and Corresponding Levels

Reflexes are used to test the integrity of the spinal cord at their corresponding levels (Table 6-16).

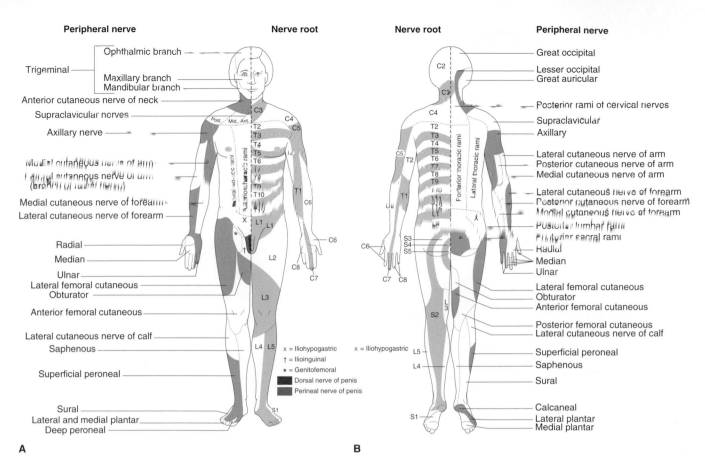

Peripheral nerve   **Nerve root**   **Nerve root**   **Peripheral nerve**

FIGURE 6-32. **Cutaneous innervation (anterior and posterior views).** (A) Cutaneous innervation (anterior view). The segmental or radicular (nerve root) distribution is shown on the left side of the body, and the peripheral nerve distribution on the right side of the body. (B) Cutaneous innervation (posterior view). The segmental or radicular (nerve root) distribution is shown on the left side of the body, and the peripheral nerve distribution on the right side of the body.

Cross-Section of the Spinal Cord

- Gray matter: Central "butterfly" that contains the cell bodies of neurons that send projections either to the periphery or up through the spinal cord tracts.
- White matter: Myelinated tracts of the spinal cord.
- White communicating rami: Contain myelinated preganglionic sympathetic fibers. Found only from T1 to L3 in conjunction with the lateral horn and intermediolateral cell column.
- Gray communicating rami: Contain unmyelinated postganglionic sympathetic fibers.

Tracts of the Spinal Cord

The spinal cord is similar to a bundle of electrical wires with various types of information traveling along their respective paths (Figure 6-35).

- **Motor** pathways travel **away** from the brain. The names of motor pathways begin with the brain structure and end with **-spinal** (ie, rubro**spinal** tract).
- **Sensory** pathways travel **toward** the brain. The names of sensory pathways begin with **spino-** and end with the brain structure (ie, **spino**thalamic tract) except the dorsal columns (cuneate and gracile fasciculi).

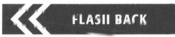

FLASH BACK

The **intermediolateral cell column** contains neuron cell bodies for the entire sympathetic system. It appears as the **lateral horn** from T1 to L3. Fibers arising from the intermediolateral cell column exit the spinal cord via the **white communicating rami** from T1 to L3.

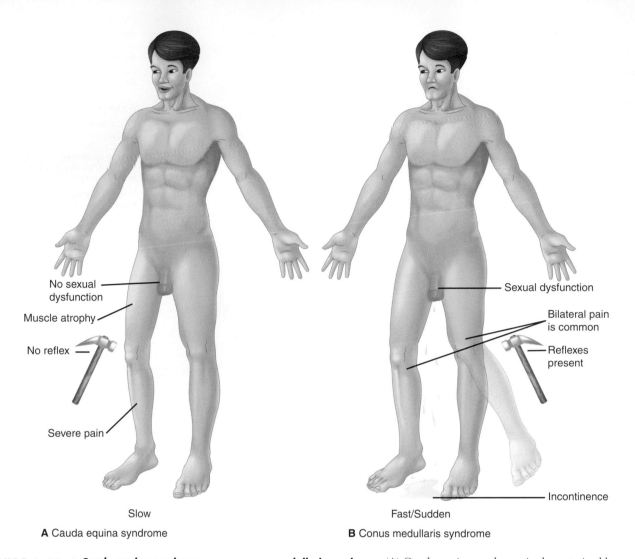

A Cauda equina syndrome

Slow

No sexual dysfunction

Muscle atrophy

No reflex

Severe pain

B Conus medullaris syndrome

Fast/Sudden

Sexual dysfunction

Bilateral pain is common

Reflexes present

Incontinence

FIGURE 6-33. Cauda equina syndrome versus conus medullaris syndrome. (A) Cauda equina syndrome is characterized by preservation of sexual function, muscle atrophy, unilateral pain and areflexia, and a slow progression. (B) Conus medullaris syndrome is characterized by sexual dysfunction, bilateral mild pain, incontinence, and preservation of reflexes.

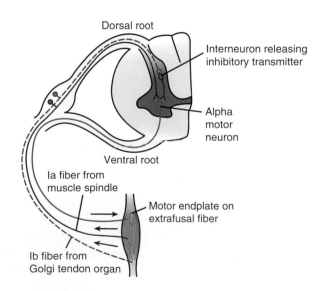

Dorsal root

Interneuron releasing inhibitory transmitter

Alpha motor neuron

Ventral root

Ia fiber from muscle spindle

Motor endplate on extrafusal fiber

Ib fiber from Golgi tendon organ

FIGURE 6-34. Myotatic reflex pathway. Diagram of the myotatic/stretch reflex. The Ia fibers transmit information on muscle length, and the Ib Golgi tendon organ fiber transmits information about tension in the tendon. (Modified with permission from Waxman SG. *Clinical Neuroanatomy*, 25th ed. New York: McGraw-Hill, 2003.)

TABLE 6-16.   **Deep Tendon Reflexes**

MUSCLE STRETCH REFLEX	CORD SEGMENT	MUSCLE
Ankle jerk	S1	Gastrocnemius
Knee jerk	L2–L4	Quadriceps
Biceps jerk	C5–C6	Biceps
Forearm jerk	C5–C6	Brachioradialis
Triceps jerk	C7–C8	Triceps

CORTICOSPINAL TRACTS

The major motor tracts from the cortex. Conduct signals directing purposeful actions (Figure 6-36).

- **Lateral corticospinal tract:** Mediates voluntary skilled motor activity, primarily of the upper limbs.
    - Origin: Cell bodies are the **giant cells of Betz** in layer V of the cortex (see Figure 6-36).
        - Primary motor cortex (Brodmann area 4).
        - Premotor cortex (Brodmann area 6).
        - Supplementary motor cortex (Brodmann area 6).
    - Course:
        - Cortex: The axons of the cells of Betz pass through the posterior limb of the internal capsule, which then forms the crus cerebri as it enters the midbrain.
        - Brain stem: The fibers continue through the ventral part of the brain stem and decussate in the medulla, forming the medullary "pyramids."
        - Spinal cord: The axons travel along the corticospinal tract in the lateral aspects of the spinal cord.

KEY FACT

Before the decussation, the lateral and ventral corticospinal tracts run together. At the pyramids in the medulla, 85–90% of corticospinal fibers decussate and form the **lateral corticospinal tract;** the remaining 10–15% continue as the **ventral corticospinal tract.**

KEY FACT

The lateral corticospinal tract inhibits the **Babinski reflex.** Because myelination of the lateral corticospinal tract is not complete until the second year of life, children < 2 years old often have a positive Babinski sign. Any **upper motor neuron lesion** or lesion of the tract above the alpha motor neuron synapse (ie, spinal cord, cortex) can also result in a positive Babinski sign.

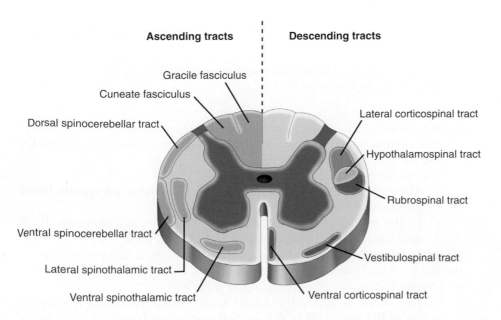

Ascending tracts | **Descending tracts**

- Gracile fasciculus
- Cuneate fasciculus
- Dorsal spinocerebellar tract
- Ventral spinocerebellar tract
- Lateral spinothalamic tract
- Ventral spinothalamic tract
- Lateral corticospinal tract
- Hypothalamospinal tract
- Rubrospinal tract
- Vestibulospinal tract
- Ventral corticospinal tract

FIGURE 6-35.   **Tracts of the spinal cord.**

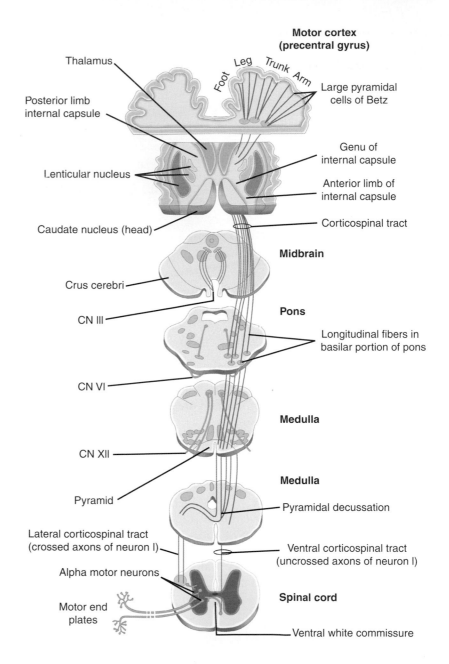

FIGURE 6-36. **Lateral and ventral corticospinal tracts.** The lateral and ventral tracts deviate from each other at the level of the medulla.

- Termination: The fibers synapse onto interneurons within the adjacent gray matter, which then synapse onto alpha motor neurons within the ventral horn of the spinal cord.
- Transection:
  - Above the decussation, injury results in **contralateral spastic hemiparesis and Babinski sign.**
  - In the spinal cord (below the decussation), transection results in **ipsilateral spastic hemiparesis and Babinski sign.**
- **Ventral corticospinal tract:** Mediates posture and gross movements involving the neck and trunk and lower limbs.
  - Origin: Premotor cortex (Brodmann area 6).
  - Course: Same as that of the lateral corticospinal tract **until the decussation of the pyramids** in the **medulla,** where the ventral corticospinal

tract does not decussate and continues ipsilaterally along the ventral white matter of the spinal cord.

- Termination: The fibers then terminate **bilaterally** near the level of exit of the corresponding alpha motor neurons. Decussating fibers contribute to the **ventral white commissure.** Axons then synapse on alpha motor neurons in the ventral horn of the ipsilateral and contralateral spinal cord. These motor neurons innervate axial muscles used in balance and posture.
- Transection results in axial/truncal instability (transection in the brain stem and spinal cord have the same manifestation because this tract is uncrossed). Unilateral transection results in more subtle defects because the axial muscles have bilateral innervation.

- **Hypothalamospinal tract:** Carries autonomic information from the hypothalamus.
  - Origin: Hypothalamus.
  - Course: Travels from the hypothalamus through the lateral tegmentum of the brain stem and down through the dorsolateral quadrant of the lateral funiculus.
  - Termination: Ciliospinal center of the intermediolateral cell column at T1–T2.
  - Transection causes **Horner syndrome:** Ipsilateral miosis, ptosis, hemianhidrosis, and apparent enophthalmos.
- **Other motor tracts:** Mediate coordination of movements and balance. The specific functions are beyond the scope of this text.
  - Vestibulospinal tract
  - Rubrospinal tract

SENSORY PATHWAYS

- **Dorsal column–medial lemniscus pathway:** Mediates light touch discrimination, vibration sensation, form recognition, and conscious proprioception (joint and muscle position sense; Figure 6-37).
- **Sensory receptors:** Pacinian corpuscles, Meissner corpuscles, Merkel discs, Ruffini corpuscles, joint capsule receptors, muscle spindles, Golgi tendon organs (Table 6-17).
- **First-order neurons:** Cell bodies are located in the dorsal root ganglia. Dendrites terminate as receptors in the periphery. Axons project to the spinal cord and give rise to the following:
  - The **gracile fasciculus** (medial) arises from sensory axons in the lower extremities and ascends the spinal cord and synapses on the gracile nucleus.
  - The **cuneate fasciculus** (lateral) arises from sensory axons in the upper extremity and ascends the spinal cord and synapses on the cuneate nucleus.
  - Spinal reflex collaterals that branch off the main axon and synapse on Ia fibers (see "myotatic reflex," Figure 6-34).
- **Second-order neurons:**
  - Cell bodies: Gracile and cuneate nuclei of the caudal medulla.
  - Axons: Decussate in the medulla as **internal arcuate fibers,** form the **medial lemniscus,** and then ascend in the contralateral brain stem.
  - Termination: Synapse on neurons of the **ventral posterolateral (VPL) nucleus** of the thalamus.

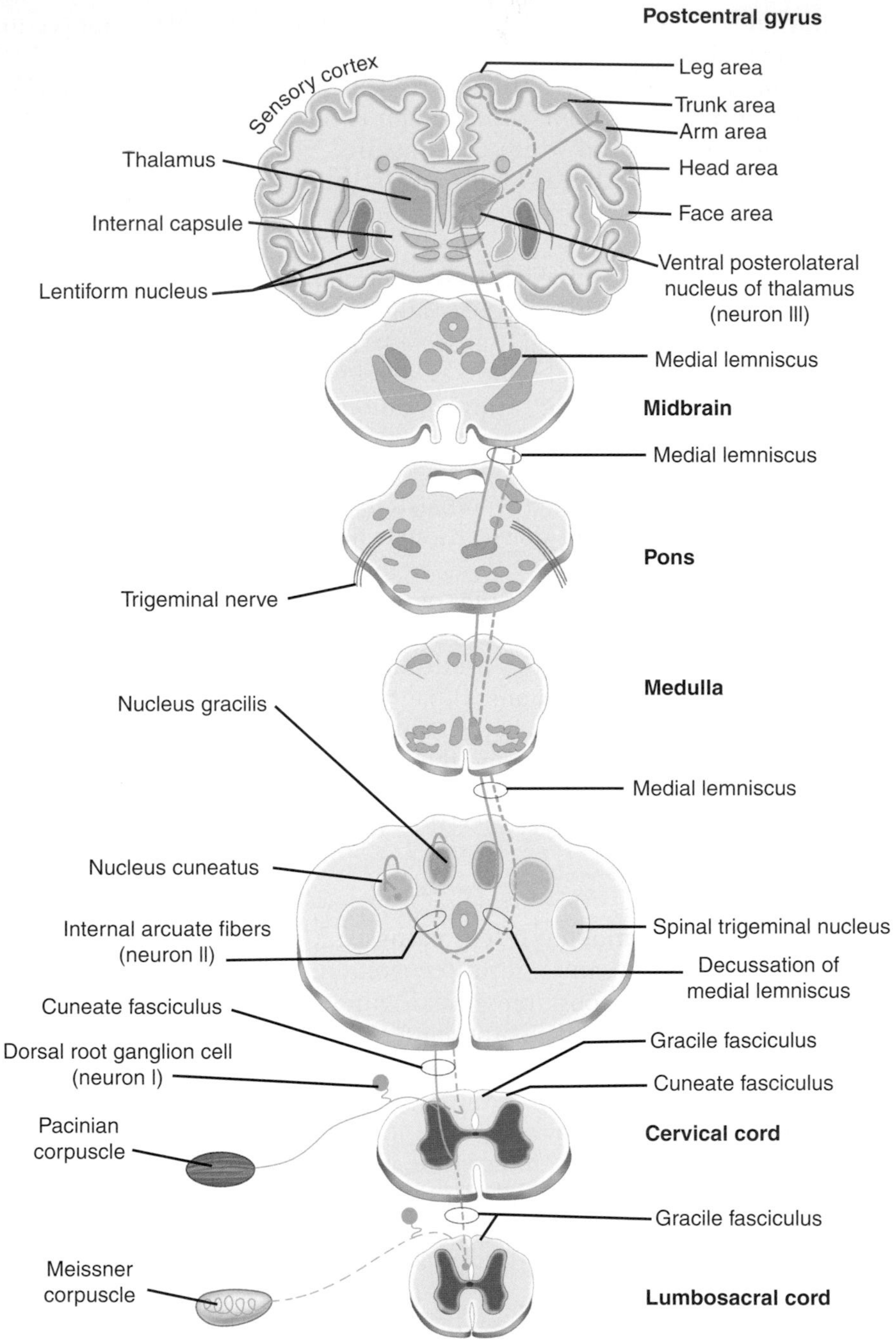

FIGURE 6-37. **Dorsal column–medial lemniscus pathway.** Impulses from light touch, pressure, and vibration travel along this pathway.

KEY FACT

Since the **cuneate fasciculus** carries sensory axons from the upper extremity to the spinal cord, it does not exist below T2, the most inferior level of nerves supplying the upper extremity.

- **Third-order neurons:** Located in the VPL nucleus of the thalamus. Axons project through the posterior limb of the internal capsule to the **primary somatosensory cortex** (Brodmann areas 1, 2, 3) in the postcentral gyrus.
    - Transection:
        - **Above the decussation** of the internal arcuate fibers leads to **contralateral** loss of light touch, vibration, and proprioception.
        - In the **spinal cord (below the decussation)** results in **ipsilateral** loss of the above modalities.

TABLE 6-17.   Major Sensory Corpuscles

Sensory Corpuscle	Meissner Corpuscle	Pacinian Corpuscle and Ruffini Corpuscle	Merkel Corpuscle	Golgi Tendon Organ	Muscle Spindle
Mediates	Light touch, pressure (dynamic)	Deep pressure, vibration, stretching of skin	Light touch, pressure (static)	Muscle tension	Muscle stretch
Description	Small encapsulated	Large encapsulated	Tactile disks associated with peptide-releasing cells			
Location	Between dermal papillae	Dermis	Dermis	Within tendon (in series with muscle fibers)	Within muscle fiber (in parallel with muscle fibers)
Location in the body	Glabrous skin, palms, and soles	Skin, joint capsules, ligaments, serous membranes, and mesenteries	Fingertips, hair follicles, and hard palate	Within tendon	Within muscle fiber

- Lateral spinothalamic tract: Mediates pain and temperature sensations (Figure 6-38).
  - Receptors: Free nerve endings divided into **fast-** and **slow-conducting pain fibers** (Aδ and C fibers, respectively).
    - First-order neurons: Cell bodies are found in the dorsal root ganglia. Dendrites terminate as free nerve endings. Axons project to the spinal cord and ascend or descend a few levels within the **tract of Lissauer** (lateral root entry zone) before synapsing ipsilaterally on second-order neurons in the dorsal horn (**substantia gelatinosa**).
    - Second-order neurons: Cell bodies are found in the dorsal horn (substantia gelatinosa). Axons decussate in the **ventral white commissure** and ascend in the contralateral **lateral funiculus**. Axons terminate in the VPL nucleus of the thalamus.
    - Third-order neurons: Like those of the dorsal column-medial lemniscus tract, third-order neurons are located in the VPL nucleus of the thalamus. Axons project through the posterior limb of the internal capsule to the **primary somatosensory cortex** (Brodmann areas 1, 2, 3) in the postcentral gyrus.
    - Transection causes ipsilateral loss of pain and temperature sensation for a few levels above and below the lesion along the Lissauer tract and **contralateral** loss of pain and temperature sensation for all levels **below** the decussation.

KEY FACT

Both the dorsal column–medial lemniscus and the spinothalamic tract follow the same rule: Primary afferents synapse ipsilaterally; secondary afferents synapse, then cross. However, the decussations occur at different levels: brain stem for the former and spinal cord for the latter.

BROWN-SÉQUARD SYNDROME

Hemisection of the spinal cord or the brain stem results in Brown-Séquard syndrome. Brown-Séquard syndrome is characterized by its striking clinical manifestation of **ipsilateral** hemiparesis, **ipsilateral** loss of vibratory and tactile sensation, and **contralateral** loss of pain and temperature (Figure 6-39). Additionally, it also involves **ipsilateral** loss of pain and temperature sensation within two levels of the lesion because the first-order neurons of the lateral

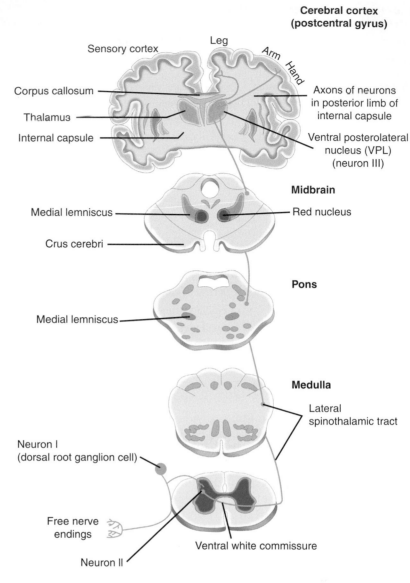

FIGURE 6-38. **Spinothalamic tract.** Impulses from pain and temperature travel along this pathway.

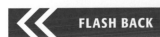

KEY FACT

Fasciculations are coordinated spontaneous depolarizations of a group of muscle fibers innervated by one motor neuron. Manifests as twitches.

Fibrillations are small spontaneous depolarizations of a single muscle fiber that has been denervated.

FLASH BACK

The **nucleus pulposus** is the remnant of the notochord.

spinothalamic tract traverse within the **Lissauer tract** a few levels up or down the spinal cord before synapsing on second-order neurons in the substantia gelatinosa, which then cross the midline via the ventral white commissure. A hemisection at or above the level of T1 also causes ipsilateral Horner syndrome.

Lesions of the Spinal Cord

These result in various symptoms, depending upon which tracts are affected (Table 6-18 and Figures 6-40 and 6-41).

CRANIAL NERVES

Twelve cranial nerves innervate the head and neck. Symptoms of lesions of the cranial nerves are important in localizing pathology within the complex anatomy of the head and neck (Figures 6-42 and 6-43 and Tables 6-19 and 6-20).

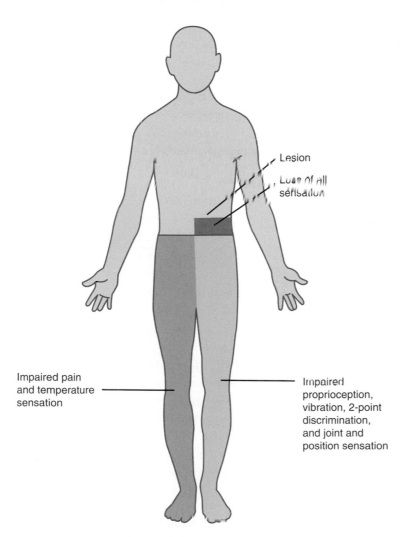

Lesion

Loss of all sensation

Impaired pain and temperature sensation

Impaired proprioception, vibration, 2-point discrimination, and joint and position sensation

FIGURE 6-39. **Brown-Séquard syndrome.** (Modified with permission from Waxman SG. *Clinical Neuroanatomy*, 25th ed. New York: McGraw-Hill, 2003: Figure 5-25.)

TABLE 6-18. **Lesions of the Spinal Cord**

CATEGORY	LESION	MECHANISM	CLINICAL MANIFESTATION	EXAMPLES/OTHER FACTS
Motor pathway lesions	Upper motor neuron (UMN)	Transection of or damage to the corticospinal tract or cortical motor neurons.	Spastic paresis with a positive Babinski sign.	Stroke, ischemic/ traumatic injury to brain stem or spinal cord.
	Lower motor neuron (LMN) (see Figure 6-40A)	Damage to alpha motor neurons.	Flaccid paralysis, areflexia, atrophy, fasciculations, and fibrillations of the muscle fibers.	Poliomyelitis, Werdnig-Hoffman disease ("floppy baby").
	Combined UMN and LMN (see Figure 6-40C)	Damage to both corticospinal tracts and alpha motor neurons.	Both UMN and LMN symptoms.	Amyotrophic lateral sclerosis (ALS).

(continues)

TABLE 6-18. Lesions of the Spinal Cord (continued)

CATEGORY	LESION	MECHANISM	CLINICAL MANIFESTATION	EXAMPLES/OTHER FACTS
Sensory pathway lesions	Dorsal column (see Figure 6-40E)	Destruction of the dorsal column.	Loss of tactile discrimination and position and vibration sensation; shooting pain and paresthesias; **Romberg sign.**	Tabes dorsalis in **tertiary syphilis.**
Combined motor and sensory lesions	Spinal cord hemisection (Brown-Séquard syndrome, see Figure 6-39)	Damage to: • Dorsal columns. • Lateral corticospinal tract. • Lateral spinothalamic tract. • Ventral (anterior) horn.	Gives rise to: • Ipsilateral loss of tactile discrimination, position, vibration. • Ipsilateral loss of pain and temperature sensation (within 2 segments of lesion). • Ipsilateral spastic paresis (below lesion). • Contralateral loss of pain and temperature sensation (below lesion). • Ipsilateral Horner (lesion T1 or above). • Ipsilateral flaccid paralysis (at segment of the lesion).	Trauma.
	Ventral/anterior spinal artery occlusion (see Figure 6-40D)	Infarction of anterior two-thirds of spinal cord; damage may be unilateral or bilateral; characteristically spares dorsal columns and Lissauer tract.	**Preserved** tactile, position, and vibration sense; **loss** of pain and temperature sense; paresis; urinary and stool incontinence; Horner syndrome (lesion T1 or above).	Embolus, aortic dissection.
	Subacute combined degeneration (see Figure 6-40G)	Damage to: • Dorsal columns. • Lateral corticospinal tract. • Spinocerebellar tracts.	• Bilateral loss of tactile discrimination, position, vibration sense. • Bilateral spastic paresis. • Bilateral upper and lower ataxia.	**Vitamin B$_{12}$ deficiency,** pernicious anemia, **Friedreich ataxia** (autosomal recessive, no treatment, 40-year life span).
	Syringomyelia (see Figures 6-40F, 6-41)	Central cavitation of the **cervical** cord (C8–T1) of unknown cause; damage to: • Ventral white commissure. • Ventral horns.	Results in: • Bilateral loss of pain and temperature sensation of upper extremities. • Bilateral flaccid paralysis of intrinsic muscles of the hands.	Commonly seen with Arnold-Chiari syndrome type II; referred to as the sensation of wearing a "cape over the shoulders."

TABLE 6-18. **Lesions of the Spinal Cord** *(continued)*

CATEGORY	LESION	MECHANISM	CLINICAL MANIFESTATION	EXAMPLES/OTHER FACTS
Combined motor and sensory lesions *(continued)*	Multiple sclerosis (see Figure 6-40B)	Random, asymmetrical autoimmune-mediated demyelination of cervical segments of the spinal cord and brain; pathology shows destruction of oligodendrocytes and **reactive gliosis.**	**Charcot triad:** ■ Scanning speech. ■ Nystagmus (MLF syndrome). ■ Intention tremor. Also spastic paresis and sensory loss.	See text discussion.
PNS lesions	Guillain–Barré syndrome	Demyelination and edema of motor fibers of ventral roots and peripheral nerves.	Facial diplegia, papilledema from elevated protein levels, ascending lower extremity weakness, LMN symptoms, **paresthesias,** life-threatening **respiratory paralysis.**	See text discussion.
Intervertebral disk herniation	90% L4–S1 10% C5–C7	Prolapse, herniation of the **nucleus pulposus** through defective annulus fibrosus and into vertebral canal, impinging on spinal roots.	Paresthesias, pain, sensory loss, hyporeflexia, muscle weakness.	Other clues: History of heavy lifting, positive leg-raise test, no relief with sitting.
Terminal cord syndromes	Cauda equina syndrome (see Figure 6-33)	Tumor impingement, spinal stenosis, or inflammation at L3–Co.	Results in: ■ **Gradual** and **unilateral** onset. ■ Radicular **unilateral** pain. ■ Loss of sensation in unilateral saddle-shaped area. ■ Unilateral muscle atrophy and **absent** patellar (L4) and ankle (S1) jerks. ■ **Mild** incontinence and sexual dysfunction.	Treat with emergency surgery.
	Conus medullaris syndrome (see Figure 6-33)	Impingement of S3–Co from intramedullary tumor (ependymoma).	Results in: ■ **Sudden** and **bilateral** onset. ■ **Bilateral** mild pain. ■ Loss of sensation in **bilateral** saddle-shaped area. ■ **Mild** muscle weakness, **preserved** reflexes. ■ **Severe** incontinence and sexual dysfunction.	Nonurgent treatment with corticosteroid injection or radiation.

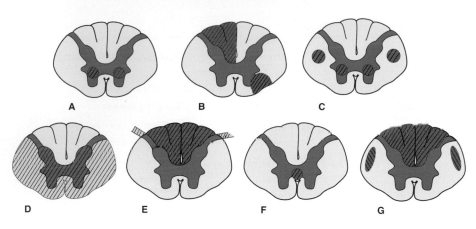

FIGURE 6-40. Patterns of spinal cord lesions. Shaded areas demarcate areas commonly lesioned in specific diseases. (A) Poliomyelitis and Werdnig-Hoffmann disease: Lower motor neuron lesions only due to destruction of anterior horns; flaccid paralysis. (B) Multiple sclerosis: Mostly white matter of cervical region; random and asymmetrical lesions, due to demyelination; scanning speech, intention tremor, nystagmus. (C) Amyotrophic lateral sclerosis: Combined upper and lower motor neuron deficits with no sensory deficit; both upper and lower motor neuron signs. (D) Complete occlusion of ventral artery; spares dorsal columns and tract of Lissauer. (E) Tabes dorsalis (tertiary syphilis): Degeneration of dorsal roots and dorsal columns; impaired proprioception, locomotor ataxia. (F) Syringomyelia: Crossing fibers of corticospinal tract damaged; bilateral loss of pain and temperature sensation. (G) Subacute combined degeneration (eg, vitamin B_{12} neuropathy, Friedreich ataxia): Demyelination of dorsal columns, lateral corticospinal tracts, and spinocerebellar tracts; ataxic gait, hyperreflexia, impaired position and vibration sense.

 KEY FACT

Spinal artery infarction (anterior/ventral arteries are more susceptible because of sparse collaterals) presents with:
- Bilateral loss of pain and temperature (STT).
- Bilateral spastic paresis (CST).
- S2–S4: loss of bladder control.
- Above T2: Horner syndrome.
- The dorsal columns and tract of Lissauer (tract in which the STT travels superior and inferior) are spared.
- Flaccid paralysis (LMN).

 KEY FACT

Romberg sign is a test for proprioception, *not* cerebellar dysfunction. The patient stands with her feet together and closes her eyes. The sign is positive if the patient falls or loses balance.

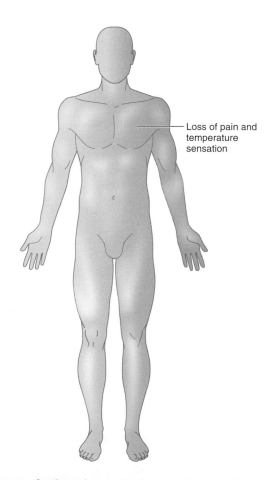

— Loss of pain and temperature sensation

FIGURE 6-41. Loss of pain and temperature sensation in syringomyelia. Involves enlargement of the central canal of the spinal cord, damaging fibers of the spinothalamic tract. Sensory loss is often described as feeling like one is wearing a cape over one's shoulders because it is most commonly found in C8–T1. Often seen in Arnold-Chiari malformation. (Modified with permission from Waxman SG. *Neuroanatomy with Clinical Correlations*, 25th ed. New York: McGraw-Hill, 2003.)

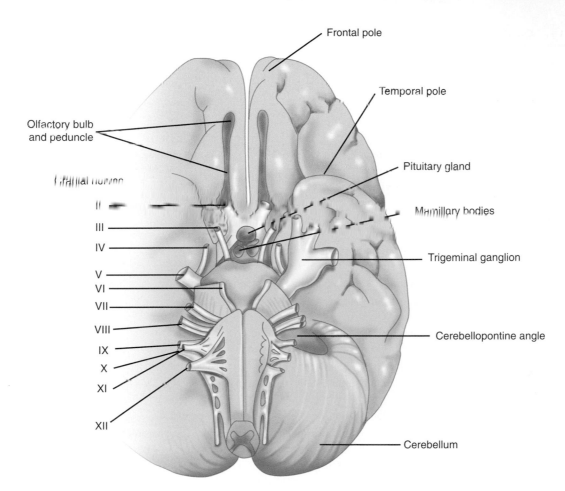

FIGURE 6-42. **Anatomic exits of cranial nerves.** The cranial nerves that are factors of 12 (II, III, IV, VI, and XII) exit near the midline, whereas the rest exit laterally. Of these that exit near the midline, III and IV exit at the level of the midbrain, VI at the level of the pons, and XII at the level of the medulla. Of note, CN IV exits posteriorly and wraps around to the anterior surface.

Cranial Nerve Lesions

Although most lesions are straightforward, some are frequently tested for peculiarities (Table 6-21).

Facial nerve lesions are divided into upper motor neuron lesions (UMN) and lower motor neuron lesions (LMN).

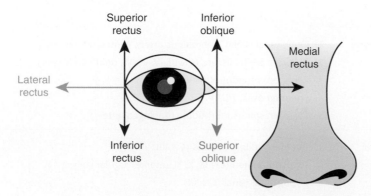

FIGURE 6-43. **Extraocular muscles and their corresponding eye motions.** All muscles are innervated by cranial nerve III with the exception of superior oblique (CN IV, in blue) and lateral rectus (CN VI, in orange). (Modified with permission from Aminoff MJ, Greenberg DA, Simon RP. *Clinical Neurology*, 6th ed. New York: McGraw-Hill, 2005: Figure 4-5C.)

TABLE 6-19. **Cranial Nerves**

NERVE	CN	FUNCTION	TYPE	MNEMONIC
Olfactory	I	Smell.	Sensory	Some
Optic	II	Sight.	Sensory	Say
Oculomotor	III	Eye movement, pupil constriction, accommodation, eyelid opening.	Motor	Marry
Trochlear	IV	Eye movement (superior oblique).	Motor	Money
Trigeminal	V	Muscles of mastication, facial sensation.	Both	But
Abducens	VI	Eye movement (lateral rectus).	Motor	My
Facial	VII	Facial movement, taste from anterior 2/3 of tongue, lacrimation, salivation (submandibular and sublingual glands), eyelid closing.	Both	Brother
Vestibulocochlear	VIII	Hearing, balance.	Sensory	Says
Glossopharyngeal	IX	Taste from posterior 1/3 of tongue, swallowing, salivation (parotid gland), monitoring carotid body and sinus chemo- and baroreceptors.	Both	Big
Vagus	X	Taste from epiglottic region, swallowing, palate elevation, talking, thoracoabdominal viscera, monitoring aortic arch chemo- and baroreceptors.	Both	Brains
Accessory	XI	Head turning, shoulder shrugging.	Motor	Matter
Hypoglossal	XII	Tongue movement.	Motor	Most

- UMN lesion (Figure 6-44):
  - Lesion in the motor cortex or connection between the cortex and the facial nucleus.
  - Leads to paralysis of the **contralateral lower face only,** sparing the forehead.

TABLE 6-20. **Cranial Nerve and Vessel Exits from the Skull**

Cribriform plate (CN I)	
Middle cranial fossa (CN II–VI) through sphenoid bone	1. Optic canal (CN II, ophthalmic artery, central retinal vein) 2. Superior orbital fissure (CN III, IV, V_1, VI, ophthalmic vein) 3. Foramen rotundum (CN V_2) 4. Foramen ovale (CN V_3) 5. Foramen spinosum (middle meningeal artery)
Posterior cranial fossa (CN VII–XII) through temporal or occipital bone	1. Internal auditory meatus (CN VII, VIII) 2. Jugular foramen (CN IX, X, XI, internal jugular vein) 3. Hypoglossal canal (CN XII) 4. Foramen magnum (spinal roots of CN XI, brain stem, vertebral arteries)

TABLE 6-21.   Frequently Tested for Cranial Nerve Lesions

CRANIAL NERVE	NOTE ON LESION
III	Triad of ptosis, blown pupil, and "down and out" eyes.
VII	Paralysis of **both** the upper and lower face (eg, Bell palsy).
VIII	Sensorineural hearing loss. Weber test: normal > affected. Rinne test: air > bone (see Auditory System section).
X	Uvula deviates away from the side of lesion.
XI	Weakness turning head to **contralateral** side of lesion.
XII	Tongue deviates **toward** the side of lesion ("lick your wounds").

- LMN lesion (see Figure 6-44):
  - Lesion of the facial nucleus or facial nerve.
  - Leads to paralysis of the ipsilateral **upper and lower face.**
  - Idiopathic facial nerve palsy is referred to as **Bell palsy.**

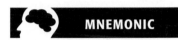

Facial nerve palsy is seen in ALexander Bell with STD:
AIDS
Lyme disease
Bell palsy (idiopathic)
Sarcoid
Tumors
Diabetes

SENSORY PATHWAYS

Visual System

The visual system performs several important functions, including vision, pupillary reflex, near and far accommodation, and coordination of eye movements or gaze (see Figure 6-43).

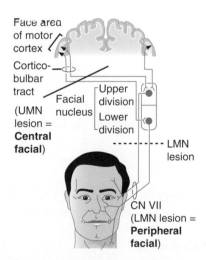

FIGURE 6-44.   Facial lesions. Notice how the upper face receives input from the cortex on both sides, thus a unilateral upper motor neuron (UMN) lesion spares the upper face due to sparing of the contralateral fibers that are innervating the ipsilateral facial nucleus. However, a unilateral lower motor neuron (LMN) lesion disrupts all fibers from the facial nucleus, producing complete paralysis of one side of the face.

MNEMONIC

Divisions of CN V exit owing to Standing Room Only:
CN V₁: **S**uperior orbital fissure
CN V₂: Foramen **R**otundum
CN V₃: Foramen **O**vale

KEY FACT

Lesions of the **afferent pathway** or CN II result in loss of the direct pupillary reflex with preservation of the indirect papillary reflex **(relative afferent pupillary defect, or Marcus Gunn pupil).**
Lesions of the **efferent pathway** or CN III result in complete paralysis of the ipsilateral pupil.

KEY FACT

Argyll Robertson pupil (pupillary light-near dissociation) is the lack of pupillary constriction in response to light, with preservation of pupillary constriction by accommodation to near stimulus. It was formerly referred to as **"prostitute's pupil"** because it "accommodates, but doesn't react." Seen in tertiary **syphilis** and **diabetes.**

KEY FACT

Adie tonic pupil is a large pupil caused by damage to the parasympathetic cillary ganglion; similar to the **Argyll Robertson pupil,** it has impaired reaction to light, retains accommodation to near vision, but reacts very slowly. Seen in women with diminished knee and ankle reflexes.

VISUAL PATHWAY

- **Photoreceptors** of the retina: **Rods** mediate black and white vision; **cones** mediate color vision.
- **Ganglion cells** of the retina: Receive input from the rods and cones via other intermediary cells and send information down axons that form the **optic nerve** (CN II). Ganglion cells from the **nasal** hemiretina project to the **contralateral** lateral geniculate nucleus (LGN), and those from the **temporal** hemiretina project to the **ipsilateral** LGN. Thus, vision from the right visual field of both eyes is projected to the left LGN and vice versa (Figure 6-45).
- The **optic nerve** projects from the optic cup at the posterior aspect of the eye through the optic canal to the optic chiasm, where the fibers split.
- **Papilledema:** Results from congestion of the optic disc and pressure on the root of the optic nerve from increased intracranial pressure (ICP). Results in **enlarged blind spots** with **preserved visual acuity.** Commonly due to mass-occupying lesions in the brain, severe hypertension, or noncommunicating hydrocephalus.

The visual pathway begins at the retina. The **optic tract** is formed from fibers from the ipsilateral temporal hemiretina and contralateral nasal hemiretina. These nerve fibers travel from the optic chiasm to the ipsilateral **LGN, pretectal nuclei,** and **superior colliculus.** Fibers from the LGN then project to the primary visual cortex (Brodmann area 17) through the **geniculocalcarine tract** or **visual radiation.** The **geniculocalcarine tract (visual radiation)** projects through two divisions: the **upper division** and the **lower division (Meyer loop).** The upper division passes through the parietal lobe, and Meyer loop passes through the temporal lobe. Both converge at the **visual cortex.** The posterior area of the visual cortex receives **macular input,** or central vision, the intermediate area receives **perimacular input,** or peripheral vision, and the anterior area receives **monocular input.** Lesions at the various locations of the pathway create different visual defects (Table 6-22).

The **pupillary light reflex pathway** is mediated by the parasympathetic nervous system. It relies on an afferent pathway through CN II and an efferent pathway through CN III (Figure 6-46).

The **pupillary dilation pathway** is mediated by the sympathetic nervous system. Lesions result in ipsilateral **Horner syndrome.**

The **near reflex and accommodation pathway** allows pupils to constrict and focus on near objects.

Auditory System

The auditory system can detect frequencies of **20–20,000 Hz.** The afferent of the auditory system is CN VIII, the cochlear nerve.

AUDITORY PATHWAY (FIGURE 6-47)

Hair cells of the **organ of Corti** transmit to the:

- Bipolar cells of the **spiral ganglion,** that in turn stimulate the
- Cochlear nerve (enters the brain stem at the **cerebellopontine angle**) ascends to the cochlear nuclei, which sends off fibers that
- Decussate via the **trapezoid body,** and travel to the
- **Superior olivary nucleus** bilaterally,
- Ascends via the **lateral lemniscus** to the
- **Nucleus of the inferior colliculus,** which projects to the

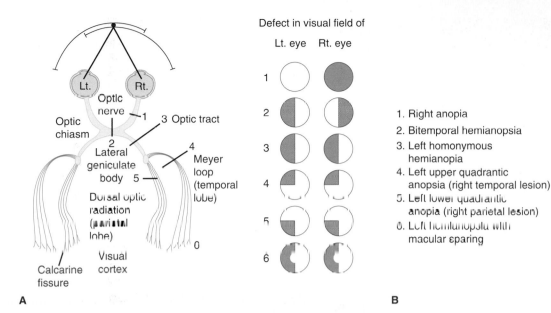

Defect in visual field of

Lt. eye   Rt. eye

1. Right anopia
2. Bitemporal hemianopsia
3. Left homonymous hemianopia
4. Left upper quadrantic anopsia (right temporal lesion)
5. Left lower quadrantic anopia (right parietal lesion)
6. Left hemianopsia with macular sparing

A   B

FIGURE 6-45. **Visual pathways and associated lesions with clinical manifestations.** (A) Visual pathway leading from retina to visual cortex. (B) Lesions along the pathway and corresponding clinical manifestations. Note that lesions proximal to the chiasm can be associated with monocular and ipsilateral defects, and lesions distal to the chiasm lead to contralateral and binocular defects.

TABLE 6-22. **Lesions of the Visual Pathway**

SITE	LESION	COMMENT
Optic nerve (see Figure 6-45, lesion 1)	Optic nerve	Ipsilateral monocular loss of vision. Loss of ipsilateral pupillary reflex (light in ipsilateral eye does not induce pupillary constriction of either eye).
Optic chiasm (see Figure 6-45, lesion 2)	Midsagittal	Bitemporal hemianopia, usually from an enlarging pituitary tumor in adults and a craniopharyngioma in children.
	Bilateral lateral	Binasal hemianopia, usually from calcified internal carotid arteries.
	Unilateral lateral	Contralateral nasal hemianopia, usually from a calcified internal carotid artery.
Optic tract (see Figure 6-45, lesion 3)	Optic tract	Contralateral homonymous hemianopia.
Geniculocalcarine tract	Lower division: Meyer loop (see Figure 6-45, lesion 4)	Contralateral upper quadrantanopia, "pie in the sky." If bilateral, it is called upper altitudinopia.
	Upper division (see Figure 6-45, lesion 5)	Contralateral lower quadrantanopia. If bilateral, it is called lower altitudinopia.
Visual cortex	Perimacular (see Figure 6-45, lesion 6)	Contralateral homonymous hemianopia with macular sparing.
	Macular	Central scotoma.

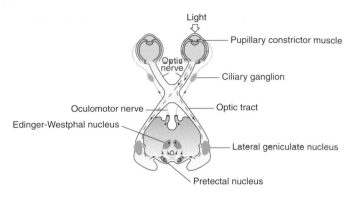

FIGURE 6-46. **Pupillary light reflex pathway.** Retinal ganglion cells → CN II (afferent pathway) → pretectal nucleus of the midbrain → bilateral Edinger-Westphal nucleus of CN III (preganglionic parasympathetic fibers) → CN III (efferent pathway) → ciliary ganglion (postganglionic parasympathetic fibers) → sphincter muscle of the iris.

- **Medial geniculate nucleus (MGN)** via the **brachium of inferior colliculus,** which radiates by way of the **sublenticular part of the internal capsule** to the
- **Transverse temporal gyri of Heschl/primary auditory cortex** (Brodmann areas 41 and 42).

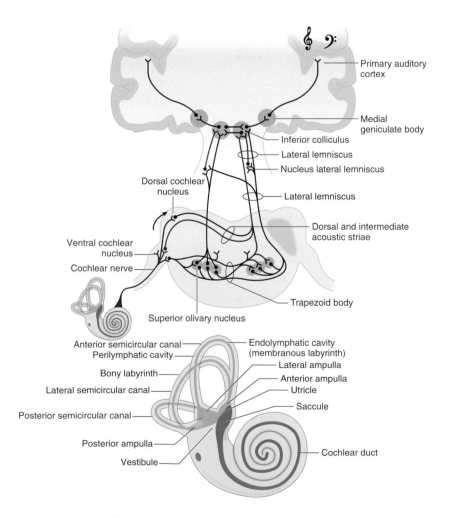

FIGURE 6-47. **Auditory pathway.** The enlarged drawing of the inner ear shows the details of the vestibular system. (Modified with permission from Noback CR. *The Human Nervous System*, 3rd ed. New York: McGraw-Hill, 1981: Figure 15-2.)

HEARING DEFECTS

- **Conduction deafness:** Caused by anything that prevents sound waves from reaching the organ of Corti. The defect is in the **external** or **middle** ear. May be due to **obstruction** (ie, wax), **otosclerosis,** or **otitis media.**
- **Sensorineural deafness:** Caused by disease of the cochlea, cochlear nerve, or central auditory pathways. Usually due to degeneration of the organ of Corti. May also be due to tumors that disrupt the cochlear nerve (eg, **acoustic neuroma**).
- Two major tests of hearing can be done at the bedside to differentiate between conduction and nerve deafness:
    - **Weber test:** Place a vibrating tuning fork on the top of the skull. Ask the patient which side sounds louder. A normal patient hears the sound equally in both ears.
    - **Rinne test:** Place a vibrating tuning fork on the mastoid process behind the ear until the patient can no longer hear the sound. The patient is using **bone conduction** during this phase of the test. Once the patient no longer hears the sound, the tuning fork is held in front of the ear. Normally, the patient still hears the sound using **air conduction.** Therefore, air conduction > bone conduction in a normal patient.
        - In **conduction deafness,** the sound is louder on the affected side in the Weber test. Bone conduction is greater than air conduction in the Rinne test (abnormal).
        - In **sensorineural deafness,** the sound is louder on the unaffected side in the Weber test. Air conduction is greater than bone conduction in the Rinne test (normal).

Vestibular System

The vestibular system maintains balance and coordinates head and eye movements. **Vertigo** results from disruption of the vestibular system (see Figure 6-47).

LABYRINTH

- **Kinetic labyrinth:** Consists of three semicircular canals (superior, lateral/horizontal, and posterior) that are filled with a fluid called **endolymph.** Provides information on **angular acceleration and deceleration** of the head. **Hair cells** lie in the **ampulla** and are activated by endolymph flow.
- **Static labyrinth:** Consists of the **utricle** and **saccule** and responds to **linear acceleration** of the head, including **gravity** (head position). **Hair cells** reside on the otolithic membrane, and bending toward the longest cilium (**kinocilium**) results in activation.

VESTIBULAR PATHWAYS

Hair cells of labyrinth structures → vestibular ganglion → vestibular nuclei in brain stem → cerebellum, MLF, spinal cord, thalamus.

Olfactory System

The olfactory system mediates the sense of smell and involves CN I, the olfactory nerve. It is the only sensory modality that is not relayed by the thalamus before reaching the cortex. Thus, it is thought to be one of the most primal sensory systems.

KEY FACT

Strachan syndrome results from vitamin B_1 (thiamine) intoxication. It produces the following set of symptoms:
- Sensorineural deafness
- Optic atrophy
- Spinal ataxia

KEY FACT

Foster Kennedy syndrome occurs when a meningioma of the olfactory groove compresses the olfactory and optic nerves, producing the following set of symptoms:
- Ipsilateral anosmia (inability to detect smells)
- Ipsilateral optic atrophy
- Contralateral papilledema

KEY FACT

Bilateral acoustic neuroma is a typical manifestation in neurofibromatosis type 2 (NF2). In these patients, the Rinne test is normal because the lesion causes nerve deafness. However, the Weber test may be normal also if the nerve deafness affects both ears equally.

KEY FACT

Kallmann syndrome results from lack of proper formation of the olfactory tract during development. Hypothalamic neurons rely on the olfactory tract to migrate to their destinations. In Kallmann syndrome, the gonadotropin-releasing hormone (GnRH) neurons do not migrate properly from the olfactory placode to the hypothalamus. It produces the following set of symptoms:

- Anosmia
- Hypogonadism
- Infertility

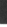

KEY FACT

Proteins and other substances are transported anterograde (away from the cell body) or retrograde (toward the cell body) along microtubules via **kinesins** and **dyneins,** respectively.

KEY FACT

Myelination of neurons in the CNS occurs by oligodendrocytes. Each oligodendrocyte myelinates multiple axons.
Myelination in the periphery occurs by Schwann cells. Each Schwann cell myelinates only one axon.

KEY FACT

Local anesthetics such as lidocaine work by blocking Na^+ channels in the axon on the cytoplasmic side and impeding the conduction of APs triggered by painful stimuli.

OLFACTORY PATHWAY

Olfactory receptor cells → mitral cells of the olfactory bulb → olfactory tract/nerve → primary olfactory cortex (piriform cortex) and amygdala.

Gustatory System

The gustatory system mediates taste and is carried by two major nerves: the special sensory division of CN VII (facial nerve), which supplies the anterior two-thirds of the tongue, and CN IX (glossopharyngeal nerve), which supplies the posterior one-third of the tongue.

GUSTATORY PATHWAY

- Taste buds of the anterior two-thirds of the tongue → intermediate nerve (CN VII) and chorda tympani (CN VII) travel with the lingual nerve (branch of CN V_3) → geniculate ganglion (cell bodies of the taste buds) → solitary tract and nucleus → ventral posteromedial nucleus of the thalamus → gustatory cortex (parietal operculum, insular cortex).
- Taste buds of the posterior one-third of the tongue → glossopharyngeal nerve (CN IX) → petrosal (inferior) ganglion → solitary tract and nucleus → ventral posteromedial nucleus of the thalamus → gustatory cortex (parietal operculum, insular cortex).

Histology

CELLS OF THE NERVOUS SYSTEM

Neurons

The basic subunits of the CNS and PNS. Several variants (sensory, motor, and interneuron) of these cells all share similar basic components (Figure 6-48):

- Cell body (**soma**): Contains the nucleus, organelles, and prominent clusters of rough endoplasmic reticulum, the latter visualized as **Nissl bodies.**
- Dendrites: Afferent single or multiple extensions of the cell membrane that receive signals from other neurons or the environment of the neuron. They also contain Nissl bodies. In some instances, dendrites can also transmit efferent signals.
- Axons: Efferent extensions of the cell membrane that send signals **away** from the cell body to other neurons or end organs. They may be myelinated or unmyelinated.

Neurons may have any number of dendrites and axons, which can be used for classification purposes:

- **Unipolar** neurons have one dendrite or one axon.
- **Pseudounipolar** neurons have one process that branches into a dendrite and an axon.
- **Bipolar** neurons have one dendrite and one axon.
- **Multipolar** neurons have many dendrites and axons.

Neuronal axons contain both areas that are myelinated and those that are unmyelinated.

- **Myelin:** Multiple layers of membranous phospholipid that form a sheath around an axon. Myelination permits fast transmission of action potentials (APs) along the axon.

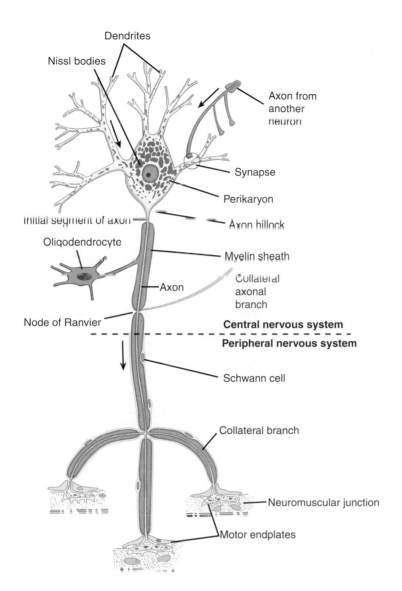

FIGURE 6-48.   Central and peripheral neurons. Basic structure of neurons. Note that in the PNS, axons are myelinated by Schwann cells, whereas in the CNS, axons are myelinated by oligodendrocytes. (Modified with permission from Waxman SG. *Clinical Neuroanatomy*, 25th ed. New York: McGraw-Hill, 2003.)

■ **Nodes of Ranvier:** Areas of naked axon in between areas encased by myelin. Contain a high density of ion channels such as voltage-gated Na^+ channels that allow current to flow across the axon membrane. Allows rapid saltatory conduction of APs along the axon.

Neuroglia

Neurons are maintained by supportive cells known as neuroglia. Neuroglia come in several forms:

■ Astrocytes: Cells that repair and provide nutritional support to neurons, maintain the blood-brain barrier (BBB), and regulate the composition of CSF. They contain the intermediate filament glial fibrillary acidic protein (**GFAP**); stains for GFAP are used to assist in the differential diagnosis of neurologic lesions.
■ Ependymal cells: Form a single layer of cells lining the ventricles and produce CSF.

KEY FACT

Wallerian degeneration occurs in a segment of axon after it has been disconnected from the cell body. In the periphery, degradation and phagocytosis of the axon and myelin is followed by proliferation of Schwann cells.

Chromatolysis occurs in a cell body when an axon has been cut off. It is characterized by:

■ Disruption and dispersion of Nissl bodies
■ Rearrangement of the cytoskeleton with neuronal swelling
■ Marked accumulation of intermediate filaments

KEY FACT

HIV-infected microglia form multinucleated giant cells. Characteristic of **HIV encephalitis.**

- Microglia: Phagocytes of mesodermal origin with irregular nuclei and little cytoplasm. They proliferate around injured nerve tissue and transform into large ameboid phagocytic cells in response to tissue damage.
- Oligodendroglia: Each cell may myelinate up to 30 neurons in the CNS. Destroyed in central demyelinating diseases such as **multiple sclerosis.**
- Schwann cells: Each cell myelinates one PNS axon. Gaps between Schwann cells constitute the nodes of Ranvier. They assist in axonal regeneration by creating a pathway for axon growth and secreting growth factors. Mutation of the tumor suppressor gene neurofibromatosis type 2 (NF2) may give rise to **schwannomas,** commonly located in the internal acoustic meatus (**acoustic neuroma**). Destroyed in peripheral demyelinating diseases such as **Guillain-Barré syndrome.**

INTERCELLULAR COMMUNICATION

Synapses

Neurons communicate with each other through **synapses.** Synapses involve the following structures (Figure 6-49):

- Presynaptic membrane: Contains voltage-gated calcium (Ca^{2+}) channels that open in response to APs.

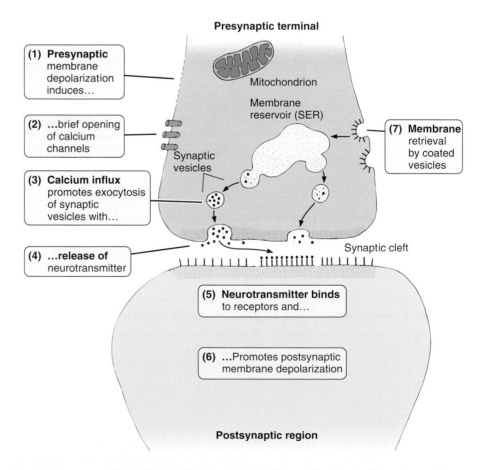

Presynaptic terminal

(1) Presynaptic membrane depolarization induces…

Mitochondrion

Membrane reservoir (SER)

(7) Membrane retrieval by coated vesicles

(2) …brief opening of calcium channels

Synaptic vesicles

(3) Calcium influx promotes exocytosis of synaptic vesicles with…

Synaptic cleft

(4) …release of neurotransmitter

(5) Neurotransmitter binds to receptors and…

(6) …Promotes postsynaptic membrane depolarization

Postsynaptic region

FIGURE 6-49. Steps of synaptic transmission. The small spikes on the postsynaptic membrane represent receptors for neurotransmitters. SER, smooth endoplasmic reticulum. (Reproduced with permission from Junqueira LC, Carneiro J. *Basic Histology*, 11th ed. New York: McGraw-Hill, 2005: 158.)

- Secretory vesicles: Contain the neurotransmitter and rest in the cytoplasm, until Ca^{2+} influx recruits them to the presynaptic axon terminal for exocytosis.
- Synaptic cleft: Site where exocytosed neurotransmitter molecules diffuse across to the postsynaptic membrane.
- Postsynaptic membrane: Contains receptors for various neurotransmitters.
- Receptors: Bind the neurotransmitter and facilitate depolarization of the postsynaptic membrane by activating Na^+ channels.
- Ion channels: Include Na^+, potassium (K^+), and Ca^{2+} channels. Sodium channels are responsible for depolarization (AP); K^+ channels are responsible for repolarization (termination of the AP) and maintenance of the resting potential; and Ca^{2+} channels are responsible for permitting increased intracellular calcium concentration that allows for muscle contraction in the PNS.

Neuromuscular Junction

Neurons communicate with muscle fibers through the neuromuscular junction (NMJ), which resembles a synapse except that the postsynaptic membrane is the membrane of a muscle fiber, also known as an **endplate.** The neurotransmitter is always acetylcholine (ACh). The following lists the sequence of events that takes place during activation of the NMJ (Figure 6-50):

- A wave of depolarization propagates down the axon toward the axon terminal, promoting exocytosis of ACh (similar to the process in the synapse, described earlier).
- Nicotinic ACh receptors (ligand-gated ion channels) lie on the postsynaptic membrane and permit Na^+, K^+, and Ca^{2+} (certain subtypes) to traverse the sarcolemma when activated by ACh.
- Calcium channels on the surface of the sarcolemma (dihydropyridine-type) interact with voltage-gated Ca^{2+} channels (ryanodine-type) on the surface of the sarcoplasmic reticulum (SR). The interaction causes a surge of calcium from the SR into the cytosol in a process called **calcium-induced calcium release.**
- Calcium binds troponin C, which moves tropomyosin off myosin-binding sites on actin, allowing myosin heads to bind to actin and generate muscle contraction.
- Meanwhile, acetylcholinesterase (AChE) degrades any ACh that remains in the synaptic cleft.

KEY FACT

In **neuroleptic malignant syndrome** and **malignant hyperthermia,** muscles of the body involuntarily contract, causing a dangerous elevation of body temperature and damage to muscle fibers. **Dantrolene** can be used to treat these conditions (blocks the ryanodine receptors, inhibiting calcium-induced calcium release).

DISEASES OF THE NEUROMUSCULAR JUNCTION

Myasthenia gravis is an autoimmune disease in which antibodies attack the nicotinic ACh receptors, decreasing their numbers partly through the endocytic pathway (Table 6-23). If left untreated, myasthenia gravis can lead to respiratory failure. Diagnosis is via the **Tensilon test:** Administration of **edrophonium,** a short-acting AChE inhibitor rapidly improves symptoms in myasthenia gravis but not in Lambert-Eaton syndrome.

Lambert-Eaton syndrome is an autoimmune disease in which antibodies attack presynaptic voltage-gated Ca^{2+} channels of the neuromuscular junction (see Table 6-23).

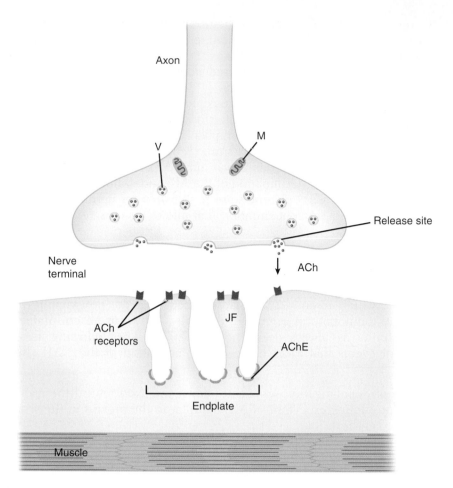

FIGURE 6-50. **Neuromuscular junction.** The "nerve terminal" is the presynaptic bouton. ACh, acetylcholine; AChE, acetylcholine esterase; JF, junctional fold; M, mitochondria; V, vesicles containing ACh.

Sensory Corpuscles

Neurons receive sensory signals through the skin via specialized sensory organs: Meissner, Pacinian, Merkel, and Ruffini corpuscles, muscle spindles, and Golgi tendon organs. Other sensory organs include joint receptors, stretch receptors, baroreceptors, and hair cells of the inner ear (see Table 6-17).

- Pacinian corpuscles: Mediate discrimination of coarse spatial differences.
- Meissner and Merkel corpuscles: Mediate discrimination of fine spatial differences.

TABLE 6-23. **Diseases of the Neuromuscular Junction**

MYASTHENIA GRAVIS (MG)	LAMBERT-EATON SYNDROME
Antibodies attack postsynaptic **ACh receptors**	Antibodies attack presynaptic **Ca^{2+} channels.**
Associated with **thymoma**	Associated with **small-cell lung cancer.**
Muscles are **weaker with repetition**	Muscles are **stronger with repetition.**
Manifests with ptosis, diplopia, muscle weakness **at the end of the day**	Manifests with difficulty rising from a chair and weakness of large muscles especially **in the morning**. Respiratory and ocular muscle involvement not as severe as in MG.

- Joint capsule receptors: Sense flexion/extension of the joints.
- Muscle spindles (in parallel with muscle fibers): Sense muscle length.
- Golgi tendon organs (in series with muscle fibers): Sense tension of tendons and muscles.

Organization of Peripheral Nerves

Nerve fibers consist of axons and their myelin sheaths and are bundled together into peripheral nerves. From outermost to innermost, the three layers of a nerve are:

- **Epineurium** (dense connective tissue) surrounds the entire nerve.
- **Perineurium** (permeability barrier) surrounds a fascicle of fibers; must be rejoined in limb attachment surgery.
- **Endoneurium** surrounds a single nerve fiber (Figure 6-51).

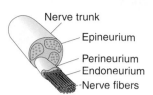

FIGURE 6-51. Layers of the nerve fiber.

Pathology

NEURAL TUBE DEFECTS

Congenital failure of the neural folds and coverings to fuse in the midline leads to deformities in the developing nervous system (see Figure 6-3). Clinical presentation varies in severity depending on which layer is defective (see Table 6-1). The development of these defects is associated with low maternal folic acid levels early in pregnancy. Therefore, babies of mothers taking folate supplements prior to conception have a decreased risk of neural tube defects. Elevated α-fetoprotein in amniotic fluid and maternal serum is diagnostic. In utero ultrasound can confirm the presence of a deformity.

VENTRICULAR SYSTEM MALFORMATIONS

Disruption in the flow of CSF in the cerebral ventricles and subarachnoid space may lead to hydrocephalus and an increase in ICP (Figure 6-52). Malformations may occur anywhere along the pathway and result in a decrease in CSF flow from either **direct blockage of the foramina** or **decreased resorption by the arachnoid granulations.**

PRESENTATION

Hydrocephalus can often manifest with an enlarged calvarium if the cranial bones have not yet fused (ie, the fontanelles are still present). Patients with increased ICP present with the cardinal signs of headache, vomiting without nausea, and papilledema.

DIAGNOSIS

- Made by imaging studies (ultrasound, CT, or MRI) showing abnormalities in CSF flow and ventricle dilation.
- Malformations leading to hydrocephalus can be categorized according to whether they are communicating or noncommunicating.
  - **Communicating:** No anatomic block of CSF flow between the ventricles and the subarachnoid space. Examples include meningitis and subarachnoid hemorrhage.
  - **Noncommunicating:** Blockage of CSF flow from the ventricles to the subarachnoid space at any point in the ventricular system.

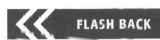

FLASH BACK

Early formation of the neural tube is complete by day 28 of pregnancy. This is important with respect to maternal folate levels because folate is necessary for DNA synthesis, which is essential for dividing cells.

KEY FACT

Carbamazepine and valproic acid have been strongly associated with the development of neural tube defects. Valproic acid is a folate antagonist. Both drugs inhibit intestinal folate absorption.

KEY FACT

α-Fetoprotein is also elevated in hepatocellular carcinoma and yolk sac (endodermal sinus) tumors.

KEY FACT

The three markers tested in the triple screen test, done at 15–18 weeks of gestation, are human chorionic gonadotropin (hCG), estriol, and α-fetoprotein. High hCG coupled with low levels of estriol and α-fetoprotein indicates an increased risk of having a child with **Down syndrome.**

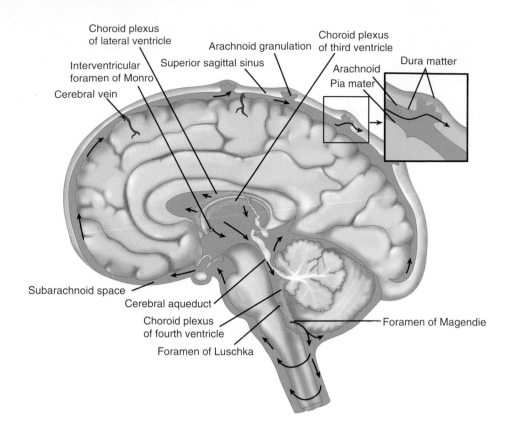

FIGURE 6-52. **Diagram of cerebrospinal fluid flow (*arrows*) through the ventricles.**

KEY FACT

In patients thought to have increased ICP, inspection for papilledema and loss of venous pulsations in the retina on physical exam as well as CT scan should be performed prior to lumbar puncture because of the danger of precipitating tonsillar herniation due to the sudden drop in pressure.

KEY FACT

Riboflavin inhibitors (isotretinoin), posterior fossa trauma, and viral infection (rubella, cytomegalovirus [CMV]) have been implicated in the development of **Dandy-Walker malformation.**

TREATMENT

Ventricular-peritoneal shunt.

NONCOMMUNICATING HYDROCEPHALUS

Blockage of CSF flow can lead to increased ICP, which causes dilation of the ventricles proximal to the blockage.

Dandy-Walker Malformation

Dilation of the fourth ventricle, often secondary to atresia of the foramina of Luschka and Magendie, results in hypoplasia of the midline portion (vermis) of the cerebellum and enlargement of the posterior fossa (see Dandy-Walker syndrome in the section on Congenital Malformations under Brain Development earlier in this chapter).

Congenital Aqueduct of Sylvius Stenosis

The most common cause of hydrocephalus in newborns is obstruction of CSF flow between the third and fourth ventricles. This results in dilation of the ventricles proximal to this obstruction, namely, the third and lateral ventricles.

PRESENTATION

Dilation of the third and lateral ventricles along with clinical signs of papilledema, vomiting, and headache.

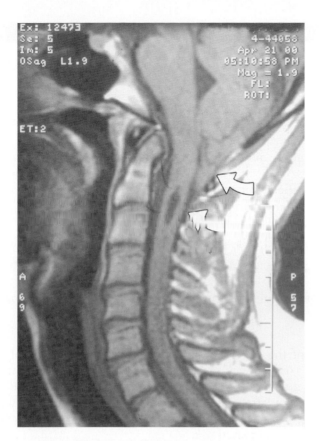

FIGURE 6-53. **Arnold-Chiari malformation and developmental syringomyelia.**
T_1-weighted MRI of the low-lying cerebellar tonsils below the foramen magnum and behind the upper cervical cord (*upper arrow*) and the syrinx cavity in the upper cord (*lower arrow*). (Reproduced with permission from Ropper AH, Brown RH. *Adams and Victor's Neurology*, 8th ed. New York: McGraw-Hill, 2005: 862.)

DIAGNOSIS

MRI or CT showing enlarged third and lateral ventricles, signs of increased ICP can be seen in clinical exam (eg, papilledema).

TREATMENT

Shunt, cerebral aqueductoplasty.

PROGNOSIS

Simple aqueduct stenosis is associated with a very good outcome, with more than half of patients expected to complete normal schooling.

Arnold-Chiari Malformation

Caudal extension of the medulla and cerebellar vermis through the foramen magnum leads to noncommunicating hydrocephalus (Figure 6-53). This malformation is strongly associated with **cervical syringomyelia** (segmental amyotrophy and sensory loss, with or without pain) and lumbar **meningomyelocele.** A more thorough review of Arnold-Chiari malformation is provided in the section on Congenital Malformations under Brain Development earlier in this chapter.

COMMUNICATING HYDROCEPHALUS

Normal CSF flow with abnormal absorption into the dural sinuses leads to dilation of all ventricles.

Hydrocephalus Ex Vacuo in the Elderly

PRESENTATION

Ventricular dilation after significant neuronal loss (eg, Alzheimer disease, stroke). CSF passively fills the vacant space. Results in symptoms of hydrocephalus with deficits in cognition.

DIAGNOSIS

Imaging studies (MRI, CT) showing significant neuronal loss.

TREATMENT

Shunts are not helpful, as the underlying defect is loss of brain parenchyma.

Meningitis

Inflammation of the meninges in the CNS (brain and spinal cord) results from bacterial, viral, fungal, or parasitic infection. The consequent postmeningeal scarring and interstitial edema lead to decreased resorption of CSF at the arachnoid granulations and an increase in ICP. The elderly (> 60 years), the very young (< 3 years), and those living in close quarters (military barracks, dorms) are at increased risk.

PRESENTATION

Meningismus (patient cannot touch chin to chest), nuchal rigidity, headache, and fever, as well as signs of elevated ICP.

DIAGNOSIS

CT prior to lumbar puncture if focal neurologic deficits are present (risk of tonsillar herniation if ICP is elevated), CSF profile.

TREATMENT

Empiric antibiotic therapy.

PROGNOSIS

Viral < 1% mortality rate except in neonates; bacterial 25% mortality rate.

Subarachnoid Hemorrhage

Blood in the subarachnoid space (same space as the CSF) may derive from a ruptured berry aneurysm at the bifurcation of the anterior communicating artery or from congenital arteriovenous malformation. This results in communicating hydrocephalus because the blood clogs the arachnoid granulations, thereby preventing proper CSF resorption. Five percent of the U.S. population has berry aneurysms.

PRESENTATION

Sudden-onset "worst headache of my life," bloody/xanthochromic spinal tap (yellow discoloration from degradation of RBCs), isolated CN III palsy, as well as decreased level of consciousness preceding signs of hydrocephalus.

DIAGNOSIS

Xanthochromic CSF is highly sensitive (> 90%). CT scan showing blood covering the surface of the brain (through the subarachnoid space) and angiogram to determine whether it is of spontaneous or traumatic origin.

TREATMENT

Surgical excision of the aneurysm or filling with metal coil (prior to rupture).

PROGNOSIS

Forty-five percent die within 1 month following hospitalization.

>> **FLASH FORWARD**

Berry aneurysms (see Figure 1-43) are associated with autosomal dominant polycystic kidney disease, Ehlers-Danlos syndrome, and Marfan syndrome. Additional risk factors include old age, hypertension, smoking, and race (higher rates in African Americans).

Normal-Pressure Hydrocephalus

Causes include meningitis, subarachnoid hemorrhage, and atherosclerosis. Results from decreased resorption of CSF at the arachnoid granulations. In 50% of cases, no clear cause can be identified, and an idiopathic intermittent increase in ICP causes the ventricles to slowly enlarge.

PRESENTATION

Classic triad of bladder incontinence, dementia, and slowly developing ataxia. Note that no papilledema or headaches occur because ICP is not increased. The gait is described as a "magnetic gait" in which the patient attempts to initiate each step several times before taking a small step.

DIAGNOSIS

Clinical signs, with CT/MRI showing ventriculomegaly without proportional sulcal atrophy (parenchymal loss) or increased CSF (Figure 6-54).

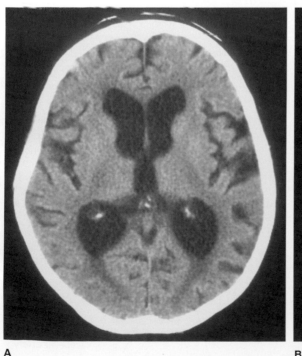
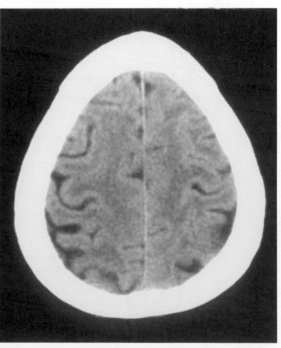

A   B

FIGURE 6-54. **CT scan of a patient with normal-pressure hydrocephalus.** (A) The frontal horns of the lateral ventricles are greatly enlarged. (B) Normal sulci on another image in the same sequence, suggesting disproportionate enlargement of ventricles relative to cortical atrophy. (Reproduced with permission from Ropper AH, Brown RH. *Adams and Victor's Neurology*, 8th ed. New York: McGraw-Hill, 2005: 536.)

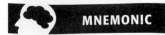

Normal-pressure hydrocephalus manifests with a "wet, wacky, and wobbly" triad: incontinence, dementia, and ataxia.

TREATMENT

Shunt.

PROGNOSIS

Normalization of ventricle size is typically associated with reversal of symptoms.

CEREBROVASCULAR DISORDERS

Cerebrovascular disorders arise from any pathologic disorder in the blood vessels supplying the brain, such as occlusion by thrombus or embolus, increased vascular permeability, and vessel rupture (Figure 6-55). The pathologic processes underlying these conditions manifest themselves clinically as ischemia (with or without infarction) or hemorrhage. Strokes are the third leading cause of death behind myocardial infarctions and cancer.

PRESENTATION

Depends on the location of the cerebral lesion; see following discussion of the different types.

DIAGNOSIS

CT to detect hemorrhage/blood, diffusion tensor MRI to detect infarction.

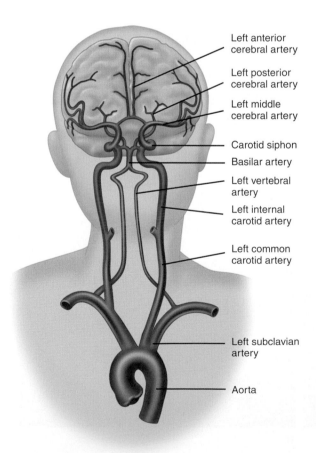

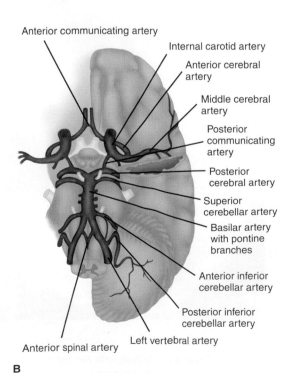

A

B

FIGURE 6-55. **Schematic representation of cerebral vasculature.**

Thrombotic Stroke (Pale Infarction)

The most common type of stroke results from a platelet thrombus that forms over an inflammatory plaque in the middle cerebral artery (MCA) or internal carotid artery. This causes liquefactive necrosis that usually remains pale because of the lack of reperfusion. The brain exhibits a wedge-shaped area of infarction that develops at the periphery of the cerebral cortex; 1–2 days after infarction, edema develops with loss of demarcation between the gray and white matter; myelin breakdown also occurs. A cystic area and reactive gliosis (astrocytic proliferation at the margin of the infarct) occur in the weeks following the infarct.

PRESENTATION

Sudden onset focal neurologic deficits such as unilateral weakness (face, upper extremities, lower extremities), slurring of speech, trouble walking, or visual disturbances, followed by slow improvement over time. Alternatively, patients may wake up in the morning with these symptoms. Transient ischemic attacks, or TIAs (similar symptoms that last < 24 hours), may precede the stroke.

DIAGNOSIS

Symptoms consistent with middle or internal carotid artery distribution indicate where the infarct occurred. Noncontrast head CT is almost universally obtained in suggested strokes to look for any signs of cerebral hemorrhage.

TREATMENT

IV tissue plasminogen activator (tPA) within 3 hours of the onset of symptoms to dissolve the thrombus and enable reperfusion of the ischemic region. Most important side effect is bleeding. IV tPA is not given if CT shows existing cerebral hemorrhage, or if the time of initial onset is unclear.

Long-term management with aspirin, statin, and rehabilitation therapy.

Embolic Stroke (Hemorrhagic Infarction)

Hemorrhagic infarction is thought to result from lysis of embolic material following arterial occlusion and ischemic necrosis that leads to partial restoration of blood flow, which causes blood extravasation through the damaged vessel (reperfusion injury). Emboli originate most often from the heart or proximal atherosclerotic plaques in the carotid arteries.

PRESENTATION

Grossly hemorrhagic infarcts extend to the periphery of the cerebral cortex in the distribution of the arterial supply. Clinically indistinguishable from a thrombotic stroke.

DIAGNOSIS

CT or MRI.

TREATMENT

Treat underlying conditions predisposing to emboli: atrial fibrillation, bacterial/nonbacterial endocarditis, or rheumatic heart disease. Anticoagulants (eg, warfarin) are preventive. Rehabilitation therapy.

KEY FACT

MRI is the imaging modality of choice for detection of ischemic brain injury, whereas CT is optimal for detecting hemorrhage rapidly.

KEY FACT

Vomiting at the onset of intracerebral hemorrhage occurs much more frequently than with infarction and suggests bleeding as the cause of acute hemiparesis.

Intracranial Hemorrhage

These types of hemorrhage are best understood by their anatomic location and typical clinical presentation (Table 6-24, Figure 6-56).

Binswanger Disease

A variant of multi-infarct dementia. Widespread degeneration of cerebral white matter occurs secondary to a vascular lesion (hypertension, atherosclerosis of small vessels, and multiple strokes).

TABLE 6-24. Types of Intracranial Hemorrhage

HEMORRHAGE	ETIOLOGY	PRESENTATION	TREATMENT/PROGNOSIS
Epidural (Figure 6-56A)	Rupture of MMA following blunt trauma at pterion (temporoparietal junction).	Characteristic loss of consciousness followed by lucid interval, which can last minutes to hours.	Without urgent hematoma clot evacuation and cauterization of the MMA, death can result from increased ICP, uncal herniation, and respiratory arrest.
		Bradycardia with increased systolic pressure (Cushing effect).	Permanent brain damage prior to surgical intervention correlates with higher mortality rate.
		Noncontrast CT is diagnostic and shows bright biconvex disc hematoma is between dura and bone and does not cross suture lines (Figure 6-56A).	
		Pressure on CN III parasympathetic portion results in blown pupil.	
Subdural (Figure 6-56B)	Rupture of bridging (emissary) veins between dural sinuses and arachnoid.	Venous bleeding with a delayed onset of symptoms; low-pressure venous system causes slow expansion and delayed onset of symptoms (days to weeks).	Removal of the hematoma by craniotomy is the treatment of choice.
	Seen in brain atrophy (eg, alcoholics, the elderly) or abrupt deceleration (eg, shaken baby syndrome, whiplash).	Fluctuating level of consciousness that develops slowly, crescent-shaped hemorrhage that covers convexity of brain and crosses suture lines.	Without treatment, severe cerebral compression and displacement with temporal lobe–tentorial herniation can result in death.
Subarachnoid (Figure 6-56C, D)	Rupture of aneurysm (usually saccular/berry aneurysm) or an arteriovenous malformation that results in blood moving into the same spaces as the CSF (see Figure 1-43).	"Worst headache of my life," sudden-onset severe occipital headache.	Hemorrhage tends to recur at same site.
		Isolated CN III palsy with aneurysm at the junction of the PCA and PComA.	Hemorrhage can be prevented with surgical excision of aneurysm or fill with metal coil prior to rupture.
		No single large clot and blood fills convexities and cisterns.	Level of consciousness at time of arteriography best index of prognosis.

TABLE 6-24. **Types of Intracranial Hemorrhage** *(continued)*

HEMORRHAGE	ETIOLOGY	PRESENTATION	TREATMENT/PROGNOSIS
Subarachnoid *(continued)*		Bloody/xanthochromic spinal tap.	
		Impaired CSF resorption at the arachnoid granules resulting in communicating hydrocephalus (Figure 6-56C, D).	
		Carotid and vertebral angiography only means of demonstrating aneurysm.	
Parenchymal (Figure 6-56E, F)	Hypertension, amyloid angiopathy, diabetes mellitus, and tumors.	Lateral striate artery hemorrhage secondary to hypertension affects the basal ganglia (putamen), thalamus, and internal capsule (Figure 6-56F), leading to hemiplegia, contralateral sensory loss; also affects pons/cerebellum, causing vomiting, inability to sit/stand/walk.	70-35% patients die within 30 days.
	Hypertension leads to stress on penetrating vessels (lenticulostriate vessels), causing Charcot-Bouchard macroaneurysm with vessel wall thickening; most frequently affects the deep cerebral structures (eg, basal ganglia, thalamus, internal capsule).		Location largely affects the prognosis along with the size of the hemorrhage.
	Ruptured aneurysms lead to intracerebral hemorrhage, which creates a clot that pushes the brain parenchyma aside.		Maintain adequate ventilation, monitor ICP.
			With sustained mean BP > 110 mm Hg, give β-blockers, ACE-inhibitors.
			Surgical evacuation of cerebellar hematomas.

ACE = angiotensin-converting enzyme; BP = blood pressure; ICP = intracranial pressure; MMA = middle meningeal artery; PCA = posterior cerebral artery; PComA = posterior communicating artery.

PRESENTATION

Dementia, gait disorder, and a pseudobulbar state, alone or in combination with long-standing hypertension in older patients.

DIAGNOSIS

Clinical findings and imaging.

TREATMENT

Treat the underlying hypertension and atherosclerosis.

PROGNOSIS

Depends on the location of the infarction.

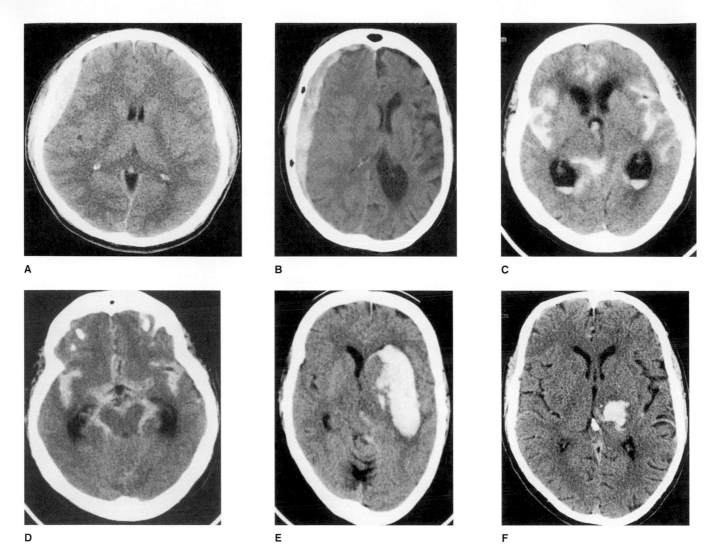

FIGURE 6-56. CT scans of intracranial hemorrhages. (A) Epidural hemorrhages are often a result of blunt trauma to the head and rupture of the middle meningeal artery. The convex lens appearance that does not cross suture lines is classic. (B) Subdural hemorrhages are often secondary to rupture of the bridging veins. Bridging veins are put under tension by sudden deceleration (trauma), cortical atrophy (elderly), or repeated shaking ("shaken babies"). The hemorrhage can cross suture lines and appears as a crescent. (C, D) Subarachnoid hemorrhage is often characterized by a "thunderclap headache" from a ruptured aneurysm. Patient history may include polycystic kidney disease or connective tissue disease. (E) Intraparenchymal hemorrhage that drains into the left lateral ventricle. Intraparenchymal hemorrhage often results from uncontrolled hypertension (Charcot-Bouchard aneurysms), ruptured aneurysms, vascular malformations (eg, arteriovenous malformation), or amyloid angiopathy. (F) Intraparenchymal hemorrhage often occurs in the deep nuclei of the brain. Here hemorrhage is seen in the left thalamus. (Part A reproduced with permission from Kasper DL, Braunwald E, Fauci AS, et al. *Harrison's Principles of Internal Medicine*, 16th ed. New York: McGraw-Hill, 2005: 2450. Parts B–F reproduced with permission from Ropper AH, Brown RH. *Adams and Victor's Neurology*, 8th ed. New York: McGraw-Hill, 2005: 711, 713, and 719.)

Lacunar Infarcts

Cystic areas of microinfarction result from hyaline arteriolosclerosis (small vessels) secondary to hypertension or diabetes mellitus (DM). Lacunar infarcts often occur in the distal end of small cerebral vessels, causing a number of classic clinical presentations.

PRESENTATION

- Pure sensory stroke when the infarct is in the thalamus; characterized by numbness, tingling, pain, or burning sensation without motor symptoms.
- Pure motor hemiparesis from an infarct in the posterior limb of the internal capsule or basis pontis; the face, arm, and leg are almost always

involved as opposed to occlusion of the MCA (face and arm worse than the leg) or anterior cerebral artery (ACA) (leg worse than the face and arm).
- Ataxic hemiparesis from an infarct in the base of the pons; characterized by a combination of cerebellar and motor symptoms.
- Dysarthria and a clumsy hand or arm due to infarction in the base of the pons or in the genu of the internal capsule.
- Pure motor hemiparesis with "motor (Broca) aphasia" due to thrombotic occlusion of a lenticulostriate branch supplying the genu and the anterior limb of the internal capsule and adjacent white matter of the corona radiata.

DIAGNOSIS

Clinical signs and symptoms, imaging studies to exclude hemorrhage, X-ray cerebral angiography.

TREATMENT

Reduction in BP (statins, angiotensin-converting enzyme [ACE] inhibitors), well-controlled DM, and aspirin.

PROGNOSIS

Generally fair to good. Depends on the location and extent of damage (as determined by positron emission tomography [PET] scan, MR diffusion with MR perfusion to identify the ischemic penumbra—the area of ischemic tissue on the periphery of the infarct that will likely infarct as well).

Stroke Presentation According to Cerebral Location of Occlusion
- Middle cerebral artery:
  - Parietal lobe results in contralateral hemianesthesia (face and arm worse than leg).
  - Frontal lobe results in contralateral hemiplegia (face and arm worse than leg).
  - Temporal lobe results in homonymous quadrantanopia.
  - If the **dominant hemisphere** is affected (usually left), aphasia will also develop.
  - If the **nondominant hemisphere** is affected (usually right), sensory neglect and apraxia will develop (no complex movements, inability to follow commands).
- Anterior cerebral artery:
  - Parietal results in contralateral hemianesthesia (leg worse than face and arm).
  - Frontal lobe results in contralateral hemiplegia (leg worse than face and arm).
  - Medial frontal (midline) causes urinary incontinence, reemergence of the grasp reflex.
- **Posterior cerebral artery:** Occipital causes homonymous hemianopia with macular sparing.
- **Anterior inferior cerebellar artery (lateral pontine syndrome):**
  - **Ipsilateral:** Paralysis of facial movement (CN VII), paralysis of conjugate gaze to side of lesion (CN VI), facial pain/temperature loss (spinal trigeminal nucleus/tract), Horner syndrome (descending sympathetics), hearing loss/vertigo/nausea and vomiting/nystagmus away from lesion (CN VIII/cochlear nucleus), dystaxia (inferior/middle cerebellar peduncle), which is difficulty controlling voluntary movements.
  - **Contralateral:** Loss of pain and temperature sensation in the body (spinothalamic tract).

MNEMONIC

Chorea = dancing (think **choreo**graphy).

KEY FACT

Athetos = not fixed (think snake-like writhing).

KEY FACT

If a right-handed patient presents with aphasia, it can be confidently assumed that the lesion is in the left hemisphere; the same is true for most left-handed patients, though the language areas of a small proportion of left-handed patients are on the right hemisphere. Imaging (CT/MRI) confirms the clinical suspicion.

KEY FACT

Most individuals learn to read by transforming the printed word into the auditory form. Patients with Wernicke aphasia may present with alexia because the auditory center for language (Wernicke area) is damaged.
Wernicke aphasia is distinct from Wernicke-Korsakoff syndrome, a disease arising from thiamine deficiency (typically due to chronic alcohol abuse) that manifests with encephalopathy, amnesia, confabulation, ophthalmoplegia, and ataxia.

MNEMONIC

Broca's **Bro**ken **Bo**ca (Boca is Spanish for "mouth")
Wernicke is **W**ordy.

- **Posterior inferior cerebellar artery (Wallenberg syndrome/lateral medullary syndrome):**
  - **Ipsilateral:** Limb ataxia and intention tremor (inferior cerebellar peduncle), vertigo/nausea and vomiting/nystagmus away from lesion (vestibular nuclei), paralysis of larynx/pharynx/palate (nucleus ambiguus), facial pain/temperature loss (spinal V), Horner syndrome (descending hypothalamics).
  - **Contralateral:** Loss of pain and temperature sensation in the body (spinothalamic tract).

DYSKINESIAS

Disorders of movement involve disturbance of voluntary movement or the presence of involuntary movements, commonly referred to as **extrapyramidal** diseases because there is no muscle weakness (as is the case in UMN lesions). May arise from basal ganglia lesions and manifest as resting tremor, chorea, or athetosis. Other regions involved are the cerebellar hemisphere, cerebellar vermis, and subthalamic nucleus. Dyskinesias are symptoms that may be part of a syndrome or disease.

Chorea

Chorea is characterized by involuntary, jerky, purposeless movements that arise from **basal ganglia lesions.**

DISEASES CHARACTERIZED BY CHOREA

- **Inherited disorders:**
  - Huntington disease
  - Neuroacanthocytosis
  - Wilson disease
- **Infectious:** Streptococcal infection (rheumatic fever)
- **Drug-induced chorea:**
  - Neuroleptics (phenothiazines, haloperidol)
  - Phenytoin
  - Oral contraceptives in women with systemic lupus erythematosus (SLE) and antiphospholipid antibodies
  - Excessive dosage of L-dopa and dopamine agonists
  - Cocaine

Athetosis

An inability to maintain a body part in one position that usually manifests as slow, writhing movements (especially in the fingers) that alternate between extension and flexion. **Characteristic of basal ganglia lesions and antipsychotics (eg, haloperidol).**

Hemiballismus

Sudden, uncontrolled flailing of one limb results from a lesion in the **contralateral subthalamic nucleus.**

PRESENTATION

A lesion in the subthalamic nucleus interrupts the inhibitory indirect pathway (see Figure 6-20) and releases the thalamus from inhibition by the globus pallidus internus results in sudden uncontrolled flailing of the contralateral limb (continuous/intermittent).

DIAGNOSIS

MRI showing signal changes in the **contralateral subthalamic nucleus**.

TREATMENT

Haloperidol, phenothiazine.

PROGNOSIS

Hemiballismus that persists for weeks without treatment may result in exhaustion and death.

APHASIAS

The muscles involved in generating speech, chewing, and swallowing are intact. Therefore, patients with aphasia do not have a peripheral motor problem, but rather one that arises from a cortical lesion. Speech therapy is recommended for all patients with aphasia (Table 6-25 and Figure 6-18).

KEY FACT

Vascular dementia may be caused by:

- Multiple infarcts: Large-artery atherosclerosis in the circle of Willis (see Figure 6-11) and carotids.
- Binswanger leukoencephalopathy: Loss of white matter secondary to hypertension-related atherosclerosis.
- Lacunar infarcts: Small < 1-cm infarcts of the striatum and thalamus related to arteriolosclerosis.

TABLE 6-25.   Perisylvian Types of Aphasias

LOCATION	PRESENTATION	PROGNOSIS/TREATMENT
Broca area (inferior frontal gyrus, Brodmann area 44)	▪ Motor/nonfluent/expressive aphasia with good comprehension, thus patients are aware of problem, and therefore can be extremely frustrated, cannot say what they are thinking, and use mainly short monosyllabic words. ▪ Often accompanied by contralateral weakness (hemiparesis often on the right side) of the lower face and arm.	▪ May improve over time, excellent potential for functional recovery. ▪ Prognosis depends on the size of the lesion, the age of the patient, and the status of the contralateral hemisphere.
Wernicke area (superior temporal gyrus, Brodmann area 22)	▪ Sensory/fluent/auditory aphasia with impaired comprehension, neologisms, paraphasic errors, and impaired repetition. ▪ Speech is fluent but nonsensical ("word salad"). ▪ Unaware of defect. ▪ Often with contralateral visual defects (right upper quadrant loss because optic radiations from Meyer loop are affected), alexia.	▪ May improve over time. ▪ Prognosis depends on the size of the lesion, the age of the patient, and the status of the contralateral hemisphere. ▪ Patient less likely than those with injury to Broca area to return to normal social life because of severe comprehension defect.
Arcuate fasciculus	▪ Conduction aphasia because this structure connects Wernicke and Broca areas; poor repetition with intact comprehension and fluent speech. ▪ Cannot name objects.	▪ Prognosis depends on the size of the lesion, the age of the patient, and the status of the contralateral hemisphere.
Global	▪ Both speech and comprehension affected due to large perisylvian or separate frontal and temporal lesions. ▪ Often accompanied by right hemiplegia, hemianesthesia, and homonymous hemianopia.	▪ May regain degree of comprehension. ▪ Clinical picture may resemble Broca aphasia over time.

DEGENERATIVE DISEASES

Degenerative diseases, as with other CNS disorders, are best understood by recognizing the functions associated with the specific region(s) in which the lesion develops. Lesions along the corticospinal tract cause motor deficits (Table 6-26).

Generally, symptoms associated with diseases affecting the cerebrum include personality changes, memory loss, seizures, and cognitive dysfunction (Table 6-27).

Basal ganglial injuries generally manifest as movement disorders (Table 6-28).

Spinocerebellar lesions affect the spinocerebellar tracts or the cerebellum (or both) and manifest with ataxia (Table 6-29).

MNEMONIC

Treatment for Parkinson is BALSA:
Bromocriptine
Amantadine
Levodopa (with carbidopa)
Selegiline (and catechol-*O*-methyltransferase inhibitors, eg, entacapone)
Anticholinergics (eg, benztropine)

TABLE 6-26. **Motor Neuron Lesions**

TYPES	PRESENTATION	PATHOLOGY	PROGNOSIS/ TREATMENT
Amyotrophic lateral sclerosis (ALS)	Associated with both LMN and UMN signs with sparing of sensation; onset at 40–60 years of age; most common motor neuron disease; rare inherited form in 40- to 60-year-olds (chromosome 21, *SOD1* mutation).	UMN signs (spasticity, positive Babinski sign).	Rapidly fatal due to respiratory failure. Riluzole delays the onset of ventilator-dependence or tracheostomy and may increase survival by 3–5 months. Its mechanism of action includes blockade of TTX-sensitive Na^+ channels (associated with damaged neurons) and glutamate receptor blockade (reduced excitotoxicity).
	Thenar atrophy first sign (LMN lesion), fasciculations, hyperreflexia (UMN lesion, lateral corticospinal tract).	LMN signs (muscle weakness, denervation atrophy).	
Werdnig-Hoffman disease	Autosomal recessive inheritance that manifests at birth as floppy baby syndrome, tongue fasciculations, LMN disease.	Degeneration of anterior horns; **no** UMN/corticospinal tract degeneration; congenital variant of ALS with only LMN signs. Defect in gene that normally "turns off" perinatal programmed cell death.	Median age of death 7 years, rapidly fatal.
Poliomyelitis	Follows infection (fecal-oral) with poliovirus; first replicates in oropharynx and small intestine before hematologic spread to CNS, presenting with LMN signs.	Degeneration of anterior horns of spinal cord.	Hospitalize with strict bed rest to reduce rate of paralysis. Ventilation to treat respiratory muscle weakness. May develop new muscle weakness after recovery from acute paralytic poliomyelitis.
	CSF with lymphocytic pleocytosis and slight elevation of protein.		
	Virus recovered from stool or throat.		

CNS = central nervous system; TTX = tetrodotoxin.

TABLE 6-27. **Cerebral Cortex Lesions**

Types	Presentation	Pathology	Prognosis/Treatment
Alzheimer disease	Slow, progressive mental deterioration with loss of short-term memory, anosmia, difficulties with language and planning skills, decline in executive function.	Senile plaques (β-amyloid core surrounded by dystrophic neuritis in extracellular space); neurofibrillary tangles (intracellular, abnormally phosphorylated tau protein forming flame-shaped paired helical filaments twisted around each other), (silver stain positive).	AChE inhibitors that penetrate the BBB (eg, donepezil) increase ACh levels in the brain and alleviate symptoms, but have no effect on disease progression. NMDA receptor antagonists (eg, memantine) reduce glutamate-mediated excitotoxicity (also not disease-modifying).
	Spares primary sensory and motor areas.	β-Amyloid is toxic when deposited in neurons and cerebral blood vessel walls (cerebral amyloid angiopathy), leading to weakening of vessel walls and intracranial hemorrhage.	Survival 50% of expected rate secondary to cardiovascular and respiratory causes and starvation.
	Generalized cerebral atrophy beginning in temporal lobe and hippocampus leads to widened sulci and enlarged ventricles (hydrocephalus ex vacuo).	Decreased ACh due to loss of cholinergic nuclei in the forebrain (nucleus basalis of Meynert).	
	The most common cause of dementia in elderly.		
	Familial form (10%) associated with onset at < 40 years. Known genetic causes include mutations in presenilin 1 and 2 on chromosomes 1 and 14, respectively (leads to hyperphosphorylated tau and neurofibrillary tangles), *APOE4* allele on chromosome 19, and p-*APP* on chromosome 21.		
	p-*APP* increases amount of amyloid precursor protein. Trisomy 21 (Down syndrome) is associated with early-onset Alzheimer (near 100% prevalence at age 30–40 years).		
Pick disease	First sign is personality changes (disinhibition, dementia, impaired judgment) with language disturbance (aphasia).	Swollen neurons with Pick bodies (intracellular aggregated tau protein); straight filaments observed with silver staining.	Limited treatment options targeting neurotransmitters, similar to Alzheimer.
	Aspects of Alzheimer (memory loss) except with earlier age of onset (< 50 years), descent into the "sea of mindlessness."	Loss of white matter underlying atrophic cortex with gliosis, specific for frontal-temporal lobes.	

(continues)

TABLE 6-27. **Cerebral Cortex Lesions** *(continued)*

TYPES	PRESENTATION	PATHOLOGY	PROGNOSIS/TREATMENT
Multi-infarct (vascular) dementia	Second most common cause of dementia.	Secondary to atherosclerosis.	Vascular prophylaxis and stroke prevention.
	A progressive, *stepwise* decline in functioning, which differentiates it from the gradual course of Alzheimer.		

ACh = acetylcholine; AChE = acetylcholine esterase; BBB = blood-brain barrier; NMDA = *N*-methyl-D-aspartate.

TABLE 6-28. **Basal Ganglia Lesions**

TYPES	PRESENTATION	PATHOLOGY	PROGNOSIS/TREATMENT
Huntington disease	Autosomal dominant with complete penetrance and development of progressive athetoid chorea in all four limbs (writhing), dementia, and emotional disturbances. Onset at 35–45 years with anticipation.	Atrophy of striatum leads to loss of medium spiny (GABAergic) neurons.	Symptomatic treatment with haloperidol effective in suppressing movement disorder (care must be taken not to superimpose tardive dyskinesia; prescribe only for chorea that is functionally disabling).
	Atrophy of the caudate (head) and putamen may make lateral ventricles appear enlarged when imaging ("bat-wing" frontal horns). Hydrocephalus ex vacuo.	Expansion of CAG triplet repeats (polyglutamine) in *huntingtin* gene on chromosome 4 results in aggregation of mutant *huntingtin* protein (toxic to neurons).	Incurable; steadily progressive course and death 15–20 years after onset with ↑ rate of suicide; requires supportive therapy and genetic counseling.
	Spared memory, increased blinking, impaired initiation, and slowness of both pursuit and volitional saccadic movements and an inability to make a volitional saccade without movement of the head.		Length of repeat determines age of onset and severity (worse when inherited from affected father; allele more unstable during spermatogenesis leading to paternal expansion).
Parkinson disease	Clinically defined by **TRAPS: T**remor at rest (eg, pill-rolling), cogwheel **R**igidity, **A**kinesia/bradykinesia, **P**ostural instability, **S**huffling gait, flat affect.	Lewy body inclusions (eosinophilic with halo, aggregate of α-synuclein representing damaged neurofilaments) diffusely in cortical neurons with few tangles or plaques.	Disease course 10–25 years.
	Rarely, linked to MPTP exposure (meperidine derivative [synthetic heroin]).	Depigmentation of the substantia nigra pars compacta (secondary to loss of dopaminergic neurons).	Dopamine agonists, eg, levodopa, carry risk of drug-related dyskinesias.

TABLE 6-28. Basal Ganglia Lesions *(continued)*

TYPES	PRESENTATION	PATHOLOGY	PROGNOSIS/TREATMENT
Parkinson disease *(continued)*	Arises from any insult that damages basal ganglia, including antipsychotics that are dopamine antagonists, ischemia, chronic carbon monoxide poisoning, Wilson disease, encephalitis.		Surgical intervention when inadequate response to levodopa; ablation/functional blockade (deep brain stimulation) of subthalamic nucleus effective at treating symptoms with no risk of drug-induced dyskinesias associated with long term dopamine replacement therapy.
Wilson disease	Onset at age 20–30 years with asterixis, dystonia, tremor, and dementia preceded by liver cirrhosis, greenish brown pigmentation around iris (**Kayser-Fleischer rings** in cornea).	Excessive copper accumulation occurs predominantly in: (1) liver; (2) lenticular nucleus of the basal ganglia; and (3) eyes, causing a ↓ in ceruloplasmin and ↑ urinary copper.	Zinc, penicillamine (copper chelator) + pyridoxine to prevent anemia effective at preventing progression of neurologic symptoms; low-copper diet.
		Liver biopsy and copper quantification is gold standard.	Liver transplantation curative for underlying metabolic defect.
Dementia with Lewy bodies (DLB)	Extrapyramidal Parkinsonian features because of loss of dopaminergic neurons, dementia. The following symptoms are more characteristic of DLB: episodic delirium (visual/auditory hallucinations), visuospatial impairment, varying attention, and undulating clinical course.	Widespread formation of Lewy bodies (α-synuclein aggregates) in substantia nigra, limbic system, and nucleus basalis of Meynert.	Selegiline and other MAO inhibitors may be helpful.
			Mortality eventually results from complications of immobility, poor nutrition, and swallowing difficulties.

MAO = monoamine oxidase; MPTP = 1-methyl-4-phenyl-1,2,3,6-tetrahydropyridine.

Progressive Supranuclear Palsy

Disease is characterized by widespread neuronal loss and subcortical gliosis that notably spares the cerebral and cerebellar cortices.

PRESENTATION

Onset in the sixth decade presenting with difficulty in vertical movement of gaze, pseudobulbar palsy (dysarthria, dysphagia, hyperactive jaw jerk and gag reflexes, and uncontrollable laughing or crying unrelated to emotional state), axial dystonia with repeated falls, and bradykinesia without resting tremor ("atypical Parkinsonism"). Memory and intellect intact.

DIAGNOSIS

Exclusion of other causes, prominent neurofibrillary tangles.

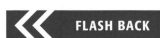

FLASH BACK

Wilson disease (hepatolenticular degeneration) results from autosomal recessive mutations in a membrane-bound copper transporter that overwhelms copper capacity because of an inability to excrete copper into bile. Copper is deposited in the putamen and globus pallidus, as well as many other organs, including the liver (see Table 6-28).

TABLE 6-29. Spinocerebellar Lesions

TYPES	PRESENTATION	PATHOLOGY	PROGNOSIS/TREATMENT
Olivopontocerebellar atrophy	Ataxia (broad-based gait), dysarthria, intention tremor, generalized rigidity, and dementia.	Loss of cerebellar Purkinje cells (GABAergic in cerebellar cortex). MRI shows flattening of pons, enlarged fourth ventricle. Alzheimer disease inheritance.	Progressive neurodegeneration with no definitive treatment. Falls and aspiration pneumonia contribute to morbidity and mortality.
Friedreich ataxia	Autosomal recessive trinucleotide repeat disease (GAA) involving *frataxin* gene, with onset of symptoms in the first decade of life. Loss of proprioception, decreased deep tendon reflexes, positive Babinski sign.	"Atrophy of spinal cord," diffuse damage to dorsal columns, spinocerebellar tracts, and lateral corticospinal tracts.	Poor prognosis, no definitive treatment.
	Most common hereditary ataxia; autosomal recessive inheritance.	Pathology mimics subacute combined degeneration of the spinal column (see Figure 6-40G).	
	Associated with myocarditis, hypertrophic cardiomyopathy, scoliosis, hearing/vision impairment, and high plantar arches (pes cavus).		

TREATMENT

No definitive treatment. Treatment with L-dopa yields poor results because dopaminergic neurons and receptors are lost.

PROGNOSIS

Death within 6–10 years.

DEMYELINATING DISEASES

Disease is characterized by the destruction of normal myelin (eg, multiple sclerosis) or the production of abnormal myelin (eg, leukodystrophy).

Multiple Sclerosis

Multiple sclerosis (MS) is defined as an inflammatory autoimmune disorder characterized by autoantibodies directed against the myelin basic protein of oligodendrocytes in the CNS, which leads to periventricular demyelination of axons of the brain and spinal cord. There is an increased prevalence in people who lived at higher latitudes north of the Equator for the first decades of their lives. It most often affects Caucasian women 20–30 years of age and is associated with HLA-DR2. MS is second only to trauma as a leading cause of neurologic disability in early to middle adulthood.

KEY FACT

Cerebellar lesions (unilateral) present with ipsilateral ataxia with negative Romberg sign, intention/movement tremor (difficulty smoothing out movements), and dysarthria (loss of complex movements of speech if lesions in the lateral hemispheres).

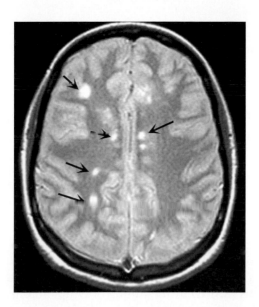

FIGURE 6-57. **Multiple sclerosis.** Axial first-echo image from T2-weighted sequence demonstrates multiple bright signal abnormalities in white matter (*arrows*), typical for MS. These demyelinating lesions may sometimes mimic brain tumors because of the associated edema and inflammation. (Reproduced with permission from Kasper DL, Braunwald E, Fauci AS, et al. *Harrison's Principles of Internal Medicine*, 16th ed. New York: McGraw-Hill, 2005: 2465.)

PRESENTATION

Classic triad of scanning speech, intention tremor, and nystagmus, as well as UMN lesion signs (hyperreflexia, positive Babinski sign). Is often relapsing-remitting. Also common are optic neuritis, MLF syndrome/internuclear ophthalmoplegia (see discussion on MLF), paraplegia, hemiparesis, and hemisensory paresthesias.

DIAGNOSIS

The diagnosis is made on the basis of the history and physical exam and must show evidence of multiple lesions occurring or worsening over numerous episodes. Labs may show increased polyclonal IgG (oligoclonal bands on electrophoresis), myelin basic protein, and leukocytes in the CSF. MRI shows multifocal plaques of periventricular demyelination in the white matter and correlates with future disease severity (Figure 6-57). The acute lesion shows perivenular cuffing with activated T cells (mostly CD4+ and some CD8+) and macrophages. The chronic lesion is characterized by gliosis (scarring).

TREATMENT

Interferon beta and immunosuppressive therapy have proven effective at reducing disease severity and relapse rates.

PROGNOSIS

Untreated patients typically develop severe physical disability within 20–25 years of onset. Early treatment may help counteract progressive brain atrophy.

Progressive Multifocal Leukoencephalopathy (PML)

A fatal subacute progressive demyelinating disease resulting from reactivation of latent John Cunningham (JC) virus infection of B lymphocytes (especially in AIDS patients) that passes through the BBB and cause eventual infection of oligodendrocytes. This leads to widespread destruction of white matter.

KEY FACT

Cerebellar hemispheres are located laterally and control the lateral limbs; the vermis is centrally located, and lesions affect the central (axial) muscles. Therefore, cerebellar vermis lesions manifest with truncal ataxia, whereas hemispheric lesions manifest with intention tremor and limb ataxia.

FLASH BACK

Poliovirus is a naked, icosahedral picornavirus with single-stranded RNA.

MNEMONIC

Triad of MS is a SI(I)N:
Scanning speech
Intention tremor
Internuclear ophthalmoplegia/
 Nystagmus

KEY FACT

Internuclear ophthalmoplegia results from a lesion of the MLF and is therefore also called MLF syndrome. With a complete lesion of the left MLF, the left ipsilateral eye fails to adduct when the patient looks to the right and vice versa. A second component is nystagmus that is limited to or most prominent in the contralateral abducting eye.

FLASH BACK

JC virus is a papovavirus that causes PML in 1% of AIDS patients.

KEY FACT

Only white matter is affected in **PML,** in contrast to **subacute sclerosing panencephalitis,** which affects both white and gray matter, and **rabies,** which only affects gray matter.

KEY FACT

Viral infection of oligodendrocytes is the key feature of subacute sclerosing panencephalitis (measles paramyxovirus) and progressive multifocal leukoenccphalopathy (JC virus).

KEY FACT

Think of Guillain-Barré as MS of the PNS.

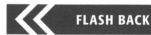

FLASH BACK

Metachromatic leukodystrophy is an autosomal recessive lysosomal storage disease (arylsulfatase A deficiency; accumulation of sulfatides) that is fatal in the first decade and manifests with progressive paralysis, dementia, and ataxia.

FLASH BACK

Krabbe disease (globoid cell leukodystrophy) is an autosomal recessive disorder associated with defective galactocerebrosidase that leads to an accumulation of galactocerebroside in large, multinucleated histiocytic cells in the CNS. This results in optic atrophy and a classic manifestation of blindness and peripheral neuropathy.

PRESENTATION

Weakness (hemiparesis), speech disturbance (aphasia), cortical blindness, and conjugate gaze abnormalities. No change in mental status.

DIAGNOSIS

MRI for white matter lesions. Eosinophilic intranuclear inclusions in abnormal giant oligodendrocytes.

PROGNOSIS

Severe dementia, often progressing to death within 6 months to 1 year. Prognosis may be better in patients with higher CD4+ lymphocyte counts.

Acute Disseminated (Postinfectious) Encephalomyelitis

Demyelinating disease follows infection with measles, mumps, rubella, or chickenpox, with a notable febrile prodrome. Distinct from **subacute sclerosing panencephalitis (SSPE)** by the timing of symptom onset. Specifically, the onset of acute postinfectious encephalomyelitis is much sooner than the onset of the SSPE.

PRESENTATION

Seen in children and adolescents with a history of recent infection or immunization presenting with abrupt onset of irritability and lethargy, mental status changes, and seizures.

DIAGNOSIS

MRI, CSF to exclude other diagnoses; history of recent vaccination or exanthematous illness.

TREATMENT

High-dose corticosteroids. Plasmapheresis or IV immunoglobulin therapy may be used in resistant cases.

PROGNOSIS

Complete recovery without apparent pathologic sequelae; degree of recovery is unrelated to severity of illness.

Guillain-Barré Syndrome

Inflammatory autoimmune demyelination of peripheral motor ventral roots and cranial nerves often associated with infections. Guillain-Barré syndrome is associated with previous inoculation or infection (1–3 weeks earlier) by herpesvirus, *Campylobacter jejuni*, *Mycoplasma pneumoniae*, and possibly with flu vaccination. Notably, males and females are equally at risk. The autoimmune reaction is presumed to result from an immune response to nonself-antigens that become misdirected against host nerve tissue.

PRESENTATION

Manifests **without fever.** Patients have diminished lower extremity reflexes, with rapidly evolving symmetrical ascending muscle weakness and paresthesias that begin in the distal lower extremities. History of antecedent infection/inoculation. Significant risk of respiratory muscle paralysis over time. May have autonomic dysfunction, resulting in cardiac dysrhythmias, hypertension, hypotension. Facial diplegia (bilateral facial paralysis in 50% of cases). Deep, aching pain in weakened muscles.

DIAGNOSIS

Clinical presentation, elevated CSF protein with normal cell count, papilledema. Abnormalities of nerve conduction by electromyography (EMG).

TREATMENT

Respiratory support is critical, as the disease ascends to involve the diaphragm. Treatment also includes plasmapheresis and IV immunoglobulins once the diagnosis is made.

PROGNOSIS

Death (< 5%) secondary to pulmonary complications within days; therefore, respiratory support is important. Most patients make a full recovery with supportive care. Prognosis is worse if axonal damage is evident.

Central Pontine Myelinolysis (CPM)

During prolonged hyponatremia, neurons compensate by reducing intracellular osmolytes to prevent cellular swelling. Upon rapid correction, the neurons are hypotonic relative to the suddenly normal serum osmolality. Fluid moves out of neurons into the extracellular compartment, leading to demyelination.

PRESENTATION

Rapid-onset quadriparesis with dysarthria/dysphagia.

DIAGNOSIS

MRI shows a diamond-shaped, or "bat wing," region of demyelination in the basis pontis that spares neurons and axons. Lack of inflammation distinguishes CPM from MS.

TREATMENT

Avoid by **slow** correction of hyponatremia (to avoid absolute and relative hypernatremia).

PROGNOSIS

Maximum recovery within months; death is common.

SEIZURES

Seizures are characterized by focal or global neuronal hyperactivity that causes a sudden change in behavior. This change manifests differently, depending on the region of the brain affected (Table 6-30).

CEREBRAL EDEMA

An increase in intracranial pressure (ICP; ie, intracranial hypertension) can occur 2–4 days postinfarction. Edema may be:

- **Cytotoxic:** Secondary to hypoxia and hyponatremia.
- **Vasogenic:** Increased vascular permeability secondary to inflammation, metastasis, trauma, respiratory acidosis → space-occupying lesions that cause mass effect on underlying brain tissue.

MNEMONIC

Krabbe (crabs) cannot see and have poor sensation with their pincers (blindness and peripheral neuropathy).

KEY FACT

Adrenoleukodystrophy is an X-linked recessive enzyme deficiency in β-oxidation of fatty acids in peroxisomes that causes a build-up of long-chain fatty acids. This causes generalized loss of myelin in the brain, coupled with adrenal insufficiency.

KEY FACT

Physiologic myoclonus is characterized by sudden jerking movements while falling asleep.

FLASH FORWARD

Eating undercooked pork infected with *Taenia solium* may lead to neurocysticercosis. This is the leading cause of seizures in Mexico.

KEY FACT

Status epilepticus: A seizure or series of seizures lasting more than 20 minutes without regaining consciousness. Typically tonic-clonic, characterized by sudden loss of consciousness, tonic contraction, and loss of postural muscle tone, followed by rhythmic contractions in all four limbs. Immediate treatment with fast-acting benzodiazepines (eg, lorazepam) is needed to stop seizures, phenytoin to reduce the risk of another epileptic attack; phenobarbital and then pentobarbital or general anesthetics (eg, propofol) may be needed to fully abort seizure.

TABLE 6-30. Types of Seizures

Type	Presentation	Treatment/Prognosis	Etiology by Age
Partial (one area of the brain)	**Simple:** Consciousness intact with motor, sensory, autonomic, and psychic components.	Rx: Carbamazepine, valproic acid, gabapentin, lamotrigine, topiramate, phenobarbital, tiagabine, vigabatrin, levetiracetam. Can secondarily generalize.	
	Complex: Components of simple but with alteration of consciousness.	Rx: Same drugs as for simple seizures, especially carbamazepine.	
Generalized	**Absence** (petit mal). 2 years old to puberty with blank stare. No postictal confusion.	Rx absence: Ethosuximide, valproic acid.	**Children:** Genetic, infection, trauma, congenital, metabolic.
	Myoclonic. Quick, repetitive jerks.	Rx myoclonic: Valproic acid. Rx Tonic-clonic: Phenobarbital, phenytoin, carbamazepine (only for secondary generalized, but not primary), valproic acid, topiramate, lamotrigine, gabapentin.	**Adults:** Tumors, trauma, stroke, infection.
	Tonic-clonic (grand mal). Tonic phase characterized by limb stiffening followed by Clonic phase characterized by rhythmic jerking. Postictal phase characterized by lethargy and disorientation.	Note: Do not treat absence seizures with sodium channel blockers, as they worsen the seizure.	**Elderly:** Stroke, tumors, trauma, metabolic, infection.
	Tonic. Stiffening (usually in children).	Valproic acid should be avoided in pregnant women as it inhibits folate absorption.	
	Atonic. "Drop" seizures; commonly mistaken for fainting.		
May-White syndrome	Familial progressive myoclonic epilepsy accompanied by lipoma, ataxia, and deafness.		

KEY FACT

An electroencephalographic (EEG) spike-and-wave complex signifies hypersynchronicity and provides a useful tool for diagnosing seizures.

PRESENTATION

Classic signs of increased ICP: papilledema (swelling of the optic disc), projectile vomiting, sinus bradycardia, hypertension, and decreased level of consciousness.

TREATMENT

Address the underlying cause if possible and manage ICP (shunt).

PROGNOSIS

Potential for herniation, which carries a poor prognosis.

CEREBRAL CONTUSION

Permanent damage to small blood vessels and the parenchyma of the brain, typically due to acceleration-deceleration injuries.

PRESENTATION

Coup (at the site of impact) and contrecoup (opposite the site of impact, usually at the tips of the frontal and temporal lobes) injuries. Contrecoup injuries are typically more devastating because of the increased forces necessary to transmit energy across the brain, resulting in diffuse axonal damage as well.

DIAGNOSIS

CT or MRI.

TREATMENT

Rarely treated surgically.

PROGNOSIS

May progress to herniation as edema develops.

PRIMARY BRAIN NEOPLASMS

Neoplasms may result in mass effect, which presents as seizures, dementia, focal lesions, increased ICP (headache worse in the morning, nausea, vomiting, and bradycardia with hypertension). Primary brain tumors seldom undergo metastasis. Most adult primary tumors are supratentorial, whereas the majority of childhood primary tumors are infratentorial (Figure 6-58 and Table 6-31). Half of adult brain tumors are metastases from, in order of decreasing prevalence: lung, breast, skin (melanoma), kidney, GI tract, and thyroid cancers. Metastatic brain lesions present as multiple spherical lesions at the gray-white junction that frequently bleed.

KEY FACT

Patients with head trauma are intentionally hyperventilated to produce **respiratory alkalosis,** which causes cerebral vessel constriction by decreasing P_{CO_2}. This decreases cerebral blood volume and vessel permeability, thereby reducing the risk of cerebral edema. Note that respiratory *acidosis* causes vasodilation and increased vessel permeability, which enhances cerebral edema.

KEY FACT

Cushing reflex: Bradycardia + hypertension secondary to increased ICP. Both arms of the autonomic system are activated: the sympathetic nervous system drives more blood centrally with concomitant activation of baroreceptors (parasympathetic) to decrease the heart rate.

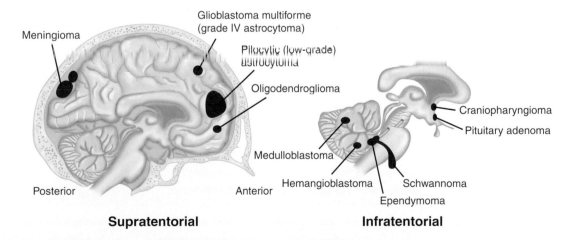

FIGURE 6-58.   Location of adult and childhood primary brain neoplasms.

TABLE 6-31.   **Primary Brain Neoplasms**

	TYPE	PRESENTATION AND PATHOLOGY	PROGNOSIS/TREATMENT
Adult peak incidence	Glioblastoma multiforme	"Pseudopalisading" tumor cells border central areas of **necrosis** and **hemorrhage,** with ring-enhancing appearance in imaging; found in cerebral hemispheres (frontal lobes most commonly) and may cross corpus callosum; ill-defined mass; **most common primary brain tumor;** high-grade astrocytoma.	< 1 year life expectancy, poor prognosis; seed neuraxis via CSF.
	Meningioma	Occurs in convexities of hemispheres and parasagittal region, leading to **spastic paresis and urinary incontinence;** arises from arachnoid cells external to the brain, may be resectable; symptoms arise from mass effect rather than infiltration of brain; spindle cells concentrically arranged in whorled pattern, **psammoma bodies** (laminated calcifications); **most common benign primary CNS tumor in adults;** common cause of new-onset focal seizures.	Resectable.
	Schwannoma-neurofibroma	Third most common primary brain tumor, benign; Schwann cell origin often localized to CN VIII at the cerebellopontine angle (vestibular schwannoma); may arise from any spinal root or CN except I and II (myelinated by oligodendrocytes); densely, uniformly enhancing on MRI; manifest with progressive unilateral tinnitus, hearing loss, ataxia with positive Romberg sign (because localized at cerebellopontine angle); commonly occurs in **neurofibromatosis II.**	Resectable; may preserve hearing if small and prevent compression of cerebellum, pons, and facial nerve; patient usually deaf at presentation.
	Oligodendroglioma	**Slow growing,** rare tumor most often in frontal lobes; **"fried egg" cells** with round nuclei and clear cytoplasm; often calcified.	Surgical resection.
	Pinealoma	Fifty percent are germinomas that occur more often in males < 30 years old with symptoms similar to pure pineal gland tumor without melatonin abnormalities; pineal gland tumors compress the superior colliculus **(Parinaud syndrome),** pretectal area, and cerebral aqueduct (obstructive hydrocephalus); also interrupt melatonin production, leading to disruption of circadian rhythm and insomnia; may calcify with age; precocious puberty.	Surgical resection.
	Pituitary adenomas (see section above)		
Childhood peak incidence	Pilocytic astrocytoma	Diffusely infiltrating benign glioma most often seen in posterior fossa (cerebellar); **Rosenthal fibers** (eosinophilic corkscrew fibers resulting from accumulation of intermediate filament proteins specific to astrocytes); cyst with mural nodule.	Good prognosis.
	Medulloblastoma	Highly malignant tumor with rosettes or perivascular pseudorosette pattern of cells; arises in cerebellar vermis; small round blue cells; presents with ataxia, projectile vomiting, nuchal rigidity; can compress fourth ventricle, leading to hydrocephalus and increased ICP.	Radiosensitive, may progress to cerebellar herniation without surgery.

TABLE 6-31. Primary Brain Neoplasms (continued)

	TYPE	PRESENTATION AND PATHOLOGY	PROGNOSIS/TREATMENT
Childhood peak incidence (continued)	Ependymoma	Ependymal cell tumors most commonly found in fourth ventricle; characteristic perivascular pseudorosettes (ependymal cells around small vessels); rod-shaped blepharoplasts (basal ciliary bodies) found near nucleus; can cause hydrocephalus (nausea, vomiting, nuchal rigidity, increased ICP).	Poor prognosis.
	Hemangioblastoma	Associated with **von Hippel-Lindau syndrome** when found with retinal angiomas; foamy cells and high vascularity are characteristic; may produce erythropoietin, causing secondary polycythemia; mesodermal origin.	Resection.
	Craniopharyngioma	Most common childhood supratentorial tumor, benign; derived from remnants of **Rathke pouch** (ectoderm resembling tooth enamel [tooth bud]); distinguish from pituitary adenoma by histology (nests of uniform granular cells); present with growth failure, papilledema; compression of pituitary stalk leads to hypopituitarism, whereas compression of optic chiasm leads to bitemporal hemianopsia.	Resection.
	Retinoblastoma	Malignant retinal tumor of childhood; sporadic cases are generally unilateral, whereas bilateral cases suggests *Rb* gene deletion; two-hit hypothesis prototype.	Radiotherapy, cryotherapy, chemotherapy, or enucleation.

CNS = central nervous system; CSF = cerebrospinal fluid; ICP = intracranial pressure.

Pituitary Adenomas

Benign neoplasms that arise from one of the five anterior pituitary cell types, and are generally monoclonal. Prolactin-secreting adenoma (prolactinoma) is the most common form.

PRESENTATION

See Table 6-32.

DIAGNOSIS

MRI, endocrine studies. Transsphenoidal surgery confirms the results of clinical and lab studies (determine local levels of relevant pituitary hormones).

TREATMENT

Transsphenoidal surgery, normalization of excess pituitary secretion (dopamine agonist bromocriptine for prolactinomas). Hormone replacement may be necessary depending on patient's age, sex, and presentation.

PROGNOSIS

If the lesion is resectable with preservation of pituitary function, then the prognosis is good.

KEY FACT

Astrocytomas account for 70% of neuroglial tumors and are typically located in the frontal lobe of adults and the cerebellum of children.

KEY FACT

Glioblastoma multiforme is associated with Turcot intestinal polyps.

MNEMONIC

Bitemporal hemianopsia resulting from sella turcica mass lesions, differential by age:
Adults → Pituitary **A**denoma
Kids → **(K) C**raniopharyngioma

TABLE 6-32. **Clinical Features of Pituitary Adenomas**

CATEGORY	HORMONE	PRESENTATION	TREATMENT
Hypersecretion	Prolactin	Men: Hypogonadism, infertility, impotence, ↓ libido, galactorrhea, gynecomastia. Women: If premenopausal → menstrual irregularities, oligomenorrhea or amenorrhea, ↓ libido, dyspareunia, vaginal dryness, galactorrhea, anovulation, and infertility. Potential mass effects (eg, bitemporal hemianopia, headaches) in both men and women.	Dopamine agonists (eg, bromocriptine); surgical resection
	GH	Acromegaly (gigantism prior to epiphyseal plate closure).	Surgical resection
	ACTH	Classic symptoms of Cushing disease (see Chapter 2).	Surgical resection, radiation therapy
	TSH	Classic symptoms of hyperthyroidism (see Chapter 2).	Surgical resection
Hypopituitarism		Compression of hypothalamic-pituitary stalk, leading to decreased production of other pituitary hormones; GH deficiency (lag in growth), hypogonadotropic hypogonadism, etc.	Surgical resection followed by hormone replacement

ACTH = adrenocorticotropic hormone; GH = growth hormone; TSH = thyroid-stimulating hormone.

KEY FACT

PSaMMoma bodies are associated with:
- **P**apillary adenocarcinoma (thyroid)
- Papillary **S**erous cystadenocarcinoma (ovary)
- **M**eningioma
- **M**esothelioma

KEY FACT

Astrocytes can be visualized by staining for glial fibrillary acidic protein (GFAP), an intermediate filament.

KEY FACT

Meningiomas are associated with neurofibromatosis (NF). NF2 is also associated with bilateral schwannomas.

SPINAL CORD AND PERIPHERAL NERVE LESIONS

See Tables 6-33, 6-34, and 6-35 and Figure 6-59.

Brown-Séquard Syndrome

Brown-Séquard syndrome results from hemisection of the spinal cord that interrupts conduction through the lateral corticospinal tract (CST, motor), lateral spinothalamic tracts (STT, pain and temperature sensation), and dorsal columns (DC, proprioception and tactile sensation).

TABLE 6-33. **Comparison of Lower and Upper Motor Neuron Lesions**

MOTOR NEURON SIGNS	UPPER MOTOR NEURON (UMN)	LOWER MOTOR NEURON (LMN)
Weakness	+	+
Atrophy	−	+
Fasciculation	−	+
Reflexes	↑	↓
Tone	↑	↓
Babinski	+	−

TABLE 6-34. Upper Extremity Nerve Injury

NERVE	SITE OF INJURY/DEFICIT IN MOTION	DEFICITS IN SENSATION/COURSE
Radial (C5–C8)	**Shaft of humerus,** leading to loss of triceps brachii, brachioradialis, and extensor carpi radialis.	Posterior brachial cutaneous; also involved in lateral epicondylitis ("tennis elbow").
Median (C5–T1)	**Supracondylar region of humerus,** leaving arm muscle function intact with impaired forearm pronation, wrist flexion (with ulnar deviation), finger flexion, thumb abduction and opposition. Thenar atrophy.	Loss of sensation over the lateral palm, thumb and lateral 2.5 fingers, and thumbnail bed.
	Carpal tunnel syndrome (repetitive use injury).	Passes through pronator teres, under flexor retinaculum in carpal tunnel.
	Slashing the wrist causes loss of thenar muscle innervation, so all thumb movement is lost except for adduction (ulnar).	*Tinel sign* (shock-like pain when lightly tapped on palmar side of wrist) and *Phalen sign* (wrist in flexion reproduces painful symptoms).
Ulnar (C8–T1)	**Medial epicondyle,** causing impaired wrist flexion (radial deviation) and adduction, thumb adduction, flexion of the medial two fingers (claw-hand deformity), and wasting of hypothenar eminence and PAD/DAB interosseous muscles.	Loss of sensation over medial palm and medial 1.5 fingers.
		Passes through carpi ulnaris, at elbow; passes between medial epicondyle and two heads of flexor carpi ulnaris.
Axillary (C5 and C6)	**Surgical neck of humerus** or **anterior shoulder dislocation** causes loss of deltoid action (failure to abduct arm > 15 degrees).	**On physical exam,** palpable depression under acromion.
Musculocutaneous (C5–C6)	Loss of function of coracobrachialis, biceps, and brachialis muscles, along with decreased supination	Passes through coracobrachialis and continues as lateral cutaneous nerve of forearm below elbow.

PAD/DAB mnemonic: Palmar adducts/Dorsal abducts.

Nerves that run from the motor cortex to the spinal cord are referred to as upper motor neurons (UMNs); nerves that run from the anterior horn of the spinal cord to the periphery are referred to as lower motor neurons (LMNs).

PRESENTATION (SEE FIGURE 6-39, TABLE 6-18)

- **Ipsilateral** UMN signs below the lesion (CST).
- **Ipsilateral** loss of tactile, vibration, and proprioception (DC) at and below the lesion.
- **Contralateral** loss of pain and temperature below the lesion (because of crossing fibers, STT).
- **Ipsilateral** loss of pain and temperature a few levels above and below the lesion.
- LMN signs at the level of the lesion.
- If the lesion is above T1, patient may present with Horner syndrome.

DIAGNOSIS

History and physical exam.

KEY FACT

Ependymoma arises in the cauda equina in adults.

KEY FACT

Choroid plexus papillomas occur in the lateral ventricles of boys.

TABLE 6-35. **Lower Extremity Nerve Injury**

NERVE	DEFICIT IN MOTION	DEFICITS IN SENSATION/COURSE
Common peroneal (L4–S2) (divides into superficial and deep *branches at the neck of fibula*)	Deep peroneal: Innervates muscles of anterior leg compartment. Loss of dorsiflexion, causing foot drop.	**Anterior compartment syndrome** results from increased pressure that causes compression of the deep peroneal nerve and vasculature, causing foot drop and weak dorsalis pedis pulse. Deep peroneal: First web space.
	Superficial peroneal: Innervates lateral leg compartment muscles. Loss of eversion.	Superficial peroneal: Dorsal surface of foot except first web space.
Tibial (L4–S3) (courses posterior to the medial malleolus)	Loss of plantarflexion because the tibial nerve innervates the posterior compartment of the thigh and leg.	Plantar surface of foot.
Femoral (L2–L4)	Loss of knee extension/knee jerk.	Paresthesias of anterior/medial thigh and medial leg.
Obturator (L2–L4) (exits through the obturator canal to enter the thigh)	Loss of hip adduction.	

KEY FACT

CNS lymphomas usually result from metastasis of high-grade non-Hodgkin lymphoma of B-cell origin.

FLASH BACK

Primary CNS lymphoma is associated with AIDS. Epstein-Barr virus (EBV)-mediated B-cell lymphoma is the most common cerebral tumor in AIDS patients. MRI showing a single ring-enhancing lesion suggests this diagnosis although toxoplasmosis (more often multiple lesions) must be ruled out.

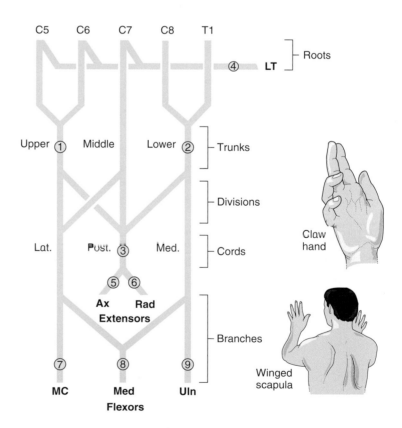

FIGURE 6-59. **Diagram of the brachial plexus and associated presentation of lesions.** Rad, radial nerve; Ax, axillary nerve; LT, long thoracic nerve; MC, musculocutaneous nerve; Med, median nerve; Uln, ulnar nerve. ① Waiter tip (Erb palsy); ② Claw hand (Klumpke palsy); ③ Wrist drop; ④ Winged scapula; ⑤ Deltoid paralysis; ⑥ Saturday night palsy (wrist drop); ⑦ Difficulty flexing elbow, variable sensory loss; ⑧ Decreased thumb function, Pope blessing; ⑨ Intrinsic muscles of hand, claw hand.

TREATMENT

Early treatment with high-dose steroids has shown benefit, as have physical therapy and surgery.

PROGNOSIS

Poor; depends on the cause of the syndrome (trauma, infection, disk herniation).

Poliomyelitis

Destruction of the anterior horn of the spinal cord occurs secondary to fecal-oral infection by poliovirus (a picornavirus), leading to LMN destruction (see Figure 6-40, Table 6-26). Poliovirus replicates in the oropharynx and small intestine before spreading through the bloodstream to the CNS.

PRESENTATION

Malaise, headache, fever, nausea, abdominal pain, and sore throat characterize the acute infection. **Signs of LMN lesion** include muscle atrophy, flaccid paralysis, and hyporeflexia, with preserved sensation.

DIAGNOSIS

CSF with lymphocytic pleocytosis and slight elevation of protein. Virus is recovered from stool or the throat.

TREATMENT

Prevention with vaccine (Salk inactive parenteral vaccine). Oral (Sabin) vaccine carries small risk of disease but confers mucosal immunity in contrast to inactive vaccine. Bed rest decreases the incidence of paralysis; intensive care is needed if respiratory muscle weakness occurs.

PROGNOSIS

High mortality rate if bulbar involvement; persistent muscle weakness may develop years after acute infection.

Tabes Dorsalis (Tertiary Syphilis)

Degeneration of the dorsal roots and columns (mainly lumbosacral) that develops 15–20 years after the onset of *Treponema pallidum* infection. Primarily affects the fasciculi gracilis bilaterally.

PRESENTATION

Ataxia, bilaterally impaired proprioception (positive Romberg sign), paresthesias (shooting pains), Argyll Robertson pupils (accommodate, but do not react to light), and absence of deep tendon reflexes. Purely sensory deficit; muscular power is retained. Associated with Charcot joints (insensitivity to pain in the joint, leading to increased susceptibility to joint injury).

DIAGNOSIS

Clinical and CSF analysis (pleocytosis [> 5 WBC/mm^3], increased protein concentration [> 45 mg/dL], and/or VDRL reactivity). Note that the Venereal Disease Research Laboratory (VDRL) test may be positive in autoimmune diseases, mononucleosis, or hepatitis; so follow with specific treponemal tests, such as fluorescent treponemal antibody absorption (FTA-Abs) or micro-hemagglutination serology to confirm.

FLASH BACK

In contrast to **craniopharyngiomas** (which arise from the remnant Rathke pouch and create symptoms by interruption of the infundibulum connecting the hypothalamus to the pituitary), **pituitary adenomas** arise from cells within the pituitary gland itself, with symptoms resulting from a combination of aberrant tumor cell hormone secretion and mass effect.

KEY FACT

Subependymal giant-cell astrocytoma is pathognomonic for **tuberous sclerosis** (also with cardiac myomas and renal angiomyolipomas).

MNEMONIC

Randy Travis Drinks Cold Beer (proximal to distal):
Roots
Trunks
Divisions
Cords
Branches

KEY FACT

Familial syndromes associated with pituitary adenomas include multiple endocrine neoplasia (MEN 1), McCune-Albright syndrome, and familial acromegaly.

MNEMONIC

Lower motor neuron lesion = everything **lowered** (↓ muscle mass, ↓ tone, ↓ reflexes, downgoing toes = negative Babinski sign).
Upper motor neuron lesion = everything **up** (↑ tone, ↑ reflexes, and upgoing toes = positive Babinski sign).

KEY FACT

Diabetic polyradiculopathy mimics tabes dorsalis.

KEY FACT

The sciatic nerve (L4–S3) emerges at the midpoint between the greater trochanter and the ischial tuberosity, then branches into the tibial and common peroneal nerves at the short head of the biceps femoris. All gluteal injections should target the superolateral quadrant to avoid damage to the gluteal nerves and sciatic nerve (superomedial quadrant).

KEY FACT

Vitamin B_{12} deficiency may also be caused by **pernicious anemia,** an autoimmune disorder that involves antibodies against *intrinsic factor* or gastric parietal cells (or both). In addition to subacute combined degeneration, vitamin B_{12} deficiency can result in megaloblastic anemia (large, abnormal RBCs).

FLASH BACK

Methylated B_{12} (methylcobalamin) is an essential cofactor for the conversion of homocysteine to methionine, so deficiency results in impairment of DNA synthesis. High levels of homocysteine is a risk factor for cardiovascular disease.

KEY FACT

The patient with **syringomyelia** classically presents after repeatedly burning their hand on the stove due to loss of pain and temperature sensation.

TREATMENT

Penicillin; treat symptoms.

PROGNOSIS

If untreated, may progress to paralysis, blindness, and dementia. Residual symptoms may persist after treatment.

Subacute Combined Degeneration (Vitamin B_{12} Deficiency)

Most commonly results from a failure to absorb vitamin B_{12} across the intestinal mucosa, which leads to a functional vitamin B_{12} deficiency and results in build-up of methylmalonyl-CoA and its precursor, propionyl-CoA. Propionyl-CoA displaces succinyl-CoA in fatty acid synthesis, resulting in anomalous insertion of odd-chain fatty acids into lipids, such as myelin. Demyelination of the dorsal columns and lateral CST may occur with patients presenting with proprioceptive and motor symptoms.

PRESENTATION

Dementia, ataxic gait, symmetrical spastic paresis (demyelinated CST leads to UMN loss) and impaired position and vibration sense (bilateral demyelination of dorsal columns).

DIAGNOSIS

- Serum cobalamin.
- MRI.
- Schilling test:
    1. Give patient oral radiolabeled B_{12} [rB_{12}] plus intramuscular injection of unlabeled vitamin B_{12} and measure urine rB_{12} (should be high).
    2. If the first test is abnormal, give rB_{12} and intrinsic factor (to determine if a malabsorption problem exists), and then measure urine rB_{12}.
    3. If still no rB_{12} in urine, give rB_{12} and antibiotics (to rule out bacteria overgrowth) and measure urine rB_{12}.
    4. If still no rB_{12} in urine, then give rB_{12} and pancreatic enzymes (to rule out pancreatitis) and then measure urine rB_{12}.

TREATMENT

Vitamin B_{12} supplements (oral, intramuscular).

PROGNOSIS

Best prognosis is in those with gait disturbance < 3 months prior to commencement of treatment.

Syringomyelia

Enlargement of the central canal of the spinal cord leads to damage of the STT fibers as they cross in the anterior commissure. May also erode the anterior horn, resulting in LMN defects. Often presents in patients with Arnold-Chiari type II malformation (herniation of the cerebellar vermis through the foramen magnum, causing hydrocephalus, meningomyelocele, and syringomyelia).

PRESENTATION

Bilateral loss of pain and temperature sensation in the upper extremities (most often at C8–T1 ["cape and shawl" distribution; see Figure 6-41]) with preservation of touch sensation. LMN signs of flaccid paralysis if the anterior horn cells are affected, causing combined sensory and motor defects. Atrophy of hand interossei (ulnar nerve). Note that amyotrophic lateral sclerosis (ALS, thenar atrophy) can be distinguished from syringomyelia by clinical presentation: ALS patients have motor, but not sensory deficits.

DIAGNOSIS

MRI is diagnostic.

TREATMENT

With Arnold-Chiari malformation, place shunt to treat hydrocephalus before correction of syrinx (posterior fossa decompression).

PROGNOSIS

Poor.

Thoracic Outlet Syndrome (Klumpke Palsy)

An embryologic defect in the cervical rib can result in compression of the subclavian artery and the inferior trunk of the brachial plexus (C8, T1). Also observed in weightlifters (hypertrophy of the anterior scalene muscle compresses the neurovascular bundle that runs between the anterior and middle scalene muscles) or hyperabduction of the arm (as in falling, breech birth).

PRESENTATION

Thenar and hypothenar eminence (median and ulnar nerves) atrophy, atrophy of the interosseous muscles (ulnar nerve), and sensory deficits on the medial side of the forearm and hand (ulnar nerve, medial cutaneous nerve of the forearm). Disappearance of the radial pulse when the head is rotated toward the opposite side due to compression of the subclavian artery.

DIAGNOSIS

History, physical exam, and chest X-ray demonstrating cervical rib.

TREATMENT

Anterior scalenectomy (careful to avoid the phrenic nerve that runs on the anterior scalene deep to the prevertebral fascia); surgical removal of cervical rib if present and implicated; physical therapy.

PROGNOSIS

Symptoms may return following treatment secondary to scarring and fibrosis around the nerve roots.

PERIPHERAL NEUROPATHY

Two types occur:

- Demyelination often presents segmentally with sensory changes (discrete sensory loss following the distribution of one or more nerves).
- Axonal degeneration of motor nerves presents as muscle fasciculations and atrophy. Axonal degeneration of sensory nerves occurs first (small fibers are more prone to damage) and presents with a **"stocking-and-glove"** distribution (longer fibers are more prone to damage).

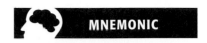

MNEMONIC

Radial nerve Innervates the BEST:
Brachioradialis
Extensors
Supinator
Triceps

KEY FACT

Patients with diabetes mellitus (DM) may develop peripheral neuropathy secondary to osmotic damage to Schwann cells. This is the most common cause of peripheral sensory and motor axonopathy; for this reason, it is extremely important to check the feet of diabetic patients!

KEY FACT

Toxin-associated peripheral neuropathy results from alcohol abuse, exposure to heavy metals, or diphtheria.

Charcot-Marie-Tooth Disease

The most common hereditary neuropathy (autosomal dominant). Primarily affects the peroneal nerve. Onset is typically in the first or second decade.

PRESENTATION

Peroneal nerve neuropathy leading to atrophy of the lower leg muscles. This results in an "inverted bottle" appearance of the legs.

DIAGNOSIS

History and physical exam.

TREATMENT

No therapy to prevent onset or delay progression; patients may benefit from physical therapy and surgery for contractures.

PROGNOSIS

No cure; progressive peripheral neuropathy.

CRANIAL NERVE PALSY

Cranial nerves arise from their nuclei in the brain stem and course toward their targets, primarily in the face. Muscles of facial expression, mastication, autonomic functions, and sensory fibers are supplied by these nerves. Defects result either when the nucleus or the fibers are damaged and may be bilateral or unilateral, depending on the degree of damage to the cortical collateral pathways; unilateral defects commonly present with lesions closer to the periphery (Table 6-36).

Defects in Eye Movement

CN III LESION

PRESENTATION

Lesion causes the eye to point "down and out" (only the lateral rectus and superior oblique muscles are functional), dilation of pupil, and severe ptosis (as opposed to Horner syndrome, which is characterized by mild ptosis).

ETIOLOGY

- Posterior cerebral artery aneurysm compresses the nerve, which causes a fixed, dilated pupil because parasympathetic fibers run along the periphery of the nerve bundle.
- Weber syndrome: Midbrain tegmentum lesion causing ipsilateral CN III palsy and contralateral body hemiplegia.
- Diabetic CN III palsy involves the oculomotor muscles but spares the pupil because it is an ischemic rather than a compressive lesion. Parasympathetic fibers run on the surface of the nerve, so they are the first to be involved in compression and the last to be involved in ischemia. Oculomotor muscle fibers run along the interior of CN III.
- Mass effect (eg, brain tumor, epidural hematoma), leading to herniation of brain tissue with compression of CN III.

DIAGNOSIS

Physical exam.

KEY FACT

Bilateral facial nerve paralysis is almost always the result of Lyme disease.

KEY FACT

Fibers to the upper facial muscles receive bilateral corticobulbar innervation, which explains why UMN lesions of CN VII present only with lower facial paralysis. Fibers to the lower facial muscles are only innervated by the contralateral cortex.

KEY FACT

Trigeminal neuralgia (tic douloureux) presents as severe stabbing pain in the sensory distribution of CN V. If present in a young person, it almost always indicates multiple sclerosis (MS).

TABLE 6-36.   Cranial Nerve Palsies

Type/Location	Presentation	Etiology/Notes
CN III	Oculomotor paralysis (eg, in transtentorial herniation) leads to denervation of the levator palpebrae muscle, causing ptosis; denervation of the extraocular muscles innervated by CN III, causing "down and out" orientation of eyes; and interruption of ophthalmic parasympathetic innervations, leading to internal ophthalmoplegia (dilated, fixed pupil and impairment in accommodation [cycloplegia]).	(See text).
CN IV	Extorsion of the eye, weakness of downward gaze, vertical diplopia (worse when looking down), and characteristic compensatory head tilting (pseudotorticollis).	
CN V motor lesion	Jaw deviates toward side of lesion.	If lesion is at trigeminal motor nucleus, then ipsilateral loss.
		If lesion is higher up in thalamus and cortex, then contralateral signs.
CN VII (Bell palsy if idiopathic)	Drooping corner of mouth with drooling; loss of buccinator muscle function.	
	Difficulty speaking, inability to close eye.	
	Loss of taste in anterior two-thirds of tongue (chorda tympani).	Seen in AIDS, Lyme disease, sarcoidosis, tumors, and diabetes.
	Loss of lacrimation and salivation.	
	Peripheral lesions: paralysis of upper and lower face. Central (nuclear) lesions: paralysis of lower face only (see Figure 6-44).	
CN X lesion	Uvula deviates away from side of lesion.	Brain stem infarct.
CN XI lesion	Weakness turning head to side contralateral to lesion; shoulder droop on side of lesion.	Sternocleidomastoid (SCM) contraction normally moves head to contralateral side.
		Loss of SCM and trapezius innervation accounts for presentation.
CN XII lesion (LMN)	Tongue deviates toward side of lesion ("lick your wounds").	Anterior spinal artery infarct.
Parinaud syndrome	Bilateral paralysis of upward gaze.	Midbrain dorsal tectum lesion (eg, **pineal gland tumor**) that compresses superior colliculus, pretectal area, and cerebral aqueduct (obstructive hydrocephalus); also interrupts melatonin production, leading to disruption of circadian rhythm, insomnia; may calcify with age, cause precocious puberty.

KEY FACT

CN IV (trochlear nerve) is the only cranial nerve to exit the brain stem dorsally and cross the midline; therefore, a lesion at the nucleus results in the contralateral eye deviating superiorly and laterally.

KEY FACT

Cavernous sinus syndrome results from internal carotid aneurysm (mass effect) that presents as ophthalmoplegia and ophthalmic and maxillary sensory loss (CN V_1 and V_2).

KEY FACT

Signs suggestive of brain stem lesions: vertigo (CN VIII), diplopia (CN III, IV, VI), ataxia (cerebellar), perioral numbness (CN V), loss of consciousness (reticular activating system).

KEY FACT

Argyll Robertson pupil, seen in tertiary syphilis, systemic lupus erythematosus (SLE), and DM: accommodation to near objects is intact, but the pupil does not react to light by constricting.

MNEMONIC

Argyll Robertson pupil is seen in the 3 S's:
Syphilis
SLE
Sugar (DM)

TREATMENT

Watchful waiting or treatment of the underlying condition (eg, surgical clipping of an aneurysm).

PROGNOSIS

Most cases resolve within 6–8 weeks.

CN IV LESION

Eye rotated superior and lateral because of unopposed action of the inferior oblique.

ETIOLOGY

Compression within the cavernous sinus (as with an internal carotid aneurysm).

DIAGNOSIS

Physical exam, imaging to detect underlying cause.

TREATMENT

Surgical intervention.

PROGNOSIS

Most cases resolve completely within 6 months.

CN VI LESION

Affected eye fails to abduct; unaffected eye develops nystagmus when the patient tries to abduct the affected eye.

ETIOLOGY

Lesion within the cavernous sinus or pontomedullary junction; increased ICP, causing a downward shift in the posterior fossa.

DIAGNOSIS

Physical exam and imaging.

TREATMENT

Watchful waiting or treat underlying cause if known.

PROGNOSIS

Most cases resolve within 6 months.

Facial Lesions

UMN LESION

Lesion of the motor cortex or the connection between the cortex and the facial nucleus results in contralateral paralysis of the lower face only (see Figure 6-44).

LMN LESION

Ipsilateral paralysis of the upper and lower face.

Visual Field Defects

Lesions occurring anywhere from the retina to the visual cortex result in defects in the visual field (see Figure 6-45). The specific intervention depends on the underlying cause and whether the lesion is a severed tract or a parenchymal injury.

Uveitis

PRESENTATION

Blurry vision (resulting from inflammation of the iris, ciliary body, and choroids) may lead to retinal detachment and acute glaucoma.

Associated with:

- **Autoinflammatory disease:** Ankylosing spondylitis, Reiter syndrome, sarcoidosis, ulcerative colitis.
- **Infection:** Toxoplasmosis, cytomegalovirus (CMV), toxocariasis (ocular larval migrans), histoplasmosis, tuberculosis (TB), syphilis.

Internuclear Ophthalmoplegia (Medial Longitudinal Fasciculus Syndrome)

Lesion of the medial longitudinal fasciculus (MLF) results in medial rectus palsy on attempted lateral gaze. This lesion is distinguished from CN III palsy by preserved convergence, in contrast to the "down and out" appearance of CN III palsy. Most common cause is MS.

PRESENTATION

When the affected eye is adducting, nystagmus is seen in the abducting opposite eye (Figure 6-60). Normal convergence ("finger to nose" eye test), but loss of conjugate gaze (Figure 6-61). In patients with MS, internuclear ophthalmoplegia (INO) results from demyelination of the MLF.

DIAGNOSIS

Clinical; if bilateral, high suspicion that MS is the cause. Need to exclude myasthenia gravis in patients with isolated medial rectus palsy

TREATMENT

Underlying condition needs to be managed for MLF syndrome to resolve.

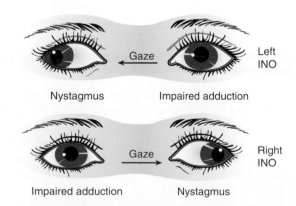

FIGURE 6-60. A clinical exam for medial longitudinal fasciculus (MLF) syndrome.
When looking left, the left nucleus of CN VI fires, which contracts the left lateral rectus and stimulates the contralateral nucleus of CN III via the right MLF to contract the right medial rectus. INO, internuclear ophthalmoplegia.

 KEY FACT

Marcus Gunn pupil results from a deficit in the afferent light reflex pathway (eg, CN II lesion, retinal detachment). The affected pupil appears to expand when light is switched from the unaffected eye to the affected eye (pupil is actually returning to baseline from a constricted state). Diagnosed by swinging a light from pupil to pupil; usually seen in the context of MS.

 KEY FACT

Xerophthalmia (dry eyes) may be caused by vitamin A deficiency (desquamation of conjunctival cells) or Sjögren syndrome (keratoconjunctivitis sicca).

 KEY FACT

Macular degeneration occurs secondary to disruption of the retinal membrane, leading to slow-onset loss of central vision with preserved peripheral vision. Most common cause of premature vision loss in the elderly.

 KEY FACT

Cataracts (opacification of lens) are seen in the elderly and in those with DM, rubella, and corticosteroid use.

 KEY FACT

Amaurosis fugax is a sudden unilateral loss of vision due to embolization of atheromatous plaque material to the ophthalmic artery. Associated with carotid bruit and atherosclerosis. Classic visual sign of transient ischemic attack (TIA, "ischemia of the eye") that presents like a shade being pulled over the eye.

KEY FACT

Lens dislocation is seen in homocystinuria (inferior), Marfan syndrome (superior), and Alport syndrome (glomerulonephritis with blindness and deafness).

KEY FACT

Optic neuritis (inflammation of CN II) results in loss of vision and Marcus Gunn pupil. Causes include MS and methyl alcohol (methanol) poisoning.

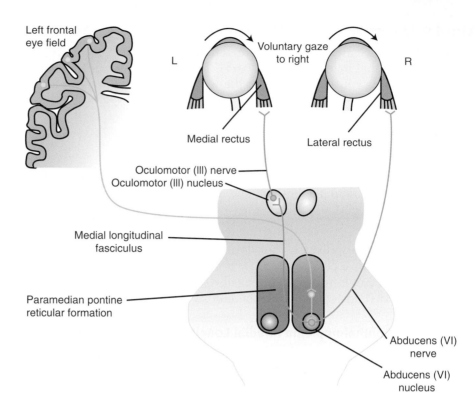

FIGURE 6-61. **Schematic illustrating pathway for conjugate horizontal gaze.** (Modified with permission from Aminoff MJ, Greeberg DA, Simon RP. *Clinical Neurology*, 6th ed. New York: McGraw-Hill, 2005: 130.)

KEY FACT

Glaucoma develops as a result of increased intraocular pressure that leads to optic nerve atrophy. Increased intraocular pressure may be a consequence of decreased flow of aqueous humor through the canal of Schlemm with or without narrowing of the anterior chamber angle.

CENTRAL NERVOUS SYSTEM INFECTIONS

Infections that arise in the CNS can be divided into those that affect immunocompetent individuals and those that affect immunocompromised patients, with some specific exceptions. AIDS-defining lesions (fungal, JC viral infection, and *Mycobacterium tuberculosis*) typically occur in immunocompromised patients. Table 6-37 details the types of patients affected and the typical disease course of various CNS infections.

Meningitis

Inflammation of the pia mater covering the brain may be bacterial, viral, or fungal in origin. Usually occurs secondary to hematogenous spread.

HERNIATION SYNDROMES

Under increased intracranial pressure, portions of the brain are displaced through openings of dura partitions or into openings of the skull (eg, foramen magnum) (Figure 6-62). Therefore, treatment is aimed at removing the insult that generated the increased pressure (eg, shunt for hydrocephalus, control of intracranial hemorrhage). Treat with hyperosmotic therapy such as mannitol or hypertonic saline; can use dexamethasone to mitigate cerebral edema (reduce ICP) if that is the underlying cause.

Cingulate/Subfalcine

The cingulate cortex herniates under the falx cerebri and may compress the anterior cerebral artery, leading to symptoms detailed earlier in the cerebro-

TABLE 6-37. Central Nervous System Infections According to Type of Microbe

TYPE	PRESENTATION	CAUSATIVE MICROBE
Viral	Acute	Echovirus is most common cause of aseptic meningitis.
	Acute or subacute	Herpes encephalitis.
	Subacute	Progressive multifocal leukoencephalopathy (JC virus), subacute sclerosing panencephalitis (measles).
Bacterial (meningitis)	1 month	Group B streptococci, *Escherichia coli*, *Listeria monocytogenes*.
	1 month to 18 years	*Neisseria meningitidis* (*Haemophilus influenzae* is now rare because of vaccine).
	> 18 years	*Streptococcus pneumoniae*.
	Immunocompromised	*Mycobacterium tuberculosis* (complication of primary TB).
	Liver/renal disease, aseptic meningitis (Weil syndrome)	*Leptospira interrogans*.
Fungal	Immunocompromised (subacute meningitis)	*Cryptococcus neoformans*.
	DKA, leukemia	Mucormycosis (*Mucor, Rhizopus*).
Parasitic	Rapidly fatal (immune-competent)	*Naegleria fowleri*.
	Rapidly fatal (immunocompromised)	*Acanthamoeba*.
	Neurocysticercosis	*Taenia solium*.
	AIDS	*Toxoplasma gondii*.
	Malaria with CNS infection	*Plasmodium falciparum*.
Brain abscess	Bacterial	Streptococci, *Staphylococcus aureus*, Enterobacteriaceae, *Bacillus fragilis*, *Peptostreptococcus*.
	Helminthic	*Taenia solium*, *Schistosoma*, hydatid cyst (*Echinococcus granulosus*).

CNS = central nervous system; DKA = diabetic ketoacidosis.

vascular section. The falx cerebri normally separates the two cerebral hemispheres along the midline of the skull (see Figure 6-62, arrow 1).

Uncal

DEFINITION AND EPIDEMIOLOGY

The medial temporal lobe (uncus) compresses the crus cerebri by herniating through the tentorium cerebri. Results from a mass lesion that forces the

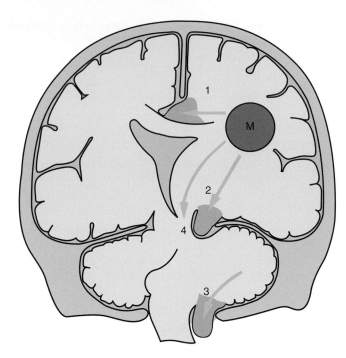

FIGURE 6-62.   Way in which mass effect may result in any of the four types of herniation syndromes. Types include (1) subfalcine or cingulate, (2) uncal, (3) cerebellar tonsillar, and (4) transtentorial. (Modified with permission from Ropper AH, Brown RH. *Adams and Victor's Neurology*, 8th ed. New York: McGraw-Hill, 2005: 310.)

medial aspect of the temporal lobe under the tentorium cerebri (see Figure 6-62, arrow 2).

PRESENTATION

- Stretching CN III leads to ipsilateral dilated pupil, ptosis, oculomotor muscle dysfunction (loss of pupillary light reflex proceeds to loss of motor function).
- Compression of the ipsilateral posterior cerebral artery leads to contralateral homonymous hemianopia secondary to hemorrhagic infarct of the occipital lobe.
- Compression of the ipsilateral crus cerebri (lateral CST) leads to contralateral paresis.
- Compression of the contralateral crus cerebri (lateral CST, Kernohan notch) leads to ipsilateral paresis.
- Caudal displacement of the brain stem (compression of the midbrain) leads to Duret hemorrhages, paramedian artery rupture, and midbrain hemorrhage.

Cerebellar Tonsillar

Herniation of the cerebellar tonsil into the foramen magnum results in cardiorespiratory arrest by compression of the medulla (see Figure 6-62, arrow 3).

Transtentorial

Coma and death result when these herniations compress the brain stem (see Figure 6-62, arrow 4).

Pharmacology

OVERVIEW

CNS pharmacology is a vast and complicated field. From the use of ether and chloroform in surgery in the 1840s to the purification of barbiturates at the turn of the 20th century, nervous system medications have defined many aspects of modern medicine. Although these drugs have been heavily studied, much remains unknown. Yet, elucidating their properties has become a useful tool in the understanding of CNS physiology as well as the pathophysiology of common diseases.

CENTRAL NERVOUS SYSTEM NEUROTRANSMITTERS

An increase or decrease of certain neurotransmitters or their receptors has been implicated in many neurologic disorders. Certain therapies therefore target neurotransmitters or their receptors. There are multiple subtypes of dopamine, serotonin, and noradrenergic receptors throughout the CNS and the rest of the body. Because no two medications in a class of drugs (eg, anti-depressants, atypical antipsychotics) have the same action on the same combination of receptors, patents experience differences in the clinical effect and side effects. A very basic example of a synaptic neurotransmission site is shown in Figure 6-63.

Acetylcholine

Acetylcholine (ACh) is a neurotransmitter of both the peripheral (PNS) and central (CNS) nervous systems. This molecule has two classes of receptors: nicotinic

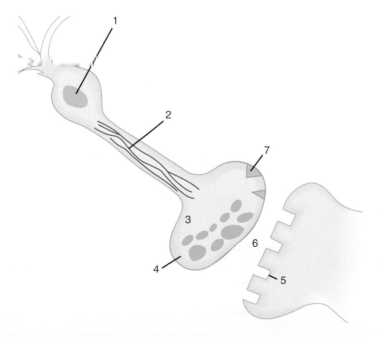

FIGURE 6-63. **Synaptic neurotransmission site.** (1) Cell body. (2) Microtubules. (3) Site of precursor or neurotransmitter uptake for presynaptic storage vesicles. (4) Presynaptic storage vesicles. (5) Postsynaptic neurotransmitter receptors. (6) Reuptake of the released neurotransmitter back into the presynaptic terminal. (7) Presynaptic neurotransmitter receptors. (Modified with permission from Ebert MH, Loosen PT, Nurcombe B. *Current Diagnosis & Treatment in Psychiatry.* New York: McGraw-Hill, 2000: 30.)

KEY FACT

The **nucleus basalis of Meynert** is an important site for the production of ACh in the brain.

KEY FACT

The **substantia nigra pars compacta** and the **ventral tegmental area** are important sites of dopaminergic neurons in the brain.

and muscarinic. It is formed in the nerve terminal by *choline acetyltransferase* (Figure 6-64). A decrease in levels of ACh is implicated in Alzheimer dementia. Like histamine receptors, muscarinic ACh receptors are subject to off-target blockade by **antipsychotics** and **tricyclic antidepressants,** resulting in dry mouth, blurred vision, and urinary hesitancy.

Dopamine

A neurotransmitter synthesized from tyrosine, dopamine serves as a precursor to norepinephrine (NE) and epinephrine (Figure 6-65). Dopamine is implicated in psychosis ($\uparrow$ levels), mania ($\uparrow$ levels), schizophrenia ($\uparrow$ levels), and Parkinson disease ($\downarrow$ levels).

γ-Aminobutyric Acid (GABA)

The major inhibitory neurotransmitter in the CNS, GABA is associated with anxiety ($\downarrow$ levels) and epilepsy ($\downarrow$ levels). Anxiolytics (eg, alcohol, benzodiazepines, and barbiturates) are agonists of the $GABA_A$ receptor (see sections on anxiolytics and hypnotics for further explanation of benzodiazepines and barbiturates).

Glutamate

The major excitatory neurotransmitter in the CNS, glutamate is implicated in epilepsy ($\uparrow$ levels), schizophrenia ($\uparrow$ levels), and Alzheimer disease ($\uparrow$ levels).

Glycine

Glycine is an inhibitory neurotransmitter that controls/modulates glutamate activity in the brain and spinal cord.

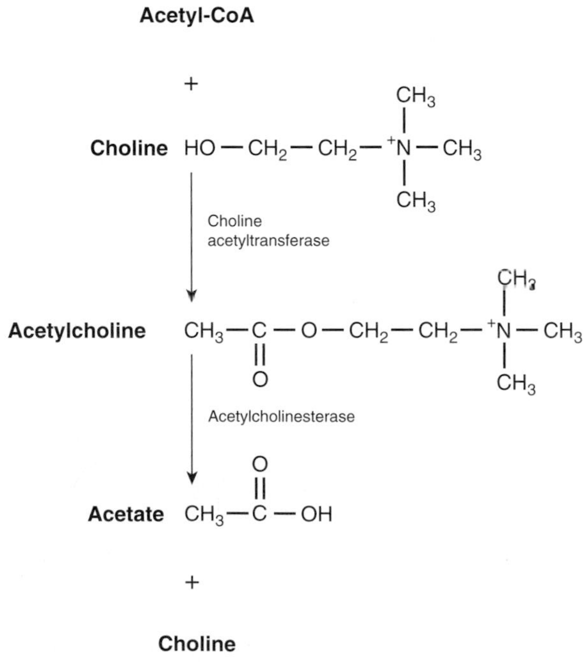

Acetyl-CoA

+

Choline $HO - CH_2 - CH_2 - {}^+N - CH_3$ (with CH_3 groups)

Choline acetyltransferase

Acetylcholine $CH_3 - C - O - CH_2 - CH_2 - {}^+N - CH_3$

Acetylcholinesterase

Acetate $CH_3 - C - OH$

+

Choline

FIGURE 6-64. **Synthesis and degradation of acetylcholine.** Acetyl-CoA and choline combine with help from the enzyme choline acetyltransferase to form acetylcholine. Acetylcholinesterase is responsible for breaking down the neurotransmitter into acetate and choline.

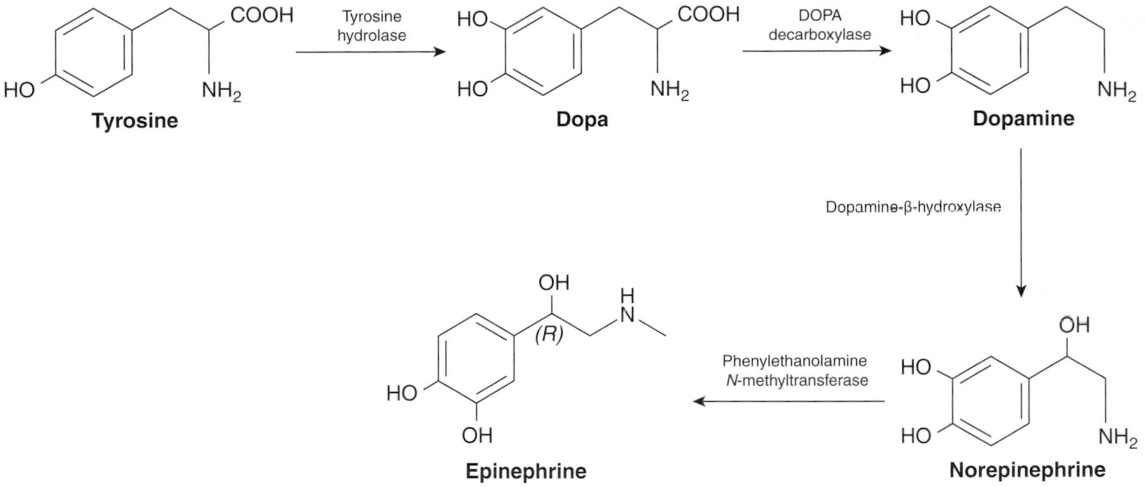

Figure showing synthesis pathway.

FIGURE 6-65. **Synthesis of dopamine, norepinephrine, and epinephrine.** Dopa, dopamine, norepinephrine, and epinephrine are all derivatives of the amino acid tyrosine. (Modified with permission from Ebert MH, Loosen PT, Nurcombe B. *Current Diagnosis & Treatment in Psychiatry.* New York: McGraw-Hill, 2000: 31.)

Histamine

Histamine is a ubiquitous chemical that, in the CNS, is responsible for sleep modulation and satiety. Antipsychotics and tricyclic antidepressants can cause histamine (H_1)-receptor blockade, leading to side effects such as sedation and increased appetite, leading to weight gain.

Norepinephrine

A catecholamine (precursor to epinephrine), norepinephrine (NE) is found at sympathetic postganglionic terminals (see Figure 6-65). It is implicated in major depressive disorder (↓) and anxiety (↑).

Serotonin (5-Hydroxytryptamine)

Serotonin is a monoamine neurotransmitter that regulates mood, body temperature, sexuality, and sleep. It is converted from tryptophan in a critical reactions (Figure 6-66) and is degraded by the enzyme monoamine oxidase. It is implicated in major depressive disorder (↓), bipolar disorder (↓), anxiety disorder (↓), and schizophrenia (↑).

AUTONOMIC DRUGS

Autonomic drugs are chemical agents that act within the autonomic nervous system at sympathetic and parasympathetic nerve terminals (Figure 6-67). These drugs interact with preexisting neurotransmitters in order to achieve desired effects at the junction of the CNS and the PNS.

Neuromuscular Junction Blocking Agents

Neuromuscular junction (NMJ)-blocking agents are drugs used for skeletal muscle relaxation. These agents work at the NMJ, as opposed to inhaled anesthetics or regional nerve blocks, which act at different sites (see Figure 6-50). Because they work only at the NMJ, these agents do not cause analgesia or

KEY FACT

Histaminergic neurons are located in the **ventral posterior hypothalamus (tuberomammillary nucleus).**

KEY FACT

The **locus ceruleus,** found in the upper pons is the primary site of norepinephrine synthesis in the brain.

KEY FACT

The **raphe nucleus** in the brain stem releases serotonin to projections throughout the brain.

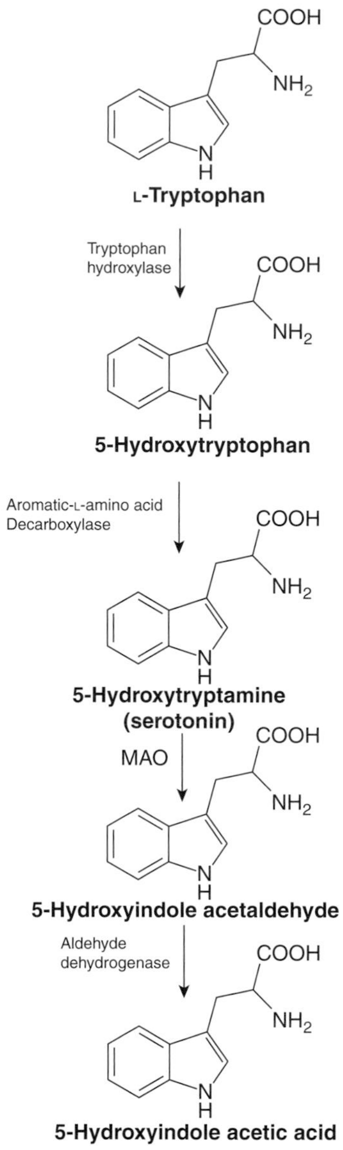

FIGURE 6-66. **Synthesis of serotonin.** Serotonin is a derivative of the amino acid tryptophan and is converted by monoamine oxidase to yield 5-hydroxyindole acetaldehyde. (Modified with permission from Ebert MH, Loosen PT, Nurcombe B, *Current Diagnosis & Treatment in Psychiatry*. New York: McGraw-Hill, 2000: 34.)

unconsciousness, **only paralysis.** They are similar in structure to ACh, allowing them to bind to ACh receptors on the muscle membrane. The two classes of NMJ-blocking agents work differently at the ACh receptor; **depolarizing** agents behave as ACh receptor **agonists,** and **nondepolarizing** agents behave as ACh receptor **competitive antagonists.**

Depolarizing Agents

DRUG NAME

Succinylcholine (short-acting).

MECHANISM

In general, depolarizing agents, such as succinylcholine, work as ACh receptor agonists. They achieve their desired effect in two distinct phases. In phase

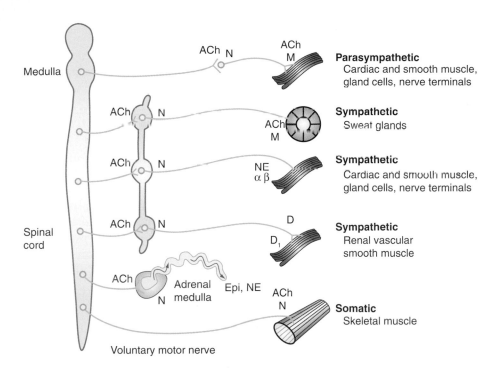

FIGURE 6-67. **The autonomic and somatic nervous systems.** ACh, acetylcholine; D, dopamine; D_1, type 1 dopamine receptor; Epi, epinephrine; N, nicotinic receptor; NE, norepinephrine; M, muscarinic receptor; α, alpha-adrenergic receptor; β, beta-adrenergic receptor. (Modified with permission from Katzung BG. *Basic & Clinical Pharmacology*, 10th ed. New York: McGraw-Hill, 2007: 76.)

I, the drug binds aggressively to the ACh receptor and triggers depolarization of the motor endplate. However, it is resistant to AChE and remains bound to the ACh receptor. Sodium channels found at the motor endplate that initially closed after depolarization remain closed since the drug remains bound to the receptor and prevents repolarization of the motor endplate. Phase II block occurs after the drug remains bound to the ACh receptor over time, inducing a conformational change at the NMJ. This leads to a nondepolarizing neuromuscular block that cannot be reversed. The effects of succinylcholine are evident within 30 seconds and last for 10 minutes (duration of action is limited by diffusion away from the NMJ). **Pseudocholinesterase** metabolizes succinylcholine before the drug reaches the site of action.

USES

Succinylcholine is the only depolarizing agent approved for clinical use in the United States. It is used to effect temporary muscle paralysis (eg, surgery, intubation).

SIDE EFFECTS

- Cardiovascular:
    - Low dose: Negative chronotropic and inotropic effects.
    - High dose: Positive chronotropic and inotropic effects; raises catecholamine levels.
- Fasciculations (visible motor unit contractions in phase I).
- Myalgia.
- Hyperkalemia (can ↑ serum potassium levels by 0.5 mEq/L, which is a concern in the setting of burns/trauma, spinal cord injury, cardiac disease, and/or metabolic abnormalities).
- Malignant hyperthermia.

Nondepolarizing Agents

DRUG NAMES

Mivacurium (short-acting), vecuronium (intermediate-acting), rocuronium (intermediate-acting), atracurium (intermediate-acting), pancuronium (long-acting), doxacurium (long-acting).

MECHANISMS

Nondepolarizing agents operate as ACh receptor competitive antagonists. The drug binds to the ACh receptor, but does not cause the motor endplate to depolarize. By binding to the receptor, it prevents ACh from binding, thereby preventing depolarization of the motor endplate and causing paralysis. Most nondepolarizing agents depend on hepatic or renal elimination to terminate their effect. An exception is mivacurium, which is metabolized by pseudocholinesterase and is safe for patients with hepatic or renal dysfunction. Reversal of nondepolarizing block depends on metabolism of the drug or administration of a reversal agent (eg, AChE inhibitor).

USES

Nondepolarizing agents are similar to depolarizing agents in causing muscle paralysis and can substitute for depolarizing agents as a muscle relaxant. Such uses include intubation, prevention of fasciculations (especially important in patients who may be sensitive to variations in serum potassium levels), decreasing the amount of required inhalational agents, and maintenance of paralysis.

SIDE EFFECTS

- Respiratory failure due to diaphragmatic paralysis.
- Tachycardia (pancuronium).
- Histamine release (mivacurium).

Cholinesterase Inhibitors

DRUG NAMES

Neostigmine, pyridostigmine, edrophonium, physostigmine.

MECHANISMS

These drugs inactivate AChE by electrostatic or covalent binding. They are used to reverse the effects of a nondepolarizing neuromuscular drug. They prevent degradation of ACh at the NMJ and therefore increase the available ACh to compete for ACh receptors, causing the nondepolarizing agent to "wash out." Reversal agents are contraindicated when depolarizing agents are used because they inhibit cholinesterase and pseudocholinesterase, thereby prolonging the phase I block.

USES

They are used to reverse nondepolarizing neuromuscular drugs (eg, pancuronium) during surgery; they can also be used to diagnose (edrophonium) and treat myasthenia gravis (eg, neostigmine).

SIDE EFFECTS

- Bradycardia
- Bronchospasm

- Excitation (physostigmine)
- Intestinal spasm
- Increased bladder tone
- Pupillary constriction

Anticholinergic Drugs

DRUG NAMES

Atropine, scopolamine, benztropine, glycopyrrolate.

MECHANISMS

These drugs competitively block ACh receptors and therefore prevent the endogenous neurotransmitter from acting (similar to the way nondepolarizing neuromuscular agents work at the NMJ).

USES

These drugs are primarily used in anesthesiology. However, they have many uses outside of anesthesiology, as they affect many organ systems.

- Glycopyrrolate is a charged molecule and cannot cross the blood-brain barrier (BBB) to cause CNS effects.
- Scopolamine is generally administered for its CNS effects (eg, antiemetic).
- Atropine is generally administered for it cardiovascular effects; it is also the first-line treatment for organophosphate poisoning (with pralidoxime):
  - Reversing vagal-stimulated bradycardia.
  - Decreasing respiratory tract secretions.
  - Bronchial smooth muscle relaxation.
  - Reversal of antipsychotic extrapyramidal side effects.

SIDE EFFECTS

- CNS stimulation.
- Cutaneous blood vessel dilation.
- Urinary retention.
- Cycloplegia (paralysis of ciliary muscle of the eye, leading to an inability to accommodate).
- Decreased secretions.

MNEMONIC

Adverse side effects of anticholinergic drugs: "blind as a bat, dry as a bone, red as a beet, mad as a hatter, and hot as a hare."

ANXIOLYTICS AND HYPNOTICS

Both benzodiazepines and barbiturates target $GABA_A$ receptors. Typically, activation of the $GABA_A$ receptor causes a chloride ion channel to open, allowing chloride to enter and hyperpolarize the cell. With both types of medications, there are concerns about tolerance (decreased responsiveness after repeated doses) and withdrawal (physical dependence; adverse symptoms in absence of medication).

Barbiturates

DRUG NAMES

Phenobarbital, pentobarbital, thiopental, secobarbital.

MECHANISMS

Barbiturates increase the duration of chloride channel opening on $GABA_A$ receptors, resulting in enhanced GABAergic transmission. Barbiturates can block excitatory glutamate receptors in addition to targeting GABA receptors. They also induce CYP-450 microsomal enzymes in the liver so that other drugs that are metabolized by this system are eliminated more quickly.

Phenobarbital is 75% inactivated in the liver and 25% excreted in the urine unchanged.

USES

Barbiturates have many clinical uses. Certain short-acting agents (eg, thiopental, methohexital) are used during anesthesia. Other agents, like phenobarbital, are used as anticonvulsants in the long-term management of tonic-clonic seizures, status epilepticus, and eclampsia. Anxiolytic properties of barbiturates make them applicable for use as mild sedatives that relieve anxiety. Furthermore, clinicians can use barbiturates in the treatment of insomnia but this is typically not recommended because barbiturates suppress REM sleep more than other stages of sleep.

SIDE EFFECTS

- High risk of dependence.
- Synergistic effects with alcohol and benzodiazepines (cross-tolerance).
- Respiratory, cardiovascular, CNS depression sufficient to cause coma and death.
- Induction of cytochrome P450.
- Contraindicated in patients with **acute intermittent porphyria** because barbiturates activate *ALA synthase*, the enzyme that catalyzes the rate-limiting step in heme synthesis.

Treatment of overdose consists of managing symptoms (ABCs) and hemodialysis in severe cases. Alkalinization of urine can aid in the elimination of phenobarbital.

WITHDRAWAL

Barbiturate withdrawal can mimic alcohol withdrawal. The withdrawal syndrome includes:

- Anxiety.
- Irritability.
- Elevated heart and respiration rate.
- Muscle pain.
- Nausea.
- Tremors.
- Hallucinations.
- Confusion.
- Seizures.
- Death is possible if untreated.

Barbiturate withdrawal syndrome is dangerous and must be treated in the hospital. Gradual administration of phenobarbital can be used to treat withdrawal symptoms.

Benzodiazepines

DRUG NAMES

Diazepam, lorazepam, triazolam, temazepam, oxazepam, midazolam, chlordiazepoxide, alprazolam.

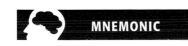

MNEMONIC

Barbi**DURAT**e increases the **DURAT**ion of opening of the GABA$_A$ receptor chloride channel.

MECHANISMS

Increased frequency of chloride channel opening is associated with binding of benzodiazepines on the GABA$_A$ receptor. The entry of chloride hyperpolarizes the cell, making it more difficult to depolarize; therefore, it reduces neural excitability. The effects of this class of drugs are terminated through both redistribution and excretion (metabolized by the hepatic microsomal system into active metabolites). Benzodiazepines can cross the placental barrier.

USES

Benzodiazepines have a number of clinical uses. They can be used as anxiolytics (via inhibition of neuronal circuits in the limbic system), as muscle relaxants to treat muscle spasms, as amnesic agents for endoscopic procedures (eg, upper endoscopy, colonoscopy), and as anticonvulsant agents.

SIDE EFFECTS

- Synergistic effects with alcohol and barbiturates (cross-tolerance).
- Respiratory depression and coma (much less than with barbiturates).
- Drowsiness and confusion.
- Tolerance.
- Dependence.

It is possible to reverse the effects of a benzodiazepine with **flumazenil**, a competitive antagonist at the benzodiazepine binding site of the GABA$_A$ receptor.

WITHDRAWAL

Long-term use of benzodiazepines can lead to tolerance and dependence. Withdrawal is similar to barbiturate withdrawal, but rarely as severe. Signs of benzodiazepine withdrawal include:

- Confusion
- Anxiety
- Agitation
- Restlessness
- Insomnia
- Tension

Opioids

DRUG NAMES

Morphine, hydromorphone, oxymorphone, methadone, meperidine, fentanyl, sufentanil, alfentanil, remifentanil, codeine, hydrocodone, oxycodone, buprenorphine.

MECHANISMS

Opioids are analgesics that act on the CNS. Opioids are either endogenous (endorphins, met- and leuenkephalins, and dynorphins) or exogenous (derived from opium or synthetically created). Endogenous endorphins are formulated from proopiomelanocortin (POMC), which is also the precursor for the formation of adrenocorticotropic hormone (ACTH), melanocyte-stimulating hormone (MSH), and lipotropin (LPH). Synthetic opioids are structurally similar to endogenous opioids, but have been altered to achieve distinct properties. Most opioids provide analgesia by acting as agonists on the μ-opioid receptor, although different formulations have varying strengths (full

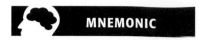

MNEMONIC

For short-acting benzodiazepines, think—

TOM Thumb
Triazolam
Oxazepam
Midazolam

KEY FACT

Benzodiazepines decrease latency to sleep onset and increase stage 2 of non-REM sleep. Both REM sleep and slow-wave sleep (stages 3 and 4) are decreased.

MNEMONIC

Benzodiazepines should be called **FRE**nzodiazepines because they increase the **FRE**quency of chloride ion entry through the GABA$_A$ receptor.

agonist vs. partial or weak agonist). By activating these receptors, the ascending pain pathways are modulated.

USES

Common uses of opioids include local analgesia (eg, regional nerve blocks, epidural nerve blocks, spinal nerve blocks), systemic pain relief (eg, patient-controlled analgesia), and chronic pain management (eg, transdermal patches). They are also used in antitussives (eg, dextromethorphan). Opioids are frequently substances of abuse for IV drug users (heroin).

SIDE EFFECTS

- Tolerance
- Dependence
- Overdose potential

Buspirone

MECHANISM

Buspirone is a partial agonist to serotonin 1A (5HT-1A) receptors in the CNS. Because it does not affect GABAergic receptors, it is does not interact with ethanol, nor does it have as profound sedating properties, risk of dependence, and associated euphoria as benzodiazepines and barbiturates.

USES

Buspirone is used to treat **generalized anxiety disorder** (see Chapter 7).

SIDE EFFECTS

- May stimulate the locus ceruleus, increasing NE release (causing increased anxiety).
- May not work in patients with a history of benzodiazepine use or severe anxiety.

ANTIDEPRESSANTS

Antidepressants target imbalances in endogenous serotonin, NE, and/or dopamine. Heterocyclic agents (HCAs), selective serotonin reuptake inhibitors (SSRIs), monoamine oxidase (MAO) inhibitors, and atypical antidepressants modulate the effects of endogenous neurotransmitters. Extended treatment with antidepressants leads to downregulation of postsynaptic neurotransmitter receptors. There are multiple target receptors; no two antidepressants have the same receptor profile.

Selective Serotonin Reuptake Inhibitors

DRUG NAMES

Citalopram, fluoxetine, paroxetine, sertraline, fluvoxamine.

MECHANISMS

SSRIs are the current first-line treatment for depressive and anxiety disorders. They prevent reuptake of serotonin by the presynaptic terminal, allowing for increased availability of serotonin to the postsynaptic membrane. It can take 3–6 weeks to see a desired effect clinically. Mood is not elevated in nondepressed patients, and mania may be precipitated in patients with bipolar disorder (see Chapter 7). SSRIs can be used in pregnant patients and the elderly because they have relatively few side effects.

USES

SSRIs are also used in illnesses other than depressive disorders. They can be used in the specific treatment of panic disorder, generalized anxiety disorder, and obsessive-compulsive disorder. Also, they can be used in the treatment of social anxiety disorder, posttraumatic stress disorder, eating disorders (eg, fluoxetine in bulimia), and trichotillomania (impulsive hair pulling). In addition, SSRIs have been shown to decrease poststroke depression and morbidity/mortality even in the absence of depression.

SIDE EFFECTS

- Diarrhea.
- Sexual dysfunction (↓ libido, erectile dysfunction, anorgasmia).
- Weight gain.
- Fatigue.
- Discontinuation syndrome (worse with short-acting medications).
- Birth defects (absolute risk is small with all SSRIs, but greatest risk is with paroxetine).

Monoamine Oxidase Inhibitors

DRUG NAMES

Phenelzine, tranylcypromine, isocarboxazid.

MECHANISM

Monoamine oxidase-A (MAO-A) is an enzyme that breaks down NE (see Figure 6-66). Irreversibly inhibiting this breakdown increases the amount of available NE. MAO-A is also responsible for the breakdown of serotonin and tyramine (see side effects).

USES

MAOIs are used to treat depressive disorders, including atypical depression (presenting with psychotic, polyphagic, or phobic features), anxiety, and hypochondriasis. MAO inhibitors are used less often since the introduction of SSRIs because of their dangerous interaction with foods containing tyramine (see side effects).

SIDE EFFECTS

- Use with tyramine causes potentially fatal side effects and the following symptoms:
  - Hypertensive crisis
  - Diaphoresis
  - Headache
  - Vomiting
- Use with SSRIs can cause **serotonin syndrome**, characterized clinically as:
  - Confusion
  - Hyperthermia
  - Myoclonus
  - Diaphoresis
  - Hyperreflexia

KEY FACT

SSRI discontinuation syndrome consists of dizziness, vertigo, nausea, fatigue, headaches, insomnia, shock-like sensations, paresthesias, visual disturbances, muscle pain, chills, irritability, agitation, and suicidal thoughts.

KEY FACT

The most common congenital anomaly associated with SSRI use is ventral septal defect (VSD).

KEY FACT

Tyramine-rich foods include:
- Cheese (pizza)
- Pepperoni
- Beer
- Wine
- Smoked or pickled meat
- Liver
- Spoiled foods

Tricyclic Antidepressants

DRUG NAMES

Amitriptyline, imipramine, amoxapine, clomipramine, desipramine, doxepin, nortriptyline, protriptyline.

MECHANISMS

Tricyclic antidepressants (TCAs) increase the synaptic concentration of serotonin and NE in the CNS. They achieve this effect by inhibiting serotonin and NE reuptake by the presynaptic terminal, resulting in the availability of more neurotransmitter to bind to postsynaptic neuronal receptors.

USES

TCAs can be used to treat chronic pain, major depression, and anxiety disorders. Historically, TCAs have been used in children for the treatment of enuresis. However, due to the incidence of sudden death, it is not a first-line treatment.

SIDE EFFECTS

- **Constipation**
- **Cardiac arrhythmias**
- **Coma** (overdose potential)
- Sudden death in children (imipramine and desipramine)
- Sedation
- Tremor
- Insomnia
- Orthostatic hypotension
- Psychosis
- Seizures
- Weight gain

Nontricyclic Heterocyclic Antidepressants

DRUG NAME

Bupropion.

MECHANISM

Bupropion is a heterocyclic antidepressant that can be used for smoking cessation. Although the mechanism of bupropion is not fully understood, it is generally considered to work by inhibiting the reuptake of dopamine and NE, allowing for increased amounts of both neurotransmitters to bind their respective receptors in the CNS. This allows the drug to be useful in patients in whom TCAs are not tolerated due to side effects (eg, orthostatic hypotension). The mechanism for smoking cessation is also unknown, but it is believed to be mediated by nicotinic ACh receptor antagonism.

USES

Nontricyclic heterocyclic antidepressants are second- and third-line medications used in the treatment of major depression and smoking cessation. They are also used as substitutes in patients who do not tolerate TCAs.

SIDE EFFECTS

- Stimulant effects.
- Tachycardia.

- Insomnia.
- Headaches.
- Seizure risk is greater than with other antidepressant drugs.

Contraindicated in the following conditions:

- Anorexia.
- Bulimia.
- Seizure disorders (lowers seizure threshold).
- MAO inhibitor treatment within the past 2 weeks.

DRUG NAMES

Venlafaxine, duloxetine.

MECHANISMS

Both venlafaxine (which is converted to an active metabolite O-desmethylvenlafaxine) and duloxetine work through a similar mechanism to achieve their antidepressant effects. Both medications inhibit the presynaptic reuptake of serotonin > NE.

USES

These serotonin and NE reuptake inhibitors are used to treat major depression including melancholia (venlafaxine), anxiety disorders, chronic pain associated with depression, and diabetic peripheral neuropathic pain (duloxetine).

SIDE EFFECTS

- Sedation
- Nausea
- Constipation
- Elevated blood pressure
- Sweating

DRUG NAMES

Nefazodone, trazodone, mirtazapine.

MECHANISMS

These medications are serotonin modulators. They block the $5\text{-}HT_2$ receptor and inhibit reuptake of 5-HT and NE. Mirtazapine also antagonizes histaminic H_1 receptors and weakly blocks peripheral α_1-adrenergic and muscarinic receptors. Trazodone can antagonize serotonin at low doses and behaves like a serotonin agonist at high doses. In addition to blocking presynaptic serotonin reuptake, trazodone is thought to effect histamine blockade, allowing it to be useful in the treatment of insomnia.

USES

These medications are used to treat major depression and anxiety disorders. In addition, trazodone may be used for insomnia.

SIDE EFFECTS

- Sedation (especially low-dose mirtazapine)
- Increased appetite
- Weight gain
- Dry mouth

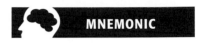

MNEMONIC

Both **VE**nlafaxine and **DUAL**oxetine are **VE**ry good **DUAL** inhibitors.

- Hepatotoxicity (nefazodone)
- Priapism (trazodone)
- Visual trails (nefazodone)
- Postural hypotension

DRUG NAME

Maprotiline.

MECHANISMS

Maprotiline is a tetracyclic antidepressant that selectively prevents the reuptake of NE. Maprotiline differs from tricyclic antidepressants and other heterocyclic antidepressants in that it does not prevent the reuptake of serotonin.

USES

Maprotiline is used in the treatment of major depression.

SIDE EFFECTS

- Sedation
- Orthostatic hypotension

NEUROLEPTICS

Neuroleptics (classified as first- and second-generation antipsychotics) block type 2 dopamine receptors (D_2). These drugs are most effective against the positive symptoms of schizophrenia, such as hallucinations and delusions.

First-Generation Antipsychotics

DRUG NAMES

Chlorpromazine and thioridazine (low potency), haloperidol, trifluoperazine, pimozide, perphenazine (high potency).

MECHANISMS

First-generation antipsychotics work in the mesolimbic system by blocking postsynaptic D_2 receptors. The low-potency drugs (eg, chlorpromazine, thioridazine) also have an affinity for muscarinic ACh receptors, α-adrenergic receptors, and histaminergic receptors (see side effects). High-potency drugs (eg, haloperidol) have greater affinity for D_2 receptors.

USES

First-generation antipsychotic drugs are useful in the treatment of acute psychosis and schizophrenia as well as in bipolar disorder. Haloperidol can be used in Tourette syndrome (to control tics) and Huntington disease (to combat choreiform movements associated with advanced disease).

SIDE EFFECTS

- Extrapyramidal signs (Parkinsonism, akathisia, tremor); (high-potency antipsychotics).
- Movement disorders (tardive dyskinesia, dystonias); (high-potency antipsychotics).
- Sedation (low-potency antipsychotics).
- Neuroleptic malignant syndrome.
- Hyperprolactinemia (amenorrhea, galactorrhea, gynecomastia).

- Anticholinergic side effects (low-potency antipsychotics).
- Sudden death from prolongation of the QT interval, leading to torsades de pointes (thioridazine).
- Irreversible retinal pigmentation (thioridazine).
- Deposits in the lens and cornea (chlorpromazine).

Second-Generation (Atypical) Antipsychotics

DRUG NAMES

Clozapine, risperidone, olanzapine, quetiapine, ziprasidone, aripiprazole.

MECHANISMS

Atypical antipsychotics have effects on the serotonergic, dopaminergic (with affinity for D_2), and noradrenergic systems. Each medication has a different neuroreceptor profile, accounting for differences in therapeutic action and side effects. Atypical antipsychotics have several advantages over typical antipsychotics. Second-generation antipsychotics are more effective with negative and chronic symptoms of schizophrenia (eg, avolition, alogia, flattened affect). In addition, the risk of tardive dyskinesia, neuroleptic malignant syndrome, and extrapyramidal signs is lower with atypical antipsychotics.

USES

These medications are used to treat schizophrenia, psychosis, bipolar disorder, and for antidepressant augmentation (risperidone).

SIDE EFFECTS

- Cardiotoxicity.
- Neuroleptic malignant syndrome.
- Extrapyramidal signs (see previous Side Effects section).
- Agranulocytosis (clozapine).
- Increased chance of seizures.
- Weight gain (clozapine, olanzapine).
- Insulin intolerance, leading to type 2 diabetes (for some second-generation agents, this side effect may be unrelated to weight gain).
- Hyperlipidemia.
- Electrocardiogram (ECG) abnormalities (prolongation of QT and PR intervals may occur with ziprasidone).
- Increase in prolactin levels (gynecomastia, galactorrhea, and amenorrhea, seen especially with risperidone).

Ziprasidone and aripiprazole have fewer metabolic side effects than do the other second-generation antipsychotics.

MOOD STABILIZERS AND ANTICONVULSANTS

Mood Stabilizers

DRUG NAME

Lithium.

MECHANISMS

The exact mechanism of this mood stabilizer is unknown. However, it is believed that lithium interferes with monoamine synthesis, release, and reuptake.

KEY FACT

Blockade of muscarinic receptors causes:
- Facial flushing
- Dry mouth
- Urine retention
- Constipation

Blockade of histamine receptors causes:
- Weight gain
- Sedation
- Orthostatic hypotension
- Tremor
- Sexual dysfunction

USES

Lithium is used in the treatment of bipolar disorder and to augment antidepressants in major depressive disorder. The effects of lithium may take 2–3 weeks to manifest, and because of its low therapeutic index, its blood level must be followed and kept to the minimum therapeutic level. Creatinine (renal function) and thyroid-stimulating hormone (TSH, thyroid function) must also be followed regularly.

SIDE EFFECTS

- **Hypothyroidism,** goiter.
- Thirst.
- Tremor.
- Diarrhea.
- Renal dysfunction (**nephrogenic diabetes insipidus** results in increased creatinine and eventual kidney failure).
- Increased appetite and weight gain.
- Cardiac conduction problems.
- Mild cognitive impairment.
- CNS depression (at toxic levels).
- Congenital abnormalities.

Anticonvulsants

Anticonvulsants are agents that suppress uncontrolled neuronal discharge in epileptic seizures. Seizures are characterized as either partial or generalized. Within the category of partial seizures, a patient can have a simple seizure, a complex seizure, or a partial seizure with secondarily generalized tonic-clonic seizure. Within the category of generalized seizures, a patient can have an absence seizure, myoclonic seizure, tonic-clonic seizure, atonic seizure, or status epilepticus. Anticonvulsants inhibit neuronal firing through three different mechanisms to reduce the likelihood that a seizure will occur: (1) increasing GABAergic activity, (2) blocking voltage-activated sodium channels, or (3) blocking voltage-activated calcium channels (see Figures 6-68, 6-69, and 6-70, respectively).

DRUG NAME

Valproic acid.

MECHANISM

Valproic acid, or valproate (its dissociated or ionized form), works via binding to voltage-gated sodium channels and favoring the inactivated state (see Figure 6-69). It also has a role in decreasing calcium influx across the cell membrane through T-type calcium channels, reducing the calcium current in thalamic neurons (see Figure 6-70).

USES

Valproic acid is used for the treatment of partial and generalized tonic-clonic seizures, bipolar disorder (mood-stabilizing properties), and intermittent explosive disorder (a behavioral disorder characterized by extreme expression of anger that is disproportionate with inciting cause). Also, it can be used as prophylaxis for migraines and is the second-line treatment for generalized absence seizures after ethosuximide. Use of this drug is decreasing due to the higher number of side effects and its lower efficacy compared with other medications.

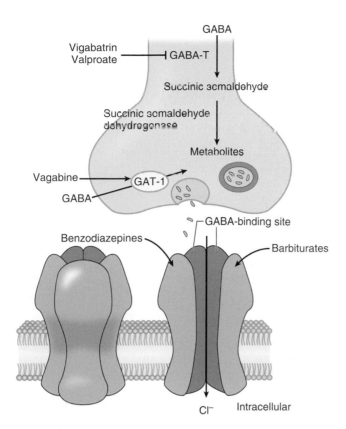

FIGURE 6-68. **Anticonvulsants that target presynaptic and postsynaptic γ-aminobutyric acid (GABA) and the GABA receptor.** Vigabatrin, valproate, tiagabine, barbiturates, and benzodiazepines all target GABA and its receptor to inhibit central nervous system activity. (Modified with permission from Katzung BG. *Basic & Clinical Pharmacology*, 10th ed. New York: McGraw-Hill, 2007: 506.)

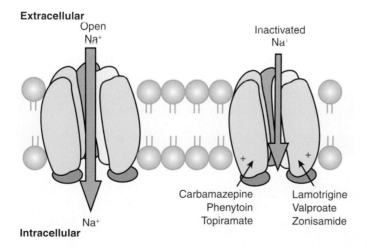

FIGURE 6-69. **Anticonvulsants that target and extend sodium channel inactivation.** Carbamazepine, phenytoin, topiramate, lamotrigine, valproate, and zonisamide all target voltage-gated sodium channels and aim to prolong their inactivation in the treatment of seizures. (Modified with permission from Katzung BG. *Basic & Clinical Pharmacology*, 10th ed. New York: McGraw-Hill, 2007: 505.)

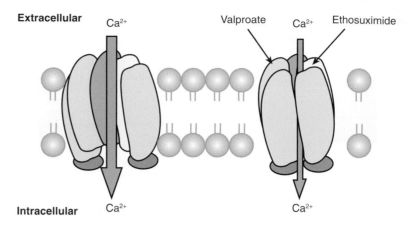

FIGURE 6-70. Anticonvulsants that target and reduce current through calcium channels. Only valproate and ethosuximide target and reduce current through T-type calcium channels in the treatment of generalized absence seizures.

SIDE EFFECTS

- GI upset, with stomach pain, nausea, and diarrhea.
- Increased appetite, leading to weight gain.
- Tremor.
- Sedation.
- Alopecia.
- Hepatotoxicity.
- Decreased platelet count.
- Possible polycystic ovarian syndrome.
- Congenital neural tube defects (folate antagonist).

DRUG NAME

Ethosuximide.

MECHANISMS

Ethosuximide, like valproic acid, works by reducing the calcium current in thalamic neurons. The thalamus is responsible for the generation of the 3-Hz spike-and-wave rhythms seen in absence seizures. By reducing these T-type currents in the neurons of the thalamus, ethosuximide can stop the rhythmic discharge associated with an absence seizure (see Figure 6-70).

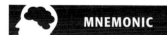 **MNEMONIC**

E**TH**osuximide targets the **TH**alamus.

USES

Ethosuximide is the first-line treatment for **absence seizures**.

SIDE EFFECTS

- GI distress
- Lethargy
- Headache
- Urticaria
- Stevens-Johnson syndrome

DRUG NAME

Phenobarbital.

MECHANISMS

A member of the barbiturate drug class, phenobarbital acts on the $GABA_A$ receptor. By doing so, it increases CNS inhibition and raises the seizure threshold (see Figure 6-68).

USES

Phenobarbital has many uses; however, its role in anticonvulsive therapy is specific to treating patients in **status epilepticus.**

SIDE EFFECTS

- Sedation
- Tolerance
- Dependence
- Induction of cytochrome P450 system

DRUG NAME

Carbamazepine.

MECHANISMS

Carbamazepine reduces the rate of recovery of voltage-activated sodium channels, blocking the rapid successive firing of action potentials that is classically associated with partial seizures and generalized tonic-clonic seizures (see Figure 6-69).

USES

Carbamazepine is used to treat partial seizures and tonic-clonic seizures (first line) as well as bipolar disorder and **trigeminal neuralgia.**

SIDE EFFECTS

- Aplastic anemia.
- Agranulocytosis.
- Hyponatremia.
- Induces cytochrome P450 enzymes, causing increased metabolism of many drugs, including itself and oral contraceptives.

DRUG NAME

Phenytoin.

MECHANISMS

Like carbamazepine, it acts by slowing the rate of recovery of voltage-activated sodium channels (see Figure 6-69).

USES

Phenytoin is used to treat all types of partial and generalized seizures (except absence seizures). It is also the first-line treatment for prophylaxis against status epilepticus.

SIDE EFFECTS

Toxicity (at high levels):

- Nystagmus
- Diplopia

- Ataxia
- Sedation
- Gingival hyperplasia
- Megaloblastic anemia
- SLE-like syndrome
- Induction of cytochrome P450
- Fetal hydantoin syndrome

DRUG NAME

Lamotrigine.

MECHANISMS

Lamotrigine has a mechanism similar to that of phenytoin and carbamazepine (see Figure 6-69). In addition to prolonging inactivation of voltage-gated sodium channels, it may be associated with reducing the amount of released glutamate.

USES

It is used to treat partial seizures, generalized tonic-clonic seizures, focal epilepsy, Lennox-Gastaut syndrome, and bipolar disorder.

SIDE EFFECTS

- Dizziness.
- Nausea.
- Headache.
- Skin rash (hypersensitivity reaction).
- Stevens-Johnson syndrome (avoided by increasing the dose very slowly).

DRUG NAME

Pregabalin.

MECHANISMS

Its antinociceptive and antiseizure effects may be due to binding to the α_2-δ subunit of high-voltage-activated Ca^{2+} channels. Pregabalin increases the density of the GABA transporter protein and increases the rate of functional GABA transport. It also decreases presynaptic release of glutamate, NE, and substance P.

USES

Pregabalin is used to treat neuropathic pain associated with diabetic neuropathy and postherpetic neuralgia and in the adjunctive treatment of partial seizures and fibromyalgia.

SIDE EFFECTS

- Dizziness
- Somnolence
- Weight gain

DRUG NAME

Gabapentin.

MECHANISMS

Although designed to be a GABA analog, gabapentin does not modulate GABA receptors. It binds avidly to the α_2-δ subunit of high-voltage-activated Ca^{2+} channels, thereby modulating their function. Like pregabalin, gabapentin also acts presynaptically to decrease the release of glutamate.

USES

Since it is a highly lipid-soluble drug, gabapentin is used for sedation as well as to treat partial seizures, pain (including neuropathic), peripheral neuropathy, bipolar disorder, and anxiety.

SIDE EFFECTS

- Sedation
- Weight gain

TREATMENTS FOR NEURODEGENERATIVE DISEASE

Drugs Used to Treat Alzheimer Disease

The decrease in ACh levels and the increase in the excitatory neurotransmitter glutamate are a notable part of Alzheimer disease. One strategy to manage symptoms of Alzheimer disease is to block the N-methyl-D-aspartate (NMDA) receptors that are activated by excess glutamate. Likewise, since acetylcholinesterase (AChE) breaks down ACh into choline and acetate (see Figure 6-64), blocking the action of AChE may aid in improving cognition. To date, no FDA-approved drug modifies disease progression.

DRUG NAME

Memantine.

MECHANISM

During depolarization of neuronal cells, the magnesium blockade of NMDA receptors is relieved and calcium enters the cell. Over time, the influx of calcium leads to neuronal damage. Memantine noncompetitively blocks NMDA receptors in the CNS, preventing stimulation by glutamate. This results in less intracellular calcium. In essence, lowering intracellular calcium levels spares the neurons from further damage.

USES

Memantine is used to treat moderate to severe Alzheimer disease. It may also have a role in the treatment of vascular dementia.

SIDE EFFECTS

- Agitation
- Urinary incontinence
- Insomnia
- Diarrhea

DRUG NAMES

Tacrine, donepezil, rivastigmine, galantamine.

MECHANISMS

All of these medications are selective inhibitors of AChE in the CNS. By selectively inhibiting AChE in the CNS, levels of ACh increase, which has been shown to improve cognition. The benefits of having centrally acting AChE inhibitors are improved efficacy and decreased peripheral side effects.

USES

These drugs are generally used in the treatment of Alzheimer disease because they are centrally acting (cross the BBB) unlike other AChE inhibitors used for myasthenia gravis (eg, neostigmine).

SIDE EFFECTS

■ Nausea
■ Vomiting
■ Diarrhea
■ Insomnia

Drugs Used to Treat Parkinson Disease

Parkinson disease is caused by a loss of dopaminergic neurons in the substantia nigra pars compacta, which results in lower levels of dopamine in the CNS. Decreased dopamine manifests clinically with mask-like facies, bradykinesia, resting tremor, muscle rigidity, shuffling gait, and postural instability. Several strategies are used to increase the levels of CNS dopamine: (1) increase endogenous dopamine by preventing its degradation, (2) add an exogenous precursor of dopamine (levodopa) that is converted to dopamine centrally, or (3) give dopamine agonists that directly stimulate D_2 receptors (Figure 6-71).

DRUG NAMES

Bromocriptine, pergolide, ropinirole, pramipexole.

MECHANISMS

Broadly, these drugs work as dopamine receptor agonists. However, each drug has different effects on the different types of dopamine receptors. For example, pergolide is an agonist of both D_1 and D_2 receptors, ropinirole and pramipexole act only at D_2 receptors, and bromocriptine is a D_2 receptor agonist and

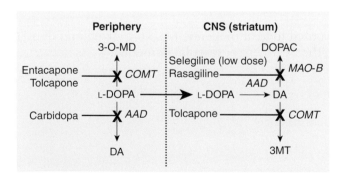

FIGURE 6-71. **Relationship between peripheral and centrally acting drugs used to treat Parkinson disease.** AAD, amino acid decarboxylase; COMT, catecholamine O-methyltransferase; DA, dopamine; DOPAC, dihydroxyphenylacetic acid; MAO-B, monoamine oxidase-B; 3-O-MD, 3-ortho-methyldopa; 3MT, 3-methyoxytyramine. (Modified with permission from Brunton LL, Lazo JS, Parker KL. *Goodman and Gilman's The Pharmacological Basis of Therapeutics*, 11th ed. New York: McGraw-Hill, 2006: 536.)

D_1 receptor antagonist. Bromocriptine also has properties that allow it to antagonize D_1 receptors in the hypothalamus.

USES

These medications are used to treat Parkinson disease. Bromocriptine can be used to reduce the rate of growth of pituitary adenomas (eg, prolactinoma) and to treat acromegaly.

SIDE EFFECTS

- Headache.
- Nausea.
- Vomiting.
- Epigastric pain.
- Hypotension/syncope initially, leading to hypertension over time.

DRUG NAME

Levodopa (L-dopa).

MECHANISMS

Levodopa is a metabolic precursor of dopamine that enters the brain through an L-amino acid transporter. Dopamine itself cannot cross the BBB. Once in the CNS, it is further decarboxylated to dopamine. Levodopa appears in the urine as the metabolites homovanillic acid (HVA) and dihydroxyphenylacetic acid (DOPAC).

USES

First-line medication in the treatment of Parkinson disease. Given with carbidopa to reduce peripheral conversion of L-dopa to dopamine, which decreases side effects and increases availability of L-dopa for the CNS.

SIDE EFFECTS

- Nausea and vomiting
- Tachycardia
- Atrial fibrillation
- Dyskinesias
- Depression
- Agitation
- Confusion

Levodopa is contraindicated in psychosis and closed-angle glaucoma.

Monoamine Oxidase Inhibitors

Two types of monoamine oxidase have been distinguished in the nervous system:

- Monoamine oxidase A (MAO-A) metabolizes NE and serotonin (discussed previously).
- Monoamine oxidase B (MAO-B) metabolizes dopamine.

DRUG NAMES

Selegiline, rasagiline.

MECHANISMS

Selegiline is an irreversible selective inhibitor of MAO-B. MAO-B is found in the striatum and metabolizes dopamine in the brain.

USES

Parkinson disease. A selegiline preparation (Emsam) is available in a skin patch that allows the drug to bypass the GI tract. Its low dose does not have the tyramine food interactions seen with other MAO inhibitors.

SIDE EFFECTS

Serotonin syndrome (can occur when taken in combination with meperidine, TCAs, or SSRIs).

Catechol-*O*-Methyltransferase Inhibitors

DRUG NAMES

Tolcapone (central and peripheral), entacapone (peripheral).

MECHANISMS

The catechol-O-methyltransferase (COMT) inhibitors tolcapone and entacapone can prolong the action of levodopa by diminishing its peripheral and central metabolism. Entacapone is preferred to tolcapone (less hepatotoxicity) even though it only has peripheral activity.

USES

Used to increase the levels of levodopa in the treatment of Parkinson disease.

SIDE EFFECTS

- Dyskinesias
- Nausea
- Confusion

CLINICAL ANESTHETICS AND ANALGESICS

General Anesthetics

General anesthetics are essential to surgery because they cause analgesia, amnesia, and unconsciousness. They also cause muscle relaxation and suppression of reflexes.

Stages of Anesthesia

Four sequential stages:

- Stage 1—Analgesia: "Conscious and conversational."
- Stage 2—Disinhibition: Autonomic variations (changes in blood pressure, heart rate, and respiratory rate).
- Stage 3—Surgical anesthesia: Unconscious with relaxed muscles.
- Stage 4—Medullary depression: Respiratory and vasomotor center depression.

Method of Delivery

Inhaled agents are volatile, halogenated hydrocarbons that were derived from early research and clinical experience with ether and chloroform. On the other hand, IV drugs are typically used for their common property of rapid induction.

Inhaled Anesthetics

Depth of anesthesia can be rapidly altered by changing the inhaled concentration of the drug, making it suitable for maintaining anesthesia. The speed of induction of inhaled anesthetics depends on the alveolar gas and venous blood partial pressures, the solubility of the anesthetic agent in the blood, and the alveolar blood flow. The minimum alveolar concentration (MAC), which is very similar to ED_{50}, is equal to the alveolar concentration of an inhaled anesthetic that stops movement in 50% of patients in response to incision.

In order to cross the selectively permeable BBB, drugs must penetrate through membrane lipids (lipophilic) or must be actively transported.

DRUG NAMES

Halothane, isoflurane, sevoflurane, desflurane.

MECHANISMS

The mechanism of inhaled anesthetics is poorly understood.

USES

Inhaled anesthetics are used in the maintenance of anesthesia.

SIDE EFFECTS

- Respiratory depression
- Nausea
- Emesis
- Hypotension

TOXICITY

- Hepatotoxicity (halothane).
- Nephrotoxicity (methoxyflurane, no longer used in the United States)
- Convulsions (enflurane).
- Malignant hyperthermia (all agents except nitrous oxide).

Intravenous Anesthetics

Used to rapidly induce anesthesia, with propofol having the ability to both induce and maintain anesthesia.

TYPES

- Barbiturates
- Benzodiazepines
- Ketamine
- Opiates
- Propofol
- Etomidate

BARBITURATES (THIOPENTAL)

Highly lipid-soluble agents that enter the brain rapidly, making them suitable for induction of anesthesia and short surgical procedures. Redistribution from the brain to other tissues causes loss of effects. They are not analgesic and

KEY FACT

Drugs with **low** solubility in blood have rapid induction and recovery times. Drugs with **high** solubility in oil or lipids have increased potency. Anesthetics with greater solubility in oil tend to also have greater solubility in blood and vice versa, implying that there is frequently a tradeoff between **potency** and **speed of induction.**

KEY FACT

Dantrolene is used to treat malignant hyperthermia because it interferes with calcium release from the sarcoplasmic reticulum of muscle cells by binding to ryanodine receptors.

KEY FACT

Anesthetic concentrations of pentobarbital block high-frequency sodium channels.

KEY FACT

Opioids are reversed with naloxone or naltrexone, which antagonize the μ-opioid receptor.

MNEMONIC

B. B. King on OPIATES PROPOses FOOLishly:
Barbiturates
Benzodiazepines
Ketamine
Opiates
PROPOFOL

therefore require a supplementary analgesic. IV barbiturates can cause severe hypotension in patients who are hypovolemic or in shock.

BENZODIAZEPINES (MIDAZOLAM)

Most common drug used for endoscopy; it is used with inhalational anesthetics and narcotics. Midazolam can cause severe postoperative respiratory depression and amnesia.

KETAMINE (ARYLCYCLOHEXYLAMINE)

A PCP analog that acts as a dissociative anesthetic (very high affinity for NMDA receptors). It causes sedation, amnesia, immobility, disorientation, and hallucinations.

OPIOIDS (MORPHINE, FENTANYL, SUFENTANIL)

Used with other CNS depressants during general anesthesia. Toxicity involves hypotension, respiratory depression, and muscle rigidity.

PROPOFOL

Used for rapid induction of anesthesia and short surgical procedures. An excitatory phase may occur, causing muscle twitching, spontaneous movements, and hiccups. It also can reduce ICP. Propofol is used in the resection of spinal tumors. Since it has much less effect than volatile anesthetics on CNS-evoked potentials, it can be used when assessing spinal cord function.

CHAPTER 7

Psychiatry

Basic Definitions and Concepts

DEFINING PSYCHIATRIC ILLNESS

FLASH FORWARD

Olfactory hallucinations often occur as part of the aura before a seizure.

Visual hallucinations are more commonly associated with medical disorders.

Auditory hallucinations are most consistent with schizophrenia.

Tactile hallucinations are common in delirium tremens (alcohol withdrawal) and in cocaine abusers (during intoxication).

Mental illness, also called psychiatric illness, is defined by abnormalities in thought, perception, mood, or behavior that deviate from the social norm for an individual's culture and impair social functioning. Although many advances have been made in the diagnosis and treatment of psychiatric illnesses, some patients with psychiatric illness face social stigmatization.

As with other areas of medicine, accurate diagnosis of psychiatric illness requires that a patient's subjectively described **symptoms** and objectively observable **signs** be properly identified. Important terms used to describe signs and symptoms of psychiatric illnesses are defined in Table 7-1.

Disordered **thought process, thought content, perception, mood, affect,** and/or **motor activity** are the main hallmarks of psychiatric illness. Refer to Table 7-2 for descriptions and examples of symptoms of disorders within five of these areas. Abnormal mood is discussed in the section on mood disorders.

Observed collections of signs and symptoms that often occur together are grouped into **syndromes.** Specifically recognized syndromes are referred to as **psychiatric disorders. Psychopathology** is the study of mental disorders.

CLASSIFICATION OF PSYCHIATRIC DISORDERS

The fourth edition of the American Psychiatric Association's *Diagnostic and Statistical Manual of Mental Disorders, Text Revision* (DSM-IV-TR), published in 2000, is the standard diagnostic text used by American medical and research professionals. Recognizing that our understanding of the etiologies and underlying pathophysiology of many psychiatric disorders is incomplete, the DSM-IV-TR defines mental disorders by a series of inclusion and exclusion criteria.

Therefore, DSM-IV-TR provides the field with a consistent classification system and nomenclature that can be used by clinicians and researchers to more effectively communicate patient information and conduct research on mental illness. The fifth edition of *Diagnostic and Statistical Manual of Mental Disorders* (DSM-5) will be published in May 2013.

TABLE 7-1.   **Important Terminology for Describing Psychiatric Signs and Symptoms**

TERM	DEFINITION
Affect	Outward display of a patient's feelings or emotions, which can be objectively observed. A patient's affect can reflect a normal range of emotions or be flat, blunted, broad, or inappropriate.
Mood	Subjective feelings or emotions experienced and expressed by the patient.
Psychosis	Significant transient or persistent impairment in reality testing.
Reality testing	Process of comparing thoughts or ideas to information gathered from the external world.
Thought disorder	Abnormal thinking affecting a patient's language, communication, thought content, or thought process.

TABLE 7-2. Definitions and Examples of Symptoms of Disordered Thought, Perception, Affect, Behavior, and Motor Activity

Symptom	Definition	Patient Example
Disorders of Thought Process		
Thought blocking	Sudden cessation of thought or speech.	During an interview, a patient with schizophrenia appears to lose the ability to express thoughts.
Short attention span	Inability to complete an act or thought.	A man begins to answer a question and rapidly forgets what he is answering.
Clang associations	A type of thinking in which the sound of a word, rather than its meaning, provides the impetus for subsequent associations.	During a manic episode a woman approaches a man and says, "Hey, man is your name Dan? Plan fans, ban pans!"
Flight of ideas	Rapid succession of thoughts.	While answering a question, a man abruptly and repeatedly switches to unrelated topics.
Concrete thinking	One-dimensional thought.	A schizophrenic patient interprets a parable in a literal way.
Tangential thought	Patient gets lost on an unrelated thought and does not return to the original concept.	When asked about his childhood, a man describes riding his bike with friends but soon begins a lengthy recollection of President Kennedy.
Circumferential thought	Patient veers from the original idea, but eventually returns to it.	When answering a question, a man frequently digresses to related topics before answering the question.
Disorders of Thought Content		
Delusions	Fixed, false beliefs that are not shared by the general population. Maintained in spite of proof to the contrary. Can be bizarre (eg, involving supernatural forces) or nonbizarre (eg, fear that organized crime is targeting someone in the family).	A man tells his doctor that his landlord is poisoning him with toxic gas.
Phobias	Extreme, irrational fear of a situation or an object.	A student with agoraphobia becomes extremely anxious when leaving his dorm room.
Obsessions	Intrusive and repetitive thoughts.	A man believes that his hands remain dirty although he has adequately washed them.
Suicidal/homicidal thoughts	Strong desire or preoccupation to kill oneself or others.	A patient with schizophrenia plans to kill herself because she fears that she cannot avoid being tortured by her neighbor.

(continues)

TABLE 7-2. **Definitions and Examples of Symptoms of Disordered Thought, Perception, Affect, Behavior, and Motor Activity** *(continued)*

SYMPTOM	DEFINITION	PATIENT EXAMPLE
Disorders of Thought Content *(continued)*		
Poverty or overabundance of thoughts	Too few or too many ideas.	A person does not answer most of a doctor's questions and only speaks one or two words at a time (poverty of thoughts). A person has many different answers to a single question (overabundance of thoughts).
Disorders of Perception		
Illusion	Misperception of real external stimuli.	An anxious woman interprets the sound of a door slamming as a shot being fired from a gun.
Idea of reference	False belief of being referred to by others.	A woman states that a radio show host is talking about her.
Hallucination (visual, auditory, olfactory, tactile, gustatory)	False sensory perception.	A cocaine abuser feels bugs crawling under his skin (formication, or "cocaine bugs").
Disordered Affect, Behavior, or Motor Activity		
Flat affect	Diminished range of emotional expression.	A patient appears to be staring far into the distance and displays no discernable emotion.
Compulsions	Repetitive behaviors; often associated with temporary relief from obsessions.	After using the bathroom, a man washes his hands five times.
Stereotyped movement	Repetitive purposeless movement.	A person experiencing amphetamine intoxication repetitively moves her hand in a similar fashion.
Hyperactivity	Increase in activity above a normal level.	During a manic episode, a man begins intensely cleaning the entire house.
Hypoactivity	Decreased activity.	During a major depressive episode, a woman sits in a chair all day without moving.
Catatonia	A syndrome characterized by excited or retarded movement and posturing.	A patient with schizophrenia maintains an awkward, rigid pose for hours and ignores all external stimuli.

TABLE 7-3. **Major DSM-IV-TR Diagnostic Classes**

GROUPING	DSM-IV-TR DIAGNOSTIC CLASS
Disorders grouped based on typical age of onset	Disorders usually first diagnosed in infancy, childhood, or adolescence
Disorders grouped based on common etiology	Mental disorders due to a general medical condition not elsewhere classified Substance-related disorders Adjustment disorders
Disorders grouped according to common presenting symptoms	Delirium, dementia, amnesia, and other cognitive disorders Schizophrenia and other psychotic disorders Mood disorders Anxiety disorders Somatoform disorders Factitious disorders Dissociative disorders Sexual and gender identity disorders Eating disorders Sleep disorders Impulse-control disorders not elsewhere classified Personality disorders

The DSM classification system is "axis-based."

- Axis I—Psychiatric disorders other than personality disorders
- Axis II—Personality disorders, mental retardation
- Axis III—Pertinent medical conditions
- Axis IV—Psychosocial and environmental stressors
- Axis V—Global assessment of function

All of the disorders described in the DSM-IV-TR are grouped into diagnostic categories, which are organized based on typical age of onset, cause, or common presenting symptoms (Table 7-3). Since the DSM-IV-TR is used as the standard for diagnosis of mental disorders in the United States, information about the diagnosis of specific psychopathologic disorders in the following sections is based on the DSM-IV-TR criteria.

DISORDERS WITH KNOWN BIOLOGICAL CAUSES

As more is learned about the biological causes of psychiatric disorders and the pathophysiologic basis for their manifestations, the distinction between psychiatric disorder and general medical condition becomes artificial and increasingly misleading. Furthermore, many general medical conditions can manifest with signs or symptoms of mental illness. Therefore, to correctly describe a patient's condition it is important to understand the terms **secondary** and **substance-induced** (Table 7-4).

TABLE 7-4. **Classification of Mental Illness With a Known Cause**

TERM	DEFINITION	CLASSIFICATION	EXAMPLE
Secondary	A mental disorder, sign, or symptom that is caused by an identified, specific medical disorder.	Classified phenomenologically with related disorders.	A mood disorder caused by hypothyroidism is classified in the mood disorders section of the DSM-IV-TR.
Substance-induced	A sign or symptom of a mental disorder that is primarily the result of substance intoxication or withdrawal.	Classified as a substance-related disorder.	Psychosis related to LSD intoxication is classified as a substance-related disorder.

TRANSFERENCE AND COUNTERTRANSFERENCE

During the evaluation and treatment of a psychiatric patient it may be important to understand the concepts of transference and countertransference:

- **Transference:** A patient unconsciously projects feelings or attitudes from a person or situation in the past onto a person or situation in the present (eg, the patient's physician). For example, a patient may project a parent-like quality onto the doctor and expect that the doctor will provide solutions for all of his problems.
- **Countertransference:** A physician unconsciously projects feelings or attitudes onto the patient. This may be the physician's unconscious response to transference. For example, while treating a patient, a physician may begin to think and act like the patient's parent.

PSYCHOLOGICAL MOTIVATORS

Reporting of symptoms by a patient may be influenced by psychological motivators that can be categorized into primary versus secondary gain. **Primary gain** refers to internal motivations. For example, a patient who is unable to deal with an internal psychological conflict may unconsciously convert the conflict to somatic symptoms (**conversion disorder**). **Secondary gain** refers to external motivators. For example, a patient's disease may allow him/her to garner sympathy or qualify for workers' compensation. The patient may or may not recognize these gains.

DEFENSE MECHANISMS

Defense mechanisms are automatic and unconscious reactions to psychological stress. They function by keeping conflicts out of the conscious mind, thereby helping to alleviate potential anxiety caused by these conflicts. Defense mechanisms can be categorized as immature or mature (Table 7-5). Immature defense mechanisms are developmentally primitive (seen first during early stages of development) and are characterized by the patient reverting back to childlike behavior in response to psychological stress. Although also unconscious reactions, mature defense mechanisms reflect a more developed understanding of the conflict.

TABLE 7-5.   Defense Mechanisms

DEFENSE MECHANISM	CHARACTERISTICS	EXAMPLE
Mature Defense Mechanisms		
Altruism	Negative feelings about oneself are alleviated by assisting other people.	A man who has negative feelings about being abandoned by his parents as a child works at an orphanage.
Humor	Focusing on the humorous aspect of an uncomfortable or adverse situation.	A nervous patient jokes about an upcoming operation.
Sublimation	Replacing a socially unacceptable desire with an action that is similar, but is socially acceptable.	A man who has violent thoughts decides to pursue a career as a butcher.
Suppression	Voluntarily pushing uncomfortable ideas or feelings out of the conscious mind.	A student consciously chooses not to think about upcoming exams until a few days prior to the exams.
Immature Defense Mechanisms		
Acting out	Unacceptable thoughts or feelings are expressed through attention-seeking actions.	A 16-year-old whose parents are going through a divorce begins to skip classes.
Dissociation	Temporary change in memory, personality, or consciousness.	A soldier who witnessed the murder of a friend has no memory of the incident.
Denial	Refusing to acknowledge the reality of a painful experience or situation.	A woman refusing to believe that she was recently diagnosed with cancer.
Displacement	Transferring an undesirable or unacceptable idea or feeling for one person onto another person.	A man who is angry at his boss comes home and yells at his children.
Fixation	Becoming obsessed with and attached to a person, animal, object, or event.	An adult avoids obligations by obsessively watching the sports channel.
Identification	Unconsciously mimicking someone else's behavior.	An abused child grows up to abuse his own children.
Isolation	Exhibiting a lack of emotion associated with a stressful situation.	A woman who witnesses a murder describes the incident with no emotion.
Projection	Attributing one's own personally unacceptable feeling(s) onto another person.	A woman who has desires to cheat on her husband is convinced that her husband is cheating on her.
Rationalization	Giving logical reasons for a negative situation in an attempt to convince oneself that the situation is a reasonable one; superficial insight.	A man who did not get the job that he wanted told his friends that it was a good thing because it would have been a very stressful position.
Reaction formation	Replacing a personally unacceptable emotion with the opposite attitude.	A woman who unconsciously resents her marriage constantly showers her husband with affection and gifts.

(continues)

TABLE 7-5. Defense Mechanisms *(continued)*

DEFENSE MECHANISM	CHARACTERISTICS	EXAMPLE
Immature Defense Mechanisms *(continued)*		
Regression	Regressing back to child-like behaviors.	A 10-year-old boy who recently moved to a new state begins to have enuresis.
Repression	A desire is involuntarily excluded from a person's consciousness.	A woman has a phobia of spiders but cannot remember the first time she was afraid of them.
Splitting	Labeling people or situations as either purely bad or purely good. Difficulty tolerating ambiguity.	A patient believes that his primary care physician is a terrible person while his therapist is the most wonderful person in the world.

PSYCHIATRIC TREATMENT APPROACHES

Treatment approaches in psychiatry include those that are psychosocial, pharmacologic, or somatic in nature, although several different approaches are often used together to treat a patient's illness. Important examples of specific treatments within these three categories are summarized here and will be mentioned in subsequent sections during the discussion of specific psychiatric disorders.

Psychosocial

Psychosocial treatments include certain forms of psychotherapy, counseling, as well as social and vocational training. Two important psychosocial treatment approaches are psychodynamic therapy and cognitive behavioral therapy.

- **Psychodynamic therapy:** A form of psychotherapy that evolved from psychoanalysis. This type of therapy focuses on the unconscious processes that influence a person's thinking and behavior.
- **Cognitive behavioral therapy (CBT):** A form of psychotherapy that is based on the idea that a person's thoughts, not the external world, are the basis of his feelings and behaviors. In contrast to psychodynamic therapy, this form of therapy can be shorter in duration and is less centered on the therapeutic relationship between physician and patient.

Pharmacologic

Psychopharmacotherapy involves the use of psychoactive medications in the treatment of psychiatric disorders. Important categories of psychiatric drugs include anxiolytics, antipsychotics, antidepressants, and mood stabilizers (Table 7-6).

Somatic

Somatic treatments are a class of psychiatric nonpharmacologic treatment modalities that are centered on a patient's physical body rather than her mind. Electroconvulsive therapy (ECT) is a notable example of somatic treatment. In ECT electric currents are passed through the brain. ECT can be effective

TABLE 7-6. Summary of Psychiatric Drugs

Class of Drugs (Common Examples)	Mechanism	Common/Notable Adverse Effects
Anxiolytics		
Benzodiazepines (diazepam, lorazepam, midazolam, clonazepam)	Potentiate $GABA_A$-mediated inhibition.	Ataxia, dizziness, somnolence, fatigue, memory difficulties.
Barbiturates (phenobarbital)	Potentiate $GABA_A$-mediated inhibition.	Sedation, ataxia, confusion, dizziness, decreased libido, depression.
Buspirone	Serotonin 5-HT_{1A} receptor partial agonist.	Dizziness, confusion, headache, blurred vision, nervousness.
Antipsychotics		
Typical antipsychotics (chlorpromazine, haloperidol)	Antagonize dopamine D_2 receptors.	Parkinsonian symptoms, neuroleptic malignant syndrome, tardive dyskinesia, anticholinergic symptoms.
Atypical antipsychotics (risperidone, clozapine, olanzapine, aripiprazole, others)	Antagonize dopamine D_2 and serotonin 5-HT_2 receptors. Clozapine and olanzapine also antagonize dopamine D_4 receptors. Note: in contrast, aripiprazole is a D_2 and 5-HT_1 partial agonist.	Mild extrapyramidal symptoms, anticholinergic symptoms, sedation, weight gain.
Antidepressants		
Selective serotonin reuptake inhibitors (SSRIs: sertraline, paroxetine, fluoxetine, citalopram, escitalopram)	Increase synaptic serotonin levels by inhibiting presynaptic uptake.	Serotonin syndrome (when used concomitantly with an MAOI), sexual dysfunction, gastrointestinal distress.
Serotonin-norepinephrine reuptake inhibitors (SNRIs: venlafaxine, duloxetine)	Inhibit serotonin reuptake and norepinephrine reuptake at the synapse.	Hypertension, sweating, weight loss, gastrointestinal distress, blurred vision, sexual dysfunction, neuroleptic malignant syndrome.
Atypical antidepressants (bupropion)	Weakly inhibit uptake of serotonin, norepinephrine, and dopamine.	Tachyarrhythmia, pruritus, sweating, rash, dyspepsia, constipation, dizziness.
Tricyclic antidepressants (TCAs: amitriptyline, clomipramine, others)	Inhibit serotonin and norepinephrine reuptake.	Heart block, bloating, constipation, xerostomia, dizziness, somnolence, urinary retention.
Monoamine oxidase (MAO) inhibitors (MAOIs: iproniazid, moclobemide, befloxatone, brofaromine, others)	Increase serotonin and norepinephrine levels in presynaptic neurons and synapses by inhibiting their breakdown.	Tyramine toxicity, dizziness, somnolence, orthostatic hypotension, weight gain.

(continues)

TABLE 7-6.   Summary of Psychiatric Drugs *(continued)*

CLASS OF DRUGS (COMMON EXAMPLES)	MECHANISM	COMMON/NOTABLE ADVERSE EFFECTS
Mood Stabilizers		
Lithium	Inhibits adrenergic, muscarinic, and serotonergic neurotransmission in the brain. Alters serotonin, norepinephrine, and dopamine neurotransmission.	Acute lithium intoxication (nausea, vomiting, diarrhea, renal failure, ataxia, tremor), bradyarrhythmia, hypotension, hyperkalemia, nephrogenic diabetes insipidus, hypothyroidism, goiter, ECG and EEG abnormalities, acne.
Lamotrigine	Inhibit neurotransmission by blocking neuronal sodium channel.	Rash, ataxia, somnolence, blurred vision.
Stimulants		
Amphetamine, methylphenidate	Increase catecholamine release from the synaptic terminal, block catecholamine reuptake, weakly inhibit MAO.	Hypertension, tachyarrhythmia, restlessness, loss of appetite, addiction potential.

MNEMONIC

Causes of delirium—

I'M DELIRIOUS

Impaired delivery (eg, infarction, hemorrhage)
Metabolic
Drugs (eg, alcohol, anticholinergics, benzodiazepines, antihypertensive medications)
Endocrinopathy
Liver disease
Infrastructure (of cortical neurons; eg, postictal state)
Renal failure (eg, electrolyte imbalance, uremia)
Infection (eg, meningitis)
Oxygen (lack of)
Urinary tract infection
Sensory deprivation

KEY FACT

Delirium is more likely to affect the visual system, whereas psychosis is more likely to affect the auditory system.

in treating certain severe psychiatric disorders and is often used for patients who cannot tolerate or have not responded adequately to other treatments.

Pathology

COGNITIVE DISORDERS

Cognitive disorders are categorized into delirium, dementia, and amnestic disorders (Table 7-7). They are the result of central nervous system (CNS) impairment and affect memory, attention, orientation, and judgment. The Mini-Mental State Examination is used to determine the severity of the disorder. This test determines a patient's mental state by testing orientation, registration, attention, recall, language, and calculation.

Delirium

Characterized by variation in a patient's level of consciousness throughout the day. Patients are easily distracted, disoriented with respect to time and place, have language disturbances, and can experience illusions and hallucinations. Elderly patients often experience symptoms when "sundowning" (delirium worsening at night).

Delirium can be caused by a variety of medical disorders, including infection, trauma, hypoxia, substance withdrawal (eg, alcohol), medications, and toxins (eg, heavy metals). It is commonly seen in ICUs and in association with acute medical illness.

Symptoms of delirium can last for days or weeks, and if left uncorrected, the condition is associated with a high-mortality rate. Correction of the underlying medical disorder resolves the delirium.

TABLE 7-7.   Difference Between Delirium and Dementia

	DELIRIUM	DEMENTIA
Onset	Acute (from hours to days)	Gradual
Duration	Days to weeks	Months to years
Level of consciousness	Fluctuates (varies throughout the day)	Normal (does not change throughout the day)
Symptoms	Fluctuates (worse at night)	Stable
Orientation	Impaired	Not impaired in early stages of disease
Memory	Dramatic decline in a short period of time	Gradual decline over a longer period of time (recent and remote memory are impaired)
Awareness	Reduced	Normal
Medical status	Usually reversible (after correction of underlying medical disorder)	Most are irreversible (only 15% are reversible if caused by an underlying medical disorder)
Hallucinations	Visual hallucinations common	Hallucinations less common
EEG changes	Present (fast waves/generalized slowing)	None
Causes	Impaired delivery of substrates/blood to the brain, metabolic disturbances, drugs (eg, alcohol, opiates, barbiturates), endocrinopathy (eg, thyroid storm), liver disease, loss of cortical neurons, renal failure, CNS infection, hypoxemia, urinary tract infection, neurosensory disturbance	Alzheimer disease, microvascular disease (vascular dementia), Pick disease/frontotemporal dementia, Huntington disease, Parkinson disease, Creutzfeldt-Jakob disease, normal pressure hydrocephalus

EEG = electroencephalograph.

DSM-IV-TR DIAGNOSTIC CRITERIA

- Acute change in consciousness.
- Level of consciousness varies throughout the day (ie, waxes and wanes).
- Change in cognition (eg, disorientation, deficits of memory, language disturbance).
- Evidence that the change in consciousness is secondary to an underlying medical disorder.

Delirium can be categorized into two groups: quiet and agitated. Patients with quiet dementia may appear depressed.

TREATMENT

- Rule out anticholinergic drug use.
- Correct the underlying medical disorder.
- Pharmacologic therapy: Antipsychotics, benzodiazepines (can also cause delirium; be cautious with their use because they can cause respiratory depression and an increased risk of falls).

- The patient should be placed in a well-lit and quiet environment and in a place where there can be close observation by nurses.
- Constantly reorient patient (eg, tell patient what time it is and where she is).
- Limit the amount of sedation given to the patient (to minimize the amount of napping).

Dementia

Characterized by progressive and usually irreversible impairment of cognitive function and memory. It is a debilitating disorder that affects mainly the elderly. Unlike delirium, the level of consciousness does not vary throughout the day, and the signs and symptoms of dementia generally appear progressively. The incidence increases with age, and 20% of people older than age 80 years suffer from severe dementia. Depression is relatively common in elderly patients and should be ruled out in patients with so-called quiet dementia. Causes of dementia include increasing age, Alzheimer disease (50–60%), and vascular dementia (10–20%).

DIAGNOSIS

A treatable and reversible cause may underlie the symptoms of 15% of patients with dementia. It is important to rule out these treatable causes of dementia. Such causes include hypoxia, hypothyroidism, lead toxicity, Lyme disease, meningitis, neurosyphilis, and medications. Malnutrition can cause vitamin B_{12} or thiamine deficiencies, which can manifest with dementia-like symptoms. Folate deficiency is not a malnutrition-related cause of dementia, although emerging evidence suggests that it may be associated with the development of dementia in the elderly.

TREATMENT

There is no cure for dementia unless it is caused by a treatable medical condition (eg, vitamin B_{12} deficiency). Treatment, therefore, usually involves palliative care. Patient and family should be educated, and long-term care should be discussed. In patients with behavioral or emotional symptoms, low-dose antidepressants or neuroleptics can be used. Antipsychotics can be used for paranoia or hallucinations, and benzodiazepines can be used to treat anxiety and agitation.

Amnestic Disorders

These disorders lead to memory impairment without impaired consciousness or other cognitive functions. Like delirium, amnestic disorders are often caused by an underlying medical disorder, including cerebrovascular accident, brain trauma or tumor, hypoxia, hypoglycemia, systemic illnesses, seizures, multiple sclerosis, herpes simplex encephalitis, and substance use (eg, alcohol, medications). Amnestic disorders can be temporary or permanent depending on the underlying cause.

Amnesia can be categorized into two types:

- **Anterograde:** Unable to make new memories and remember things that occur after the CNS insult (eg, alcohol intoxication).
- **Retrograde:** Inability to recall old memories from before the CNS insult. Often seen transiently with electroconvulsive therapy (ECT).

Note that patients may experience a combination of the two types of amnesia. Moreover, a patient may lose only certain classes of memories. For example, a person may be able to remember how to brush his teeth but can't remember his name (procedural vs. semantic memory).

TREATMENT

If amnesia is caused by a reversible medical disorder (eg, seizures, hypoglycemia), then the disorder will resolve following treatment of the medical condition. However, when the amnesia is permanent, it is important to discuss the patient's limitations with the patient and his family.

SCHIZOPHRENIA AND OTHER PSYCHOTIC DISORDERS

Psychosis is defined as a disconnect from reality in which patients experience **delusions, hallucinations,** and **disordered thinking.** It can be caused by psychotic disorders, substance abuse, or medical illness. It is important to note that patients with psychotic symptoms can have intact reality testing despite ongoing hallucinations. For example, a patient might complain of hearing voices but know that it is his psychotic disorder.

Schizophrenia

A chronic psychiatric disorder characterized by episodes of psychosis and abnormal behavior lasting > 6 months. There are several subtypes of schizophrenia and they are defined by particular associated features (Table 7-8).

This psychiatric disorder affects about 1% of the population across all ethnic groups and countries studied. Most often, schizophrenia begins to appear in young adult patients; the age of onset generally ranges from 15 to 25 years in males and 25 to 35 years in females, with a slight increase in diagnoses for women during the perimenopausal period. Men with schizophrenia are often less responsive to antipsychotic medications than women and show more social and cognitive deficits.

Genetic factors likely contribute to the development of schizophrenia, as there is an increased rate of diagnosis seen in monozygotic twins relative to dizygotic twins. Three neurologic findings have been associated with some patients:

- Hyperactivity of dopaminergic, serotonergic, and noradrenergic systems; there is also increasing evidence for disordered glutamate utilization.
- Enlargement of the lateral and third ventricles of the brain.
- Abnormalities of the frontal lobes.

TABLE 7-8. Subtypes of Schizophrenia

SUBTYPE	CHARACTERISTICS
Catatonic	Motor disturbances with strange posturing, incoherent speech; can involve extreme motion or no motion.
Paranoid	Delusions (eg, persecutory), but with better social functioning than other types and best prognosis.
Disorganized	Inappropriate emotional responses (eg, emotional blunting), disheveled appearance. Severe impairment and poor prognosis.
Undifferentiated	Characteristics of multiple subtypes.
Residual	One or more psychotic episodes in the past, residual flat affect, withdrawal, odd behavior or thinking, but no severe psychotic symptoms.

PRESENTATION

Patients demonstrate psychosis and disordered thinking or behavior. These patients generally have normal memory and are oriented to person, place, and time. The symptoms are divided into positive and negative. **Positive symptoms** are thoughts, sensory perceptions, or behaviors in a person with a psychiatric disorder that are abnormal within the person's culture. **Negative symptoms** are thoughts, sensory perceptions, or behaviors that are present in a normal person but are absent in a patient with mental illness (see following lists of symptoms).

The differences between schizophrenia and type A personality disorders can be subtle and a source of confusion (see Table 7-17). **Schizotypal personality disorder** is considered part of the spectrum of schizophrenic disorders, whereas there is little association between schizophrenia and **schizoid personality disorder**. These disorders are discussed in the personality disorders section. Also, schizophrenia should not be confused with dissociative identity disorder (multiple personality disorder), which is categorized as a dissociative disorder.

> **KEY FACT**

Schizophrenic patients with predominantly negative symptoms have a poorer prognosis. Patients with a more rapid onset of illness have a better prognosis.

- Positive symptoms:
  - **Delusions:** Can be bizarre (eg, there is an alien living inside the patient's body) or not bizarre (eg, the FBI is secretly investigating his activities).
  - **Loose associations:** Patient repeatedly talks about topics completely unrelated to what she was talking about before.
  - **Strange behavior.**
  - **Hallucinations:** Typically auditory (eg, hearing voices when no one is really there).
- Negative symptoms:
  - **Social withdrawal.**
  - **Flat affect:** Patient talks in a monotone voice and does not show any emotion.
  - **Lack of motivation** (avolition).
  - **Thought blocking:** Patient starts talking about a topic but stops in mid-sentence and is unable to continue with what he was saying.
  - **Poverty of speech** (alogia).

DSM-IV-TR DIAGNOSTIC CRITERIA

A diagnosis of schizophrenia requires that two or more of the following five symptoms have been present for at least 1 month:

- Hallucinations
- Delusions
- Disorganized speech
- Disorganized behavior
- Negative symptoms

Furthermore, the following statements must also be true.

- Symptoms cause significant impairment in daily living.
- Symptoms are not due to any other medical condition or substance abuse.

TREATMENT

Antipsychotic agents (ie, dopamine receptor blockers) and psychosocial interventions (eg, family, individual, and behavioral therapy). Haloperidol decanoate is an example of a long-acting injectable medication that can be useful for noncompliant or poorly compliant psychotic patients. There are long-acting formulations of other antipsychotics as well. The advent of atypical antipsychotics increased the utility of these agents for the treatment of patients with psychotic symptoms because they lack the side effects associated with earlier antipsychotics (Parkinsonism and tardive dyskinesia). Atypical antipsychotics, such as risperidone and clozapine, are combined dopamine and serotonin receptor antagonists.

PROGNOSIS

A continued downward spiral can occur over several years that is associated with frequent treatment noncompliance and recurrent psychotic episodes. Earlier onset of schizophrenia may impair normal brain development and lead to a poorer prognosis. Better prognosis is highly associated with community support, low expressed emotion in immediate family, and absence of comorbid substance abuse. Suicide is common, with more than 50% attempting and 10% of those succeeding.

Other Psychotic Disorders

Patients presenting with psychosis, delusions, or hallucinations may not meet the diagnostic criteria for schizophrenia, but may in fact be suffering from one of several other psychotic disorders, which include: **brief psychotic disorder, schizophreniform disorder, schizoaffective disorder,** and **substance-induced psychotic disorder** (Table 7-9).

MOOD DISORDERS

Mood is defined as one's internal emotional state, which is affected by internal and external stimuli. Normally, people have some control over their mood, but patients with mood disorders lose this control. Uncontrollable, disruptive emotional states cause significant distress as well as impairment in occupational and social functioning for patients with mood disorders.

There are no ethnic differences in the prevalence of mood disorders. However, due to disparities in health care availability, patients in lower socioeconomic classes often come to the attention of health care providers later and may be misdiagnosed as having schizophrenia. The most common and severe mood disorders are **bipolar disorder** and **major depressive disorder.** The lifetime prevalence for major depressive disorder is about two times higher in women, whereas bipolar disorder is about equal across the sexes.

KEY FACT

Positive symptoms respond well to typical antipsychotics, but negative symptoms respond better to atypical agents.

KEY FACT

If a patient is not oriented or has memory deficits, consider a cognitive disorder (see section on Cognitive Disorders).

TABLE 7-9.   Characteristics of Other Psychotic Disorders

DISORDER	CHARACTERISTICS
Brief psychotic disorder.	Similar symptoms to schizophrenia but lasts **< 1 month** and is often preceded by stressful psychosocial events or factors.
Schizophreniform disorder.	Same presentation as brief psychotic disorder but psychotic and residual symptoms **last 1–6 months.**
Schizoaffective disorder.	Schizophrenia with **mood disorder** symptoms (see the rest of the section on Mood Disorders). Psychotic symptoms must at times be present without mood disorder symptoms (vs. mood disorder with psychotic features).
Substance-induced psychotic disorder.	Related to the use of stimulants, hallucinogens, or withdrawal from sedatives; usually visual or tactile hallucinations and delusions.

It is believed that a complex interplay of biological and psychosocial factors leads to the development of a mood disorder. Pathophysiologic changes that are thought to occur in mood disorders include the following:

- Altered neurotransmitter activity.
- Depression is associated with **decreased** levels of serotonin, norepinephrine, and possibly dopamine. Note, however, that simply increasing these neurotransmitter levels in the brain does not show therapeutic utility. Current research suggests that improvements in mood associated with increasing these neurotransmitters pharmacologically or behaviorally result from downstream effects on the cell nucleus and possibly the increased secretion of trophic factors.
- Mania is associated with **increased** norepinephrine levels.
- Limbic-hypothalamic-pituitary-adrenal axis abnormalities.

The major mood disorders are divided into two broad syndromes: bipolar disorder, which is characterized by the presence of at least one manic or hypomanic episode, and major depressive disorder (Table 7-10).

Major Depressive Disorder

With a lifetime prevalence of about 5.8%, it is one of the most common and disabling psychiatric illnesses. Major depressive disorder is characterized by the occurrence of one or more major depressive episodes. It is important to note that a patient who has experienced a manic or hypomanic episode in addition to a major depressive episode should receive a diagnosis of bipolar disorder, not major depressive disorder, as treatment with SSRI drugs can precipitate mania in a bipolar patient.

PRESENTATION

Patients with major depressive disorder generally present with a history of a sustained, depressed mood with anhedonia (a loss of interest or pleasure in one's typical activities of daily life) and may also exhibit substantial feelings of guilt and worthlessness.

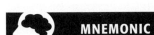

MNEMONIC

Depressive symptoms are SIG E CAPS + depressed mood:

Sleep disturbances (eg, hypersomnia or insomnia; early morning awakenings)

Loss of **I**nterests (ie, anhedonia)

Guilt or feelings of worthlessness

Loss of **E**nergy

Loss of **C**oncentration

Appetite changes/weight changes (usually decreased except in atypical depression)

Psychomotor retardation or agitation (ie, abnormally slow or restless)

Suicidal ideation

TABLE 7-10. **Comparison of Mania and Depression**

DEPRESSION	MANIA
Sleep disturbances	Decreased need for sleep
Appetite changes	Self-destructive pleasure-seeking activities (eg, sex, drugs, spending, gambling)
Weight changes	Agitation
Reduced libido	Flight of ideas
Fatigue	Pressured speech
Concentration difficulties	Grandiosity
Feeling of worthlessness	Distractible
Suicidal ideation	Increased goal-directed activities

DIAGNOSIS

The diagnosis of major depressive disorder is made when a patient has experienced two or more instances of a major depressive episode as specified by the DSM-IV-TR criteria. DSM-IV-TR criteria for a major depressive episode state that a patient must exhibit five or more of the symptoms described in the "SIG E CAPS" mnemonic, including either depressed mood or anhedonia for a period longer than 2 weeks. These symptoms must result in clinically significant distress or impairment in functioning.

In addition to major depressive disorder, there are several other distinct depressive disorders with specific features and DSM-IV-TR diagnostic criteria (Table 7-11).

KEY FACT

In atypical depression, patients have hypersomnia along with weight gain and leaden paralysis.

TREATMENT

Major depressive disorder (MDD): Pharmacotherapy includes antidepressants (eg, serotonin reuptake inhibitors [SSRI], tricyclic antidepressants [TCAs], monoamine oxidase [MAO] inhibitors) (Figure 7-1). Psychotherapy (eg, cognitive behavioral therapy) has also been shown to be effective in some patients. Electroconvulsive therapy (ECT) is the preferred treatment for depression that is refractory to other treatments. The patient must be hospital-

TABLE 7-11. Features of Depressive Disorders

DISORDER	FEATURES
Major depressive disorder (MDD)	Recurrent depressive episodes (two or more), each lasting > 2 weeks along with a symptom-free period lasting at least 2 months.
MDD with melancholic features (melancholia)	Depression with profound anhedonia and dysphoria. Other associated features may include worse mood in the morning, early morning waking, psychomotor abnormality (agitation or retardation), weight loss or decreased appetite, or excessive or inappropriate guilt.
MDD with atypical features	Depression that manifests with features that are not considered typical for MDD, including mood reactivity (mood improves in response to positive events), weight gain or increased appetite, hypersomnia, or leaden paralysis. Associated with sensitivity to rejection.
Chronic MDD	The criteria for a major depressive episode have been met for > 2 years.
Postpartum-onset depression	Depressive, manic, or mixed episode occurring within the first 4 weeks after delivery. Not synonymous with subclinical postpartum "blues," which occurs commonly after delivery. High risk of recurrence in subsequent deliveries (30–50%).
MDD with catatonic features	Patient displays catatonic features similar to those observed in schizophrenia, including posturing, waxy flexibility, catalepsy, negativism, and mutism. Generally observed in patients at the severe and psychotic end of the spectrum of mood disorders.
Dysthymic disorder	Mild depression most of the time for > 2 years but not meeting the criteria for MDD. These patients cry frequently.
Seasonal affective disorder	Depression for at least 2 consecutive years during the same season and periods of depression are followed by nondepressed seasons.

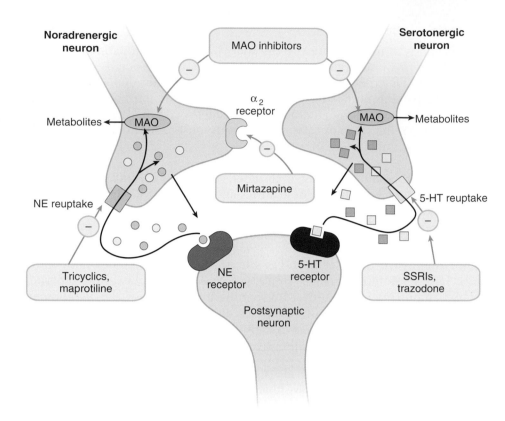

FIGURE 7-1. **Antidepressant sites of action.** (Adapted with permission from Katzung BG, Trevor AJ. *USMLE Road Map: Pharmacology*, 1st ed. New York: McGraw-Hill, 2003: 80.)

ized if he is at a significant risk for suicide, homicide, or is unable to take care of himself.

- **Melancholia:** Research suggests that patients with this specific form of MDD may respond well to treatment with antidepressants and ECT.
- **MDD with atypical features:** May be difficult to treat and require a combination of medications and psychotherapy. MAO inhibitors have been used successfully for patients with this form of MDD.
- **Chronic MDD:** This condition is generally relatively refractory to existing treatments.
- **Postpartum-onset depression:** Pharmacologic or psychotherapy (or both).
- **Dysthymic disorder:** The most effective treatment is insight-oriented psychotherapy; however, antidepressants can also be used.
- **Seasonal affective disorder:** Broad-spectrum light therapy, antidepressants, or psychotherapy.

Bipolar Disorder

The second major syndrome of disordered mood is bipolar disorder, which is characterized by the occurrence of at least one manic or hypomanic episode. The lifetime prevalence of bipolar disorder is about 1%, and its incidence peaks between the ages of 25 and 30. It is a strongly familial disorder—the concordance rate in monozygotic twins is approximately 60%.

PRESENTATION

Patients with bipolar disorder present with a history of a manic or hypomanic episode. A **manic episode** is commonly described as a period during which the patient exhibits an abnormally elevated or irritable mood, rapid speech,

MNEMONIC

Manic symptoms are DIG FAST + excessively elevated or irritable mood:

Distractibility
Insomnia (decreased need for sleep)
Grandiosity
Flight of ideas
Increased **A**ctivity/psychomotor agitation
Pressured **S**peech (nonstop flow of speech)
Thoughtlessness/pleasure seeking/ decreased judgment

TABLE 7-12. Features of Bipolar Disorders

Disorder	Features
Bipolar I disorder	Episodes of **mania** and depression. Associated with suicidality.
Bipolar II disorder	Episodes of **hypomania** and depression.
Cyclothymic disorder	Cyclic mood shifts between dysthymia and hypomania for at least 2 years.

hyperactivity, and possibly psychotic symptoms. Note that any episode of increased activity that results in hospitalization is by definition manic. A **hypomanic episode** is similar to a manic episode but is less severe, does not cause marked impairment in social or occupational functioning, and is not associated with psychotic symptoms. In either case, the patient typically also experiences periods of depressed mood, although some bipolar patients do not. In fact, patients with bipolar disorder often are more disturbed by the periods of depression than they are by the periods of mania/hypomania.

DIAGNOSIS

The diagnosis of bipolar disorder is made when a patient has experienced at least one manic (type I) or hypomanic (type II) episode that meets the DSM-IV-TR criteria. The DSM-IV-TR criteria for a manic episode require that a patient experience a period of elevated or irritable mood lasting at least 1 week during which the patient displays three or more of the symptoms described in the "DIG FAST" mnemonic. These symptoms must result in clinically significant distress or impairment in functioning.

Features of the bipolar disorders are summarized in Table 7-12.

TREATMENT

Medications for treatment of these disorders include lithium (a mood stabilizer), anticonvulsants, and antipsychotics (eg, olanzapine). Psychotherapy and ECT have also been shown to be effective in some patients.

ANXIETY DISORDERS

Anxiety is defined as a state of apprehension, terror, and fear in response to an external threat.

Anxiety becomes pathologic when:

- Reaction is out of proportion to the severity of the threat.
- Anxiety interferes with daily living.

Collectively, the anxiety disorders—generalized anxiety disorder, posttraumatic stress disorder, panic disorder, phobias, and obsessive-compulsive disorder—are very common (44% combined U.S. lifetime prevalence), although specific phobias and social phobias are roughly twice as prevalent as each of the other anxiety disorders. In general, anxiety disorders are more common in women than in men.

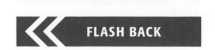

FLASH BACK

Anxiety involves the amygdala and is associated with increased activity of norepinephrine and decreased activity of γ-aminobutyric acid (GABA) and serotonin.

Generalized Anxiety Disorder

Patients with generalized anxiety disorder (GAD) experience excessive anxiety about various aspects of their daily lives, causing severe impairment of their daily activities. GAD, often described as "free-floating anxiety," has a lifetime prevalence of 5.7%, and affects women more commonly than men (2:1). Two-thirds of patients with GAD have comorbid major depression, and an equally high proportion have an additional anxiety disorder. Typically, symptoms of GAD begin before age 20. Although the cause is not well defined, genetic and psychosocial factors are believed to play a role.

DSM-IV-TR Diagnostic Criteria

- Excessive anxiety about various aspects of life.
- Symptoms have to be present for more than 6 months and severely affect daily life.
- The patient is unable to ease the anxiety.
- The anxiety has to be accompanied by at least three of the following:
  - Feeling of being on edge
  - Fatigue
  - Difficulty concentrating
  - Irritability
  - Sleep disturbance (ie, difficulty falling asleep, restless sleep)
  - Muscle tension

Treatment

- **Cognitive-behavioral therapy.**
- **Pharmacotherapy:**
  - Benzodiazepines (short-term and low-dose)
  - Buspirone
  - SSRIs
  - SNRIs: venlafaxine (extended-release)

Patients should be started first on benzodiazepines and then switched to buspirone to avoid dependency; however, the effects of buspirone take 2 weeks to manifest.

Posttraumatic Stress Disorder

Posttraumatic stress disorder (PTSD) occurs in individuals who have experienced or witnessed a traumatic situation, the memory of which they continue to relive. They commonly avoid anything that reminds them of the experience. Some patients become emotionally detached and have a restricted affect. The trauma experienced by males usually is related to combat, whereas that of women tends to be due to physical or sexual abuse. PTSD can be preceded by acute stress disorder, which is characterized by anxiety symptoms occurring within 1 month of the trauma and lasting for < 1 month. If the symptoms last > 1 month, then the patient is diagnosed with PTSD. Although almost 90% of patients who have experienced a traumatic event will suffer an acute stress disorder, only about 30% of these patients will go on to manifest PTSD.

DSM-IV-TR Diagnostic Criteria

The patient witnessed or experienced a situation in which he felt that his well-being or the well-being of others were threatened, and this experience brought about feelings of extreme fear and helplessness.

KEY FACT

Patients with PTSD are at a greater risk for developing depression and substance abuse.

- Patient continually relives the experience in one of the following ways:
    - Recurrent and intrusive thoughts.
    - Dreams.
    - Objects or situations that symbolize or resemble an aspect of the traumatic experience.
- The patient goes to great lengths to avoid anything that will trigger the anxiety.
- Emotionally detached/restricted affect.
- Signs of increased arousal (ie, difficulty falling or staying asleep or concentrating; irritable; inappropriate outbursts of anger).
- Daily functioning is severely affected by anxiety.
- Symptoms present for at least 1 month.

TREATMENT

- **Psychosocial therapy:**
    - Exposure therapy (treatment of choice): The patient is gradually exposed to the situation that elicits anxiety and is then taught techniques to ease the anxiety.
    - Relaxation techniques.
    - Support groups.
    - Psychotherapy.
- **Pharmacologic therapy:**
    - SSRI.
    - MAOI.
    - TCA (imipramine and amitriptyline).
    - Benzodiazepines (for acute attacks).
    - Anticonvulsants, prazosin (for nightmares and flashbacks).

Panic Disorder With or Without Agoraphobia

The defining feature of panic disorder (PD) is unexpected and recurrent episodes (twice or more per week) of panic attacks that develop abruptly and last ~30 minutes (reaching a peak in 10 minutes). There is a strong genetic component; first-degree relatives of patients with PD have a four to eight times greater risk of developing the disorder. Patients with PD have dysregulation of the autonomic nervous system, CNS, and cerebral blood flow.

PANIC ATTACKS

PRESENTATION

- Shortness of breath.
- Chest pain/discomfort.
- Palpitations/increased heart rate.
- Sweating, shaking.
- Nausea/abdominal discomfort.
- Feelings of choking, going crazy, losing control, or dying.
- Constantly afraid of having additional attacks.
- Numbness/tingling.
- Chills/hot flashes.
- Light-headedness.
- Depersonalization.

DSM-IV-TR DIAGNOSTIC CRITERIA

Recurrent panic attacks occur in which the trigger is unknown. At least one of the attacks has been followed by more than 1 month of at least one of the following:

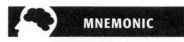

MNEMONIC

Having **PTSD** is **HARD:**
Hyperarousal
Avoidant of triggers
Reexperience traumatic event
  continually
Distress that interferes with daily
  functioning

KEY FACT

Many of the symptoms of panic attacks are similar to those of myocardial infarction (MI), and the possibility of MI must be ruled out. If the symptoms are due to a panic attack, the patient's electrocardiogram (ECG) and cardiac enzymes will be within normal limits.

MNEMONIC

Criteria for panic attack—

PANIC
Palpitations
Abdominal distress
Numbness, nausea
Intense fear of death
Choking, chills, chest pain

- Constant worry about having additional attacks.
- Substantial concerns about the implications/consequences of attacks (eg, "going crazy," losing control).
- Impairment of daily functioning due to symptoms. Significant change in behavior related to the attacks.

The panic attacks must not be due to the direct physiologic effects of a substance or general medical condition (eg, hyperthyroidism) and should not be better accounted for by another mental disorder.

AGORAPHOBIA

PD can occur with or without agoraphobia. Agoraphobia is extreme fear of being in a place where escape is difficult. Both PD with and without agoraphobia are more common in women, with average age of onset of 25. The condition is chronic, and attacks can be triggered by psychosocial stressors.

DSM-IV-TR DIAGNOSTIC CRITERIA

Great anxiety about being in a situation where escape is difficult in the event of a panic attack. The patient avoids the situation, endures it with great anxiety, or needs someone to accompany him or her. Symptoms cannot be attributed to another mental disorder.

TREATMENT

- **Psychosocial therapy:**
  - Relaxation techniques.
  - Cognitive-behavioral therapy (ie, exposure/desensitization therapy).
  - Psychotherapy.
- **Pharmacologic therapy:**
  - Antidepressants: SSRI, TCA, or MAO inhibitor (an SSRI is first-line treatment for agoraphobia).
  - Benzodiazepines.

Phobias (Social and Specific)

Social phobia is an extreme fear of social situations in which an individual has to interact with unknown people or is subject to scrutiny by others, thus resulting in embarrassment or humiliation. The lifetime prevalence of social phobia among adults in the United States is 12.1% and occurs with equal incidence in males and females. The most common types of social phobia are public speaking and public washroom use.

Specific phobia is characterized by an extreme and irrational fear of a specific object or situation. Among U.S. adults, specific phobias have the highest 1-year prevalence, although its lifetime prevalence is comparable to or less than that of social phobia, major depressive disorder, and alcohol abuse.

The object or situation that elicits the fear can be placed in one of the following categories:

- Situational (eg, closed spaces)
- Animal/insect/environmental (eg, cats, spiders, heights)
- Other (eg, injections, blood)

Women are twice as likely as men to have specific phobias.

KEY FACT

Patients with PD with or without agoraphobia also have a higher risk of developing depression, substance abuse, phobias, and obsessive-compulsive disorder (OCD).

KEY FACT

Social phobia is fear of embarrassment in a certain setting, whereas avoidant personality disorder is an overall fear of rejection and sense of inadequacy. Patients can have both disorders concurrently.

Both social and specific phobias may have a genetic component, as they tend to run in families. Specific phobias may be connected to a traumatic event, and overproduction of adrenergic neurotransmitters may also be a contributing factor.

DSM-IV-TR DIAGNOSTIC CRITERIA

- **Social phobia:**
  - Intense fear that is triggered by social situations in which the patient might be humiliated or embarrassed.
  - The anxiety response is immediately elicited by the situation.
  - The patient is aware that his or her reaction is excessive.
  - The patient goes to great lengths to avoid the situation.
- **Specific phobia:** Symptoms are similar to those of social phobia, with the exception that intense fear is triggered by a specific object or situation (eg, fear of spiders [arachnophobia]).

TREATMENT

- **Social phobia:**
  - SSRI (eg, paroxetine).
  - β-Blockers (for acute situations such as public speaking).
  - Cognitive-behavioral therapy.
- **Specific phobia:** Cognitive-behavioral therapy (ie, exposure/desensitization therapy).

Obsessive-Compulsive Disorder

Obsessions are persistent and recurrent thoughts that cause great anxiety. The patient realizes that the thoughts are a product of her mind and that the response to these thoughts is exaggerated (ie, ego-dystonic). Note, that in contrast to obsessive-compulsive disorder (OCD), the symptoms of the cluster C personality disorder known as obsessive-compulsive personality disorder (OCPD) are ego-syntonic (OCPD is discussed in the section on personality disorders).

Compulsions are repetitive and inflexible actions that are done by the patient in an attempt to eliminate anxiety. The actions are not necessarily logically connected to the anxiety-triggering thoughts (ie, obsessions).

The prevalence of OCD is 2–3% and affects men and women equally. First-degree relatives of patients with Tourette disorder have a greater risk of developing OCD. Genetics, psychosocial factors, and an imbalance in serotonin levels all contribute to OCD. It is also thought that there is a psychosocial aspect to OCD. In 60% of patients, the symptoms are triggered by a stressful situation.

DSM-IV-TR DIAGNOSTIC CRITERIA

- Symptoms of obsession and/or compulsion as defined earlier.
- Symptoms are ego-dystonic.
- Daily living is severely affected by the disorder.

TREATMENT

- **Cognitive-behavioral therapy:** Exposure and response prevention.
- **Pharmacotherapy:** SSRI (first-line treatment); TCA (clomipramine).

KEY FACT

Phobias are common psychiatric disorders in the United States. The 1-year adult prevalence rate of specific phobias is 8.7%.

KEY FACT

Patients do not need to have both obsessions and compulsions to be diagnosed with OCD, but 75% of OCD patients have both obsessions and compulsions.

SOMATOFORM DISORDERS

These are characterized by physical symptoms that occur in the absence of an identifiable physical pathology and are not being intentionally exhibited by the patient (Table 7-13). These disorders are thought to be unconscious expressions of unacceptable feelings. Although the physical symptoms are brought on by psychosocial factors, patients believe that their symptoms are medical in nature. Primary and secondary gain are associated with the somatic symptoms, but patients are unaware of the gains and do not consciously seek them out. Except for hypochondriasis, somatoform disorders are more prevalent in women. It is estimated that 10–30% of primary care visits for somatic complaints may be attributed to somatoform disorders.

Somatization Disorder

Patients have numerous doctor visits complaining of recurrent and multiple physical symptoms that significantly affect their daily lives. Their physical symptoms are related to multiple organ systems but have no underlying organic pathology. It is very important to rule out any medical causes of these complaints while balancing the cost, risk, and possible benefits of diagnostic tests performed. This disorder can be chronic, and potentially lifelong; symptoms can worsen when the patient is exposed to certain stressors.

TABLE 7-13. Key Characteristics of Somatoform Disorders

TYPE OF SOMATOFORM DISORDER	KEY CHARACTERISTICS	BUZZWORDS
Somatization disorder	▪ Physical symptoms related to multiple organ systems, which cannot be explained by known general medical conditions. ▪ Numerous visits to the doctor. ▪ No cure.	Multiple organ systems.
Conversion disorder	▪ Acute onset of neurologic symptoms brought on by a stressor with no identifiable organic cause. ▪ Patient is not concerned about the condition. ▪ Tend to recover spontaneously.	Neurologic symptoms.
Hypochondriasis	▪ Patient is convinced that she has a severe disease. ▪ Unsatisfied by assurances from her physician. ▪ Visits many different physicians.	Fixed belief that one has severe disease.
Pain disorder	▪ Pain at more than one site that begins abruptly. ▪ Pain cannot be explained medically.	Medically unexplained pain.
Body dysmorphic disorder	▪ Patient is obsessed about a perceived physical flaw. ▪ Tries to fix with make-up or plastic surgery, but is usually unsatisfied with the results.	Perceived physical imperfection.
Undifferentiated somatoform disorder	▪ One or more physical symptoms not explained by a known general medical condition. ▪ Do not meet criteria for another somatoform disorder.	Not explained by other somatoform disorder.

Females have a 5–20 times greater risk of developing a somatization disorder than males. There is also a greater prevalence of somatization disorder in low socioeconomic groups.

Somatization disorder has a genetic basis, and there is a 30% concordance rate in monozygotic twins. In addition, first-degree female relatives have a greater chance of developing somatization disorder than the general population.

DSM-IV-TR DIAGNOSTIC CRITERIA

- At least two GI symptoms.
- At least one neurologic symptom.
- At least one symptom that is sexual or related to the reproductive system.
- At least four pain symptoms.
- Onset before the age of 30 years.
- There is no organic cause of the symptoms.

TREATMENT

Patients truly believe that there is an organic cause for their symptoms and thus feel the need to see their primary care physician and are resistant to seeing a psychiatrist. As a result, the best way to "treat" such patients is to allow them to see their doctors, but secondary gain should be minimized. Great caution should be used when prescribing medications. Psychotherapy, hypnosis, and relaxation techniques have been shown to be helpful in some patients.

Conversion Disorder

Patients have either sensory or motor symptoms (most often affecting sensory organs of voluntary muscles) that are suggestive of a neurologic deficit. Patients may appear to have an inappropriate lack of concern regarding their symptoms (often termed *la belle indifference*). Work-up and physical exam are negative.

PRESENTATION

Neurologic symptoms include:

- Blindness
- Paralysis
- Paresthesias
- Pseudoseizures
- Mutism
- Globus hystericus (ie, feeling of a lump stuck in the throat)

The onset of symptoms is usually brought on by psychological stressors. Unlike somatization disorders, patients with conversion disorder appear to be unconcerned about their condition. Conversion disorder is common, but it affects women two to five times more than men. It is more common in people of low socioeconomic status, uneducated young adults, and in people who "doctor shop." Onset of symptoms can occur at any age but often appear in adolescence or early adulthood.

DSM-IV-TR DIAGNOSTIC CRITERIA

- One or more neurologic symptoms that cannot be explained medically.
- Identifiable psychological stressor that preceded the onset of symptoms.
- Symptoms are not intentional.
- Daily living is severely impaired by symptoms.
- Symptoms are not caused by other mental disorders.

KEY FACT

Half of patients with somatization disorder also suffer from another mental disorder.

KEY FACT

Levels of serum lactate can be used to differentiate a real seizure from a pseudoseizure: serum lactate is elevated after a seizure but not after a pseudoseizure.

KEY FACT

Many patients with conversion disorder also suffer from other mental disorders such as depression, anxiety disorders, and schizophrenia.

TREATMENT

Most patients recover without any therapy. However, insight-oriented psycho-therapy, relaxation techniques, and hypnosis have all been shown to be effective in some patients.

Hypochondriasis

Patients have a constant and exaggerated concern that they have a serious disease. Normal physical findings are misinterpreted by these patients to be signs of severe medical illness. Whereas hypochondriacs constantly worry that they *have* a serious illness, some patients with OCD constantly worry that they *will catch* an illness.

KEY FACT

Patients with hypochondriasis often also suffer from major depression (90%), anxiety disorder (70%), and psychotic disorder (30%).

PRESENTATION

Patients believe they might be suffering from a serious disease through misinterpretation of normal physical symptoms. They are convinced that they have a serious illness and are not reassured by their doctors. As a result, they visit many different physicians to get different opinions. Symptoms can be exaggerated at times of stress. The average age of onset is 25 years, and both women and men are equally affected.

DSM-IV-TR DIAGNOSTIC CRITERIA

- Constant and exaggerated concern about a serious illness.
- The concern persists despite a normal medical evaluation.
- Symptoms are present for 6 months or more.

TREATMENT

There is no cure, and patients are often resistant to seeing a psychiatrist. The best way to deal with these patients is to schedule frequent visits to their primary care doctor.

Pain Disorder

Patients with pain disorder complain of severe pain that cannot be explained medically.

The onset of pain occurs abruptly and increases in severity during the first few months. This disorder can be categorized as acute (< 6 months) or chronic (> 6 months). Women are twice as likely as men to have pain disorder. The average age of onset ranges from 30 to 50 years.

KEY FACT

Patients with pain disorder have higher incidence of coexisting major depression, anxiety disorder, and substance abuse.

ETIOLOGY

Psychosocial and genetic influences. Incidence is higher in first-degree relatives.

DSM-IV-TR DIAGNOSTIC CRITERIA

- Pain at one or more sites.
- Pain cannot be explained medically.
- Pain causes great distress.
- Pain is associated with psychological factors.

TREATMENT

Transient nerve stimulation, hypnosis, psychotherapy, and SSRIs have been shown to help with symptoms.

Body Dysmorphic Disorder

An obsession with a perceived imperfection of a body part. Although the imperfection is minimal or imaginary, patients feel very self-conscious and spend an excessive amount of time trying to correct the perceived imperfection, either through makeup or plastic surgery. Women are more likely than men to develop this disorder. The onset of symptoms usually begins in midadolescence.

DSM-IV-TR DIAGNOSTIC CRITERIA

- Obsession about a perceived flaw of a body part that causes great distress.
- Daily living is severely affected.

TREATMENT

Although patients use makeup or plastic surgery to correct their perceived imperfection, they are usually not satisfied with the results and continue to be preoccupied with their flaw. Fifty percent of patients respond favorably to SSRIs (fluoxetine).

KEY FACT

- Hypochondriasis: patients feel they have a **specific disease.**
- Body dysmorphic disorder: patients feel a **body part** is abnormal.
- Body image disturbance: patients feel their **whole body** is abnormal.

FACTITIOUS DISORDER AND MALINGERING

These disorders are related to the somatoform disorders in that a known general medical condition cannot be identified to explain the patient's subjective physical symptoms. However, unlike the somatoform disorders, patients with these disorders consciously mimic physical illnesses for purposes of either primary (factitious disorder) or secondary/external gain (malingering). There are critical distinctions between the somatoform disorders (eg, somatization disorder) and the somatoform-like disorders, which include **factitious disorder, malingering,** and specific types of factitious disorders (**Munchausen syndrome** and **Munchausen syndrome by proxy**) (Table 7-14).

Factitious Disorder

Patients deliberately (consciously) produce a medical or psychological symptom with the sole purpose of assuming a sick patient's role. There is primary gain associated with this disorder.

There is a higher incidence in males and in health care workers. The most common symptoms presented include hallucinations, depression, abdominal pain, seizures, and hematuria.

Some patients have a history of child abuse or neglect, which could lead to impaired sexual adjustment and a poor sense of self. As a result, these patients feel the need to play the role of a sick patient to fulfill their need to be in a comforting and safe environment (ie, hospital).

DIAGNOSTIC CRITERIA

Patient presents with a medical or psychological disorder that was deliberately produced with the intention of assuming a sick role. There are no associated monetary or other tangible incentives.

TREATMENT

There is no treatment. Primary care physicians should avoid doing any unnecessary medical procedures and maintain a good relationship with these patients.

TABLE 7-14. **Comparison of Somatoform and Related Disorders**

DISORDERS	LEVEL OF AWARENESS	TYPE OF GAIN	CHARACTERISTICS
Somatization	Unaware.	Primary and secondary	▪ A somatoform disorder. ▪ Physical symptoms are brought on by psychosocial factors. ▪ Patient truly believes that symptoms have a medical basis.
Factitious	Aware.	Primary	▪ Not a somatoform disorder. ▪ Symptoms are not real. ▪ Patient complains of vague symptoms that do not have a medical explanation.
Munchausen syndrome	Aware.	Primary	▪ A specific type of factitious disorder. ▪ Symptoms are not real or are real but intentionally induced. ▪ Patients induce symptoms in different ways (eg, take insulin to produce hypoglycemia or add blood to urine).
Munchausen by proxy	Patient is unaware, but the caregiver is aware.	Primary	▪ A specific type of factious disorder. ▪ Symptoms are not real or are real but intentionally induced. ▪ Caregivers induce symptoms in different ways (eg, deliberately make a patient sick or appear sick).
Malingering	Aware.	Secondary (tangible) gain (eg, monetary)	▪ Not a somatoform disorder. ▪ Symptoms are not real. ▪ Patients pretend to have symptoms (eg, walk around on crutches to mimic an injured leg).

MUNCHAUSEN SYNDROME

A form of factitious disorder predominated by physical symptoms. Patients have very specific demands (eg, demand certain types of medications) and are experienced at producing certain symptoms (eg, takes insulin to achieve a hypoglycemic state; mixes feces in with urine to fake a urinary tract infection).

MUNCHAUSEN SYNDROME BY PROXY

Another form of factitious disorder in which symptoms are deliberately produced in another person (eg, usually a child). It is considered to be a form of abuse, though the motivation is often unconscious.

Malingering

Unlike factitious disorders, in which external incentives (eg, monetary gains) are not the primary motivator of the patient's actions, patients who malinger intentionally produce physical or psychological symptoms for secondary (external) gains. They often complain of vague symptoms that only improve after they have achieved their desired purpose. Like factitious disorders, it is more common in men than women.

KEY FACT

Malingering is associated with tangible gain (eg, monetary reward), but factitious disorders are associated with psychological gain (ie, feelings that come with being a patient).

DISSOCIATIVE DISORDERS

Patients have sudden, temporary loss of identity or memory for personal events. These disorders are most commonly seen in women 15–30 years of age. Dissociative disorders are often preceded by a stressful life event. A high proportion of patients with dissociative disorder have a history of trauma or child abuse (Table 7-15).

PERSONALITY DISORDERS

Personality disorders are caused by patterns of enduring, inflexible, and maladaptive personality traits. These disorders cause impaired social or occupational functioning (or both). Patients are often unaware they suffer from a personality disorder (ego-syntonic); therefore they do not seek psychiatric help and do not do well in psychotherapy. The pattern of the disorder is usually established by adolescence and is associated with other complications such as violence, depression, psychotic episodes, and suicide. A significant proportion of the general population may meet criteria for one or more personality disorders (10–20%). The prevalence of personality disorders is greater among the psychiatric population; an estimated 50% of inpatients with major depression have a personality disorder. A patient must be > 18 years old to be diagnosed with a personality disorder.

Ten personality disorders are organized into **three personality clusters** (as defined by DSM-IV-TR), as summarized in Table 7-16. Note that the cluster B personality disorders generally involve outward expression of traits, whereas patients in cluster A or cluster C have disorders that tend to be inwardly directed. Additional personality disorders that do not fall into one of these traditional clusters are referred to as **personality disorder not otherwise specified (NOS)** and include **passive aggressive personality disorder, sadistic personality disorder, and sadomasochistic personality disorder.**

Cluster A

Patients with cluster A personality disorders avoid social situations and are **unable to develop meaningful relationships.** They do not have psychotic symptoms and are often viewed as weird. Characteristics of the cluster A personality disorders are presented in Table 7-17.

Cluster B

Patients with cluster B personality disorders exhibit emotional lability. They are dramatic, emotional, unstable, and have a higher incidence of substance abuse. They are often seen as "bad" or "wild." Cluster B personality disorders are often familial and have a genetic association with mood disorders. Characteristics of the cluster B personality disorders are presented in Table 7-18.

Cluster C

Patients with cluster C personality disorders appear to be anxious and are fearful. There is a genetic association with anxiety disorders. They are often seen as "worriers." Characteristics of the cluster C personality disorders are presented in Table 7-19.

MNEMONIC

Schi**zoids avoid** reality, and may daydream or be cold and introverted.
Schizo**typals** are odd, magical **types.**

MNEMONIC

Symptoms of borderline personality disorder—

PRAISE
Paranoid ideas
Relationship instability
Abandonment fears, angry outbursts
Impulsiveness
Suicidal gestures
Emptiness

KEY FACT

Patients with antisocial personality disorder commonly have a history of conduct disorder during childhood.

KEY FACT

Schizoid patients avoid social interaction because they have no desire for such interactions. Avoidant patients want to have social interactions, but their extreme fear of social humiliation prevents them from having any kind of social interaction.

TABLE 7-15. **Key Characteristics of Dissociative Disorders**

DISORDER	DSM-IV-TR CRITERIA	EPIDEMIOLOGY	COURSE	TREATMENT
Dissociative amnesia	■ ≥ 1 episode of inability to recall important personal information regarding a traumatic event. ■ Symptoms cause significant impairment in daily living.	■ Women > men. ■ Adolescents and young adults > the elderly. ■ Associated with other mental disorders (eg, major depression).	■ Most patients regain memory over a period of days. ■ Recurrences are uncommon.	■ To prevent recurrence, it is important to help patients recover lost memories. ■ Hypnosis and lorazepam are used in the interview to help patients relax and to recover memory. ■ Psychotherapy after patient recovers memory.
Depersonalization disorder	■ Recurrent episodes of feeling detached from body or mind (ie, patients feel like they are observers of their own lives). ■ Patients are aware of symptoms. ■ Symptoms cause significant distress.	■ Women > men. ■ Age of onset: 15–30 years. ■ Patients have increased incidence of other mental disorders (eg, major depression).	■ Chronic.	■ Treat associated mental disorders (eg, SSRI or antianxiety drugs for major depression or anxiety, respectively).
Dissociative fugue	■ Inability to recall past events; therefore patients are confused about personal identity or assume new identity. ■ Patients leave their place of residence and travel to another destination and can take on a new identity (ie, start a new life).	■ Onset preceded by stressful life event. ■ Predisposing factors: Substance abuse, mental illness (eg, major depression), head trauma.	■ Lasts for a few days to years. ■ When patient regains memory of old identity, he or she is unaware of loss of memory.	■ Similar to dissociative amnesia.
Dissociative identity disorder (multiple personality disorder)	■ Patient exhibits ≥ 2 distinct identities (with one personality being the dominant one). ■ Identities frequently take control of the patient's life. ■ While one personality is in control, patients are unable to recall details of other personalities.	■ Women > men. ■ Predisposing factors: Childhood abuse, sexual abuse. ■ High incidence of other mental disorders (eg, major depression).	■ Patients with earlier age of onset have a poorer prognosis.	■ Hypnosis. ■ Psychotherapy (insight-oriented).

TABLE 7-16.   **Summary of Personality Disorder Clusters**

Type	General Characteristics	Familial Association With Other Disorders	Mnemonic
Cluster A (see Table 7-17)	"Weird": odd, eccentric	Schizophrenia	**A**ccusatory, **A**loof, **A**wkward
Cluster B (see Table 7-18)	"Wild": dramatic, emotional, erratic	Mood disorders, substance abuse	"**B**ad to the **B**one"
Cluster C (see Table 7-19)	"Worried": anxious, fearful	Anxiety disorders	**C**owardly, **C**ompulsive, **C**lingy

EATING DISORDERS

Patients have a distorted body image and use different methods to try to achieve their perceived ideal body image. The etiology of eating disorders is multifactorial and includes social (eg, cultural/occupational), biological (ie, genetic), and psychosocial (eg, sense of lack of control over aspects of life or

TABLE 7-17.   **Characteristics of Cluster A Personality Disorders**

Type and Example	Etiology	Clinical Symptoms	Treatment
Paranoid	Small increased risk in relatives of schizophrenics.	■ Distrustful and suspicious; believe others are plotting to harm or deceive them. ■ Quick to interpret events or remarks as threatening (sensitive). ■ Emotionally distant. ■ Differential: Paranoid schizophrenia; paranoid personality disorder patients do not have fixed delusions and are not psychotic.	■ Psychotherapy. ■ Antipsychotics.
Schizoid	■ Increased risk in relatives of patients with schizophrenia or cluster A personality disorders. ■ There is a theory that neglectful parenting plays a role.	■ Voluntary social withdrawal—"loners." Does not have nor desire close relationships or sexual encounters. ■ Chooses to engage in solitary activities, indifferent to others, avoids personal contact. ■ Flattened affect and emotionally detached. ■ Differential: Paranoid schizophrenia (no fixed delusions in schizoid personality disorder, and no frank psychosis), schizotypal personality disorder (schizoid patients are less eccentric and do not demonstrate magical thinking).	■ Psychotherapy.
Schizotypal	■ Increased risk in first-degree relatives of schizophrenics.	■ Symptoms similar to schizophrenia but less severe. ■ Odd thought patterns, behavior, and beliefs. Magical thinking (not as severe as schizophrenics). ■ Paranoid ideation. ■ Ideas of reference. ■ Inappropriate/constricted affect. ■ Lifetime suicide rate is 10%. ■ Differential: Paranoid schizophrenia (schizotypal patients are not grossly psychotic), schizoid personality disorder (schizotypal patients have more magical thinking and are more eccentric, and schizoid patients avoid people, whereas people avoid schizotypal patients).	■ Psychotherapy. ■ Low-dose antipsychotics.

TABLE 7-18. **Characteristics of Cluster B Personality Disorders**

TYPE	ETIOLOGY	CLINICAL SYMPTOMS	TREATMENT
Borderline	■ Five times more common in first-degree relatives of borderline patients. ■ Increased risk in relatives of alcoholics and patients with mood disorders. ■ Sexual or physical abuse could play a role. ■ Childhood neglect and abuse can be predisposing factors.	■ Forms intense but unstable relationships. ■ Fear of abandonment. ■ Impulsive. ■ Feelings of emptiness or boredom and unstable sense of self. ■ Unable to control anger, impulses. ■ Suicidal gestures (no intent to commit suicide, but may take gestures to dangerous extremes). ■ Self injury (eg, cutting of arms). ■ Splitting (ie, alternating between extremes of idealization and devaluation). ■ Differential: Schizophrenia (borderline patients are not frankly psychotic), mania.	■ Psychotherapy. ■ Group therapy. ■ Dialectical behavioral therapy. ■ Cognitive-behavioral therapy. ■ Low-dose antipsychotics or antidepressants (avoid benzodiazepines because of abuse potential). ■ Medications are more effective in borderline personality disorder than any other personality disorder.
Antisocial	■ Increased risk in relatives of patients with antisocial personality disorder. ■ Violent, criminal environment leads to greater risk of developing antisocial disorder. ■ Begins in childhood as conduct disorder (eg, fire-setting, animal creulty, enuresis).	■ Does not conform to societal laws (has criminal behavior). ■ Disregard for rights of others. ■ Remorseless, reckless. ■ Deceitful, aggressive, and impulsive. ■ Differential: Drug abuse (important to consider which comes first, because behavior may be attributable to addiction).	■ Control of behavior (prison or psychiatric hospital). ■ Psychotherapy. ■ Caution with medications because of high addiction potential in these patients.
Narcissistic	■ Not known.	■ Exaggerated sense of self-worth and entitlement. Willing to exploit others for personal gain. ■ Arrogant, demands attention. ■ Lack of empathy for others. ■ Low self-esteem underlies outward inflated sense of self. ■ Differential: Antisocial personality disorder (both exploit others, but narcissistic patients want status whereas antisocial patients want material gain or subjugation of others).	■ Psychotherapy.
Histrionic	■ Genetic link to antisocial personality and somatization disorders.	■ Need to be the center of attention. ■ Inappropriately seductive and flirtatious (use physical appearance to attract attention). ■ Considers relationships to be more meaningful than they really are (assumed intimacy). ■ Unable to maintain intimate relationships. ■ Defense mechanism of regression, an immature defense in which the person returns to an earlier libidinal phase in order to avoid conflict. ■ Differential: Borderline personality disorder.	■ Psychotherapy.

TABLE 7-19. Characteristics of Cluster C Personality Disorders

Type	Etiology	Clinical Symptoms	Treatment
Avoidant	Not known	■ Extreme fear of humiliation and rejection from others, which leads them to avoid interpersonal contact. ■ Feels inferior to others. ■ Differential: Schizoid personality disorder (schizoids have no desire for companionship, but avoidants do). ■ Differential: Social phobia—**situations** are scary because of **embarrassment** vs. Avoidant personality disorder—**interpersonal contact** is scary because of **fear of rejection.** ■ Differential: Dependent personality disorder (both cling to relationships; however, avoidant patients are slow to get involved, but dependent patients aggressively seek new relationships).	■ Psychotherapy. ■ Systematic desensitization. ■ Cognitive therapy. ■ β-Blockers to control anxiety symptoms.
Dependent	Not known	■ Extreme need to be dependent on others for emotional support. ■ Unable to make own decisions (needs advice and assurance from others). ■ Poor self-confidence. ■ Fear of being deserted or alone. ■ May tolerate abuse by a partner to avoid the situation of being left alone. ■ Differential: Avoidant personality disorder. ■ Differential: Borderline and histrionic personality disorders (all three are dependent on other people, with dependent patients having long-lasting relationships, versus borderline or histrionic patients, who cannot maintain lasting relationships).	■ Psychotherapy. ■ Assertiveness training. ■ Group therapy. ■ Cognitive therapy.
Obsessive-compulsive personality disorder (OCPD)	Not known	■ Perfectionism, attention to detail. ■ Hinder ability to complete tasks. ■ Devoted to work. ■ Inflexible. ■ "Packrat." ■ Cold and rigid in intimate relationships. ■ Differential: OCD (OCD patients have **recurrent** obsessions or compulsions and are ego-dystonic). ■ Differential: Narcissistic personality disorder (both are assertive and high achievers, but narcissistic patients are motivated by status, whereas OCPD patients are motivated by work itself).	■ Psychotherapy. ■ Cognitive therapy.

history of sexual abuse) factors. Eating disorders are divided into three categories: anorexia nervosa, bulimia nervosa, and binge eating.

Anorexia Nervosa

Characterized by an obsession with staying thin. Patients believe that they are overweight when they are actually dangerously underweight. Anorexic patients restrict their eating or eat in cycles of fasting and binge eating in an attempt to lose weight (Table 7-20).

KEY FACT

Anorexic patients are underweight (> 15% below normal weight), whereas bulimic patients may maintain a normal weight.

TABLE 7-20. **Differences Between Anorexia Nervosa and Bulimia Nervosa**

	ANOREXIA NERVOSA	**BULIMIA NERVOSA**
Weight	■ Underweight (> 15% below normal).	Normal weight.
Characteristics	■ Restrictive type: Starve and exercise vigorously. ■ Binge eating/purging type: Binge then purge or use laxatives/diuretics.	■ Purging type: Similar to binge eating type of anorexia. ■ Nonpurging type: Fast or exercise excessively.
Mortality and prognosis	Mortality ~ 10%.	Better prognosis then anorexia nervosa.
Ego-dystonic or ego-syntonic	Ego-syntonic.	Ego-dystonic.

Anorexic patients are placed into two categories based on their predominant method of achieving weight loss: restrictive and binge eating/purging. Patients who are restrictive anorexics starve themselves and exercise vigorously. Binge eating/purging anorexic patients binge, then use induced vomiting, laxatives, or diuretics to help them lose weight. They also exercise excessively. Anorexia nervosa affects 4% of adolescents and young adults, and women are at 10–20 times greater risk than men. Average age of onset is 20 years. Genetics and psychosocial factors both contribute to the development of anorexia nervosa.

DSM-IV-TR DIAGNOSTIC CRITERIA

■ Distorted body image.
■ Body weight > 15% below healthy weight.
■ Obsession about gaining weight.
■ Amenorrhea in females.

ASSOCIATED MENTAL DISORDERS

The restrictive type of anorexia nervosa is associated with obsessive-compulsive traits, and many of these patients are socially withdrawn. Major depression and substance abuse are associated with the binge eating/purging type of anorexia nervosa.

MEDICAL COMPLICATIONS

Medical complications that are associated with this disorder include:

■ Amenorrhea.
■ Electrolyte abnormalities (hyperkalemia, hypochloremia, alkalosis).
■ Hypercholesterolemia.
■ Cardiac abnormalities (arrhythmias, cardiac arrest).
■ Melanosis coli (due to laxative abuse).
■ Leukopenia.
■ Osteoporosis.

TREATMENT

If body weight is < 80% of normal body weight, treatment includes inpatient monitoring of weight gain. Behavioral and family therapy have also been shown to be beneficial. Due to the high association with major depression, antidepressants should also be prescribed.

PROGNOSIS

This disorder has a variable course. Some patients have complete recovery, but others have relapses or get progressively worse. Mortality rate is ~10% due to suicide, starvation, or dehydration (resulting in elevated blood urea nitrogen [BUN] and electrolyte imbalances). Additional harmful conditions that can be associated with anorexia include endocrine abnormalities (abnormally low glucose tolerance with fasting hypoglycemia, elevated cortisol levels), osteoporosis, nonspecific ECG abnormalities, and hypothermia.

Bulimia Nervosa

Bulimic patients have a distorted body image but usually maintain normal body weight. Binge episodes are followed by vomiting, excessive exercise, or use of laxatives or diuretics. Patients can be categorized into two subtypes: purging and nonpurging. Purging bulimic patients predominantly engage in self-induced vomiting or use of laxatives or diuretics, whereas nonpurging patients exercise excessively or eat little to prevent weight gain. This disorder affects 3% of adolescents and young adults and is more common in women than men. Bulimia nervosa is associated with mood disorders, impulse control disorders, and substance abuse.

PRESENTATION

Medical complications associated with bulimia nervosa include:

- Electrolyte abnormalities (hypokalemic alkalosis and hypochloremia secondary to vomiting).
- Cardiac abnormalities (arrhythmias).
- Dental erosion and reddened knuckles (Russell sign from self-induced vomiting).
- Hypertrophy of salivary glands.

DSM-IV-TR DIAGNOSTIC CRITERIA

- Episodes of binge eating (ie, excessive eating within a 2-hour period associated with a feeling of losing control).
- Binge eating is followed by self-induced vomiting, excessive exercising, or inappropriate use of laxatives or diuretics.
- Symptoms occur at least two times a week for 3 months.
- The way in which the patient perceives self is defined by weight.

TREATMENT

Includes psychotherapy (both individual and group), cognitive-behavioral therapy, and antidepressants (SSRI, TCA).

PROGNOSIS

Bulimic patients tend to have better prognoses than anorexic patients. Patients who have onset before age 15 and are able to maintain a healthy body weight for 2 years after onset have better prognoses than patients with later age of onset and those who are hospitalized for their symptoms.

Binge-Eating Disorder

Patients have recurrent episodes of binge eating associated with severe distress. In contrast to anorexia or bulimia, however, these patients do not try to prevent weight gain through excessive exercise, vomiting, or use of laxatives and diuretics. As a result, many patients with this disorder are obese and are thus at risk for obesity-related medical conditions such as hypertension, type 2 diabetes, and cardiac disease.

KEY FACT

Some bulimic patients exhibit the Russell sign, which consists of abrasions and scars on the back of the hands due to manual attempts to induce vomiting.

KEY FACT

Bulimic patients are ego-dystonic, unlike anorexic patients, and are thus more likely to want and seek help.

FLASH BACK

Vomiting may lead to hypokalemia, hyponatremia or hypernatremia, and metabolic **alkalosis.** Diarrhea leads to similar electrolyte disturbances as well, but causes metabolic **acidosis.**

KEY FACT

Bupropion is contraindicated in patients with bulimia or anorexia nervosa because of an increased incidence of seizures.

DSM-IV-TR Diagnostic Criteria

- Recurrent episodes of binge eating that are not associated with other behaviors (eg, excessive exercise).
- Symptoms are ego-dystonic (eg, patients eat alone because they are ashamed of their eating habits; patients feel guilty and depressed about their behavior).
- Symptoms occur at least twice a week for 6 months.
- Three or more of the following symptoms are present:
  - Rapid eating.
  - Eating when not hungry.
  - Consuming an excessive amount of food.
  - Feeling embarrassed or guilty about their behavior; thus, they tend to eat alone.

Treatment

- Diet and exercise program
- Psychotherapy
- Psychosocial
  - Behavioral therapy
  - Pharmacologic therapy:
    - Stimulants to suppress appetite.
    - Sibutramine to inhibit reuptake of serotonin and NE.

SLEEP DISORDERS

The reticulate-activating system modulates arousal/wakefulness. Sleep disorders are very common and affect approximately one-third of people in the United States. Sleep disorders are classified as either primary or secondary. Secondary sleep disorders are caused by another disorder (eg, mental or medical disorder or substance abuse, see Table 7-21). Primary sleep disorders are not associated with other disorders and are categorized into either **dyssomnias** or **parasomnias.**

Dyssomnias

Dyssomnias are primary sleep disorders characterized by impairment in the amount, quality, or timing of sleep. Various disorders fall into this category: primary insomnia, primary hypersomnia, narcolepsy, circadian rhythm sleep disorder, and sleep apnea (Table 7-22).

Parasomnias

Parasomnias are also primary sleep disorders characterized by abnormal behavior during the sleep cycle. Disorders that fall into this category include nightmare disorder, night terror disorder, and somnambulism (Table 7-23).

Other Sleep Disorders

Restless Legs Syndrome

This neurologic disorder is characterized by unpleasant sensations in the legs and an uncontrollable urge to move when at rest. The sensations in the legs are often described as burning, creeping, tugging, or like insects crawling inside the legs. The symptoms can begin or worsen during periods of rest or inactivity and are partially or totally relieved by movement. They typically worsen or occur only in the evening or at night and can disturb sleep. The FDA has recently approved ropinirole (Requip), which is used to treat Parkinson disease, for the treatment of restless legs syndrome.

FLASH BACK

Elevated levels of dopamine or norepinephrine lead to decreased total sleep time. Melatonin accumulation allows for sleep onset to occur.

KEY FACT

Buzz words for narcolepsy:
- Hypnagogic hallucinations
- Hypnopompic hallucinations
- Short REM latency
- Cataplexy
- Sleep paralysis

KEY FACT

Obstructive sleep apnea: Ventilation is disrupted by physical obstruction (ie, patients have respiratory effort, but airway obstruction prevents air from getting into the lungs).
Central sleep apnea: Little or no respiratory effort is made. The medulla does not respond to increasing levels of CO_2.

KEY FACT

Eighty percent of people with restless legs syndrome also have periodic limb movement disorder.

TABLE 7-21. **Sleep Disturbances Associated With Psychiatric Disorders (Including Substance Abuse Disorders)**

DISORDER	SLEEP DISTURBANCES
Depression	▪ Normal sleep onset. ▪ Early morning awakenings (ie, waking up before the patient desires). ▪ Decreased REM latency. ▪ Increased total REM sleep. ▪ Decreased slow-wave sleep. ▪ Overall decreased sleep.
Bipolar	▪ Difficulty initiating sleep. ▪ Needs less sleep during manic episodes.
Anxiety	▪ Difficulty initiating sleep.
Caffeine	▪ Most common cause of insomnia.
Benzodiazepines	▪ Insomnia (upon discontinuation—withdrawal symptom). ▪ Nightmares and other sleep disturbances, including restless legs syndrome. ▪ Nocturnal myoclonus. ▪ Hypnagogic hallucinations.
Alcohol	▪ Difficulty initiating sleep; frequent awakenings (associated with withdrawal). ▪ Decrease in sleep quality and associated daytime fatigue (associated with abuse and dependence).

REM = rapid eye movement.

NOCTURNAL MYOCLONUS

Nocturnal myoclonus is also called periodic limb movement disorder. It is a sleep disorder in which the patient moves the limbs involuntarily during sleep and is related to restless legs syndrome.

This disorder can become worse when taking certain medications such as TCAs and MAOIs. Withdrawal from anticonvulsants, benzodiazepines, and barbiturates can also worsen the symptoms of this disorder. Treatment includes non-ergot-derived dopaminergic drugs.

SUBSTANCE-USE DISORDERS

When referring to substance-use disorders, it is important to differentiate between substance **abuse** and substance **dependence.**

Substance abuse is defined as a maladaptive pattern of substance use that leads to clinically significant impairment or distress for a period of at least 1 year. These patients have not yet met criteria for substance dependence. Substance abuse is manifested as **any one** of the following:

- Use resulting in failure to fulfill major obligations (eg, going to work).
- Substance use in potentially dangerous situations (eg, driving under the influence).

TABLE 7-22. **Key Characteristics of Dyssomnias**

	DIAGNOSIS	EPIDEMIOLOGY/ETIOLOGY	TREATMENT
Primary insomnia	▪ Problems falling asleep and/or staying asleep. ▪ Occurs ≥ 3 times/week for at least 1 month.	▪ Affects one-third of the population. ▪ Anxiety about not getting enough sleep exacerbates the condition.	▪ Maintain sleep hygiene (ie, regular sleep schedule, limit caffeine intake, no daytime naps). ▪ Diphenhydramine, zolpidem, zaleplon, trazodone (short term).
Primary hypersomnia	▪ Excessive daytime sleepiness or excessive sleep for at least 1 month.	▪ Onset often in adolescence.	▪ First-line treatment is with amphetamines (stimulants). ▪ SSRIs.
Narcolepsy	▪ Sudden sleep attacks (repeated) during the day for at least 3 months. ▪ Associated with cataplexy (sudden collapse while awake, loss of voluntary muscle tone), short REM latency, sleep paralysis, hypnagogic and hypnopompic hallucinations. ▪ Immediately go into REM sleep without passing through stages 1–4.	▪ Uncommon. ▪ Onset often during childhood or adolescence. ▪ Possible genetic association.	▪ Scheduled daytime naps. ▪ Amphetamines, methylphenidate (stimulants). ▪ SSRIs or sodium oxalate for cataplexy.
Circadian rhythm sleep disorder	▪ Disparity between circadian sleep-wake cycle and environmental sleep demands (eg, jet lag, night shifts).	▪ Seen in frequent travelers, shift workers.	▪ Remission, especially in patients suffering from jet lag (in 5–7 days). ▪ Light therapy (for shift workers). ▪ Melatonin (given 5 hours before bedtime).
Sleep apnea	▪ Abnormal sleep ventilation (central or obstructive) leading to sleep disruption and subsequently to excessive daytime sleepiness. ▪ Person stops breathing for at least 10 seconds repeatedly during sleep.	▪ 10% of population. ▪ Associated with obesity, pulmonary hypertension, arrhythmias. ▪ Obstructive sleep apnea: associated with snoring; seen more commonly in those 40–60 years old; male:female ratio is 8:1. ▪ Central sleep apnea: higher incidence in patients with heart failure, alcohol use; more common in the elderly.	▪ Obstructive: Continuous positive airway pressure (CPAP), surgery (nasal or uvulopalatopharyngoplasty), weight loss. ▪ Mechanical ventilation.

REM = rapid eye movement; SSRIs = selective serotonin reuptake inhibitors.

▪ Legal problems related to substance use.
▪ Continued use despite the knowledge that substance use results in significantly impaired social and personal life.

Substance dependence is also defined as a pattern of substance use that leads to significant impairment or distress for a period of 1 year. However, the DSM-

TABLE 7-23.   **Key Characteristics of Parasomnias**

	DIAGNOSIS	**EPIDEMIOLOGY/ETIOLOGY**	**TREATMENT**
Nightmares	▪ Repeatedly being awaken by nightmares and recalling the details of the dream, causing distress. ▪ Occurs during REM sleep.	▪ Onset during childhood. ▪ Increased episodes during times of stress.	▪ Usually not treated. ▪ Give TCAs to suppress total REM sleep.
Night terrors	▪ Patients have repeated episodes of extreme frightfulness during sleep. ▪ Patients have no recollection of these episodes. ▪ Occurs in stage 3 or 4 of the sleep cycle.	▪ More frequent in children (boys > girls). ▪ Genetic.	▪ Usually not treated. ▪ Diazepam at bedtime.
Somnambulism (sleepwalking)	▪ Patients have repeated episodes of walking during sleep. ▪ Patients have a blank stare. ▪ Can be associated with other behaviors (eg, dressing, talking). ▪ Patient can be awakened with great difficulty and often is confused when awoken (no recollection of episodes). ▪ Episodes occur during stage 3 or 4 of the sleep cycle.	▪ Onset during childhood (peak at 12 years old). ▪ Boys > girls. ▪ Genetic.	▪ None.

REM = rapid eye movement; TCAs = tricyclic antidepressants.

IV-TR criteria state that a patient has to exhibit **three or more** of the following symptoms in a 12-month period to be diagnosed with substance dependence:

▪ Physical dependence effects:
  ▪ Tolerance: Increased dosage of the substance is needed to achieve the desired effect.
  ▪ Withdrawal: Development of a specific set of symptoms after cessation or decreased dose after prolonged substance use.
  ▪ Use in larger amounts and for longer periods than intended.
▪ Psychological/social/behavioral effects:
  ▪ Desire to decrease usage.
  ▪ Spends a significant amount of time and effort to acquire the substance.
  ▪ Neglects other aspects of life due to use (eg, social and occupational life).
  ▪ Continues to use the substance despite the significant impairment it causes.

Altered pupillary responses are associated physical signs of substance intoxication or withdrawal (Table 7-24).

Substance abuse and dependence are very common and are more prevalent in men than in women.

Depressants

Depressant drugs depress the CNS by increasing the activity of GABA (an inhibitory neurotransmitter). Depressants include **alcohol, barbiturates,** and **benzodiazepines.**

FLASH BACK

GABA receptors are inhibitory; therefore alcohol, benzodiazepines, and barbiturates have a sedating effect. They also exhibit *cross-tolerance* (eg, an alcoholic will need a higher dose of benzodiazepines to achieve the same effect as a nonalcoholic).

FLASH BACK

Alcohol → acetaldehyde (via alcohol dehydrogenase).
Acetaldehyde → acetic acid (via aldehyde dehydrogenase—inhibited by disulfiram).
Excess acetaldehyde causes unpleasant "hangover" symptoms, while acetic acid is harmless.

TABLE 7-24. Review of Pupillary Response to Substance Intoxication or Withdrawal

SUBSTANCE	PUPILLARY DILATION	PUPILLARY CONSTRICTION
Amphetamines	Intoxication	Withdrawal
Cocaine	Intoxication	Withdrawal
LSD	Intoxication	
Opioids	Withdrawal	Intoxication (pinpoint pupils)
Alcohol	Withdrawal	

ALCOHOL

Alcohol is the most commonly abused substance. The prevalence of alcohol abuse in the United States is 7–10% (Table 7-25). Alcohol activates GABA and serotonin receptors in the CNS and is metabolized by alcohol dehydrogenase and aldehyde dehydrogenase in the liver. Studies have shown that women develop alcohol-related brain damage more readily than men. This theory is known as **telescoping,** which states that chronic alcohol consumption in women leads to a later onset but accelerated negative effects on the structure and function of the brain.

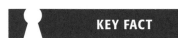

KEY FACT

Wernicke encephalopathy is reversible with thiamine therapy.

TABLE 7-25. Characteristics and Management of Alcohol Intoxication and Withdrawal

SUBSTANCE	INTOXICATION	MANAGEMENT OF INTOXICATION	WITHDRAWAL	MANAGEMENT OF WITHDRAWAL
Alcohol (serum alcohol or breathalyzer used to determine level of intoxication)	■ Dependent on blood alcohol levels (BAL). ■ Note on units: 80–100 mg/dL = 0.08–0.10% (% w/v). ■ BAL 100–150 mg/dL = ataxic gait and poor balance. ■ BAL of 400 mg/dL = respiratory depression. ■ Legal limit of intoxication in most states is 80–100 mg/dL. ■ Serum γ-glutamyltransferase (GGT) is sensitive indicator of alcohol use.	■ Check ABCs (**A**irway, **B**reathing, **C**irculation). ■ Intubate patients who are severely intoxicated. ■ Monitor electrolytes, glucose levels, and acid–base status.	■ Earliest symptoms occurs 6–24 hours after last drink. ■ Anxiety, tremor, insomnia, irritability, tachycardia, anorexia, hyperreflexia, fever, seizures, hypertension, hallucinations (tactile/ visual), delirium. ■ **Delirium tremens:** Seizures with altered mental status (a medical emergency), occur 72 hours after last drink and is associated with a high-mortality rate (15–20%). ■ ~5% of patients admitted for alcohol-related disorders (eg, detox) progress to delirium tremens.	■ Benzodiazepines (tapering doses). ■ Thiamine, folic acid, and vitamins to treat malnutrition. ■ Magnesium sulfate or carbamazepine for postwithdrawal seizures. ■ Benzodiazepines to treat delirium tremens.

PRESENTATION

Long-term alcohol abuse can lead to **Wernicke encephalopathy**, which is caused by thiamine (vitamin B_1) deficiency. Wernicke encephalopathy manifests as ataxia, confusion, and ocular abnormalities (eg, gaze palsies, nystagmus). If left untreated, it can progress to **Korsakoff syndrome**, which is chronic and irreversible. Symptoms of Korsakoff syndrome include psychosis, anterograde and retrograde amnesia, and confabulation. This syndrome is associated with periventricular hemorrhage or necrosis of the **mammillary bodies** (or both).

Alcohol withdrawal can be life threatening and is characterized by autonomic instability (tachycardia, tremulousness, anxiety, hypertension) followed by psychotic symptoms (hallucinations) and confusion. **Delerium tremens** may occur 2–3 days following the last drink and is characterized by visual and tactile hallucinations (treat with haloperidol), agitation, autonomic arousal, and seizures (treat with benzodiazepines, eg, lorazepam).

TREATMENT

Treatment of chronic dependence includes attendance at Alcoholics Anonymous meetings, disulfiram (inhibits acetaldehyde dehydrogenase, conditioning the patient negatively against alcohol consumption), psychotherapy, and naltrexone (to help reduce cravings). Alcohol withdrawal is treated with benzodiazepines (lorazepam) and haloperidol.

BENZODIAZEPINES AND BARBITURATES

Both of these drug classes are commonly abused because they are readily available, although barbiturates have become less popular. Benzodiazepines are used to treat anxiety disorders and seizures, whereas barbiturates are used as anesthetics and for epilepsy treatment. Both substances potentiate the effects of GABA and depress the CNS.

PRESENTATION

Symptoms of intoxication include drowsiness, impaired coordination and judgment, ataxia, mood lability, and nystagmus. Severe intoxication can lead to respiratory depression, coma, and even death. Symptoms of benzodiazepine and barbiturate withdrawal following heavy or prolonged use include insomnia, anxiety, delirium, hallucinations, tremor, nausea and vomiting, tachycardia, and sweating (autonomic hyperactivity).

TREATMENT

Sodium bicarbonate can be given to increase renal excretion of barbiturates (weak acid). Flumazenil (a benzodiazepine antagonist) can be used in benzodiazepine overdose. After administering flumazenil, the patient must be monitored for acute withdrawal symptoms from benzodiazepines. Treatment for withdrawal includes administration of a long-acting benzodiazepine (eg, diazepam). Seizures can be controlled with valproic acid.

Stimulants

Stimulants including cocaine, amphetamine, caffeine, and nicotine activate the CNS by increasing the concentration of dopamine. Caffeine and nicotine are the two most commonly abused stimulants.

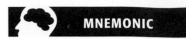

MNEMONIC

Wernicke encephalopathy (acute) and Korsakoff syndrome (chronic)—

COAT RACK
Confusion
Ophthalmoplegia
Ataxia
Thiamine deficiency
Retrograde amnesia
Anterograde amnesia
Confabulation
Korsakoff psychosis

KEY FACT

Patients with altered mental status due to alcohol should be treated with thiamine and glucose—the thiamine being given first. If glucose is given first, the mammillary bodies in the brain may become further depleted of thiamine, thus precipitating encephalopathy. Administration of glucose prior to thiamine supplementation results in thiamine depletion because glucose metabolism involves the activity of pyruvate dehydrogenase, an enzyme that utilizes the thiamine-containing cofactor thiamine pyrophosphate (TPP).

KEY FACT

Formication: Tactile hallucinations associated with alcohol withdrawal and cocaine intoxication, in which patients feel as if bugs are crawling on their skin ("cocaine bugs").
Withdrawal following alcohol intoxication can be fatal because during intoxication, CNS GABA receptors are downregulated to compensate for the CNS-depression produced by excess alcohol.

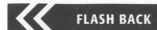

FLASH BACK

Benzodiazepines increase the **frequency** of GABA receptor opening.
Barbiturates increase the **duration** of GABA receptor opening.

KEY FACT

Cocaine can also be used as a local anesthetic. Given its vasoconstrictive properties, it maintains a high local concentration without the need for concomitant epinephrine administration, in contrast to other local anesthetics.

COCAINE

Cocaine is an alkaloid extract from the leaves of the coca plant that prevents dopamine reuptake from the synaptic cleft. Use can result in life-threatening conditions such as sudden cardiac death (coronary vasoconstriction leading to MI, arrhythmia). Maternal use can lead to placental abruption (Table 7-26).

TREATMENT

Overdose treatment consists of α-adrenergic antagonists (not β-antagonists) for cardiac symptoms, benzodiazepines for agitation, sodium bicarbonate in the case of prolonged QRS interval. Phentolamine and nifedipine can be used for severe hypertension. Haloperidol may be used to treat psychosis. Urine acidification is used because cocaine is a weak base.

Treatment for long-term dependence includes psychotherapy, group therapy, TCAs, and dopamine agonists (eg, amantadine).

AMPHETAMINES

Stimulants structurally related to catecholamine neurotransmitters can be classified into two groups: classic and substituted (designer). Classic amphetamines (eg, dextroamphetamine, methylphenidate, methamphetamine) stimulate dopamine release at the presynaptic terminal and are used in the treatment of attention deficit/hyperactivity disorder (ADHD) and narcolepsy.

TABLE 7-26. **Characteristics and Management of Stimulant Intoxication and Withdrawal**

SUBSTANCE	INTOXICATION	MANAGEMENT OF INTOXICATION	WITHDRAWAL	MANAGEMENT OF WITHDRAWAL
Cocaine (cocaine intoxication can lead to death secondary to respiratory depression and arrhythmias)	■ Increased or ↓ blood pressure, euphoria, tachycardia or bradycardia, nausea, dilated pupils, psychomotor agitation, depression, sweating, chills, respiratory depression, seizures, arrhythmias, tactile hallucinations (formication). ■ Prolonged use can lead to paranoia and psychosis. ■ Causes vasoconstriction leading to myocardial infarction ("cocaine chest-pain"), **placental abruption.**	■ Mild to moderate agitation: Benzodiazepines. ■ Severe agitation: Haloperidol. ■ Psychosis: Haloperidol. ■ Symptomatic support (eg, control of hypertension and arrhythmias).	■ Crash (occurs ~48 hours after last use): fatigue, malaise, depression, suicidality, hunger, constricted pupils, vivid dreams, psychomotor agitation/retardation. ■ Withdrawal occurs 1–10 weeks after last use.	■ Crash is not life-threatening, therefore treatment is supportive (ie, allow patients to recover on their own).
Amphetamines	■ Psychomotor agitation, impaired judgment, papillary dilation, hypertension, tachycardia, euphoria, prolonged wakefulness and attention, cardiac arrhythmias, delusions, hallucinations, fever.	■ (Similar to cocaine).	■ Crash: depression, lethargy, headache, stomach cramps, hunger, hypersomnolence.	■ (Similar to cocaine).

Designer amphetamines (methylenedioxymethamphetamine [MDMA, or "ecstasy"] and methylenedioxyethylamphetamine [MDEA, or "Eve"]) have both stimulant and hallucinogenic effects due to the release of dopamine and serotonin, respectively. The clinical presentation and treatment of amphetamine intoxication and withdrawal is similar to that of cocaine (Table 7-26).

CAFFEINE

Caffeine is the most common psychoactive agent used in the United States. It is an adenosine antagonist that also exerts a stimulant effect on the dopaminergic system.

Consumption of 250 mg of caffeine can lead to symptoms of intoxication, which include insomnia, anxiety, restlessness, twitching, rambling speech, flushed face, diuresis, and GI disturbances. If more than 1 g of caffeine (approximately 10 cups of coffee or 20 cups of tea) is ingested, symptoms such as tinnitus, severe agitation, and cardiac arrhythmia can occur. Treatment for caffeine intoxication is symptomatic and supportive.

Caffeine withdrawal also leads to symptoms including headache, anxiety, depression, and drowsiness. Treatment is symptomatic (eg, analgesics for headaches). To avoid subsequent episodes of withdrawal, the patient should slowly taper caffeine consumption.

NICOTINE

Stimulates nicotinic ACh receptors. Symptoms of intoxication include insomnia, restlessness, anxiety, and increased GI motility. The definitive treatment for nicotine intoxication is cessation.

Patients suffering from nicotine withdrawal exhibit signs of anxiety, dysphoria, increased appetite, irritability, insomnia, and intense craving. Behavioral counseling, nicotine patch or gum, and bupropion (antidepressant) have been shown to help reduce nicotine cravings.

Opiates

Opiates, such as morphine, methadone, and heroin, stimulate μ-opioid receptors and effect sedation and analgesia. Opiates also affect the dopaminergic system, thus contributing to their addictive and rewarding effects.

Methadone, L-α-acetylmethadol acetate (LAMM) and buprenorphine, all of which are synthetic opiates, can be used to treat long-term dependence on heroin (Table 7-27). All three, however, can also lead to physical dependence and tolerance. They are legally used to substitute for illegal opiates and to prevent withdrawal symptoms. Methadone is a μ-opioid receptor agonist, and buprenorphine is a partial opioid receptor agonist used for long-term maintenance therapy. It blocks the withdrawal symptoms and euphoric effects of heroin.

Hallucinogens (Phencyclidine and Lysergic Acid Diethylamide)

Phencyclidine (PCP, or "angel dust") and lysergic acid diethylamide (LSD) are both hallucinogens; however, PCP also has anesthetic and stimulant effects (Table 7-28). PCP acts on NMDA glutamate receptors and activates dopaminergic neurons, whereas LSD acts on serotonin receptors. Neither substance produces withdrawal symptoms, but patients might experience recurrence of symptoms at a later time (ie, "flash backs").

KEY FACT

Cocaine blocks the reuptake of dopamine, and amphetamine causes the release of dopamine.

FLASH BACK

Dopamine has a role in the "reward" system of the brain.

FLASH BACK

Nicotine stimulates nicotinic ACh receptors in autonomic ganglia.

FLASH BACK

Endogenous opiates include endorphins, dynorphins, and enkephalins.

KEY FACT

The classic triad of opiate overdose includes:
- Respiratory depression
- Altered mental status
- Miosis ("pinpoint pupils")

TABLE 7-27. **Characteristics and Management of Opiate Intoxication and Withdrawal**

SUBSTANCE	INTOXICATION	MANAGEMENT OF INTOXICATION	WITHDRAWAL	MANAGEMENT OF WITHDRAWAL
Opiates	■ Drowsiness, CNS depression, nausea/vomiting, constipation, constricted pupils, slurred speech, seizures, respiratory depression (leading to coma/death).	■ Overdose is life-threatening. ■ Naloxone or naltrexone for opiate overdose with respiratory depression. ■ Provide ventilatory support if needed.	■ Not life-threatening. ■ Dysphoria, insomnia, rhinorrhea, yawning, dilated pupils, lacrimation, weakness, sweating, piloerection ("cold turkey"), flulike symptoms (nausea/vomiting, fever, muscle ache).	■ Moderate symptoms: Clonidine and/or buprenorphine. ■ Severe symptoms: Methadone (tapered over 7 days).

KEY FACT

Naloxone = IV route of administration.
Naltrexone = PO route of administration.

KEY FACT

Both PCP and LSD alter a person's perception and PCP intoxication leads to impulsiveness, belligerence, psychosis, and violent, even homicidal behavior. LSD intoxication leads to anxiety or depression.

KEY FACT

Withdrawal from PCP intoxication can lead to sudden onset of random homicidal violence.

Other Substance Use Disorders

MARIJUANA

Marijuana's active ingredient is tetrahydrocannabinol (THC), which acts on the cannabinoid receptors in the brain, leading to inhibition of adenylate cyclase. Marijuana can be either smoked or eaten, and, when taken in large doses, marijuana causes euphoria, tachycardia, dry mouth, increased appetite, impaired coordination, and conjunctival injection. Only symptomatic and supportive treatment is available for intoxication.

TABLE 7-28. **Characteristics and Treatment of Hallucinogen Intoxication**

HALLUCINOGEN	SYMPTOMS OF INTOXICATION	TREATMENT FOR INTOXICATION
Phencyclidine (PCP)	■ Impulsiveness, belligerence, recklessness (eg, breaking through a pair of handcuffs), psychosis, impaired judgment, ataxia, hypertension, hyperthermia, tachycardia, **rotatory nystagmus** (pathognomonic for PCP intoxication), high tolerance to pain, agitation, **violent behavior.**	■ Check blood pressure, temperature and electrolyte levels. ■ Acidify urine with ascorbic acid (vitamin C) and ammonium chloride. ■ Diazepam for seizures and muscle spasms. ■ Benzodiazepines or dopamine antagonists for agitation. ■ Haloperidol for agitation or psychotic symptoms.
Lysergic acid diethylamide (LSD)	■ Pupil dilation, tachycardia, perceptual changes, hallucinations, sweating, palpitations, tremors, impaired coordination. ■ In high doses, paranoia (treatment involves "talking someone down"), depersonalization, anxiety.	■ For mild symptoms, patients can be reassured. ■ For severe symptoms, benzodiazepines and antipsychotics can be used (see treatment of PCP intoxication above).

CHILDHOOD DISORDERS

Diagnosing psychiatric disorders in children can be more challenging than doing so in adults because the clinical data have to be gathered from various sources. The child, the parents, teachers, and everyone else involved in the child's life should, with appropriate permission, be interviewed. Parents are often excellent sources of information and can give accurate accounts of the child's developmental progress, conduct, school performance, problems with the law, and family history. Teachers and social workers can also give valuable information about academic performance, peer relationships, and the child's social and family environment. Child psychiatric disorders can be categorized into groups depending on the dominant symptoms.

Pervasive Developmental Disorders

Pervasive developmental disorders are characterized by impairments in language and social skills. The disorder is recognized at an early age, and there is a higher incidence in males; the male:female ratio is 3:1 (with the exception of Rett syndrome, which affects females only). Pervasive developmental disorders include autistic disorder, Asperger syndrome, and Rett syndrome. Importantly, language may be normal in breadth in Asperger syndrome.

AUTISTIC DISORDER

Symptoms associated with autism are recognized early in childhood (usually before age 3) due to delayed developmental milestones. There is a high association with mental retardation, fragile X syndrome, and tuberous sclerosis. Males have a predilection for autism, and genetics have some role in its inheritance. Children with autistic disorder exhibit impairment in three different areas: social interaction, communication, and restricted and repetitive behaviors.

DSM-IV-TR DIAGNOSTIC CRITERIA

According to the DSM-IV-TR criteria, a child has to exhibit six of the following symptoms to be diagnosed with autistic disorder:

- Unable to develop peer relationships.
- Unable to express oneself through nonverbal expressions (eg, facial expressions, gestures).
- Does not initiate or reciprocate social interactions.
- Does not appropriately reciprocate emotional interactions.
- Delayed, impaired speech.
- Repetitive use of language.
- Repetitive play (eg, continually stacking three blocks in a certain way).
- Exhibit repetitive and rigid rituals.
- Obsession with parts of objects.

TREATMENT

Treatment of autism focuses on managing symptoms, which include the following:

- Behavioral management.
- Special school curriculum focused on developing social skills.
- SSRI (for control of repetitive behaviors).
- Atypical antipsychotics (for treatment of bizarre behaviors, agitation, and tics).
- Stimulants (for hyperactivity).

KEY FACT

Be sure to rule out hearing impairment during the first assessment of the child.

MNEMONIC

AUTISTICS
Again and again (repetitive behavior)
Unusual abilities
Talking (language) delay
IQ subnormal
Social development poor
Three years of age at onset
Inherited component
Cognitive impairment
Self-injury

ASPERGER DISORDER

This disorder classified as an autism spectrum disorder although unlike autism, children with Asperger disorder have normal to high intelligence. However, they may suffer deficits in social interaction, narrowed interests, and gross motor clumsiness. Asperger disorder is more prevalent in males, and its cause is not well understood.

DSM-IV-TR DIAGNOSTIC CRITERIA

According to the DSM-IV-TR criteria, patients must exhibit at least two of the following deficits in social interactions:

- Unable to develop peer relationships.
- Unable to express oneself through nonverbal expressions (eg, facial expressions, gestures).
- Does not initiate or reciprocate social interactions.
- Does not appropriately reciprocate emotional interactions.
- Exhibits repetitive behaviors or activities.
- Exhibits preoccupation with inflexible routines.

TREATMENT

Treatment is geared toward symptom management and is similar to that outlined for autism.

RETT SYNDROME

Unlike the other two pervasive developmental disorders, Rett syndrome predominates in females because it is an X-linked autosomal dominant trait. It is a very rare disorder, and onset of symptoms often occurs between the ages of 5 and 48 months. Before the onset of symptoms, patients have normal brain development. Following onset of the disease, however, there is a restriction of brain growth and a subsequent regression of development.

KEY FACT

Patients with Rett syndrome exhibit stereotyped hand movements such as clapping and wringing of hands.

DSM-IV-TR DIAGNOSTIC CRITERIA

- Brain development is normal in the first few months of life, followed by a restriction of brain growth (manifested as normal developmental milestones and head circumference initially, but impaired developmental milestones and decreasing head circumference later).
- Regression of development (ie, loss of previously learned skills).
- Exhibit stereotyped hand movements (eg, hand clapping and hand wringing).
- Loss of social interaction (could improve over time).
- Impaired gait or trunk movements.
- Impaired language and psychomotor development.

TREATMENT

There is no cure for Rett syndrome; therefore, treatment is supportive with management of symptoms.

Disruptive Behavior Disorders

Disruptive behavior disorders are characterized by behavior that does not conform to societal norms. Disruptive behavior disorder can be categorized as either conduct disorder or oppositional defiant disorder. Both disorders are more prevalent in males.

CONDUCT DISORDER

The presumed etiology of this disorder is multifactorial and includes child-rearing practices (eg, lack of parental discipline), parental or familial factors (eg, parental psychopathology), and family violence. There is an increased incidence of other mental disorders (eg, mood disorder), substance abuse, and criminal behavior in these patients.

DSM-IV-TR DIAGNOSTIC CRITERIA

Patients must exhibit the following behaviors for a period of > 1 year:

- Persistent behavior that does not conform to societal norms and violates the basic rights of others.
- Aggression toward living things.
- Destruction of property.
- Behavior causes impairment of daily functioning.

TREATMENT

Children benefit the most from early intervention. Treatment is focused on behavior modification and problem-solving skills. Parents should be involved in the treatment plan and engaged in parenting skills training and family therapy. Antipsychotics or lithium can be used for aggression management, and SSRIs can be used to treat impulsivity, mood lability, and irritability.

OPPOSITIONAL DEFIANT DISORDER

Unlike conduct disorder, patients with oppositional defiant disorder do not violate the rights of others. Onset is in early childhood, but symptoms can regress or progress to conduct disorder. Patients with this disorder have a predilection for substance abuse and have a higher incidence of comorbid mood disorders and ADHD.

DSM-IV-TR DIAGNOSTIC CRITERIA

Patients exhibit at least four of the following symptoms for ≥ 6 months:

- Frequently loses temper.
- Disobedient.
- Argues with authority figures (ie, teachers and parents).
- Exhibits anger and resentment.
- Easily annoyed.
- Annoys others on purpose.
- Spiteful.
- Refuses to take responsibility for his actions.

TREATMENT

Treatment is similar to that for conduct disorder.

Attention Deficit/Hyperactivity Disorder

The prevalence of ADHD among children is 3–5% and is more common in males than females. It is believed that the etiology of ADHD is multifactorial and involves genetic contributors, psychosocial factors, toxin exposure, prenatal trauma, and neurologic factors. The symptoms of most patients remit during adulthood, but 20% of patients ADHD have symptoms that persist into adulthood.

KEY FACT

Children who present with at least one symptom of conduct disorder before 10 years of age are more likely to develop adult antisocial personality disorder than individuals who first display symptoms later in childhood.

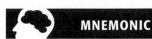

MNEMONIC

Children have **C**onduct disorder.
Adults have **A**ntisocial personality disorder.

TABLE 7-29. Symptoms of Attention Deficit/Hyperactivity Disorder

HYPERACTIVITY	INATTENTION	IMPULSIVITY
▪ Unable to stay seated.	▪ Disorganized.	▪ Interrupts or intrudes on others.
▪ Unable to play quietly.	▪ Unable to complete task.	▪ Has difficulty waiting for turn.
▪ Constantly fidgets.	▪ Forgetful.	▪ Blurts out answers.
▪ Talks excessively.	▪ Easily distracted.	
▪ Runs around.	▪ Constantly makes careless mistakes.	
	▪ Does not listen when spoken to.	

DSM-IV-TR DIAGNOSTIC CRITERIA

Patients must exhibit symptoms for 6 months and symptom onset must occur before age 7 (Table 7-29).

TREATMENT

Treatments for ADHD include psychotherapy and pharmacotherapy. Methylphenidate (Ritalin) is first-line therapy, and SSRIs and TCAs can be used as adjunctive therapy. Parents should also go for parenting skills training.

Tourette Disorder

Tourette disorder is a severe tic disorder that involves motor (eg, facial or hand tics) and vocal tics. Tics can be simple (nonpurposeful) or complex (movements or vocalizations that convey meaning). Complex vocal tics can be further categorized into either coprolalia (speaking obscene words) or echolalia (repeating words spoken to the individual). Coprolalia is uncommon in children. The onset of symptoms occurs before age 18, but symptoms can carry on into adulthood. This disorder is more common in males than females. The etiology of Tourette disorder includes genetics and impairment in dopamine regulation. Patients have a high incidence of other mental disorders (eg, OCD and ADHD).

KEY FACT

Patients must exhibit both motor and vocal tics to be diagnosed with Tourette disorder.

DSM-IV-TR DIAGNOSTIC CRITERIA

Patients exhibit symptoms for > 1 year and have an onset prior to age 18:

- Motor and vocal tics.
- Symptoms cause significant impairment in daily living.

TREATMENT

Treatment includes supportive therapy, α_2-agonists such as guanfacine, benzodiazepines, and, less commonly, antipsychotics such as haloperidol or pimozide. Importantly, patients with Tourette syndrome are not psychotic, but abnormal movement and vocalizations are likely mediated by neurotransmitters that affect the basal ganglia, hence the use of medications that block activity in this region of the brain.

Separation Anxiety Disorder

This disorder affects 4% of children with an average age of onset of 7 years. It may be preceded by a stressful life event (eg, divorce). Children with this disorder express great fear of being physically separated from their parents and avoid being physically separated (eg, the child may lie about feeling sick to avoid going to school). When they are forced to leave their parents, they express great distress and worry about not seeing their parents again. Treatment includes supportive therapy, family therapy, and low-dose antidepressants for symptom management.

Selective Mutism

This rare disorder occurs more in females than in males. The onset of symptoms is around 5 years, and it is characterized by not speaking in specific situations. Like separation anxiety disorder, it can be preceded by a stressful life event. Treatment includes supportive therapy and behavioral and family therapy.

Mental Retardation

Mental retardation affects ~2.5% of the population, and the incidence is higher in males than in females. According to DSM-IV-TR, mental retardation is defined as having an IQ of ≤ 70 in addition to having deficits in adaptive skills appropriate for the age group (Table 7-30). Mental retardation has several causes, including genetic (eg, Down syndrome, fragile X syndrome), prenatal infection or toxin exposure, prematurity, anoxia, birth trauma, malnutrition, and hypothyroidism. Mental retardation is categorized based on its severity. The majority of cases are mild.

TABLE 7-30. Classification of Mental Retardation

TYPE OF MENTAL RETARDATION	IQ
Profound	< 25
Severe	25–40
Moderate	40–50
Mild	50–70

NOTES

Renal

Embryology

RENAL DEVELOPMENT

The urinary system is derived from **intermediate mesoderm** on the posterior wall of the abdominal cavity (Table 8-1). It forms three kidney systems: the pronephros, mesonephros, and metanephros (Figure 8-1):

- **Pronephros:** Rudimentary kidneys that disappear by end of fourth week.
- **Mesonephros:** Another pair of transient kidneys that form after pronephros regression, within which lies a long epithelial duct, the Wolffian duct. This duct then fuses caudally with the cloaca.
- **Wolffian duct (WD):** Paired organ that connects the primitive **mesonephros** to the **cloaca.** The ureteric bud is an outgrowth from the caudal WD. The WD coexists with the Müllerian duct, the potential precursor of the female Fallopian tube, uterus, and upper vagina. The presence or absence of hormones secreted from the developing gonads in utero determines which adult analog will form from these ducts (eg, in male fetus, testosterone from developing gonads provides stimulus for development of epididymus and vas deferens from the WD).
- **Metanephros:** Forms the definitive kidney via reciprocal inductive signaling with the ureteric bud.

Congenital Abnormalities

POTTER SEQUENCE

Potter sequence develops as a result of malformation of the **ureteric bud,** which results in **bilateral renal agenesis** (eg, no kidneys). During normal fetal development, the fetus continuously swallows amniotic fluid, which is reabsorbed by the GI tract and then reintroduced into the amniotic cavity by the kidneys via urination. Fetuses affected with this condition are unable to eliminate the swallowed fluid, which results in **oligohydramnios** (decreased amniotic fluid). The fetus cannot float in the amniotic sac due to the decreased volume of amniotic fluid, so limb and facial deformities result from compression of the fetus against the walls of the amniotic sac throughout development.

KEY FACT

Allantois → urachus → medi**an** umbilical ligament (not the paired medi**al** umbilical ligaments, which are the remnants of the umbilical arteries).

Failure of obliteration of the allantois → **patent urachus → urachal fistula** at birth (newborn persistently draining urine from the umbilicus).

Urogenital sinus → urinary bladder and urethra.

TABLE 8-1. Renal Development

PORTION OF KIDNEY	EMBRYONIC ORIGIN	ADULT STRUCTURES
Filtration system (nephron)	Derived from *metanephric mesoderm* via reciprocal inductive signaling with the ureteric bud.	Glomerulus. Bowman capsule. Proximal convoluted tubule. Loop of Henle. Distal convoluted tubule.
Collecting system	Derived from the ureteric bud via reciprocal inductive signaling with the metanephric mesoderm.	Collecting ducts. Major/minor calyces. Renal pelvis. Ureters (splitting of the ureteric bud can result in double ureters).

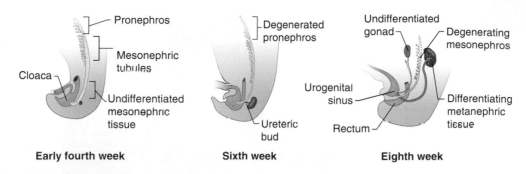

FIGURE 8-1. **Development of the nephric system.** (Reproduced with permission from Tanagho EA, McAninch JW. *Smith's General Urology*, 17th ed. New York: McGraw-Hill, 2008: Figure 2-1.)

PRESENTATION

The deformities found in Potter sequence can be divided into three groups:

- **Limb deformities:** Clubfoot, flipper hands, hyperextensible joints, and compressed thorax.
- **Facial deformities:** Sloping forehead, flattened nose, recessed chin, and low floppy ears.
- **Pulmonary hypoplasia:** Fetal lungs mature through swallowing of amnion, which allows the lungs to expand; thus, decreased amnion causes decreased expansion of the lungs.

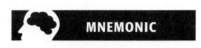

Babies with **Potter** can't go **Potty** in utero.

PROGNOSIS

Incompatible with neonatal life.

RENAL ECTOPY

During development, the embryologic kidneys ascend from the pelvis to their adult position along the posterior abdominal wall. The kidneys must pass under the *umbilical arteries* in this process. If a kidney is unable to pass beneath an umbilical artery, it will remain in the pelvis. Incidence is 1 in 100 births.

PRESENTATION

Obstructive **hydronephrosis** and **vesicoureteric** reflux can be seen in association with renal ectopy. Affected patients may present with pain or infection related to these conditions (eg, pyelonephritis and renal stones).

DIAGNOSIS

Found incidentally on routine antenatal or postnatal imaging or during evaluation for symptoms of associated anomalies.

TREATMENT

Treatment, when required, is generally surgical.

PROGNOSIS

Prognosis is related to the extent of underlying urologic disease.

HORSESHOE KIDNEY

While ascending from their position in the pelvis under the umbilical arteries, the kidneys are sometimes pushed close together, causing the lower poles

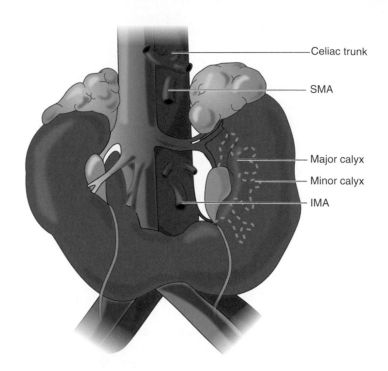

FIGURE 8-2.   **Horseshoe kidney.** IMA, inferior mesenteric artery; SMA, superior mesenteric artery. (Reproduced with permission from Tanagho EA, McAninch JW. *Smith's General Urology*, 17th ed. New York: McGraw-Hill, 2008: Figure 31-4.)

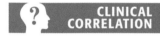

CLINICAL CORRELATION

Renal fusion can occur as a clinical feature of **VACTERL** syndrome: **V**ertebral, **A**nal, **C**ardiac, **T**racheal, **E**sophageal, **R**enal, **L**imb anomalies.

to fuse (**fusion anomaly**). The resultant horseshoe-shaped kidney continues to ascend until it is trapped under the **inferior mesenteric artery** (Figure 8-2). It is rare in females and if found should prompt work-up for Turner syndrome (7% of Turner patients have this defect).

PRESENTATION

Ninety percent are asymptomatic and found incidentally. Most common presentation is **urinary tract infection (UTI)** followed by symptoms of obstruction, hematuria, or abdominal pain. Predisposes to **nephrolithiasis.**

DIAGNOSIS

Most commonly by prenatal ultrasound.

TREATMENT

Usually not necessary unless warranted by symptoms. The renal isthmus can be surgically divided.

Anatomy

POSTERIOR ABDOMINAL WALL

The posterior abdominal wall is supported by several large muscles attached to the bony thorax, vertebral column, and pelvic bones. The retroperitoneal structures are found atop these muscles and their skeletal insertions. Table 8-2 details these muscles and their innervation, blood supply, and actions.

TABLE 8-2. **Muscles of the Posterior Abdominal Wall**

	ORIGIN/INSERTION	INNERVATION	BLOOD SUPPLY	ACTIONS
Psoas major	Vertebral column (T12–L5) to the lesser trochanter of the femur.	Ventral rami of L1–L3	Medial femoral circumflex artery.	Flexes thigh and trunk and laterally rotates the hip.
Psoas minor	Vertebral column (T12–L1) to the pectineal line.	Ventral rami of L1–L2	Various.	Flexes the trunk at the hip and stabilizes the thigh.
Iliacus	Iliac fossa to the lesser trochanter of the femur.	Femoral nerve (L3–L4)	Medial femoral circumflex artery.	Powerful hip flexor and lateral rotation.
Quadratus lumborum	Transverse processes of L3–L5 to the lower border of the 12th rib and the transverse processes of L1–L3.	Ventral branches of T12 and L1–L4	Lumbar arteries.	Extends and laterally flexes vertebral column.

RETROPERITONEAL STRUCTURES

Much of the urinary system is composed of retroperitoneal organs. Other retroperitoneal organs include the pancreas (except the tail), duodenum (second, third, and fourth parts), ascending colon, descending colon, aorta, inferior vena cava (IVC), rectum, and adrenal glands (Figure 8-3).

Kidney

The kidneys (Figure 8-4) are retroperitoneal organs located at the level of T12–L3 on the left and slightly lower on the right due to the liver. They are embedded in the Gerota fascia (loose connective tissue). The renal arteries and veins, as well as the ureters, adjoin the kidneys at the hilum.

- **Arterial supply:** Renal arteries are branches of the abdominal aorta.
- **Venous return:** Renal veins drain into the IVC.
- **Left renal vein:** Also drains blood from the left gonad and left adrenal gland; is longer than the right renal vein (must cross the aorta to join the IVC).

Lymphatic drainage is to the lumbar nodes, whereas the nerve supply is via the thoracic splanchnic nerves.

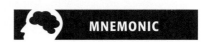

MNEMONIC

Retroperitoneal structures—

SAD PUCKER
Suprarenal glands (adrenal glands)
Aorta/IVC
Duodenum (second through fourth segments)
Pancreas (except tail)
Ureters
Colon (ascending and descending parts)
Kidneys
Esophagus
Rectum

KEY FACT

Psoas major, psoas minor, and iliacus muscles are commonly referred to collectively as the "iliopsoas muscle."

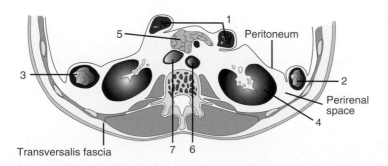

FIGURE 8-3. **Schematic representation of the retroperitoneum.** 1, Duodenum (second, third, and fourth parts); 2, descending colon; 3, ascending colon; 4, kidney and ureters; 5, pancreas (except the tail); 6, aorta; 7, inferior vena cava. The adrenal glands and rectum are not shown in this diagram.

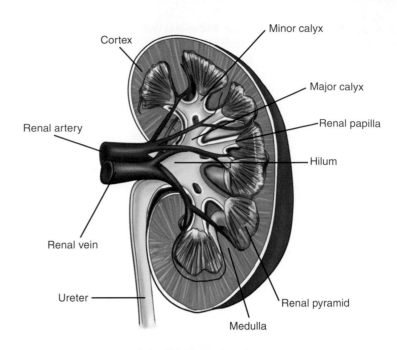

FIGURE 8-4. **Gross anatomy of the kidney sectioned.**

KEY FACT

Right gonadal vein drains into the **inferior vena cava.**
Left gonadal vein drains into the **left renal vein.**

MNEMONIC

Water **(ureters)** under the bridge **(gonadal artery, uterine artery,** and **vas deferens).**

CLINICAL CORRELATION

Ureteral stones most commonly impact at one of three sites: (1) ureter-renal pelvis junction, (2) site where external iliac artery causes a constriction in the ureter, and (3) ureter-bladder junction.

The kidney is covered by a capsule of fibrous tissue. Beneath this capsule are the cortex and medulla, which contain the functional components of the kidney. The medulla comprises the early portions of the urinary collecting system:

- Renal pyramids
- Renal papillae
- Minor calyces
- Major calyces

The major calyces join to form the renal pelvis, which then becomes the ureter.

Ureters

The ureters course distally through the retroperitoneum, first crossing under the gonadal arteries, and then entering the pelvis by passing immediately anterior to the external iliac artery where it branches off from the common iliac artery. Prior to entering the bladder, the ureter crosses under the uterine artery or vas deferens (depending on gender) (Figure 8-5).

Bladder

Situated beneath the peritoneum within the bony pelvis. The ureters join the bladder at its posterior-inferior portion, forming two points of the urinary trigone (the third is the urethral orifice). The bladder is an expandable and collapsible organ composed of several layers of smooth muscle and transitional epithelium.

Prostate

Surrounds the urethra just below the bladder. Stores and secretes an alkaline fluid constituting over 25% of semen volume. The vas deferens joins the duct of the seminal vesicle to become the ejaculatory duct, which courses through the prostate before emptying into the urethra.

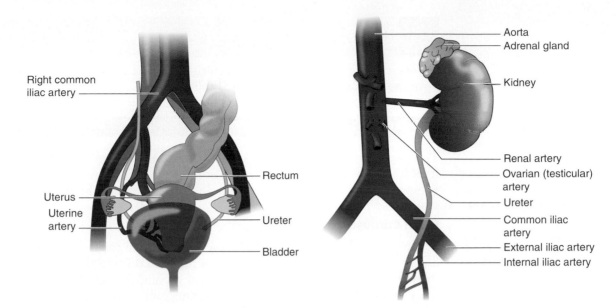

FIGURE 8-5. Course of ureter with arterial supply.

Urethra

The urethra is lined by **transitional epithelium** as it exits the bladder. It then becomes **pseudostratified columnar** epithelium followed by **stratified squamous** cells as it nears the meatus. The urethra differs in males and females.

MALE URETHRA

Four anatomic divisions, the preprostatic, prostatic, membranous, and penile. Of note:

- **Prostatic:** Passes through the prostate gland, where it receives semen from the ejaculatory ducts (union of vas deferens and duct of the seminal vesicle). The prostate gland itself also contributes prostatic fluid to the ejaculate via several prostatic ducts. Lined by transitional epithelium.
- **Membranous:** Surrounded by striated muscle, which forms the voluntary external urethral sphincter (weakness produces urinary incontinence). Viscous secretions from the bulbourethral glands enter here.
- **Penile** (including **bulbous** and **pendulous** sections): Longest segment, travels through the corpus spongiosum. Surrounded by Littre glands, which secrete mucus that is incorporated into the semen. Lined by pseudostratified columnar epithelium proximally, stratified squamous epithelium distally.

FEMALE URETHRA

Much shorter than the male urethra, which predisposes women to an increased risk of UTIs. It is lined by stratified squamous and pseudostratified columnar epithelium. At its midportion, it is surrounded by the striated muscle of the voluntary external urethral sphincter. The female urethra is also surrounded by Littre glands.

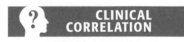

CLINICAL CORRELATION

As men age, the transitional zone of the prostate expands **(benign prostatic hypertrophy),** potentially leading to urinary retention. Most cancers of the prostate arise in the outer peripheral zone and do not cause urinary retention until relatively late in the disease progression (see Figure 9-23).

Histology

An overview of the histologic characteristics of the respective structures that form the renal system is provided in Table 8-3.

NEPHRON

The nephron is the primary functional unit of the kidney. It is the body's filtration system, removing substances from the blood and creating urine. It is composed of the **renal corpuscle** and the **tubular system** (Figure 8-6).

Renal Corpuscle

The primary filtering component of the nephron, the renal corpuscle (Figures 8-7 and 8-8) is composed of two distinct functional units: the glomerulus and the Bowman capsule. The filtration barrier is composed of (1) fenestrated capillary endothelium, (2) basement membrane, and (3) slit diaphragms between adjacent foot processes of podocytes.

GLOMERULUS

A collection of dilated capillaries with fenestrated endothelium, which emerge from the afferent arteriole and drain into the efferent arteriole.

BOWMAN CAPSULE

Double-walled epithelial capsule (visceral and parietal) that wraps around the glomerular capillaries. This is where blood is filtered.

KEY FACT

Glomerulus + Bowman capsule = Renal corpuscle.

CLINICAL CORRELATION

Damage to the filtration barrier allows larger molecules, including proteins, to cross into the urinary space, resulting in **proteinuria.**

TABLE 8-3. Histologic Characteristics of the Renal System

STRUCTURE	HISTOLOGY
Glomerulus	Fenestrated endothelium.
Bowman capsule	Epithelium with two layers: visceral layer and parietal layer.
Proximal convoluted tubule (PCT)	Simple cuboidal epithelium with brush border.
Loop of Henle	Thick descending loop; thin descending loop; thin ascending loop; thick ascending loop. Thick segments consist of simple cuboidal epithelium; thin segments consist of simple squamous epithelium.
Distal convoluted tubule (DCT)	Simple cuboidal epithelium without brush border.
Collecting tubules	Simple cuboidal epithelium.
Collecting ducts	Columnar epithelium.
Renal calyces	Transitional epithelium.
Renal pelvis	Transitional epithelium.
Ureters	Transitional epithelium.

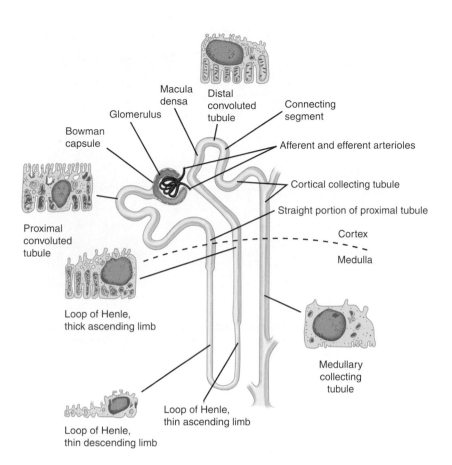

FIGURE 8-6.   Major anatomic divisions of the nephron. (Modified with permission from Morgan GE, Mikhail MS, Murray MJ. *Clinical Anesthesiology*, 4th ed. New York: McGraw-Hill, 2006, as modified from Ganong WF. *Review of Medical Physiology*, 22nd ed. New York: McGraw-Hill, 2005: 700.)

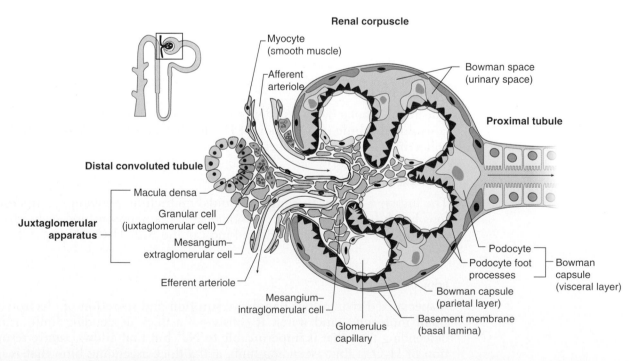

FIGURE 8-7.   Schematic drawing of the renal corpuscle.

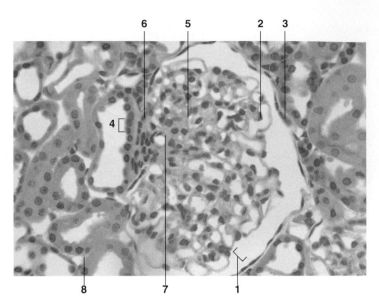

FIGURE 8-8. **Components of the renal corpuscle (hematoxylin and eosin stain, normal kidney).** 1, Bowman space; 2, Bowman capsule, visceral layer; 3, Bowman capsule, parietal layer; 4, macula densa; 5, intraglomerular mesangial cell; 6, extraglomerular mesangial cell; 7, arteriole; 8, capillary, peritubular. (Courtesy of Uniformed Services University of the Health Sciences.)

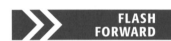

FLASH FORWARD

Heavy proteinuria is a cardinal feature of the **nephrotic syndrome.**

- The **visceral layer** is a specialized outer lining on glomerular capillaries that serves as the outermost component of the filtration barrier. The specialized lining is composed of podocytes and their interdigitating foot processes.
- The **parietal layer** does not play a role in filtration. It forms the outer covering of the renal corpuscle and is lined by a simple squamous epithelium. It is continuous with the proximal convoluted tubule (PCT).
- The **urinary space** is found between the visceral and parietal layers. Filtrate collects here after passing through the fenestrated capillary endothelium of the glomerulus, basement membrane, and the visceral layer of Bowman capsule.

Tubular System

The renal tubular system is divided into several functional units: **proximal convoluted tubule (PCT), loop of Henle, distal convoluted tubule (DCT), collecting tubules, and collecting ducts.**

PROXIMAL CONVOLUTED TUBULE

The lumen is lined with **simple cuboidal epithelium** containing a **microvillous brush border.** This is the "workhorse of the nephron" and reabsorbs all of the glucose and amino acids and most of the Na^+, H_2O, HCO_3^-, Cl^- and PO_4^{3-}.

LOOP OF HENLE

A specialized system that handles absorption and secretion of electrolytes, small molecules, and water. It consists of a thick descending limb, a thin descending limb **that is impermeable to Na^+ but that allows passive resorption of H_2O,** a thin ascending limb, and a thick ascending limb **that is impermeable to H_2O but actively pumps out Na^+ (eg, Na^+ is reabsorbed).** As described in detail in the following sections, these different permeabilities establish the solute gradient critical to the countercurrent mechanism that allows the nephron to excrete a dilute or concentrated urine.

DISTAL CONVOLUTED TUBULE

Lined with **simple cuboidal epithelium.** However, it **does not** have a **brush border,** distinguishing it from the PCT. Is considered a "diluting segment" because like the thick ascending limb, the DCT is impermeable to H_2O but actively reabsorbs Na^+.

COLLECTING TUBULES

These units are lined with **simple cuboidal epithelium.** They transport the urine from the **functional part** of the **nephron** toward the kidney's **hilum.** Here Na^+ is reabsorbed in exchange for K^+ and H^+ under the influence of aldosterone, and H_2O is reabsorbed under the influence of antidiuretic hormone (ADH).

COLLECTING DUCTS

Lined with **columnar epithelium.** Receive urine from numerous nephrons.

CORTICAL VS. JUXTAMEDULLARY NEPHRONS

Most of the kidney's nephrons are located in the renal cortex. However, the glomerulus of some nephrons is located near the junction of the cortex and medulla. These nephrons are referred to as **juxtamedullary nephrons.**

- **Juxtamedullary nephrons** are central to the filtration, absorption, and secretion of urine. Via exceptionally long loops of Henle, they establish the hypertonic gradient in the kidney, which regulates the production of concentrated urine. The loops **extend deep into the medulla** and consist of a short thick descending limb, a long thin descending limb, a long thin ascending limb, and a short thick ascending limb.
- **Cortical nephrons** have a short thin descending limb and do not have a thin ascending limb. They do not extend into the medulla.

JUXTAGLOMERULAR APPARATUS

The juxtaglomerular apparatus (JGA) consists of **macula densa** cells found in the region of the distal thick ascending limb and early DCT, and **juxtaglomerular cells** found in the walls of the afferent arterioles. The JGA functions to maintain the glomerular filtration rate (GFR) in response to blood pressure (BP) changes in the afferent arterioles.

Macula Densa

A specialized group of epithelial cells in the thick ascending limb/DCT that come in close contact with the afferent and efferent arterioles. The cells of the macula densa are sensitive to sodium concentration and rate of flow through the thick ascending limb/DCT, and regulate GFR through locally active hormones.

Juxtaglomerular (Granular) Cells

Specialized myoepithelial cells located in the afferent arterioles. These cells act as baroreceptors (they sense intrarenal pressure), which enables them to efficiently monitor BP and maintain normal GFR through the release of renin, the initial enzyme in the renin-angiotensin-aldosterone system (RAAS; see Physiology section for details).

KEY FACT

Despite large fluctuations in arterial BP (75–160 mm Hg), the GFR is maintained within a very narrow range (autoregulation).

>> **FLASH FORWARD**

Angiotensin II → cells contract → vasoconstriction and reduced glomerular flow.
Natriuretic factor → cells relax → vasodilation and increased glomerular flow.

KEY FACT

Surgeons pay special attention to ureteral peristalsis in order to identify and therefore avoid injury to the ureters.

CLINICAL CORRELATION

Micturition is controlled autonomically by the internal sphincter and voluntarily by the external sphincter. Problems with these muscles can lead to incontinence.

Intraglomerular Mesangial Cells

Specialized pericytes among glomerular capillaries that have the following properties: (1) contract to regulate blood flow of the glomerular capillaries, (2) are a major contributor to extracellular matrix, and (3) phagocytose glomerular basal lamina components and immunoglobulins.

Extraglomerular Mesangial Cells

Contractile cells with receptors for both angiotensin II and natriuretic factor, enabling them to regulate glomerular flow. Form part of the juxtaglomerular apparatus along with the macula densa and juxtaglomerular (granular) cells of the afferent arteriole.

RENAL CALYCES, RENAL PELVIS, AND URETERS

These structures are lined with **transitional epithelium.** The muscular layer of the calyces, pelvis, and ureters are composed of helically arranged smooth muscle, which becomes more longitudinal as the ureters reach the bladder. The ureters exhibit peristaltic contractions as they pass urine from the kidneys to the bladder.

BLADDER

The wall of the urinary bladder is composed of the following layers (Figure 8-9):

- **Transitional epithelium:** Lines the inner surface. Its thickness depends largely on the bladder's fullness (an empty bladder has much thicker transitional epithelium than its distended counterpart).
- **Smooth muscle:** Three layers of smooth muscle are oriented in various directions and constitute the outer wall of the bladder. The innermost of these layers becomes the involuntary urethral sphincter at the junction between the bladder and the urethra.

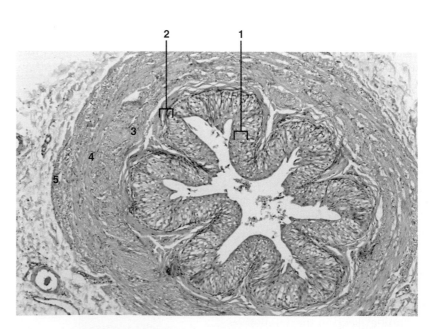

FIGURE 8-9. **Histology of the bladder.** 1, Transitional epithelium; 2, submucosa; 3, inner longitudinal smooth muscle; 4, middle circular smooth muscle; 5, outermost longitudinal smooth muscle. (Courtesy of Uniformed Services University of the Health Sciences.)

Physiology

CONCEPTS OF TRANSPORT

DEFINITIONS

- **Quantity** of a given substance in a solution is expressed through **millimoles (mmol)**, **milliequivalents (mEq)**, or **milliosmoles (mOsm)**.
- **Concentration** of a given substance in a solution reflects quantity per given volume. Commonly used units include: **mmol/L**, **mEq/L**, and **mOsm/L**.

An **equivalent** describes the **quantity of ionized (charged) molecules** in a given solution.

For example, one mole of NaCl in a solution dissociates into one equivalent of Na and one equivalent of Cl. However, one mole of $MgCl_2$ dissociates into two equivalents of Mg (ionized form has two positive charges) and two equivalents of Cl.

An **osmole** defines the number of single particles into which the solute dissociates in solution. Accordingly, **osmolarity** represents the concentration of those particles per given volume (eg, Osm/L).

Keeping in mind the previous example, the osmolarity equals molarity for nonionic substances, but they differ for ionic (charged) substances.

Forms of Transport

CONCEPTS OF TRANSPORT

There are two main types of transport: transcellular and paracellular.

- **Transcellular transport.** Substances are transported across both the apical and basolateral membranes and through the cytoplasm of the cell.
- **Paracellular transport:** The transported substances travel through the tight junctions *between* cells. This form of transport involves **simple diffusion** and/or **carrier-mediated diffusion.**

Substances can be transported via passive or active transport.

PASSIVE TRANSPORT

Relies solely on the concentration gradient across the cell membranes as the driving force (does not require energy).

- **Simple diffusion** involves net transfer of solute down the concentration gradient until the rate of transfer across the membrane becomes equal in both directions (dynamic equilibrium).
- **Facilitated diffusion** is a carrier-mediated process directed down the concentration gradient. The carriers are specific membrane proteins that exhibit a high affinity for the substance. Because the amount of carrier is limited, the transport rate does not increase indefinitely with increasing concentration gradient. Rather, the transport maximum (T_m) for a given substance is achieved when all carrier sites are saturated. Moreover, molecules with structural similarities to the substance may compete for the carrier-binding site, thus reducing the transport rate of the preferred solute; this provides the basis for competitive agonist/antagonist actions.

KEY FACT

Equivalents = net charge × molarity (not applicable to neutral molecules)
Osmolarity = number of dissociated particles × molarity

KEY FACT

Osmolarity ≠ molarity for solutes that dissociate into multiple species. For example:
10 mmol glucose = 10 mOsm/L glucose
But, 10 mmol NaCl = 20 mOsm/L NaCl
(NaCl is ionic and dissociates into Na^+ and Cl^-)

KEY FACT

Examples of substances of physiologic importance that cross the membrane by nonionic diffusion include CO_2 and NH_3. These compounds play important roles in renal regulation of acid-base balance.

- **Nonionic diffusion** is a passive process by which impermeant ions derived from the dissociation of weak acids or bases can cross cell membranes. The equation: $[HA] = [H^+] + [A^-]$ depicts the state of equilibrium between the undissociated and dissociated forms of a weak acid. Cell membranes are impermeable to ions, but permeable to the neutral, undissociated free acid form. The system's equilibrium is based on the pH gradient across the membrane.
- **Osmosis** refers to the movement of water across a semipermeable membrane from a region of low solute concentration to a region of high solute concentration. This is the only mechanism by which water is transported across the renal tubular epithelium.
- **Osmotic pressure** is the hydrostatic pressure that must be physically applied to the side of a semipermeable membrane containing high-solute concentration (low-water concentration) in order to prevent the osmotic flow of water across the membrane.

ACTIVE TRANSPORT

Substances transported against their electrochemical gradient require a specific carrier and energy source, the most important of which is ATP.

- **Primary active transport:** Requires a specific ATPase transporter. The Na^+/K^+-ATPase and the Ca^{2+}-ATPase systems are found on the basolateral membrane of the renal tubules. This allows for Na^+ to be transported in one direction only (from the tubular lumen to the renal interstitial fluid).
- **Secondary active transport:** Two different substances simultaneously bind to the same membrane carrier and are concurrently transported across the membrane; one of the substances moves down its electrochemical concentration gradient while the other moves against it. This process can occur either by co- or countertransport:
- **Cotransport (symport)** occurs when two compounds use the same protein carrier and move in the same direction across the membrane (eg, Na^+-glucose symporter).
- **Countertransport (antiport)** occurs when transported substances are moved across the membrane in opposite directions (eg, Na^+-H^+ antiporter in the proximal tubule, and the distal tubular H^+-K^+ antiporter).

KEY FACT

Potassium is the main **cation** in the **ICF.**

Proteins and **organic phosphates** are the main **anions** in **ICF.**

Sodium is the main **cation** in the **ECF.**

Cl^- and HCO_3^- are the main **anions** in **ECF.**

RATE-LIMITED TRANSPORT

The concept of T_m (transport maximum, as described previously) applies to both secretory and reabsorptive epithelial cell transport mechanisms. The different ways in which T_m applies to glucose and *para*-aminohippuric acid (PAH) are discussed later.

Fluid Compartments

COMPOSITION OF EXTRACELLULAR FLUID AND INTRACELLULAR FLUID

The ionic compositions of the extracellular (ECF) and intracellular fluid (ICF) (Figure 8-10) are remarkably different. However, the osmolarities of the compartments are virtually equal, which allows for normal cell homeostasis. These concentration gradients across cell membranes are maintained by transport mechanisms.

The fluid component of the body is divided into several compartments (Figure 8-11). Water accounts for 60% of a person's total weight (known as **total body water,** or **TBW**). Two-thirds of TBW (40% of body weight) is ICF and one-third (20% of total body weight) is ECF.

KEY FACT

TBW = ECF + ICF

KEY FACT

60-40-20 rule: TBW = 60%, ICF = 40%, and ECF = 20% of body weight.

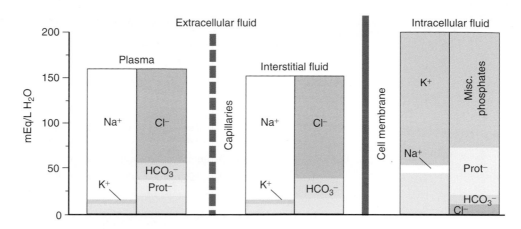

FIGURE 8-10. **Composition of body fluids.** (Modified with permission from Barrett KE, Barman SM, Boitano S, Brooks H. *Ganong's Review of Medical Physiology*, 23rd ed. New York: McGraw-Hill, 2010: Figure 1-1.)

In a 70-kg adult, assuming normal hydration, 42 L (60%) of body weight is water, of which 28 L (⅔) is in the intracellular space and 14 L (⅓) is in the extracellular space.

■ TBW varies based on age, sex, and body fat percentage. As body fat increases, the relative percentage of TBW decreases
■ **Infants and children** have higher TBW than adults due to a decreased proportion of fat. At birth, the ECF compartment consists of almost 50% of the TBW.
■ **Aging** is commonly associated with an increase in body fat (thus decreased TBW).
■ **Females,** on average, have more body fat than males, and therefore have lower TBW.

The **ECF compartment** is further divided into interstitial fluid and plasma (Table 8-4).

■ **Interstitial fluid** (75% of ECF): Water within the body but outside the cells.
■ **Plasma** (25% of ECF): Noncellular fluid of the blood.

Estimating and Measuring Fluid Compartment Volume

ESTIMATING BODY FLUID VOLUMES

The percentage of the fluid compartment multiplied by total body weight (assuming normal hydration).

> **KEY FACT**
>
> Estimating content of fluid compartments:
> TBW (L) = 0.60 × wt (kg)
> ICF = 0.40 × wt (kg)
> ECF = 0.20 × wt (kg)

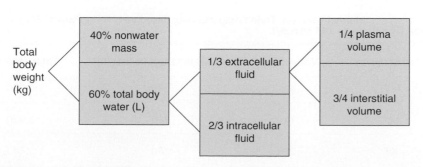

FIGURE 8-11. **Fluid compartments.**

TABLE 8-4. **Comparison of the Composition of Intracellular Fluid (ICF) and Extracellular Fluid (ECF)**

FLUID COMPARTMENT	COMPOSITION
ICF	▪ **Potassium,** magnesium, phosphate ions, organic anions, and protein ▪ Slight negative charge, due to the nature of the cell membrane
ECF	▪ **Sodium,** chloride, bicarbonate, and calcium ▪ Slight positive charge, due to the nature of the cell membrane

MEASURING BODY FLUID VOLUMES

Accomplished by injecting a known amount of a measurable molecule into the fluid space and allowing it to diffuse. The ideal molecule will enter the compartment(s) of interest and remain there without diffusing into other spaces. Normal physiologic values are depicted in Table 8-5.

The volume of the compartment of interest is calculated by applying the indicator dilution principle in which the distribution volume (V) for the indicator equals the quantity of indicator administered (Q) divided by the measured concentration (C) of indicator after equilibration has occurred.

$$V = Q/C$$

The TBW, plasma, and ECF volumes can be determined directly by using the following indicators:

- **TBW indicators:** D_2O (heavy water), ^3H_2O tritium (radioactive water), and $C_{11}H_{12}N_2O$ (antipyrine).
- **Plasma volume (PV) indicators:** Evans blue dye or radioiodinated human serum albumin (^{125}I-albumin).
- **ECF indicators:** Inulin, mannitol, and ^{22}Na.

The ICF, interstitial fluid, and blood volumes can be determined indirectly by using the following relationships:

$$ICF = TBW - ECF$$
$$Interstitial\ fluid = ECF - Plasma$$
$$Blood = Plasma / (1 - hematocrit)$$

KEY FACT

Osmolarity of ECF and ICF:
ECF osmolarity = ICF osmolarity. ECF volume changes to maintain this balance.

TABLE 8-5. **Normal Values of Fluid Compartments Based on a 70-kg Patient With a Plasma Osmolarity of 280 mOsm/L**

COMPARTMENTS	VOLUME (L)	CONCENTRATION (MOSM/L)	TOTAL (MOSM)
TBW	42	280	11,760
ECF	14	280	3,920
ICF	28	280	7,840

Intercompartmental Water Dynamics (see Figure 8-11)

Under steady-state conditions, the osmolarity of the ECF is equal to that of ICF.

- Under normal physiologic conditions, substances such as mannitol, NaCl, and $NaHCO_3$ are confined to the ECF and do not readily cross the cell membrane.
- Under certain pathophysiologic conditions, this steady state is interrupted.

Volume changes take place in the ECF; ICF changes subsequently occur to equalize osmolarity between these compartments. These compartmental disturbances can be divided into two major groups:

- **Volume contraction** refers to loss of water from the ECF.
- **Volume expansion** refers to increase in the ECF volume.

Furthermore, this can be subdivided based on the osmolarity of the ECF into **iso-osmotic, hypo-osmotic,** and **hyperosmotic** disturbances (all depicted in Figure 8-12, the Darrow-Yannet diagram), followed by practical calculations (Table 8-6).

ECF Pathophysiology Key Facts

- **Iso-osmotic volume contraction:** Prolonged watery diarrhea → hypovolemia and low flow state → activation of the RAAS → lowered urinary output (to retain Na^+ and H_2O).

> **KEY FACT**
>
> **Osmolarity = Concentration of osmotically active particles per unit volume.**
>
> Normal measured value for body fluid osmolarity (BFO) is 290 mOsm/L (for practical purposes, we can round this to 300 mOsm/L).
>
> Calculated plasma osmolarity $(P_{osm}) = 2 \times [Na^+] + [glucose]/18 + BUN/2.8$.

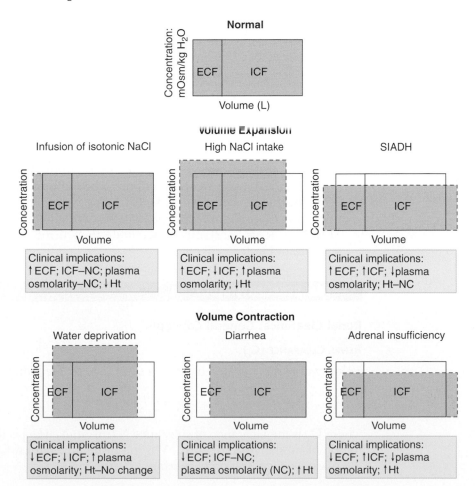

FIGURE 8-12.   **Darrow-Yannet diagram.** ECF = extracellular fluid; ICF = intracellular fluid; Ht = hematocrit; NC = no change.

TABLE 8-6. Sample Calculations

Normal physiologic conditions, normal hydration:

TBW = 0.6 × (70 kg) = 42 L

ICF volume = 0.4 × (70 kg) = 28 L

ECF volume = 0.2 × (70 kg) = 14 L

Body fluid osmolarity (BFO) = 300 mOsm/kg

Total body osmoles = (TBW) × (BFO) = (42 L) (300 mOsm/kg H_2O) = 12,600 mOsm

ICF osmoles = (ICF) × (BFO) = (28 L) (300 mOsm/kg H_2O) = 8400 mOsm

ECF osmoles = (ECF) × (BFO) = (14 L) (300 mOsm/kg H_2O) = 4200 mOsm

Example for SIADH = water intoxication = hypo-osmotic volume expansion:

Assume an extra 6 L of H_2O reabsorption:

Redistribution of H_2O, secondary to volume overload with H_2O.

TBW (L) = 0.6 × (70 kg) = 42 L + 6 L = 48 L

ICF (L) = 0.4 × (70 kg) = 28 L + 4 L (⅔ of 6 L) = 32 L

ECF (L) = 0.2 × (70 kg) = 14 L + 2 L (⅓ of 6 L) = 16 L

Compare:

Normal osmolarity: 12,600 mOsm/42 L TBW = 300 mOsm/kg

SIADH osmolarity: 12,600 mOsm/48 L TBW = 262.5 mOsm/kg

SIADH ICF volume: (ICF osm)/(SIADH osmolarity) = 8400 mOsm/262.5 mOsm/kg = 32 L

SIADH ECF volume: (ECF osm)/(SIADH osmolarity) = 4200 mOsm/262.5 mOsm/kg = 16 L

Final picture:

Increase in both ECF and ICF volumes.

Decrease in body osmolarity (plasma protein dilution).

Hematocrit does not change: decrease in concentration of RBCs is offset by increase in RBC volume (H_2O shifts into the cells).

■ **Hypo-osmotic volume expansion:** Distinguish between **psychogenic polydipsia/water intoxication** and the **syndrome of inappropriate antidiuretic hormone secretion (SIADH).** (If psychogenic polydipsia is present, urine will be dilute but will concentrate normally once fluid intake stops. SIADH patients constantly concentrate their urine and thus retain water regardless of water intake.)

GENERAL RENAL PHYSIOLOGY

Renal Clearance: General Concepts

RENAL CLEARANCE (C_x)

Volume of plasma cleared of a given substance by the kidney per unit time:

$$C_x = [U_x] \times (V/[P_x])$$

where C_x is the clearance of substance X (mL/min), $[U_x]$ is the urine concentration of substance X (mg/mL), V is the urine flow rate (mL/min), and $[P_x]$ is the plasma concentration of substance X (mg/mL).

It can be determined how a specific substance is handled by the renal tubules by comparing the clearance rate of a substance with the GFR (Table 8-7).

TABLE 8-7. Interpreting C_x

$C_x >$ GFR	Substance filtered and secreted.
$C_x <$ GFR	Substance filtered and partially reabsorbed.
$C_x =$ GFR	Substance filtered and excreted with no net reabsorption or secretion.

Inulin, a fructose polymer, is freely filtered and neither reabsorbed nor secreted, and as such can be used to determine the clearance of any substance by comparing it with the inulin clearance, expressed through the **clearance ratio.**

$$\text{Clearance ratio} = C_x/C_{inulin}$$

$C_x/C_{inulin} = 1.0$ indicates that the clearance of substance X is equal to that of inulin; the substance is neither secreted nor reabsorbed. Substances with these properties are called **glomerular markers.**

$C_x/C_{inulin} < 1.0$ indicates that the clearance of substance X is lower than that of inulin, suggesting two possibilities:

- The substance is **not filtered** (eg, albumin).
- The substance **is filtered,** but is subsequently **reabsorbed** (eg, glucose, amino acids, urea, phosphate, Na^+, Cl^-, and HCO_3^-).

$C_x/C_{inulin} > 1.0$ indicates that substance X is filtered with net secretion.

Glomerular Filtration Barrier

Glomerular filtration is closely regulated by the barrier (Figure 8-13) that separates the blood from the Bowman space and is composed of three main layers.

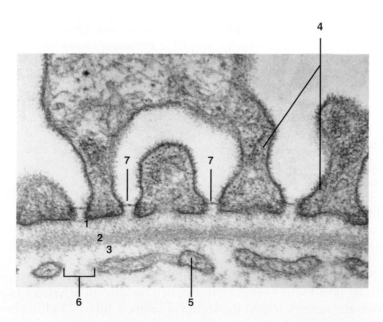

FIGURE 8-13. Electron photomicrograph of the glomerular filtration barrier. 1, Lamina rara externae; 2, lamina densa; 3, lamina rara interna; 4, pedicles; 5, capillary endothelium; 6, endothelial pore; 7, filtration slit membrane. (Courtesy of Dr. Ruth Bulger, Uniformed Services University of the Health Sciences.)

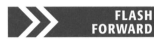

CLINICAL CORRELATION

The GBM charge barrier is lost in **nephrotic syndrome,** thereby allowing proteins to leak out of the capillaries, and leading to **albuminuria, hypoproteinemia,** and **generalized edema.** **Hyperlipidemia** is also seen in nephrotic syndrome, probably due to the stimulating effect that decreased plasma oncotic pressure has on hepatic lipoprotein synthesis.

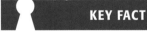

FLASH FORWARD

The α_3 chain of collagen type IV, the target antigen in **Goodpasture syndrome,** is a component of both the GBM and the alveolar basement membrane.

KEY FACT

Creatinine clearance is an estimation of GFR.

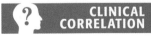

CLINICAL CORRELATION

Decreased GFR (eg, acute renal failure) leads to an elevation of both BUN and creatinine concentrations in the blood.

- **Fenestrated capillary endothelium** originates from the afferent arteriole and ends with the beginning of the efferent arteriole.
- **Glomerular basement membrane (GBM)** is composed of types IV and V collagen, laminin (glycoprotein), and heparan sulfate (proteoglycan). Laminin and heparan sulfate account for the GBM's **negative charge,** thus keeping plasma proteins, which also have a slight negative charge, from entering the Bowman space. The basement membrane is composed of **three layers:** lamina rara interna, lamina densa, and lamina rara externa.
- **Podocytes** line the outside of the GBM and form part of the visceral layer of the Bowman capsule. They form a network of interdigitating foot processes with intervening filtration slit diaphragms that regulate filtration into the urinary space.

GLOMERULAR FILTRATE

Material filtered through the glomerular filtration barrier, normally created at a rate of approximately **120 mL/min.** The glomerular filtration barrier is relatively impermeable to proteins, thus the filtrate contains little protein. Certain molecules, such as calcium and fatty acids, which are bound to plasma proteins, have a lower-than-expected concentration within the filtrate. Several other factors determine whether a substance will pass through the filtration barrier:

- Molecular size
- Shape
- Charge
- Hemodynamic conditions

GLOMERULAR FILTRATION RATE

Represents renal clearance of a substance that is **neither reabsorbed nor secreted** by the nephron.

- **Inulin** is the gold standard when measuring GFR because it is freely filtered and neither reabsorbed nor secreted (glomerular marker).
- **Creatinine** is more commonly used for GFR calculations. Creatinine is an end product of muscle metabolism and constantly released into the blood. The level of creatinine in the blood primarily depends on production by the muscle and filtration by the kidney. Creatinine clearance is an estimation of GFR and can be measured based on creatinine concentrations in the urine and blood and the urine flow (volume over time). Formulae also exist to estimate the GFR based only on serum creatinine, age, gender, and ethnicity.

Renal Blood Flow

The blood flow to the kidneys represents approximately 25% of the total cardiac output. Based on an average cardiac output of 5 L/min, the kidneys receive 1.25 L/min, or 1800 L/day. Because the kidneys handle the entire blood volume many times over each day, they play a crucial role in systemic blood circulation, as well as maintaining normal body fluid volume and composition.

The kidney contains numerous nephrons with vasculature connected in series. Blood flow to the nephrons is supplied by afferent arterioles branching off interlobular arteries within the kidney. Plasma is filtered in the glomerular capillary bed, and the filtered blood flows out into the interlobular veins via the efferent arterioles.

- The average pressure of the **afferent arteriole is 85 mm Hg.**
- The average pressure of the **efferent arteriole is 60 mm Hg.**

Regulation Mechanisms

Systemic BP and perfusion dramatically affect renal function. Physiologic changes in Starling forces and renal vascular resistance allow for regulation of renal blood flow (RBF) and function (Table 8-8, Figure 8-14).

INFLUENCING FACTORS

The sympathetic nervous system, hormones, and various drugs influence renal function.

- **Sympathetic nervous system:** Exerts its action via the catecholamines **epinephrine and norepinephrine,** via activation of α_1 **receptors,** causing vasoconstriction of the renal arterioles (afferent > efferent), and a decrease in RBF and GFR; and via β_1 receptor-mediated renin release. Moderate sympathetic stimulation does not result in a change in GFR.
- **Prostaglandins/bradykinin:** PGE_2 and PGI_2 (both produced in the kidneys) cause dilatation of afferent > efferent arterioles, thereby increasing RBF and GFR.
- **Angiotensin II:** A potent vasoconstrictor produced in response to decreased afferent arteriolar pressure from decreased renal blood flow. Angiotensin II constricts both afferent and efferent arterioles, but preferentially constricts the efferent arteriole, thus increasing or maintaining the

TABLE 8-8. Modulation of Renal Blood Flow and Filtration

EFFECT	GFR	RENAL PLASMA FLOW (RPF)	FILTRATION FRACTION (GFR/RPF)
Afferent arteriole constriction (as with norepinephrine)	↓ due to ↓ P_{GC}	↓	No change
Afferent arteriole dilation (as with PGE_2 or PGI_2)	↑ due to ↑ P_{GC}	↑	No change
Efferent arteriole constriction (as with angiotensin II)	↑ due to ↑ P_{GC}	↓	⇑
Increased plasma protein concentration (as with multiple myeloma)	↓ due to ↑ π_{GC}	No change	⇓
Decreased plasma protein concentration (as with nephrotic syndrome)	↑ due to ↓ π_{GC}	No change	⇑
Constriction of ureter or urinary tract obstruction	↓ due to ↑ P_{BS}	No change	⇓

P_{GC}, glomerular capillary hydrostatic pressure; P_{BS}, Bowman space hydrostatic pressure; π_{GC}, glomerular capillary plasma colloid osmotic pressure; π_{BS}, Bowman space interstitial colloid osmotic pressure.

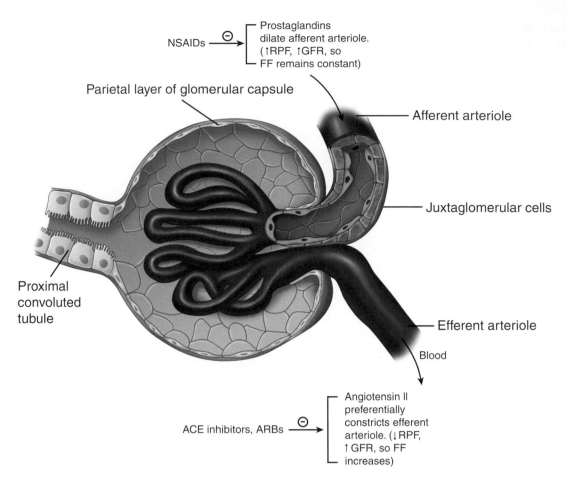

FIGURE 8-14. Effects of medications and hormones on renal plasma flow. ACE, angiotensin-converting enzyme; ARB, angiotensin receptor blocker; GFR, glomerular filtration rate; RPF, renal plasma flow.

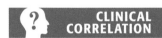

NSAIDs inhibit prostaglandin synthesis and interfere with the renal protective effects of prostaglandins (GFR and RBF are reduced).

pressure on the glomerulus. Angiotensin II maintains the GFR even in the face of decreased overall renal blood flow.

- **Dopamine** (precursor of norepinephrine) dilates the renal vessels and suppresses sodium reabsorption in the proximal tubule by inhibiting the action of the basolateral Na^+–K^+-ATPase pump. Dopamine is released directly by the proximal tubule in response to a rise in BP, resulting in increased RBF and GFR.

Autoregulation Mechanisms

Autoregulation is the process by which an organ maintains relatively constant blood flow despite variations in BP. These mechanisms typically have limits outside of which they are ineffective (eg, at systolic blood pressures < 80 mm Hg and > 200 mm Hg).

The kidney has two proposed autoregulatory mechanisms: **stretch (myogenic)** and **tubuloglomerular feedback**.

- **Stretch mechanism:** When BP increases, arterioles in the kidney are stretched. This leads to vasoconstriction of the afferent arteriole, which maintains constant RBF and GFR.
- **Tubuloglomerular feedback mechanism:** Increased arterial pressure leads to increased RBF and GFR, and increased flow to the distal tubule, which is sensed by the macula densa. Through a variety of mechanisms, the mac-

ula densa causes vasoconstriction of the afferent arteriole, thereby attenuating RBF and GFR and closing the negative feedback loop.

Measurement of Renal Plasma and Blood Flow

RENAL PLASMA FLOW

A measure of the volume of plasma delivered to the kidney in a given amount of time. If a substance could be cleared completely from the plasma, its clearance rate could be used to calculate the true renal plasma flow (RPF). However, RPF cannot be directly determined because there is no known substance that is cleared completely from the plasma.

para-Aminohippuric acid (PAH) is an endogenous substance that is 90% excreted from plasma through the kidneys via both filtration and secretion. The amount of PAH in the plasma of the renal artery is approximately equal to the amount of PAH in the urine. Therefore, the clearance rate of PAH can be used to calculate the effective renal plasma flow (ERPF).

$$ERPF = (U_{PAH} \times V)/P_{PAH} = C_{PAH}$$

where U_{PAH} is the urine concentration of PAH, V is the urine flow rate, P_{PAH} is the plasma concentration of PAH, and C_{PAH} is the clearance rate of PAH. ERPF can be used to calculate the value of true RPF and RBF

TRUE RENAL PLASMA FLOW

The ERPF is an approximation of the true RPF. Because only 90% of PAH is cleared in a single pass through the kidney, the true value of RPF is underestimated by 10%. Therefore, true RPF can be calculated as:

$$True \ RPF = ERPF/0.9$$

RENAL BLOOD FLOW

Renal plasma flow can be used to determine RBF, which represents the volume of blood delivered to the kidney in a given period of time. RBF can be determined using the equation:

$$RBF = (RPF)/(1 - hematocrit)$$

FILTRATION FRACTION

Filtration fraction (FF) is the fraction of plasma filtered across the glomerular filtration barrier. It can be calculated if the GFR and the RPF are known:

$$FF = GFR/RPF$$

Normally, the FF is approximately 0.20. Therefore, about 20% of the RPF enters the renal tubules, while the remaining 80% leaves the glomerulus via the efferent arteriole and becomes the peritubular capillary circulation.

CHANGES IN FILTRATION FRACTION

Changes in the FF alter the plasma protein concentration, and thereby the osmolarity within the peritubular capillaries. For example, an increase in FF reduces the amount and increases the osmolarity of the plasma flowing into the peritubular capillaries. The FF can be modulated by changes in either RPF or GFR.

- **Renal vascular resistance** and the **hydrostatic pressure differential** between the renal artery and vein affect the flow of blood throughout the nephrons.
- Increased vascular resistance → decreased RPF, increased hydrostatic pressure differential.
- Decreased vascular resistance → increased RPF, decreased hydrostatic pressure differential.

Changes in renal arterial and venous pressures can affect the FF; however, the autoregulatory mechanisms of the kidney ordinarily maintain the RBF and GFR within a relatively constant and narrow range.

Additionally, the rate of filtration across the glomerular capillaries is dictated by **Starling forces** (Figure 8-15). GFR can be calculated by applying the **Starling equation:**

$$GFR = K_f[(P_{GC} - P_{BS}) - (\pi_{GC} - \pi_{BS})]$$

where K_f is the filtration coefficient, P_{GC} is the glomerular capillary hydrostatic pressure, P_{BS} is the Bowman space hydrostatic pressure, π_{GC} is the glomerular capillary plasma colloid osmotic pressure, and π_{BS} is the Bowman space interstitial colloid osmotic pressure (usually π_{BS} is zero because very little protein is filtered).

Concepts of Reabsorption and Secretion

GLUCOSE

Completely reabsorbed in the **proximal tubules.** However, when serum glucose levels reach about 200 mg/dL, the reabsorption mechanism becomes overwhelmed and glucose may be excreted in the urine (this phenomenon is known as **splay,** or the excretion of a substance in small amounts before the **transport maximum** [T_m] is reached). Splay is caused by heterogeneity of nephrons and relatively low affinity of the Na⁺-glucose carriers. At serum glucose levels exceeding 350 mg/dL, the transport mechanism becomes completely saturated, resulting in clinical **glucosuria** (Figure 8-16).

AMINO ACIDS

Reabsorbed by secondary active transport in the **proximal tubules.** The transport mechanism is T_m-limited), and saturation may result in the excretion of amino acids in the urine.

KEY FACT

Glucosuria is an important clinical clue in the diagnosis of **diabetes mellitus (DM).**

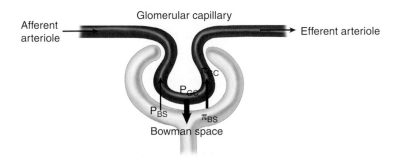

FIGURE 8-15. **Example of Starling forces acting on glomerular capillaries of a single nephron provided net pressure = 0 mm Hg and filtration equilibrium.** Average values: P_{GC} = 45 mm Hg; P_{BS} = 10 mm Hg; π_{BS} = 0 mm Hg; π_{GC} = 27 mm Hg.

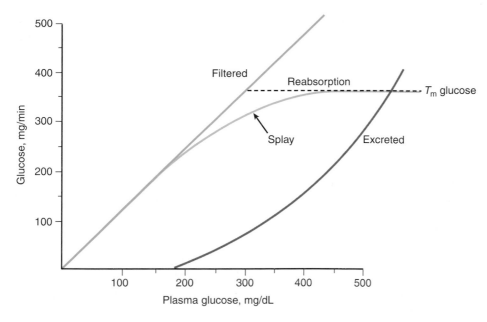

FIGURE 8-16. **Glucose titration curve.**

In general, amino acids are not found in the urine unless the individual has a genetic transport deficiency. For example, cystinuria may be observed in patients with defects in the proximal tubule protein mediating cystine reabsorption, possibly leading to formation of cystine stones.

UREA

A waste product from the metabolism of amino acids, urea is excreted in large amounts in the urine, and minimally reabsorbed. Urea contributes to the formation of **hyperosmolar urine** through its unique recirculation pathway, which helps to maintain the corticomedullary osmotic gradient (see Figure 8-21, depicting the countercurrent multiplier system, CCMS).

PARA-AMINOHIPPURIC ACID

A substance that is both freely filtered through the glomerulus and secreted from the peritubular capillaries into the tubular lumen. PAH is not reabsorbed. As a result, PAH is almost completely cleared from the plasma and is used to estimate RPF (see earlier discussion).

FREE WATER

Also referred to as solute-free water, it is produced in the thick ascending limb and the early distal tubule of the kidney. In these diluting segments of the nephron, NaCl is reabsorbed and the free water remains in the tubules to be excreted in the urine. As urine is produced, water and solutes are excreted in a somewhat independent manner. Excreted solutes can be calculated using the osmolar clearance (C_{osm}):

$$C_{osm} = \frac{(U_{osm} \times V)}{P_{osm}}$$

where U_{osm} is the urine osmolarity and P_{osm} is the plasma osmolarity. Free water clearance is equal to the difference between the urine flow rate and osmolar clearance:

$$C_{H_2O} = V - C_{osm}$$

URINE OSMOLARITY

The clearance of free water can be used to estimate the kidneys' ability to concentrate or dilute urine.

- When C_{H_2O} **is positive,** excess water is excreted and urine is dilute.
- When C_{H_2O} **is negative,** excess solutes are excreted, water is retained, and urine is concentrated.
- When C_{H_2O} **is zero,** urine is iso-osmotic to plasma.

In order to concentrate urine, high levels of ADH (vasopressin) are needed to increase the permeability of the distal tubule and the collecting ducts to water and an adequate corticomedullary osmotic gradient is required to provide the osmotic drive for water reabsorption.

- In the **presence of ADH,** urine is **concentrated** (body is conserving water).
- In the **absence of ADH,** urine is **dilute.**

Nephron Physiology and the Tubular System

The **nephron unit** is composed of the **glomerulus,** through which fluid is filtered from the blood, and the **tubular system,** where the filtered fluid is modified through reabsorption and secretion of various solutes to produce urine.

GLOMERULUS

A network of glomerular capillaries encased in the **Bowman capsule.** Blood flows from the **afferent arteriole** into the glomerular capillaries, where it is either filtered into the Bowman space or continues to flow through the **efferent arteriole** and the peritubular capillary system.

The fluid that is filtered into Bowman space flows into the tubular portion of the nephron. The tubule can be divided into several segments with different characteristics and functions. Each segment relies on the **basolateral Na⁺–K⁺-ATPase pump** to maintain low intracellular Na⁺ concentration, establishing a Na⁺ gradient for Na⁺ movement from the lumen into the cells.

PROXIMAL TUBULE

The major site of reabsorption (Figure 8-17). The cellular mechanism of reabsorption is based on the **transmembrane Na⁺ gradient,** which provides energy for numerous **secondary active transport** mechanisms. Solutes and water are reabsorbed passively and proportionally; therefore tubular fluid leaving the proximal tubule is isosmotic to plasma.

- Reabsorbs **all filtered glucose** and **amino acids,** 60–70% of the filtered electrolytes and water, and 50% of filtered urea from the tubular fluid.
- Na⁺ is reabsorbed via **cotransport** with amino acids, glucose, lactate, and phosphate, and via **countertransport** with H⁺ through the Na⁺–H⁺ exchanger, which is linked directly to the reabsorption of filtered HCO₃⁻ through the action of brush border carbonic anhydrase.

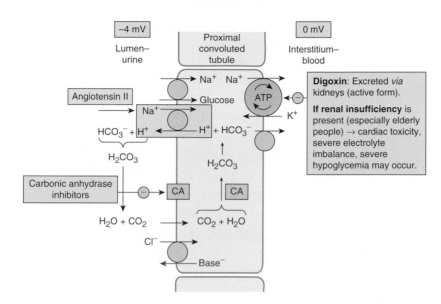

FIGURE 8-17. **Early proximal convoluted tubule, "workhorse of the nephron."** Reabsorbs all of the glucose and amino acids and most of the bicarbonate (HCO_3^-), sodium (Na^+), and water (H_2O). Secretes ammonia, which acts as a buffer for secreted H^+. Pink circles indicate transporters. CA, carbonic anhydrase.

- Ammonia secretion buffers the secreted H^+.
- Na^+ is primarily reabsorbed with Cl^- in the **late proximal tubule** as follows: Reabsorption of H_2O without significant Cl^- reabsorption in the early proximal tubule establishes a high Cl^- chemical gradient that drives Cl^- reabsorption through the cell and into the interstitium; Na^+ follows to restore the electroneutrality of the interstitium.
- Angiotensin II and also the sympathetic nervous system (eg, norepinephrine) act on the proximal tubule at the Na^+-H^+ exchanger to stimulate Na^+ reabsorption, whereas atrial natriuretic factor (ANF) released from stretched atria blocks Na^+ reabsorption.
- **Parathyroid hormone (PTH)** decreases phosphate reabsorption by activating adenylate cyclase to increase production of cAMP, which inhibits Na^+–phosphate cotransport.

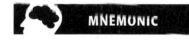

MNEMONIC

PTH puts **P**O$_4$ in the **P**ee

LOOP OF HENLE

Consists of three portions: (1) thin descending; (2) thin ascending; and (3) thick ascending limbs. The majority of action occurs in the thick ascending limb of the loop.

- **Thin descending limb** reabsorbs about 20% of the filtered water, but no solute reabsorption occurs in this segment.
- **Thin ascending limb** is impermeable to water and has no significant reabsorption.
- **Thick ascending limb** is a **diluting segment** of the tubular system (Figure 8-18). It is impermeable to water, yet reabsorbs solutes. This segment actively reabsorbs Na^+, K^+, and Cl^- via the **$Na^+-K^+-2Cl^-$ symporter.** Reabsorbed K^+ leaks back into the lumen through renal output medullary potassium (ROMK) channels, creating a slight positive charge in the lumen fluid. This positive charge indirectly induces paracellular diffusion of Mg^{2+} and Ca^{2+} into the interstitial fluid.
- The distal thick ascending limb contains the **macula densa** of the juxtaglomerular complex, which provides **tubuloglomerular feedback** for autoregulation of RBF.

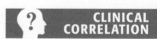

CLINICAL CORRELATION

Loop diuretics (eg, **furosemide**) act by blocking the **$Na^+-K^+-2Cl^-$ symporter.**

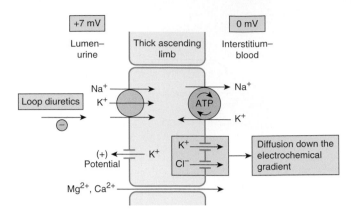

FIGURE 8-18. **Thick ascending limb of Henle.** This structure actively reabsorbs Na⁺, K⁺, and Cl⁻, and indirectly induces the reabsorption of Mg^{2+} and Ca^{2+}. It is impermeable to water. Pink circle indicates transporter.

EARLY DISTAL CONVOLUTED TUBULE

- Cortical **diluting segment** of the tubular system (Figure 8-19).
- The distal tubule transport mechanism relies on the Na⁺–Cl⁻ cotransporter (situated on the luminal membrane), which provides the basis for Na⁺, Cl⁻, K⁺, Ca^{2+}, and Mg^{2+} trafficking into and out of the lumen. This segment is impermeable to water and urea.
- **Angiotensin II** acts on the early distal tubule to stimulate Na⁺ reabsorption, while **atrial natriuretic factor (ANF)** blocks Na⁺ reabsorption.
- **PTH** acts to increase active Ca^{2+} reabsorption.

LATE DISTAL TUBULE AND COLLECTING DUCTS

Composed of two cell types, principal and intercalated cells (Figure 8-20).

- **Principal cells** reabsorb Na⁺ and water and secrete K⁺ via the basolateral Na⁺–K⁺-ATPase pump and apical ROMK channels.
- **α-Intercalated cells** are key players in acid–base regulation of body fluids, as they secrete H⁺ and reabsorb K⁺ and HCO_3^-. Carbonic acid can be formed in these cells via the catalytic action of carbonic anhydrase on H_2O and CO_2. The carbonic acid then dissociates into H⁺ and HCO_3^-. H⁺ is secreted into the tubular lumen via the H⁺-ATPase and H⁺–K⁺

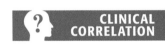
CLINICAL CORRELATION

Thiazide diuretics (eg, **hydrochlorothiazide**) act by blocking the **Na⁺–Cl⁻ cotransporter** in the early DCT.

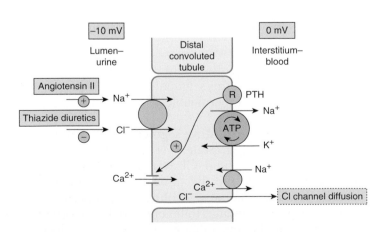

FIGURE 8-19. **Early distal convoluted tubule.** This structure actively reabsorbs Na⁺ and Cl⁻. Reabsorption of Ca^{2+} is under the control of parathyroid hormone. Pink circles indicate transporters.

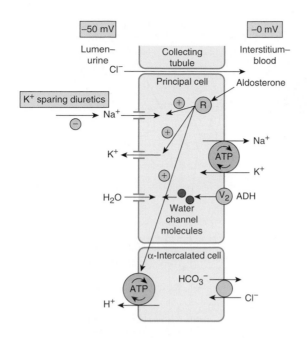

FIGURE 8-20. **Collecting tubules reabsorb Na⁺ in exchange for secreting K⁺ or H⁺ (regulated by aldosterone).** Reabsorption of water is regulated by ADH (vasopressin). Osmolarity of the medulla can reach 1200 mOsm. Pink circles indicate transporters.

exchanger. (*Note*: There are also β-intercalated cells that secrete HCO_3^- and reabsorb H^+.)

- **Aldosterone** stimulates Na^+ reabsorption and K^+ secretion in the principal cells, as well as H^+ secretion in the intercalated cells.
- In the **presence of ADH (antidiuretic hormone, aka vasopressin)**, water channels called aquaporins are recruited and inserted into the luminal membrane of the principal cells, making them **permeable to water**. In the **absence of ADH**, the late distal tubule and the collecting ducts are **impermeable to water**. The presence or absence of ADH therefore controls the concentration or dilution of urine.
- **Urea** reabsorption only occurs in the inner medullary collecting ducts (the late distal tubules, the cortical collecting ducts, and the outer medullary collecting ducts are impermeable to urea). ADH increases urea permeability in the inner medullary collecting ducts.

COUNTERCURRENT MULTIPLIER SYSTEM

The countercurrent multiplier system (CCMS) is a **U**-shaped structure that is an integral part of the nephron known as the **loop of Henle**. The CCMS comprises three loop regions (**thin descending limb, thin ascending limb, and the thick ascending limb**), which are responsible for establishing the renal medullary interstitial fluid osmotic gradient through a multistep process (see Figure 8-21). The term **countercurrent** describes the fluid movement in opposite directions in adjacent tubes.

COUNTERCURRENT EXCHANGER (VASA RECTA)

How does the water reclaimed from the filtrate make it back to the circulation? The vasa recta are **U**-shaped capillaries that are freely permeable to water and all solutes except protein. They are situated in close proximity to the loop of Henle, allowing them to equilibrate readily with the surrounding interstitial fluid. The high oncotic pressure in the vasa recta resulting from loss of protein-free filtrate in the glomerulus leads to avid water reabsorption.

KEY FACT

For each H^+ ion secreted into the lumen, one HCO_3^- can be reabsorbed across the basement membrane into the interstitial fluid.

CLINICAL CORRELATION

One effect of alcohol is the suppression of ADH, resulting in more dilute urine.

KEY FACT

In humans, the maximum osmolarity at the tip of the loop of Henle reaches about 1200–1400 mOsm/L, half of which is attributed to NaCl and the other half to urea.

KEY FACT

The role of the loop of Henle's multiplier system is to establish the hyperosmolar gradient of the renal medulla. It is this gradient that (in the presence of aquaporins) allows the osmotic flow of water out of the collecting duct and into the surrounding tissue, thus concentrating urine.

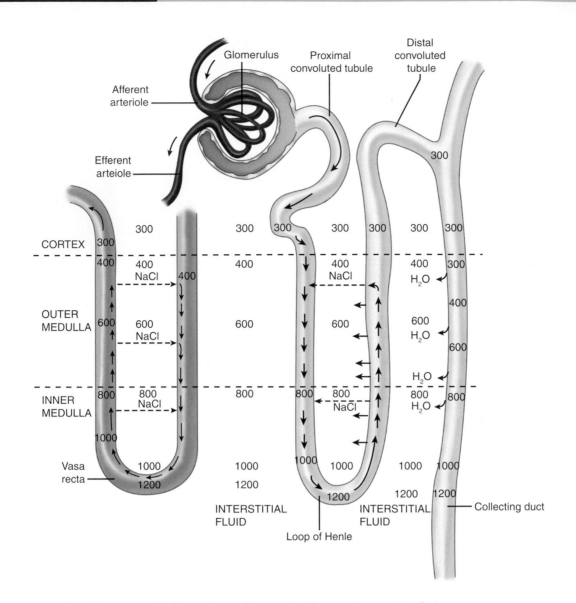

FIGURE 8-21. Countercurrent multiplier system and vasa recta, the countercurrent exchanger.

KEY FACT

The role of the vasa recta is to preserve the hyperosmolar gradient of the renal medulla while reclaiming solutes and water from the interstitial space back into the circulation.

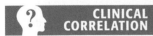
CLINICAL CORRELATION

Systemic deficiency of EPO and consequent anemia often ensue as a result of chronic kidney disease (CKD), renal malignancy, or as an adverse effect of chemotherapy.

The **U** shape of the vasa recta allows for the preservation of the corticomedullary osmolar gradient (see Figure 8-21). As the capillaries run down into the salty medulla, they lose water and gain solute. As they run back toward the cortex, they gain water and lose solute. As such, the vasa recta absorb water and excess solute without dissipating the gradient.

Kidney Endocrine Functions

The kidney performs four major endocrine functions:

- Secretion of erythropoietin (EPO).
- Formation of 1,25-dihydroxycholecalciferol.
- Production of renin (discussed in detail in the later section on the Renin-Angiotensin-Aldosterone System).
- Production of prostaglandins.

ERYTHROPOIETIN

EPO is a glycoprotein hormone released in response to hypoxia that stimulates RBC production by the bone marrow. In healthy individuals, approximately 90% of all EPO is synthesized in the kidneys. EPO exerts its action through **EPO receptors** on the surface of **proerythroblasts** in the bone marrow. This accelerates the **maturation of proerythroblasts** (to their erythroblastic stage). In the absence of EPO, few RBCs are formed by the bone marrow. Therefore, individuals with insufficient concentrations of EPO (eg, patients with severe kidney disease/failure) may become anemic because they cannot appropriately respond to hypoxia by increasing EPO and RBC production.

VITAMIN D: FORMATION OF 1,25-DIHYDROXYCHOLECALCIFEROL IN THE KIDNEYS

Vitamin D and **PTH** are critical for regulating Ca^{2+} and phosphate metabolism. Vitamin D is a fat-soluble vitamin that is mainly produced in the skin by UV-B light conversion of 7-dehydrocholesterol or ingested in the diet or dietary supplements. Vitamin D is stored in the liver in its inactive form, 25-OH-cholecalciferol; its activation depends on the plasma Ca^{2+} concentration.

Decreased plasma Ca^{2+} levels stimulate PTH secretion, which activates 1α-hydroxylase in the kidneys. This in turn enables the hydroxylation of 25-OH-cholecalciferol (C1 position) into 1,25-$(OH)_2$-cholecalciferol (physiologically active form), which increases intestinal absorption of Ca^{2+} and decreases renal Ca^{2+} and phosphate excretion.

The syndrome of **vitamin D resistance** develops if the kidneys are unable to produce its active metabolite, 1,25-$(OH)_2$-cholecalciferol, despite normal vitamin D intake and availability. This condition can be either inherited (1α-hydroxylase deficiency) or acquired (chronic kidney disease, end-stage renal failure). An extremely rare form of rickets can also result from mutations in the vitamin D receptor gene.

PROSTAGLANDINS

Prostaglandins PGE_2 and PGI_2, and **bradykinin** dilate the afferent arterioles to increase RBF and GFR. The use of NSAIDs inhibits prostaglandin production and their effects.

Hormones Acting on the Kidney

Just as the kidney produces several hormones, several others affect kidney function: ANF, PTH, aldosterone, angiotensin II, and ADH (Table 8-9).

ATRIAL NATRIURETIC FACTOR

The cardiac atria release atrial natriuretic factor/peptide (ANF/ANP) in response to increased stretching of the muscle fibers (secondary to volume overload or heart failure). ANF causes vasodilation of the afferent arterioles, vasoconstriction of efferent arterioles, and decreased sodium reabsorption in the late distal tubules and collecting ducts.

PARATHYROID HORMONE

PTH exerts three main actions on the kidneys:

- Inhibition of phosphate reabsorption in the PCT. This is accomplished by inhibition of the Na^+–phosphate cotransporter. **Phosphaturia** is followed by increased cAMP excretion (**urinary cAMP**). This action of PTH on the kidney is important for the overall Ca^{2+} availability in the ECF. Excess phosphate, resulting from decreased phosphate secretion, leads to "trapping" (complexing) of the free Ca^{2+}, thereby reducing its availability in the plasma.

KEY FACT

Human recombinant EPO is available as supportive treatment for patients with advanced chronic kidney disease, end-stage renal disease, HIV-associated anemia, and other similar conditions.
Remember: Patients must also receive proper iron supplementation.

KEY FACT

The action of 1,25-$(OH)_2$-cholecalciferol in the kidney differs from that of PTH:

- **1,25-$(OH)_2$-cholecalciferol** stimulates reabsorption of both Ca^{2+} and phosphate.
- **PTH** stimulates Ca^{2+} reabsorption, but inhibits phosphate reabsorption.

CLINICAL CORRELATION

A related peptide, brain natriuretic peptide (BNP) is released by distended ventricular myocardium under conditions of high volume and/or pressure and as such is often measured to evaluate dyspnea. High values suggest congestive heart failure (CHF) as the etiology.

TABLE 8-9. Summary of Hormones Acting on the Kidney and Their Sites of Action

HORMONE	STIMULUS	MECHANISM AND SITE OF ACTION
ADH	▪ Increased plasma osmolarity ▪ Decreased blood volume	▪ Increases H_2O permeability of principal cells in collecting ducts. ▪ Increases urea reabsorption in collecting ducts. ▪ Increases $Na^+-K^+-2Cl^-$ symporter activity in the thick ascending limb.
Aldosterone	▪ Decreased blood volume (via angiotensin II) ▪ Hyperkalemia	Late distal tubule and collecting ducts: ▪ Increases Na^+ reabsorption. ▪ Increases K^+ excretion. ▪ Increases H^+ excretion.
Angiotensin II	▪ Decreased blood volume (via renin)	▪ Contraction of efferent arteriole resulting in increased GFR. ▪ Stimulation of Na^+-H^+ exchange in the PCT. ▪ Stimulation of aldosterone synthesis by the adrenal glands.
ANF	▪ Increased atrial pressure	▪ Decreases Na^+ reabsorption; increases GFR.
PTH	▪ Decreased plasma Ca^{2+} ▪ Increased plasma PO_4^-	▪ Increases Ca^{2+} reabsorption. ▪ Decreases PO_4^- reabsorption. ▪ Increases $1,25-(OH)_2$-vitamin D production.

ADH, antidiuretic hormone; ANF, atrial natriuretic factor; GFR, glomerular filtration rate; PCT, proximal convoluted tubule; PTH, parathyroid hormone.

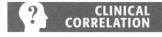
CLINICAL CORRELATION

Renal osteodystrophy results from hyperphosphatemia and hypocalcemia, both the result of little to no phosphate excretion by damaged kidneys, low vitamin D levels, and/or tertiary hyperparathyroidism. Tertiary hyperparathyroidism refers to the situation in which hyperparathyroidism, usually in the context of end-stage renal disease, becomes refractory to normal physiologic regulation and medical therapy.

▪ Stimulation of 1α-hydroxylase in the PCT to generate the active form of vitamin D: $1,25-(OH)_2$-cholecalciferol.
▪ Stimulation of Ca^{2+} reabsorption (**hypocalciuric action**) in the DCT. This occurs via the basolateral PTH receptors, which employ a second-messenger system (eg, conversion of ATP to cAMP). This further increases the availability of free Ca^{2+} in plasma.

RENIN-ANGIOTENSIN-ALDOSTERONE SYSTEM (RAAS)

The RAAS functions to allow the kidneys to regulate BP (Figure 8-22). Renin is an enzyme synthesized and stored as an inactive compound, prorenin, in the juxtaglomerular cells of the kidneys (located in the walls of the afferent arterioles proximal to the glomeruli).

Several factors affect the **release of renin** into the bloodstream:

▪ Fall in arterial BP (hypotension), which results in decreased renal perfusion. This is perceived as a decreased stretch signal by the juxtaglomerular cells, which respond by excreting renin.
▪ Increased renal parasympathetic activity.
▪ $β_1$-Adrenergic stimulation.
▪ Decreased Na^+ load/Na^+ delivery to the macula densa.

These conditions initiate the conversion of prorenin to renin in the juxtaglomerular cells, and its subsequent release into the bloodstream, where renin enzymatically cleaves angiotensinogen to release angiotensin I. **Angiotensin I** is then cleaved by angiotensin-converting enzyme (ACE), found in the endothelium of the lung vasculature and kidneys, to form **angiotensin II**.

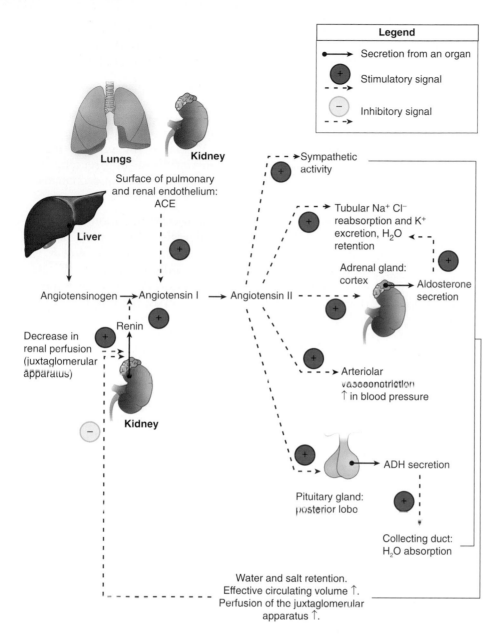

Legend

- ●——→ Secretion from an organ
- ⊕ Stimulatory signal
- ⊖ Inhibitory signal

FIGURE 8-22. **The renin–angiotensin–aldosterone system (RAAS).** ACE, angiotensin-converting enzyme; ADH, antidiuretic hormone.

There are at least three mechanisms by which circulating angiotensin II elevates arterial BP:

- **Direct vasoconstriction (fast response):** Constriction of the arterioles increases total peripheral resistance (TPR), and constriction of the veins promotes increased venous return of blood to the heart, both of which increase BP. The **efferent arterioles** of the kidney are especially affected.
- **Decreased excretion** of salt and water via stimulation of **aldosterone** synthesis in the adrenal glands (**slow response**). Aldosterone promotes Na^+ reabsorption in the distal tubules and collecting ducts, which leads to increases in the ECF and blood volumes.
- **Direct action on the kidneys:** This action is independent of its actions via the aldosterone pathway. In this case, angiotensin II stimulates Na^+–H^+ exchange at the level of the proximal tubule, thereby increasing the reabsorption of Na^+ and HCO_3^-.

 CLINICAL CORRELATION

Na^+ and Ca^{2+} reabsorption are not coupled at the level of the distal tubule as they are in the thick ascending limb. Therefore, **thiazide diuretics** can be used in cases of **idiopathic calciuria** because, though they inhibit Na^+ reabsorption, they also act to increase Ca^{2+} reabsorption.

FLASH BACK

β_1-Agonists (eg, isoproterenol) stimulate renin secretion.
β_1-Antagonists (eg, propranolol) inhibit renin secretion.

KEY FACT

Overall, angiotensin II serves to ↑ intravascular volume and ↑ BP.

CLINICAL CORRELATION

Potassium-sparing diuretics such as spironolactone inhibit the actions of aldosterone in the distal nephron.

KEY FACT

Mineralocorticoid escape is the ability of the glomerulotubular autoregulatory mechanism to override the action of aldosterone in cases of increased ECF (volume expansion). It is likely that increased ANF secondary to hypervolemia, decreased expression of thiazide-sensitive NaCl cotransporters in the distal tubule, and "pressure natriuresis" resulting from increased blood pressure all may contribute to this escape.

Angiotensin II only persists in the blood for 1–2 minutes before it is inactivated by angiotensinase. For this reason, the angiotensin II stimulation of aldosterone production is more influential in restoring arterial BP than its direct vasoconstrictive actions.

ALDOSTERONE

A mineralocorticoid synthesized in the zona glomerulosa of the adrenal cortex. Whereas adrenocorticotropic hormone (ACTH) is the primary regulator of the corticosteroid hormones, aldosterone's synthesis and secretion are mainly regulated by changes in ECF volume via the RAAS and changes in serum K^+ levels.

- **Late distal tubule:** Aldosterone exerts its action via stimulation of the mineralocorticoid receptors (MRs) on **principal cells.** This action increases the permeability of their apical (luminal) membrane to Na^+ and K^+ by adding newly synthesized proteins (epithelial sodium channels [ENaC], ROMK channels) as well as basolateral $Na^+–K^+$-ATPases and enzymes of the citric acid cycle, which stimulate ATP hydrolysis, reabsorption of Na^+ and water into the blood, and K^+ secretion into the urine.
- **Collecting duct:** Aldosterone also stimulates H^+ secretion by α-intercalated cells, thereby regulating plasma HCO_3^- levels and acid-base balance.

ANTIDIURETIC HORMONE

Also known as **vasopressin,** ADH plays a major role in determining whether the kidney produces and excretes concentrated or dilute urine (Figure 8-23). It originates in the hypothalamus/posterior pituitary gland, and is produced in response to high serum osmolarity or significantly diminished blood volume. It is also produced in response to angiotensin II as part of the RAAS, which acts to increase blood volume and BP.

- ADH acts on **V2 receptors** of **principal cells** in the **late DCT/collecting ducts.** It causes an increase in the number of functioning water channels

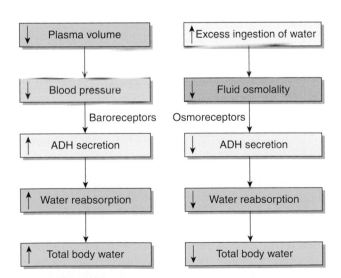

FIGURE 8-23. **Regulation of water balance.** The two major pathways for altering total body water: On the left, changes in antidiuretic hormone (ADH) release from the posterior pituitary are triggered by changes in blood volume. On the right, decreased osmolality causes swelling of osmoreceptor cells in the anterior hypothalamus, which inhibits their firing and inhibits adjacent superoptic nuclei cells, thereby reducing ADH secretion from their axonal extensions in the posterior pituitary. (Modified with permission from Eaton DC, Pooler JP. *Vander's Renal Physiology,* 6th ed. New York: McGraw-Hill, 2004: 123.)

(**aquaporins**), thereby increasing the permeability of the collecting ducts to water.

- **Presence of ADH** leads to the passive reabsorption of large amounts of water in the collecting ducts, thereby decreasing urine volume and increasing urine osmolarity (**hyperosmotic** urine).
- In the **absence of ADH**, the collecting ducts are virtually impermeable to water, and large amounts of very dilute (**hyposmotic**) urine are excreted.
- In **high levels**, ADH also acts on **V1 receptors** on arterioles to cause vasoconstriction. This is particularly important in the setting of **hemorrhage, in which ADH helps maintain systemic BP.**
- Decreased pressure leads to activation of the RAAS (see Figure 8-22), which raises total peripheral resistance and venous return and stimulates ADH release.
- Systemic baroreceptors (eg, carotid sinus) sense decreased BP, which causes ADH release from the posterior pituitary gland. ADH acts on the kidneys to retain volume, and acts on systemic arterioles to maintain pressure.

The combined efforts of the RAAS and ADH conserve fluid and maintain systemic pressure in the setting of hemorrhagic hypotension.

ACID-BASE HOMEOSTASIS

Acids and Bases

The body maintains serum pH within a tight range (approximately 7.40 ± 0.05) via a complex system that regulates acid production by metabolic processes. Importantly, most enzymes in the body function optimally within a very small pH range.

ACIDS

Molecules capable of releasing hydrogen ions into solution are known as acids.

- **Strong acids** rapidly dissociate into their ionic components in solution (eg, $HCl \rightarrow H^+ + Cl^-$).
- **Weak acids** are less likely to dissociate into their ionic components, and therefore less readily release H^+. Carbonic acid (H_2CO_3) is an example of a weak acid.

BASES

Any ion or molecule that can accept a hydrogen ion. They often have a net negative charge in solution.

- **Strong bases** readily and strongly accept hydrogen ions in solution, rapidly reducing the hydrogen ion concentration. For example, the hydroxide ion (OH^-) is a strong base.
- **Weak bases** less readily accept hydrogen ions. Bicarbonate (HCO_3^-) is an example of a weak base.

BUFFERS

Ionic compounds that resist changes in pH when acid or base is either added or removed. Buffers function along a titration curve and are most effective along the linear portion of the curve (±1.0 pH unit from the pK_a value for that

---

? CLINICAL CORRELATION

Syndrome of inappropriate ADH secretion (SIADH) → excessively concentrated urine and inappropriately dilute serum → hyponatremia.

SIADH is most commonly caused by central nervous system (CNS) or pulmonary disease, or as a paraneoplastic syndrome.

particular buffer). The pH of a buffer solution can be calculated using the **Henderson-Hasselbalch equation.**

$$pH = pK_a + \log [A^-]/[HA]$$

where A^- is the base form of the buffer and HA is the acid form of the buffer.

Acid Production

Acid production within the body is of two types: **volatile** and **nonvolatile.** Most of the acids in the body are weak acids, with the exception of hydrochloric acid (HCl^-), which is secreted in the form of gastric acid.

VOLATILE ACID

Produced in the form of CO_2 via cellular metabolism. The CO_2 produced then reacts with H_2O via the enzyme carbonic anhydrase to produce carbonic acid as shown:

$$CO_2 + H_2O \leftrightarrow H_2CO_3 \leftrightarrow H^+ + HCO_3^-$$

NONVOLATILE ACID

Protein catabolism generates sulfuric acid, and phospholipid catabolism creates phosphoric acid. Other nonvolatile acids produced by the body include salicylic acid, lactic acid, and ketones.

Physiologic Buffers

Several molecules act as a buffer system. These are categorized based on their location in relation to the cellular membrane: **intracellular** and **extracellular.**

INTRACELLULAR BUFFERS

Consist of proteins and organic phosphates.

- **Proteins:** Certain chemical moieties in amino acids, such as α-amino groups and imidazole groups, have pK_a values within the physiologic pH range and are therefore able to act as buffers. Hemoglobin is also an intracellular buffer. In the physiologic pH range, deoxyhemoglobin is a better buffer than oxyhemoglobin.
- **Organic phosphates:** These include metabolic substrates such as AMP, ADP, ATP, and 2,3-bisphosphoglycerate (2,3-BPG).

EXTRACELLULAR BUFFERS

Consist of HCO_3^- and phosphates.

- **Major:** HCO_3^- is the major extracellular buffer ($pK_a = 6.1$). It is produced via a reaction catalyzed by carbonic anhydrase (see previous formula).
- **Minor:** Phosphate is the minor extracellular buffer ($pK_a = 6.8$). Its most important function is as a buffer of urine. $H_2PO_4^-$ is referred to as a **titratable acid.**

Acid-Base Homeostasis

The body uses chemical buffer systems to regulate acid-base homeostasis.

BUFFER SYSTEMS

Consist of a pair of substances: a **weak acid** and **weak base** that undergo a reversible chemical reaction. The weak acid yields free H^+ as the hydrogen ion concentration [H⁺] starts to fall, and the weak base can bind free H⁺ when [H⁺] starts to rise.

The **Henderson-Hasselbalch equation** describes the relationship between [H⁺] and the members of a buffer pair. This equation fits the titration curve for all weak acids.

$$pH = -\log[H^+] \; pK_a + \log \frac{\text{proton acceptor}}{\text{proton donor}} = pK_a + \log \frac{[A^-]}{[HA]}$$

Inserting the values that describe the **blood bicarbonate buffer,** where (0.03 P_{CO_2}) is essentially equal to [H_2CO_3]:

$$pH = 6.1 + \log \frac{[HCO_3^-]}{0.03 \; P_{CO_2}}$$

The major chemical buffer system that the body uses to regulate extracellular acid-base balance is the carbonic acid/bicarbonate buffer system catalyzed by carbonic anhydrase:

$$CO_2 + H_2O \leftrightarrow H_2CO_3 \leftrightarrow H^+ + HCO_3^-$$

This is a reversible equilibrium reaction. The body regulates hydrogen ion concentration via CO_2 and HCO_3^- concentrations in the blood. The kidneys and lungs are the principal organs responsible for regulation of acid–base homeostasis.

PHYSIOLOGIC pH

Normal blood pH is 7.4, but it may fluctuate from 7.35 to 7.45. Values outside the range of 6.8–8.0 are typically incompatible with life due to changes in enzymatic function and protein denaturation.

- **Acidemia** versus **acidosis:**
  - **Acidemia** is a nonspecific term describing an increase in [H⁺] in the blood and is applicable when pH falls below normal (< 7.35).
  - **Acidosis** describes the specific physiologic derangement responsible for a lower than normal pH (eg, metabolic acidosis).
- **Alkalemia** versus **alkalosis:**
  - **Alkalemia** is a decrease in [H⁺] or increase in [HCO_3^-] that increases the pH above normal levels (> 7.45).
  - **Alkalosis** describes the specific physiologic derangement responsible for a higher than normal pH.

Acid-Base Homeostasis: The Kidney

Through a variety of mechanisms, the kidney is the primary regulator of [H⁺] and [HCO_3^-] in the serum over the long term. Since renal compensation occurs through chemical buffers under hormonal control, renal-mediated changes in serum pH develop relatively slowly (eg, over hours to days).

- **Renal production of H⁺ and HCO_3^-:** Proximal and distal tubule cells contain intracellular carbonic anhydrase that produces H⁺ and HCO_3^- from CO_2 and H_2O via the intermediate H_2CO_3.
- **Secretion of H⁺:** The H⁺ may be secreted as either titratable acid ($H_2PO_4^-$) or ammonium (NH_4^+).

- **Secretion as $H_2PO_4^-$:** Excretion of H^+ as titratable acid depends on the amount of urinary buffer (phosphate) present, as well as the pK_a of that buffer. HPO_4^{2-} is relatively abundant and has a favorable pK_a (6.80), making it the major urinary buffer. Once H^+ is secreted, it combines with HPO_4^{2-}, resulting in a net secretion of H^+. This accounts for the minimum pH of urine being lower than that of serum, approximately 4.5.
- **Secretion as NH_4^+:** This mechanism is a function of the amount of ammonia synthesized (from glutamine) by renal tubular cells. Secretion of NH_3 depends largely on urine pH. The lower the pH, the greater the excretion of H^+ as NH_4^+. In states of **acidosis,** there is a compensatory increase in this process in order to increase H^+ excretion.
- **Reabsorption of HCO_3^-:** Reabsorption of bicarbonate is regulated by P_{CO_2} and ECF volume. Decreased ECF volume stimulates the RAAS to produce angiotensin II, which stimulates the Na^+–H^+ exchange pump in the PCT. This in turn leads to an increase in HCO_3^- reabsorption and eventual **contraction alkalosis.** On the other hand, increased ECF volume causes decreased HCO_3^- reabsorption and **dilutional acidosis.**

Acid-Base Homeostasis: The Lungs

The lung is also a primary regulator of acid-base homeostasis. Although altered ventilatory states may be responsible for primary derangements, they may also compensate for primary metabolic derangements. Variations in ventilatory rate can change the serum pH within minutes. Therefore, the respiratory system is responsible for acid-base homeostasis in the acute setting.

- **Compensation states:** Metabolic derangements resulting in an abnormal $[HCO_3^-]$ are followed by a compensatory change in respiratory rate, which affects the carbon dioxide concentration.
  - **Metabolic alkalosis** ($\uparrow HCO_3^-$) → **decreased respiratory rate,** promoting retention of CO_2 and a decrease in pH toward the normal range.
  - **Metabolic acidosis** ($\downarrow HCO_3^-$) → **increased respiratory rate,** decreased CO_2, and an increase in pH toward the normal range.
- **Derangement states:** The lungs may also be the primary cause of either a respiratory alkalosis or acidosis.

Metabolic Acidosis/Alkalosis

METABOLIC ACIDOSIS

Occurs secondary to either a loss of HCO_3^- or an excess of H^+. Conditions that lead to metabolic acidosis can be differentiated based on the **anion gap,** defined as:

$$\text{Unmeasured serum anions} = [Na^+] - ([HCO_3^-] + [Cl^-])$$
$$(\text{normal} = 10\text{–}12 \text{ mEq/L})$$

An anion gap greater than the normal range indicates the presence of an unexpected, unmeasured serum anion (eg, lactate in lactic acidosis). In elevated anion-gap acidosis, the concentration of an unmeasured anion is increased to replace lost HCO_3^-. In contrast, in normal anion-gap (hyperchloremic) acidosis, the concentration of Cl^- is increased to replace lost HCO_3^-. See mnemonic in the margin for typical causes of metabolic acidosis. A brief explanation of some of the less obvious causes follows:

- Hyperalimentation in this context refers to total parenteral (eg, IV) nutrition (TPN). Acidosis can occur in patients receiving TPN for a variety of reasons, including insufficient thiamine in the formulation or, more commonly, coexisting renal, pulmonary, and or gastrointestinal disease.

KEY FACT

Winter's formula gives the expected P_{CO_2} based on a measured HCO_3^- and is used to determine if the respiratory compensation for a metabolic acidosis is appropriate:

$$P_{CO_2} = [(1.5 \times HCO_3^-) + 8] \pm 2$$

If the expected P_{CO_2} corresponds with the measured P_{CO_2}, then the respiratory compensation is adequate.

MNEMONIC

Anion-gap acidosis: **MUDPILES** vs. nongap (hyperchloremic) acidosis: **HARDUP**

High anion gap	Normal anion gap
Methanol	**H**yperalimentation
Uremia	**A**cetazolamide
Diabetic ketoacidosis	**R**enal tubular acidosis (Table 8-10)
Phenformin, **P**araldehyde	**D**iarrhea
Isoniazid, **I**nfection, **I**ron	**U**reteroenteric shunt
Lactic acidosis	**P**ancreatic fistula
Ethylene glycol, **E**thanol	
Salicylates	

TABLE 8-10. **Characteristics of the Different Renal Tubular Acidoses**

	Type 1	Type 2	Type 4
Defect	↓ Distal acid secretion by α-intercalated cells	↓ Proximal tubular cell HCO_3^- reabsorption	↓ Aldosterone effect
Plasma K^+	Variable	↓	↑ (cardinal feature)
Plasma HCO_3^-	Variable	12–20 mEq/L	> 17 mEq/L
Urine pH	> 5.3	Variable	< 5.3

- Ureteroenteric shunts divert urine from the urinary system to the bowel. Contact between the intestinal mucosa and urine can result in reabsorption of urinary ammonium and chloride and HCO_3^- secretion.
- Pancreatic fistulas result in loss of the bicarbonate-rich pancreatic fluid.
- Severe infections can result in shock, leading to lactic acidosis.
- Iron poisoning, though exceedingly rare, can also lead to shock. Moreover, hydration of ferric ions (Fe^{3+}) generates protons ($Fe^{3+} + 3\ H_2O \rightarrow Fe(OH)_3 + 3\ H^+$).

METABOLIC ALKALOSIS

Occurs secondary to either a loss of acid or excess of base:

- Emesis (loss of H^+ leaves HCO_3^- behind in blood; hypokalemia).
- Hyperaldosteronism (↑ H^+ secretion and new HCO_3^- formation by DCT/CD)
- Diuretics (loop and thiazide) → "contraction alkalosis" (↓ ECF volume → ↑ renin → ↑ angiotensin II → ↑ Na^+–H^+ exchange and HCO_3^- reabsorption in PCT).
- Laxative abuse. (Because intestinal secretions ordinarily contain relatively high HCO_3^- concentration, diarrhea normally results in a metabolic acidosis. The alkalosis seen in laxative abuse is not well explained, but may result from hypokalemia.)
- Hypercalcemia/milk-alkali syndrome (repeated ingestion of calcium and absorbable alkali).
- Hypokalemia (↑ NH_3 synthesis → ↑ H^+ excretion as NH_4^+; transcellular H^+–K^+ exchange: H^+ into cells, K^+ out of cells).

Respiratory Acidosis/Alkalosis

RESPIRATORY ACIDOSIS

Occurs secondary to retention of CO_2. This can result from conditions that inhibit the medullary respiratory center (↓ respiratory drive), weakening or paralysis of the muscles of respiration, or decreased CO_2 exchange (Table 8-11).

RESPIRATORY ALKALOSIS

Occurs due to low plasma concentrations of CO_2. This can result from conditions that affect the CNS, the respiratory system, or from iatrogenic causes (Table 8-12).

KEY FACT

In primary respiratory acid–base disorders, changes in pH and P_{CO_2} occur in **opposite** directions.

TABLE 8-11. Causes of Respiratory Acidosis

Mechanism	Causes
Inhibition of medullary respiratory center	- Drugs (opiates, sedatives, anesthetics) - CNS tumors/trauma - CNS hypoxia - Hypoventilation of obesity (Pickwickian syndrome)
Weakening or paralysis of muscles of respiration	- Guillain-Barré syndrome, polio, ALS, MS - Myasthenia gravis - Toxins (botulinum toxin, organophosphates) - Muscle relaxants - Scoliosis, certain myopathies, muscular dystrophy
Decreased CO_2 exchange	- COPD - ARDS
Airway obstruction	

ALS, amyotrophic lateral sclerosis; ARDS, acute respiratory distress syndrome; CNS, central nervous system; COPD, chronic obstructive pulmonary disease; MS, multiple sclerosis.

Acid-Base Clinical Implications

The key points when approaching a clinical scenario involving an acid-base disturbance (Table 8-13) are the following:

- The lungs regulate the concentration of P_{CO_2}.
- The kidneys regulate the concentration of HCO_3^-.
- Compensation is never complete (eg, pH never returns to 7.40 unless there is a second acid-base disturbance).

Respiratory compensation for metabolic acid-base disturbances is essentially instantaneous. In contrast, it takes time for the kidney to compensate for a primary respiratory disorder by excreting or retaining HCO_3^-. Thus, for primary respiratory derangements, the next step in analysis is to determine whether

TABLE 8-12. Causes of Respiratory Alkalosis

Mechanism	Causes
Central	- Head trauma - Stroke - Anxiety, stress, hyperventilation - Drugs (salicylate intoxication) - Certain endogenous compounds (eg, progesterone in pregnancy)
Pulmonary	- Pulmonary embolism - Asthma - Pneumonia - High altitude
Iatrogenic	- Increased respiratory rate while on controlled ventilation

TABLE 8-13.   Summary of Primary Acid–Base Disturbances

DISORDER	P_{CO_2}	+	H_2O	$\leftrightarrow$	H^+	+	HCO_3^-	RESPIRATORY COMPENSATION	RENAL COMPENSATION
Metabolic acidosis	↓				↑		⇓	Hyperventilation	↑ [H$^+$] excretion ↑ [HCO$_3^-$] reabsorption ↓ 1.2 mm Hg in P$_{CO_2}$ for every ↓ 1 mEq/L in [HCO$_3^-$]
Metabolic alkalosis	↑				↓		⇑	Hypoventilation	↓ [H$^+$] excretion ↓ [HCO$_3^-$] reabsorption ↑ 0.7 mm Hg in P$_{CO_2}$ for every ↑ 1 mEq/L in [HCO$_3^-$]
Respiratory acidosis	⇑				↑		↑^{a}	None	↑ [H$^+$] excretion ↑ [HCO$_3^-$] reabsorption ↑ 1 mEq/L in [HCO$_3^-$] for every ↑ 10 mm Hg in P$_{CO_2}$ (acute—ICF buffering) ↑ 3.5 mEq/L in [HCO$_3^-$] for every ↑ 10 mm Hg in P$_{CO_2}$ (chronic—renal compensation)
Respiratory alkalosis	⇓				↓		↓	None	↓ [H$^+$] excretion ↓ [HCO$_3^-$] reabsorption ↓ 2 mEq/L in [HCO$_3^-$] for every ↓ 10 mm Hg in P$_{CO_2}$ (acute – ICF buffering) ↓ 5 mEq/L in [HCO$_3^-$] for every ↓ 10 mm Hg in P$_{CO_2}$ (chronic—renal compensation)

⇑ or ⇓ — Primary disturbance.

↑ or ↓ = Effect of primary disturbance or compensation.

^{a}May be unchanged or slightly lower according to the Henderson-Hasselbalch equation:

$pH = 6.1 + \log [HCO_3^-]/[CO_2]$ Normal $[HCO_3^-]/[CO_2] = 20$.

the disturbance is an acute (ICF buffering only) or chronic (ICF buffering + renal compensation) process:

- For respiratory acidosis, we expect:
  - ↑ 1 mEq/L in [HCO$_3^-$] for every ↑ 10 mm Hg in P$_{CO_2}$ (acute—ICF buffering).
  - ↑ 3.5 mEq/L in [HCO$_3^-$] for every ↑ 10 mm Hg in P$_{CO_2}$ (chronic—renal compensation).
- For respiratory alkalosis, we expect:
  - ↓ 2 mEq/L in [HCO$_3^-$] for every ↓ 10 mm Hg in P$_{CO_2}$ (acute—ICF buffering).
  - ↓ 5 mEq/L in [HCO$_3^-$] for every ↓ 10 mm Hg in P$_{CO_2}$ (chronic—renal compensation).
- If the compensation is not appropriate, there must be another process occurring simultaneously. That is, a **mixed acid-base disorder** exists.

Signs of mixed disorders include:

- In general, suspect mixed disorders when the values observed differ substantially from those expected.

CLINICAL CORRELATION

Acidemia (pH < 7.35) produced by a primary respiratory acidosis is characterized by P$_{CO_2}$ > 40 mm Hg.

Acidemia (pH < 7.35) produced by a primary metabolic acidosis results in P$_{CO_2}$ < 40 mm Hg (respiratory compensation).

Alkalemia (pH > 7.45) produced by a primary respiratory alkalosis is characterized by P$_{CO_2}$ < 40 mm Hg.

Alkalemia (pH > 7.45) produced by a primary metabolic alkalosis results in P$_{CO_2}$ > 40 mm Hg (respiratory compensation).

- Marked change in P_{CO_2} and $[HCO_3^-]$ with little change in pH, implying offsetting abnormalities.

If a **mixed disorder** that includes an **elevated anion gap metabolic acidosis** is suspected, calculate the deviation of the anion gap from normal and the deviation of the $[HCO_3^-]$ from normal. Use these two computed values to perform **delta-delta analysis** as shown:

$$\Delta \text{ Anion gap (AG)} = \text{Calculated AG} - 12$$
$$\Delta [HCO_3^-] = 24 - \text{Measured } [HCO_3^-]$$

The delta-delta ratio is defined as

$$\Delta/\Delta = \Delta \text{ AG} / \Delta [HCO_3^-]$$

and can be interpreted using the following criteria:

- $\Delta/\Delta < 1 \rightarrow$ elevated-AG metabolic acidosis + non-AG metabolic acidosis.
- $1 < \Delta/\Delta < 2 \rightarrow$ elevated-AG metabolic acidosis **only.**
- $\Delta/\Delta > 2 \rightarrow$ elevated-AG metabolic acidosis + metabolic alkalosis.

An overview for approaching acid-base disturbances is provided in Table 8-13 and Figure 8-24.

ACID-BASE NOMOGRAM

The acid-base nomogram is a quick reference tool that can be used during clinical rotations (Figure 8-25).

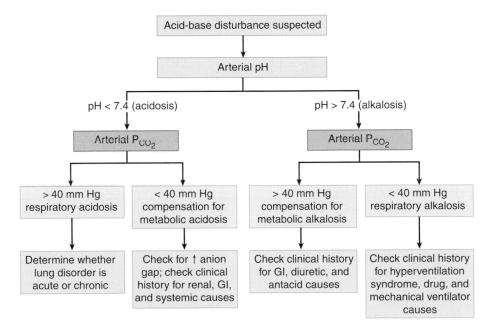

FIGURE 8-24. Flowchart describing simplified acid–base analysis. (Reproduced with permission from Stobo JD et al, ed. *The Principles and Practice of Medicine,* 23rd ed. Originally published by Appleton & Lange. Copyright © 1996 by Appleton & Lange.)

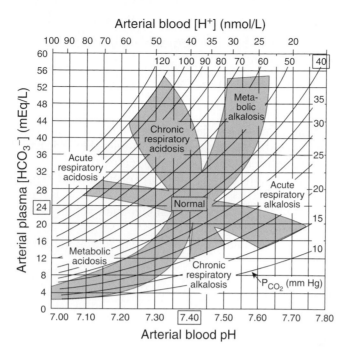

FIGURE 8-25. Acid–base (Davenport) nomogram. Note that the center of the diagram is detailed in Figure 8-26. (Modified with permission from Ganong WF. *Review of Medical Physiology*, 22nd ed. New York: McGraw-Hill, 2005: 734.)

Although the acid-base nomogram is an indispensable clinical tool, it is practically impossible to memorize for test purposes. Figure 8-26 provides a simplified version depicting the center of the nomogram. Knowing this basic setup enables you to answer the simple acid-base problems very quickly. It also helps to narrow down your answers if you do not know where to start with a more complicated mixed disorder.

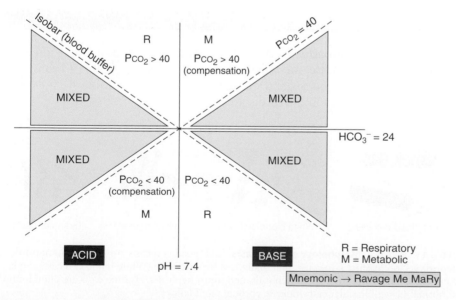

FIGURE 8-26. Center of the Davenport acid–base nomogram, simplified approach. To read this chart: Compensation is always toward the middle (eg, back to normal: pH = 7.4, $HCO_3^- = 24$, $P_{CO_2} = 40$.) Upper left octant (R) = respiratory acidosis; bottom left octant (M) = metabolic acidosis; upper right octant (M) = metabolic alkalosis; bottom right octant (R) = respiratory alkalosis. Everything in the middle octants = mixed respiratory/metabolic.

Acid-Base Problem Solving

Another approach to acid-base problem solving involves performing the same six steps for every problem:

1. Clinical scenario: What might you expect from the clinical information? (eg, loss of HCO_3^- in diarrhea vs. loss of H^+ in vomiting).
2. pH: above or below 7.4?
3. What is primary acid-base disturbance? Compare patterns of HCO_3^- above/below 24 and PCO_2 above/below 40 (eg, pH 7.25, HCO_3^- 18, PCO_2 28 is a pattern consistent with metabolic acidosis).
4. Is there compensation for the primary disturbance? (eg, in metabolic acidosis, expected $PCO_2 = 1.5 \times HCO_3^- + 8 +/- 2 = 1.5(18) + 8 +/- 2 = 33-37$). Expected PCO_2 of 33–37 is higher than actual PCO_2 of 28, thus a respiratory alkalosis is also present.
5. Anion gap: If over 20, then a high anion gap metabolic acidosis is present; consider etiologies.
6. $\Delta/\Delta = \Delta AG / \Delta [HCO_3^-]$: Look for additional metabolic alkalosis or non-gap metabolic acidosis.

KEY FACT

Presence of red blood cell or white blood cell casts indicates that hematuria or pyuria is of renal origin.

FLASH BACK

Type II hypersensitivity: Antiglomerular basement membrane (GBM) diseases (see Table 6-14 in *First Aid for the Basic Sciences: General Principles*); linear deposits of immunoglobulin G (IgG) along the GBM; consider Goodpasture syndrome and type I rapidly progressive glomerulonephritis (RPGN).

Pathology

URINARY CASTS

Casts seen on urinalysis can be an indication of tubular pathology (Figure 8-27). **Cellular casts** are formed within the tubular lumen; hence, their presence indicates that the disease process is of renal origin. **Hyaline casts,** on the other hand, are of little diagnostic significance. They can be seen in normal individuals and in volume-depleted states. All casts are made of a protein matrix primarily composed of **Tamm-Horsfall mucoprotein** secreted by renal tubular cells (Table 8-14).

GLOMERULOPATHIES

The term **glomerulopathies** applies to a group of conditions that affect the glomeruli. These entities are divided into two major groups (Table 8-15) based on their pathogenesis and clinical manifestations. Table 8-16 explains the nomenclature of glomerular disorders.

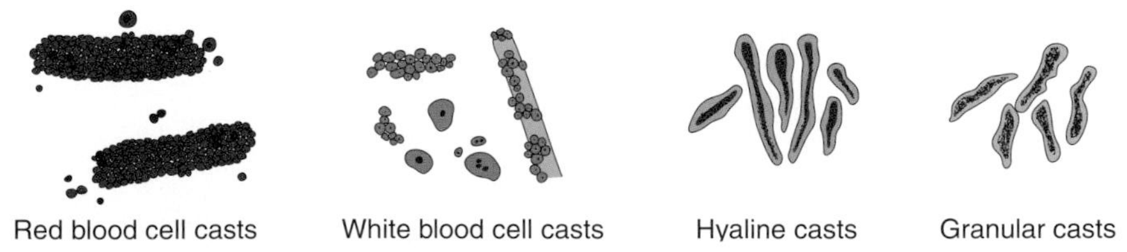

Red blood cell casts

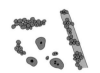
White blood cell casts

Hyaline casts

Granular casts

FIGURE 8-27. **Morphology of renal casts.** Red blood cell casts are seen in glomerulonephritis, Goodpasture syndrome, and malignant hypertension. White blood cell casts can be seen in pyelonephritis, interstitial nephritis, and lupus nephritis. Hyaline casts are often found in normal urine. Granular casts indicate chronic renal failure.

TABLE 8-14. Urinary Casts

Casts	Causes	Findings
Epithelial cell casts	▪ ATN, ethylene glycol toxicity, heavy-metal poisoning, acute rejection of transplant graft.	▪ Desquamated tubular cells in a protein matrix.
RBC casts	▪ Glomerulonephritis: IgA nephropathy, poststreptococcal glomerulonephritis, and Goodpasture syndrome. ▪ Malignant hypertension. ▪ Vasculitis. ▪ Renal ischemia.	▪ Clumps of dysmorphic RBCs with blebs and buds indicate RBCs are of glomerular origin versus bladder origin (eg, bladder cancer).
WBC casts	▪ Pyelonephritis. ▪ Interstitial nephritis. ▪ Lupus nephritis.	▪ WBC casts indicate inflammation in renal interstitium, tubules, and/or glomeruli. ▪ WBCs in urine indicate lower UTI.
Hyaline casts	▪ Often seen in normal urine. ▪ Pyelonephritis.	▪ Glassy looking. ▪ Composed of Tamm-Horsfall protein.
Granular casts	▪ ATN. ▪ Chronic renal failure. ▪ Nephrotic syndrome.	▪ Derived from the breakdown of cellular casts, especially epithelial cell casts.
Fatty casts	▪ Nephrotic syndrome.	▪ Fat droplets in hyaline matrix. ▪ **Maltese-cross configuration** due to presence of cholesterol (when viewed under polarized light).

ATN, acute tubular necrosis; UTI, urinary tract infection.

TABLE 8-15. General Division of Glomerular Diseases

Conditions That Manifest With Nephrotic Syndrome (Increased Filtration Barrier Permeability)	Conditions That Manifest With Nephritic Syndrome (Inflammatory Damage to the Glomeruli)
Minimal change disease	Acute proliferative glomerulonephritis (poststreptoccocal/infectious)
Focal segmental glomerulosclerosis	Rapidly progressive glomerulonephritis (RPGN, crescentic)
Membranous glomerulopathy	Anti-GBM disease Goodpasture syndrome
Membranoproliferative glomerulonephritis (MPGN[a])	MPGN[a]
Diabetic nephropathy associated with systemic disease	IgA nephropathy (Berger disease)
Renal amyloidosis associated with systemic disease	Hereditary nephritis (Alport syndrome)
Lupus nephritis[a]	Lupus nephritis[a]

[a]MPGN and lupus nephritis can present as either nephrotic or nephritic syndrome.
GBM, glomerular basement membrane.

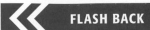

Type III hypersensitivity:
Granular deposits of IgG-antigen-complement immune complexes (see Table 6-14 in *First Aid for the Basic Sciences: General Principles*); consider poststreptococcal glomerulonephritis, type II RPGN, and membranous glomerulopathy.

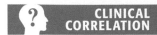

CLINICAL CORRELATION

In **nephrotic syndrome,** the excess fluid in the body may manifest as:
- Puffiness around the eyes, characteristically in the morning
- Pitting edema over the legs
- Pleural effusion
- Ascites

KEY FACT

High ratio of low- to high-molecular-weight proteins (eg, albumin to immunoglobulin) in the urine indicates **highly selective proteinuria.**

KEY FACT

Proteinuria (> 3.5 g/24 h), hypoalbuminemia, edema, hyperlipidemia, urinary fatty casts, and hypercoagulation are the hallmarks of **nephrotic syndrome.**

FLASH BACK

Patients with nephrotic syndrome are at increased risk of infection with encapsulated bacteria such as staphylococci and pneumococci due to the loss of gamma-globulins in the urine.

TABLE 8-16. Description of Glomerular Disorders

TERM	DESCRIPTION
Focal glomerulonephritis	Only a few glomeruli are affected
Diffuse glomerulonephritis	All glomeruli are affected
Proliferative glomerulonephritis	> 100 nuclei in affected glomeruli (hypercellular glomeruli)
Membranous glomerulopathy	Thick GBM but no proliferation
Membranoproliferative glomerulonephritis	Thick GBM with hypercellular glomeruli
Focal segmental glomerulosclerosis	Fibrosis of only a segment of the affected glomeruli
Crescentic glomerulonephritis	Proliferation of the parietal epithelial cell lining of Bowman capsule (forms a crescent)

GBM, glomerular basement membrane.

NEPHROTIC SYNDROME

This condition results from an **increased permeability** of the **glomerular basement membrane (GBM),** secondary to cytokines released by mononuclear cells. These cytokines induce fusion of podocytes and obliterate the negative charge of the GBM. Hence, in **nephrotic syndrome,** there is **loss of plasma proteins** (predominantly the low-molecular-weight, negatively charged **albumin**) in the urine.

Key findings in nephrotic syndrome:

- **Massive proteinuria** (> 3.5 g/24 h).
- **Hypoalbuminemia** (plasma albumin level < 3 g/dL) develops in part due to losses in urine. Albumin accounts for ~60% of total human plasma proteins and is the main mediator of the serum oncotic pressure. In the setting of massive proteinuria, the liver cannot keep up with albumin synthesis, leading to reduced serum oncotic pressure and edema.
- **Edema** develops due to lowered oncotic pressure, which leads to loss of fluid from the circulation into the interstitial space. Decreased intravascular volume leads to activation of the renin–angiotensin–aldosterone system (RAAS), increased sympathetic activity, release of vasopressin, and decreased atrial natriuretic peptide (ANP) release. All of these changes result in increased renal electrolyte and water retention, thereby exacerbating the edema.
- **Hyperlipidemia** and concomitant **lipiduria** result from an increased production of lipoproteins by the liver in an attempt to maintain the falling oncotic pressure. However, the liver is not able to synthesize sufficient quantities of lipoproteins to successfully counteract the edema. Furthermore, hypoalbuminemia triggers an increase in cholesterol synthesis by the liver through a poorly understood mechanism.

- **Hypercoagulability** secondary to loss of antithrombin III through the damaged glomeruli. There is an increased risk for renal vein thrombosis and other venous thromboses.

Many different pathologies result in a clinical presentation of nephrotic syndrome. The definitive diagnosis can only be made with a renal biopsy. However, each of the following disorders has characteristic symptoms and time courses that help to guide diagnosis and treatment.

Minimal Change Disease

Minimal change disease is the **most frequent cause** of nephrotic syndrome in **children** (> 80% of cases seen in those aged 2–3 years). It is so named due to the normal appearance of the glomeruli observed under **light microscopy.** However, **electron microscopy** shows fusion (**effacement**) of the visceral epithelial foot processes, thereby causing increased glomerular permeability. Minimal change disease is often preceded by respiratory infection or routine immunization.

Proximal tubules are often heavily laden with lipids secondary to increased tubular reabsorption of lipoproteins that passed through the injured glomeruli, hence, another name for this disease is **"lipoid nephrosis."**

PRESENTATION

Children between the ages of 2 and 3 years most frequently suffer from this disorder. Symptoms manifest as an insidious onset of nephrotic syndrome without any other obvious clinical disease (eg, no hypertension). The **proteinuria** is termed **"selective"** because primarily albumin (low-molecular-weight) is lost. Renal function is normally maintained, with only a slight decline in glomerular filtration rate (GFR) in 10–30% of patients.

DIAGNOSIS

As with all glomerulopathies, diagnosis depends on renal biopsy.

- **Light microscopy** (Figure 8-28): No obvious morphologic changes are seen in the glomeruli. Note the lipoid appearance of the cells in the proximal tubules (**lipoid nephrosis**).
- **Electron microscopy: Effacement** of visceral epithelial foot processes and increased lipoproteins in the proximal convoluted tubules (**PCTs**).

Definitive diagnosis of minimal change disease can only be made when nephrotic syndrome is accompanied by diffuse effacement of foot processes on electron microscopy.

TREATMENT

Initial therapy includes **high-dose oral glucocorticoids** (eg, **prednisone**) for up to 8 weeks. For those that fail to achieve lasting remission (defined as either relapse during steroid therapy, or recurrence more than three times per year after the steroid taper), **alkylating agents** such as cyclophosphamide or chlorambucil have been shown to be effective.

PROGNOSIS

In children, prognosis is excellent, with 90% of cases responding to treatment. In adults, prognosis is not as good, with only 50% responding to treatment.

KEY FACT

Minimal change disease is also known as **lipoid nephrosis, nil disease,** or **foot process disease.**

KEY FACT

Foot process effacement is not unique to minimal change disease. It is also seen in other glomerular diseases that present with nephrotic syndrome.

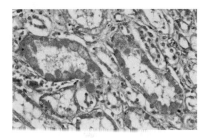
FIGURE 8-28. Histology of minimal change disease (lipoid nephrosis). Light micrograph. Note the foamy (or granular) appearance of the cells of the proximal tubules due to reabsorption of lipoproteins leaking through diseased glomeruli. (Courtesy of Uniformed Services University of the Health Sciences.)

KEY FACT

Minimal change disease is the most common cause of childhood nephrotic syndrome. Responds well to steroids. For this reason, many children with a typical presentation of MCD will be given a trial of empiric steroids without a renal biopsy.

KEY FACT

FSGS is the most common glomerular disease in HIV patients and manifests more severely in those patients. The glomeruli may appear collapsed, giving rise to the term collapsing FSGS.

KEY FACT

Children with minimal change disease = Selective proteinuria. Children with focal segmental glomerulosclerosis = Nonselective proteinuria; higher incidence of hematuria and hypertension.

Focal Segmental Glomerulosclerosis

Focal segmental glomerulosclerosis (FSGS) is considered to be a more severe form of minimal change disease due to the similar fusion of visceral epithelial foot processes. The pathologic lesion is sclerosis of < 50% of glomeruli (hence the name **focal**), with the sclerosis involving only distinct portions of the affected glomeruli (hence the name **segmental**). The cause is still unknown. This disease accounts for about 33% of nephrotic syndrome in adults and 50% of cases in African Americans.

PRESENTATION

Patients present with nephrotic syndrome. Unlike in minimal change disease, patients have **nonselective proteinuria** as well as **hypertension,** mild hematuria, and possibly decreased renal function. This disorder is associated with HIV and heroin use.

DIAGNOSIS

Definitive diagnosis is based on renal biopsy.

Light microscopy: Two distinct features are notable: **focal** accumulation of hyaline material and **segmental** sclerosis. Proper tissue biopsy is important because the prognosis of this disorder is worse than that of minimal change disease.

TREATMENT

Unlike with minimal change disease, only 20–40% of patients experience remission when treated with **oral glucocorticoids.** If there is no remission of proteinuria with steroids, **cyclophosphamide** and **cyclosporine** can be used at doses similar to those for minimal change disease.

PROGNOSIS

Generally poor, with approximately 50% of patients with this disorder developing end-stage renal disease (ESRD) within 10 years. Even following renal transplantation, there is a great risk of disease recurrence.

Diffuse Membranous Glomerulopathy

The pathogenesis of membranous glomerulopathy is not clearly established. However, immunofluorescence studies have led to a hypothesis of immune complex deposition, which is supported by its association with certain infections and systemic diseases. It is the **leading cause** of **nephrotic syndrome** in **adults,** accounting for 30–40% of cases in adults but less than 5% of cases in children. Peak incidence is from ages 30–50, and it is seen predominantly in men (2:1 ratio).

PRESENTATION

Insidious onset of **nephrotic syndrome** with **nonselective proteinuria** in otherwise healthy patients. Membranous glomerulopathy occurs in association with systemic diseases such as systemic lupus erythematosus (SLE) and rheumatoid arthritis (RA), infections such as hepatitis B and C, syphilis, schistosomiasis, malaria, and leprosy, as well as drugs such as gold and penicillamine.

DIAGNOSIS

Based on renal biopsy.

- **Light microscopy:** Diffuse GBM thickening due to subepithelial deposits nestled against the GBM.

■ **Electron microscopy:** Subepithelial deposits in a "**spike**" (extensions of GBM around deposits) and "**dome**" (deposits in the GBM) pattern. The deposits have been shown to be IgG and C3 using immunofluorescent staining.

TREATMENT

Given the high rate of spontaneous remission, only patients with severe disease should be treated with immunosuppressive therapy. Cyclophosphamide and cyclosporine when combined with glucocorticoids reduce proteinuria and slow the decline of GFR. Transplantation has been shown to be effective for patients that progress to ESRD.

PROGNOSIS

Remission is spontaneous in 40% of patients. Among those who received cyclophosphamide and glucocorticoid therapy, 40% undergo complete remission, 50% develop a chronic clinical picture with frequent relapses, and the remaining 10% go on to develop ESRD in 10–15 years.

Membranoproliferative Glomerulonephritis

Membranoproliferative glomerulonephritis (MPGN) can occur idiopathically or, more commonly, secondary to monoclonal immunoglobulin deposition diseases, autoimmune diseases such as SLE, chronic thrombotic microangiopathies, or chronic infections. There are two distinct types:

■ **Type I** (**two-thirds** of cases): Due to deposition of immune complexes (type III hypersensitivity). Associated with hepatitis B, hepatitis C, and cryoglobulinemia. Some cases have a **nephritic presentation.**
■ **Type II** (**one-third** of cases): Often associated with the **C3 nephritic factor** (**C3NeF**). It is also called **dense deposit disease**, due to the deposition of an electron-dense material between the lamina densa and subendothelial space of the GBM. Although C3 is present, there are no IgG deposits.

KEY FACT

C3NeF is a C3-convertase-specific autoantibody, which prevents its degradation. Sustained C3 activation results in low C3 levels, which is an important diagnostic feature.

PRESENTATION

Patients with **type I** disease tend to present with **nephrotic** syndrome, whereas those with **type II** can present with **either** nephrotic or nephritic syndrome, or a mix of the two.

DIAGNOSIS

Diagnosis is based on clinical presentation and renal biopsy. The disorder is characterized on tissue section by thickening of the GBM and proliferation of mesangial cells.

Electron microscopy: Generally the GBM appears to be divided by an electron-dense material.

■ **Type I** shows **subendothelial**, electron-dense deposits of IgG and C3. Ingrowth of the mesangium splits the GBM, creating a **tram-track appearance.**
■ **Type II** shows **intramembranous** deposits and increased size of glomeruli, as well as increased cellularity of the mesangial cells. The capillary wall often shows a double contour, or **tram-track appearance,** as a result of GBM splitting.

KEY FACT

MPGN = Tram-track appearance on electron microscopy and subendothelial humps (type I) or intramembranous deposits (type II).

Differentiation between types I and II is important due to differences in prognosis.

TREATMENT

There is no effective therapy for this disease, although plasma exchange with albumin has been shown to slow disease progression in some patients with circulating C3NeF.

PROGNOSIS

Differs between types I and II.

- **Type I** has a relatively benign course, with 70–85% of patients having no chronic decline in GFR.
- **Type II** tends to have a worse prognosis, with gradually deteriorating GFR. A majority of patients progress to ESRD after 5–10 years.

NEPHROPATHIES ASSOCIATED WITH SYSTEMIC DISORDERS

Many systemic disorders ultimately affect the kidneys. Specific diseases associated with nephrotic syndrome include **diabetic nephropathy, renal amyloidosis,** and **lupus nephritis.**

Diabetic Nephropathy

Diabetic nephropathy is the leading cause of ESRD in Western society, secondary to glomerular hypertension and hyperfiltration. The **first sign** of injury to the glomerulus is **microalbuminuria,** which occurs about 5–10 years before other symptoms develop (Figure 8-29). If untreated, microalbuminuria slowly progresses to nephrotic-range proteinuria. Nephropathy is generally more common in type 1 diabetes mellitus (DM-1) than DM-2, occurring in ~30% of cases.

KEY FACT

Hyaline arteriolosclerosis is a hallmark of DM; efferent arterioles are affected before afferent arterioles.

PRESENTATION

Typically, chronic renal failure (CRF) aggravated by glomerulosclerosis leads to fluid filtration abnormalities and a full spectrum of other disorders of kidney function. Cardinal symptoms include **hypertension** and **edema** (as a result of fluid retention). Other complications may include **arteriosclerosis** of the **renal artery** and the **efferent arterioles.** If left untreated, **nephrotic-range proteinuria** ultimately develops.

During its early course, diabetic nephropathy has virtually no symptoms. Late-stage diabetic nephropathy manifests as full-blown CKD.

DIAGNOSIS

Usually diagnosed on clinical grounds without the need for a renal biopsy. Should be suspected in patients with either DM-1 or DM-2 who have already developed evidence of end-organ damage from DM, such as retinopathy and neuropathy, and have dipstick-positive proteinuria.

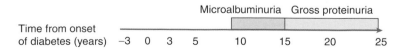

FIGURE 8-29. Time course of development of diabetic nephropathy.

Light microscopy: Thickening of the GBM and expansion of the mesangium. Classic **Kimmelstiel-Wilson lesions,** areas of nodular glomerulosclerosis, may be found (Figure 8-30).

TREATMENT

Treatment should be started for patients long before their symptoms have progressed to overt nephrotic syndrome.

- Patients who develop microalbuminuria should be started on **angiotensin-converting enzyme (ACE) inhibitors** (to counteract hyperfiltration), which have been shown to delay the progression of nephropathy in diabetic patients.
- **Good glucose control** with diet, exercise, and hypoglycemic agents has also been shown to delay the development and progression of symptoms.

PROGNOSIS

Without adequate treatment, ESRD typically arises within 5–10 years following the development of nephrotic-range proteinuria.

Renal Amyloidosis

Amyloidosis is characterized by the deposition of fibrous, insoluble proteins in a β-pleated sheet conformation in the extracellular space of organs (eg, renal glomeruli). It is a **multisystem disorder of protein folding** and can be acquired or hereditary.

The two types that affect the kidneys are **amyloid L (AL)** and **amyloid A (AA)** (see Table 8-17). When immunoglobulin light chains lacking the β-pleated configuration deposit in the kidney, the disease is called **light-chain deposition disease.**

KEY FACT

Kimmelstiel-Wilson, or "wire-loop," lesions are pathognomonic for diabetic nephropathy.

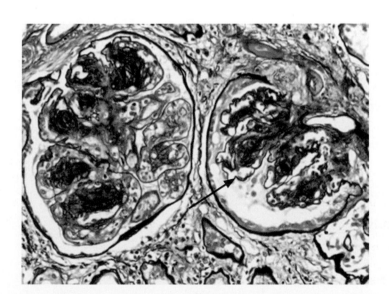

FIGURE 8-30. **Diabetic nephropathy, showing nodular glomerulosclerosis (Kimmelstiel-Wilson disease).** In the glomeruli, mesangial expansion and nodular glomerulosclerosis, so called Kimmelstiel-Wilson nodules, are evident (*arrow*). (Reproduced with permission from Kasper DL, et al, eds. *Harrison's Principles of Internal Medicine,* 17th ed. New York: McGraw-Hill, 2008.)

TABLE 8-17. Description of the Common Types of Amyloid

Amyloid Type	Description
AL	Derived from immunoglobulin light chains, eg, Bence Jones protein in the blood or urine is associated with multiple myeloma
AA	Associated with chronic inflammation, eg, RA, TB
Aβ	Main constituent of amyloid plaques in Alzheimer disease
ATTR	Found in familial amyloid polyneuropathy and senile cardiac amyloidosis
$A\beta_2M$	Derived from β_2-microglobulin, associated with long-term hemodialysis
IAPP (amylin)	Found in type 2 DM
PrP	Misfolded prion protein found in Creutzfeldt-Jakob disease

DM, diabetes mellitus; RA, rheumatoid arthritis; TB, tuberculosis.

PRESENTATION

Nephrotic-range proteinuria, severe edema, and renal insufficiency are common in renal amyloidosis. If amyloidosis is caused by a secondary disease (eg, multiple myeloma, tuberculosis, rheumatoid arthritis, etc.), the patient will also show signs and symptoms of the primary disease.

DIAGNOSIS

Definitive diagnosis is based on renal, abdominal fat pad, or rectal biopsy.

Light microscopy: Tissue stained with **Congo red** has deposits of amyloid that show **apple-green birefringence** under polarized light. In addition, mesangial expansion is present with amorphous hyaline material (amyloid) and thickening of the GBM.

KEY FACT

Congo red stain → Apple-green birefringence = amyloidosis.

TREATMENT

Some improvement has been shown with a combination of melphalan and prednisone. Treatment for **AA amyloidosis** is based on the underlying cause of the condition. Transplantation is an option for patients with both AA and AL amyloidosis, although extrarenal organ involvement may be a contraindication.

PROGNOSIS

Prognosis for renal involvement by **AL** is uniformly poor.

Lupus Nephritis

A part of the pathophysiologic spectrum of SLE.

PRESENTATION

During the early course of SLE, patients may or may not have symptoms of kidney disease. However, as the disease progresses, kidneys are almost uniformly affected, and patients present with either nephrotic or nephritic syndrome, or both, ultimately leading to ESRD. Most common symptoms resulting from glomerular pathology include weight gain, high BP, darker foamy urine, and swelling around the eyes, legs, ankles, or fingers.

DIAGNOSIS

Suspect development of lupus nephritis once a patient is diagnosed with SLE. Gold standard to confirm renal involvement is renal biopsy. According the World Health Organization (WHO), there are five classes of renal involvement:

- **Class I:** No evidence of disease, normal histology.
- **Class II:** Mesangial involvement.
- **Class III:** Focal proliferative nephritis.
- **Class IV:** Diffuse proliferative nephritis (most common type in SLE).
- **Class V:** Membranous nephritis, characterized by extreme edema and protein loss.

TREATMENT

Depends on the level of renal involvement:

- **Class I:** General SLE treatment.
- **Class II:** Typically responds well to corticosteroids.
- **Class III:** Successfully responds to high doses of corticosteroids.
- **Class IV:** Mainly treated with corticosteroids and immunosuppressant drugs.
- **Class V:** Attend to the general symptoms.

PROGNOSIS

Chiefly depends on age of onset and the overall systemic involvement and response to therapy. Lupus nephritis (especially classes II, IV, and V) ultimately leads to ESRD.

NEPHRITIC SYNDROME

The pathology of this condition is the result of **inflammation of the glomerulus** and **neutrophil-related injury.** Nephritic syndrome is characterized by a distinct set of symptoms:

- **Hematuria** secondary to destruction of glomerular capillaries and loss of RBCs into the Bowman space, resulting in dysmorphic RBCs and RBC casts on urinalysis.
- **Oliguria** secondary to the glomerular injury as a result of infiltration of inflammatory cells and immune complex deposition. This leads to obstruction of the glomerular capillary lumen, thereby decreasing the GFR and causing both oliguria (< 400 mL/day) and **azotemia** (increase of blood urea nitrogen [BUN] and creatinine).
- **Hypertension** secondary to the increased fluid retention by the kidney due to the decreased GFR. Mild **proteinuria** may be observed as a result of the glomerular capillary injury.

As with nephrotic syndrome, there are many different types of nephritic syndrome, each with a specific cause and presentation, yet all displaying the core nephritic symptoms mentioned earlier. The presumptive diagnosis is made through clinical suspicion, but the definitive diagnosis can only be made with renal biopsy. The cause of this condition is important, since as with nephrotic syndrome, it has implications for both treatment and prognosis.

KEY FACT

Hematuria, oliguria, azotemia, and **hypertension** are the hallmarks of **nephritic syndrome.**

KEY FACT

Proper diagnosis of different types of nephritic syndrome requires detailed history, serum chemistry, urinalysis, and pathology.

Important **serologic markers** to obtain when nephritic syndrome is suspected include **C3 levels, anti-GBM titer,** and **antineutrophil cytoplasmic antibody (ANCA) titer.** The corresponding patterns of these laboratory findings may obviate the need for renal biopsy in some cases.

KEY FACT

Poststreptococcal glomerulonephritis can follow either pharyngeal or skin infections, even if the initial infection is treated. In contrast, **poststreptococcal rheumatic fever** can only follow pharyngeal infection, and treatment of the initial infection can effectively prevent its development.

Acute Proliferative Glomerulonephritis (Poststreptoccocal/Infectious)

This form of nephritic syndrome most frequently develops following an infection with certain strains of **group A β-hemolytic streptococci (GABHS).** Pathogenesis is secondary to immune-complex deposition in the glomerulus with resulting complement activation and inflammation. Patients are typically children between the ages of 2 and 6 years due to the effective immunity one develops after infection, although adults occasionally develop this disease as well.

PRESENTATION

Classic presentation is **nephritic syndrome,** usually 10 days after pharyngeal infection or 2–3 weeks after skin infection with GABHS.

DIAGNOSIS

Effective diagnosis can be made based on history and clinical findings reflecting common nephritic symptoms.

- **Serum chemistry:** Antistreptolysin-O (ASO) titers or other streptococcal antibodies (anti-DNAase B) are elevated in > 90% of patients. C3 levels tend to be low; ANCA and anti-GBM antibodies are negative.
- **Urinalysis:** "Smoky brown" colored urine, RBCs and RBC casts, and in some instances proteins.
- **Pathology:** Renal biopsy if needed.
- **Light microscopy** (Figure 8-31): Hypercellular and enlarged glomeruli.
- **Electron microscopy:** Characteristic subepithelial electron-dense deposits **(humps).**
- **Immunofluorescence:** IgG and C3 coarse granular deposits, with a "lumpy–bumpy" appearance.

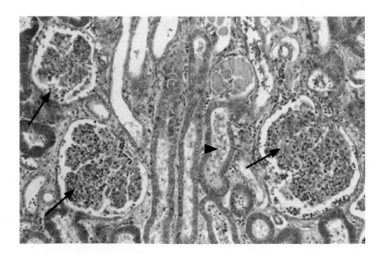

FIGURE 8-31. **Light microscopy of acute proliferative glomerulonephritis.** This low-power view shows three enlarged, hypercellular glomeruli (hypercellularity caused by proliferation of mesangial cells, endothelial cells, and global leukocytic infiltration in all lobules of the glomerulus) (*arrows*). Several tubules contain red cells and proteinaceous material (*arrowhead*). Mild interstitial edema is also evident. (Courtesy of Uniformed Services University of the Health Sciences.)

TREATMENT

Conservative therapy aimed at maintaining proper water and electrolyte balance. **Diuretics** and other **antihypertensive** drugs are used to control the hypertension and edema that may develop. Penicillin may be administered to eradicate GABHS. Although it does not prevent subsequent development of poststreptococcal glomerulonephritis, it does prevent progression to rheumatic fever.

PROGNOSIS

Excellent in **children,** with complete recovery when adequately treated. In **adults,** complete recovery can also be achieved, although the risk of developing RPGN is greater, as is progression to ESRD due to residual renal impairment.

Rapidly Progressive Glomerulonephritis (Crescentic RPGN)

RPGN is not a disease, per se, but rather is a malignant form of nephritic syndrome, in which progressive loss of kidney function occurs within weeks or months following the primary insult. The disorder is most common in adults aged 30–60 years and is slightly more common in men.

PRESENTATION

Classic nephritic syndrome; varies based on the underlying cause. There are **three distinct types of RPGN** (Table 8-18).

DIAGNOSIS

Effective diagnosis can be made based on history and histologic findings.

- **Serum chemistry:**
  - BUN and creatinine may rise rapidly.
  - Anti-GBM-antibody positive in association with Goodpasture syndrome.
  - ANCA presence varies based on the underlying cause.
  - Complement levels may be decreased in some cases.
- **Urinalysis:** Blood (RBCs), protein, WBC (monocytes), and casts.
- **Pathology:** Renal biopsy.
- **Light microscopy** confirms crescent formation (Figure 8-32). Crescents largely consist of proliferated glomerular parietal cells; Bowman space is filled with monocytes and macrophages. Large amounts of **fibrin** accumulate within the cellular layers of the crescents.

TABLE 8-18.   **Types of Rapidly Progressive Glomerulonephritis**

TYPE	DISEASES	IMMUNOFLUORESCENCE FINDINGS
I	Goodpasture syndrome	**ANCA-negative,** linear IgG and C3 deposits along the GBM
II	Poststreptoccocal GN, SLE, IgA nephropathy, Henoch-Schönlein purpura	**ANCA-negative,** granular "lumpy-bumpy" deposits
III	Wegener granulomatosis or idiopathic	**ANCA-positive,** no deposits on the GBM

ANCA, antineutrophil cytoplasmic antibody; GBM, glomerular basement membrane; GN, glomerulonephritis; SLE, systemic lupus erythematosus.

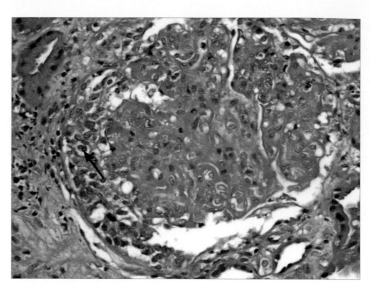

FIGURE 8-32. **Light microscopy of crescent formation.** Note the hypercellular glomerulus with a crescent of epithelial cells filling Bowman space (*arrow*), characteristic of RPGN. (Reproduced with permission from USMLERx.com.)

TREATMENT

Depends on the underlying cause.

Antiglomerular Basement Membrane Disease (Goodpasture Syndrome)

Disease characterized by **antibodies against proteins in the GBM.** Symptoms can be isolated to the kidney or may also be seen in the lung due to cross-reactivity of antigens (eg, α_3 chain of collagen type IV) that are common to both alveolar and GBMs. The underlying pathogenesis is based on a type II hypersensitivity reaction. This disease accounts for < 1% of glomerulopathies.

- **Goodpasture syndrome:** Both alveolar and glomerular symptoms occur.
- **Idiopathic anti-GBM disease:** Symptoms are isolated to the kidney.

PRESENTATION

Hematuria and other nephritic symptoms, subnephrotic range proteinuria, and rapidly progressive glomerulonephritis (RPGN) over the course of a few weeks is common. Pulmonary hemorrhage presenting with **hemoptysis** and dyspnea occurs in those patients with both glomerular and alveolar injury.

DIAGNOSIS

Gold standard is renal biopsy with immunofluorescence. Chest plain film shows bibasilar shadows in cases with pulmonary involvement.

- **Serum chemistry: Anti-GBM antibodies** are **positive** in > 90% of patients. ANCA levels are typically negative, but are occasionally mildly elevated. C3 levels are normal.
- **Urinalysis:** RBCs, RBC casts, and mild proteinuria.
- **Pathology:** Renal biopsy is the gold standard for proper diagnosis.
- **Light microscopy:** Cellular accumulation in the Bowman space; crescent formation.
- **Immunofluorescence: Linear, ribbon-like** deposits of IgG along the GBM as opposed to granular deposits characteristic of the immune complex causes detailed earlier.

KEY FACT

Hemoptysis and hematuria = **Goodpasture syndrome** or **Wegener granulomatosis.**

TREATMENT

Emergency **plasmapheresis** is performed daily until anti-GBM titers become negative.

- **Prednisone** and either **cyclophosphamide** or **azathioprine** are started simultaneously to suppress formation of new GBM antibodies.
- Patients are monitored frequently for rising titers of anti-GBM antibodies and receive plasmapheresis as needed.

PROGNOSIS

Without treatment, patients tend to develop ESRD within 1 year. When aggressive, immunosuppressive regimens are started early, > 90% of patients maintain renal function after 1 year. Although this disease is rare, the diagnosis must be made early to ensure appropriate treatment and good prognosis.

IgA Nephropathy (Berger Disease)

IgA nephropathy usually affects **children** and **young adults.** It is suspected to arise in individuals with an abnormality in IgA production and clearance (increased production of IgA in ~50% of individuals with this disease), leading to deposition of the antibodies in the mesangial matrix (Figure 8-33), which leads to glomerular injury and nephritic symptoms. It is the **most common** glomerulopathy worldwide.

IgA nephropathy can present as disease limited to the kidneys or as a component of **Henoch-Schönlein purpura.**

PRESENTATION

Episode of gross hematuria 24–48 hours after a nonspecific upper respiratory tract infection or GI infection. **Hematuria** typically lasts for several days and then spontaneously resolves, only to recur every few months. Hypertension is unusual at presentation.

DIAGNOSIS

Suspected in patients with new-onset hematuria within 1–2 days of either an upper respiratory or GI infection.

KEY FACT

The association of **Berger disease** with a recent mucosal infection suggests an exaggerated IgA response.

KEY FACT

Painless hematuria following infection suggests **Berger disease.**

FLASH BACK

Do not confuse **Berger disease** (IgA nephropathy) with **BUerger disease** (thromboangiitis obliterans), a vasculitis of small and medium vessels, which is associated with smoking.

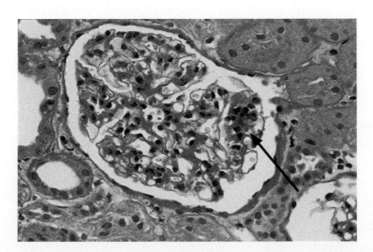

FIGURE 8-33. **Light microscopy of IgA nephropathy.** IgA nephropathy can have variable histologic findings, ranging from normal to overt crescentic glomerulonephritis. The glomerulus in this high-power view (periodic acid-Schiff [PAS] stain) shows mild changes consisting of segmental proliferation of mesangial cells and mesangial widening by matrix accumulation (*arrow*). (Courtesy of Uniformed Services University of the Health Sciences.)

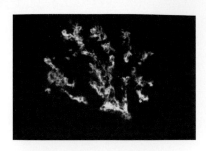

FIGURE 8-34. Immunofluorescence of IgA nephropathy. Immunofluorescent stain shows deposits of IgA primarily in mesangial regions. (Courtesy of Uniformed Services University of the Health Sciences.)

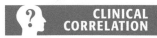

CLINICAL CORRELATION

IgA nephropathy associated with extrarenal symptoms is referred to as **Henoch-Schönlein purpura.**

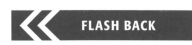

FLASH BACK

Henoch-Schönlein purpura's *extrarenal* symptoms include:

- **Skin:** Purpural lesions found on the extensor surfaces of the lower extremities, buttocks, and arms.
- **GI:** Abdominal pain, intestinal bleeding.
- **Musculoskeletal:** Joint pain.

KEY FACT

Male patients exhibit full spectrum of this disease: deafness, cataracts, and renal failure.

Female patients are carriers; symptoms are limited to mild hematuria.

- **Serum chemistry:** ANCA- and anti-GBM-negative, C3 levels are normal.
- **Urinalysis:** Painless spontaneous hematuria.
- **Pathology:** Renal biopsy.
- **Light microscopy** (see Figure 8-33): May range from normal to overt focal crescentic proliferative glomerulopathy.
- **Immunofluorescence** (Figure 8-34): Granular IgA deposits with specific distribution in mesangial cells.

TREATMENT

Glucocorticoids have been shown to be effective in cases of modest proteinuria. Patients with severe disease can be treated with plasma exchange and immunosuppression, or with high-dose immunoglobulins. ACE inhibitors and nonsteroidal anti-inflammatory drugs (NSAIDs) may retard progression to ESRD.

PROGNOSIS

Most patients have recurring episodes every few months or during mucosal infections. Between 20% and 50% of patients suffer ESRD after 20 years.

Hereditary Nephritis (Alport Syndrome)

Alport syndrome is a **hereditary form of glomerular injury** that is typically **X-linked recessive,** caused by an error in the synthesis of the α_5 **chain of type IV collagen.** This form of collagen is a major component of the GBM, and defects lead to renal dysfunction. Type IV collagen is also found in many other tissues, and therefore patients with this genetic defect tend to develop **nerve deafness, lens dislocation,** and early development of **cataracts.**

PRESENTATION

Patients are typically between 5 and 20 years old. Initially, Alport syndrome is asymptomatic. Later stages are characterized by chronic glomerulonephritis and systematic glomerular destruction, leading to hematuria and diminished GFR, and ultimately to ESRD.

DIAGNOSIS

Based on the following findings:

- **Serum chemistry:** ANCA- and anti-GBM-negative, C3 levels are normal.
- **Urinalysis:** Gross hematuria, mild proteinuria.
- **Pathology:** Renal biopsy.
- **Light microscopy:** Glomerular and mesangial proliferation. **Foam cells** may be present, which are interstitial cells with accumulation of lipids.
- **EM:** Splitting of the lamina densa (component of GBM).

TREATMENT

No specific therapy. Dialysis is used for patients who progress to ESRD. Renal transplantation is an option for those patients in renal failure, as allografts do not have similar genetic mutations so relapse does not occur. Because Alport syndrome is X-linked, this disorder is more severe in males than in females.

PROGNOSIS

Prognosis depends on the kind of mutation. Around 90% of patients develop ESRD by age 40. Patients with a large rearrangement of the α_5 chain of type IV collagen have a significantly higher chance of developing ESRD than do those with minor mutations.

Wegener Granulomatosis

Wegener granulomatosis is a systemic disease that presents as focal necrotizing vasculitis and necrotizing granulomas in both the upper and lower respiratory tract (lungs), in association with necrotizing glomerulonephritis. Renal injury occurs in up to 80% of patients with this disorder.

PRESENTATION

Patients typically present with **nonspecific symptoms,** such as fever, arthralgias, lethargy, and malaise. Renal involvement presents with **nephritic** symptoms and an occasional **mild proteinuria.**

DIAGNOSIS

Cytoplasmic staining ANCA (c-ANCA)–positive in 80% of patients with renal involvement.

Biopsy is required and demonstrates focal, segmental necrotizing glomerulonephritis with occasional crescent formation. Unlike in respiratory tract biopsies, granulomas are only rarely seen. There is a lack of immunoglobulin or complement on immunofluorescence, **anti-GBM** is **negative,** and **complement levels** are **normal.**

TREATMENT

Glucocorticoids and cyclophosphamide. Dialysis and renal transplantation are good options for those patients who progress to ESRD with little recurrence of the disorder in the allograft.

PROGNOSIS

Most patients respond well to treatment, although flare-ups occur in 25–40% of cases. A majority of patients suffer from long-term complications, such as chronic renal failure and hearing loss.

RENAL STONES (UROLITHIASIS)

Stone formation can take place anywhere in the urinary collecting system (most commonly in the collecting duct) and largely depends on sex, age, diet, climate, and genetic makeup. Their size can vary from crystals to large stones. They occur more commonly in men and in the summer due to insufficient fluid intake. There are several different types:

- **Calcium oxalate/phosphate stones** are the most common; followed by struvite, uric acid, and cystine stones (Table 8-19). They occur when calcium absorption in the gut exceeds excretion in the urine, or when there is a primary renal defect of calcium reabsorption. Less common causes are hypercalcemia secondary to hyperparathyroidism, vitamin D intoxication, and sarcoidosis. Calcium oxalate stones can result from ethylene glycol (antifreeze).
- **Struvite (magnesium ammonium phosphate) stones** occur in patients with persistently alkaline urine from urinary tract infections (UTIs) caused by **urease-positive** organisms, such as *Proteus vulgaris*, staphylococci, *Klebsiella*, and *Pseudomonas* (but **not** *Escherichia coli*). The urine pH is alkaline. When the stone creates a cast of the renal pelvis and calyceal system, it is referred to as a **staghorn kidney stone.**
- **Uric acid stones** are associated with **gout** or diseases that cause rapid cell turnover (**leukemia,** myeloproliferative diseases). They are more likely to form in **acidic urine.**

KEY FACT

Confirmation of renal involvement is necessary to make a definitive diagnosis of **Wegener granulomatosis.**

FLASH BACK

Chronic sinusitis, hemoptysis, and hematuria → Wegener granulomatosis.

CLINICAL CORRELATION

Respiratory involvement presents as paranasal sinus pain, drainage of bloody nasal discharge, hemoptysis, dyspnea, and/or chest discomfort.
Dermatologic, cardiac, and **nervous system** involvement can also be seen.

MNEMONIC

For Wegener, think **3 C's: C**-ANCA, **C**orticosteroids, **C**yclophosphamide.

CLINICAL CORRELATION

Alkalinize the urine to prevent uric acid stone formation.
Most commonly used agents are **carbonic anhydrase inhibitors** (eg, **acetazolamide**).

TABLE 8-19. Common Types of Kidney Stones

Stone Type	Frequency	Causes	Radiology	Appearance	Treatment
Calcium oxalate and calcium phosphate	Most common in adults (calcium oxalate) and children (calcium phosphate)	▪ Hypercalcemia: cancer, ↑ PTH, ↑ vitamin D, milk-alkali syndrome, idiopathic.	Radiopaque.	Colorless octahedron	Hydrochlorothiazide (to reduce hypercalciuria) Cellulose phosphate
Struvite (ammonium magnesium phosphate)	Second most common	▪ UTI with urease-positive bacteria (*P vulgaris* or *Staphylococcus*).	Radiopaque; stone creates a cast of the renal pelvis and calyceal system.	Rectangular prism, like coffin lids	Surgical removal Antibiotics to eliminate bacteria
Uric acid	Less common	▪ Hyperuricemia: gout. ▪ High cell turnover: leukemia and myeloproliferative diseases.	Radiolucent.	Yellow or red-brown, diamond or rhombus	Allopurinol Alkalinize urine
Cystine	Less common	▪ Cystinuria: genetic defects in metabolizing cystine, ornithine, lysine, and arginine.	Faintly opaque, ground glass.	Flat, yellow, hexagonal	Increase fluid intake Alkalinize urine

PTH, parathyroid hormone; UTI, urinary tract infection.

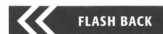
FLASH BACK

Tumor lysis syndrome can result in formation of uric acid crystals and stones. **Avoid ARF** by alkalinization of urine, allopurinol, and proper hydration.

▪ **Cystine stones** are seen in patients with genetic defects in the metabolism of cystine, ornithine, lysine, or arginine. They are more likely to form in **acidic urine.**

PRESENTATION

Kidney stones classically present with severe flank pain that **radiates to the groin** and is colicky in nature. **Hydronephrosis** and **infection** proximal to the site of obstruction can occur as a result of prolonged impediment of the urine outflow.

DIAGNOSIS

▪ **Colicky pain in flank radiating to the groin,** nausea, vomiting, patient constantly moves to relieve pain.
▪ **Abdominal radiograph** (Figure 8-35) is helpful in cases of calcium oxalate, calcium phosphate, and struvite stones (which are **radiopaque**), but are of no value for uric acid and cystine stones, which are **radiolucent** and cannot be visualized on a radiograph. Thus, noncontrast CT is valuable in diagnosing such cases.
▪ **Urinalysis** is likely to show hematuria.

TREATMENT

Mainly depends on the type and size of stones (see Table 8-19). **Increased fluid intake** and appropriate **pain management** while waiting for the stone to pass is sufficient for stones < 9 mm. Larger stones, however, require either a noninvasive approach, such as extracorporeal shockwave **lithotripsy** (ESWL)

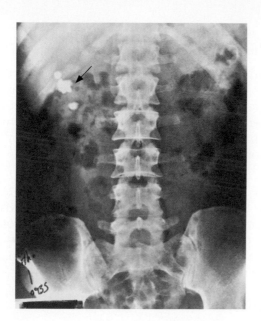

FIGURE 8-35.   Calculi (kidney stones). Note three separate deposits of calcified density confined to the right renal shadow (*arrow*). The largest one measures 2 cm in greatest diameter. (Reproduced with permission from Chen MYM, Pope TL Jr., Ott DJ. *Basic Radiology*. New York: McGraw-Hill, 2004: 204.)

or surgical treatment (**nephrolithotomy**). Prevention strategies include drinking more water, following a low-protein diet, restriction of oxalate-rich foods such as chocolate and nuts, and increasing citrate intake. Decreasing calcium intake is not advised, since doing so may lead to greater oxalate absorption.

URINARY TRACT INFECTIONS

UTIs are infections, usually bacterial, of the **lower urinary tract.** Common bacteria that cause UTIs include *E coli* and *Staphylococcus saprophyticus*. UTIs are extremely common in several different populations and settings:

- **Outpatient:** Especially common among young sexually active females and are thought to be due to the short female urethra and the small distance between the urethra and the anus.
- **Inpatient:** Very common, especially with Foley catheter use. *E coli* is the most common causal organism. *Klebsiella*, *Proteus*, *Enterobacter*, and *Serratia* are also common offenders. Likely to be asymptomatic. Have a high suspicion for UTI in any febrile inpatient.
- **Pregnancy:** Asymptomatic bacteriuria is common in pregnant women. There is a higher risk for UTIs to develop into pyelonephritis in pregnant women. UTIs also raise the risk for preterm labor and low birth weight. Bacteriuria in a pregnant woman should *always* be treated, whether or not it is symptomatic.
- **Children:** Children with recurrent UTIs should be evaluated for vesicoureteral reflux (VUR) and/or sexual abuse.

PRESENTATION

- Dysuria, frequency, urgency, suprapubic pain, and hematuria.
- In an uncomplicated UTI, there should **not** be fever, nausea, vomiting, or costovertebral angle (CVA) tenderness.

KEY FACT

Escherichia coli is the most common cause of UTIs in women, followed by *Staphylococcus saprophyticus*.

DIAGNOSIS

Can be made by history alone.

- Clean-catch urinalysis usually shows pyuria (PMNs in the urine), bacteriuria, leukocyte esterase, and nitrites (if caused by member of the Enterobacteriaceae family).
- Urine culture identifies the specific pathogen but is only indicated for inpatients, for patients who have failed antibiotic therapy, or for other complicated cases of UTI.

TREATMENT

Uncomplicated UTIs can be treated with oral antibiotics such as trimethoprim/sulfamethoxazole (TMP/SMX), ciprofloxacin, or nitrofurantoin. Around 50% of people recover without treatment within a few days to weeks. Ingestion of cranberry juice and urination immediately after sexual intercourse may decrease the incidence of UTIs.

Acute Pyelonephritis

Pyelonephritis is an infection, usually bacterial, of the upper urinary tract including the kidneys. Common bacterial causes include *E coli* and Enterococci species. It typically results from an ascending infection from the lower urinary tract. It affects the same populations as do uncomplicated UTIs but in much smaller numbers overall.

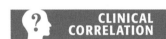

CLINICAL CORRELATION

White blood cell casts in the urine are pathognomonic for **acute pyelonephritis.**

PRESENTATION

Fever, nausea/vomiting, flank pain and CVA tenderness. Can occur in the presence or absence of typical symptoms of lower UTI (dysuria, frequency, urgency).

DIAGNOSIS

Based on history and physical exam, especially vital signs and CVA tenderness.

- **Urinalysis (UA)** and **urine culture** with **antimicrobial sensitivities** should be performed in all patients with suspected acute pyelonephritis because of the risk of serious sequelae if treatment is inappropriate. Urinalysis demonstrates **pyuria. WBC casts,** if present, are diagnostic of acute pyelonephritis.
- **Microbiology:** The pathogens responsible for pyelonephritis are the same as those responsible for uncomplicated UTIs.

TREATMENT

Oral or IV antibiotics such as TMP/SMX and ciprofloxacin.

Chronic Pyelonephritis

Recurrent or persistent infections of the kidneys ultimately lead to irreversible interstitial scarring.

Underlying factors leading to this condition are almost exclusively structural abnormalities such as **obstructions** of the urinary tract (eg, from stones or benign prostatic hypertrophy [BPH]) or **VUR** in children.

PRESENTATION

- May have asymptomatic pyuria.
- May complain of low-grade fevers, flank pain, and nausea/vomiting.
- May have evidence of renal insufficiency such as hypertension, proteinuria, or failure to thrive in children.

DIAGNOSIS

Based on the following findings:

- **Renal ultrasound** to evaluate for renal damage. A **CT scan** may offer additional information for diagnosing the underlying pathology.
- **Voiding cystourethrogram** can help diagnose VUR in children.
- Laboratory data may show **pyuria, proteinuria,** and **azotemia.**
- **Pathologic specimens:**
  - Chronic inflammation and asymmetrical corticomedullary scarring.
  - Deformities in renal pelvis and calyces.
  - **Thyroidization** of kidney.

TREATMENT

Antibiotics such as TMP/SMX and nitrofurantoin, and surgical repair of VUR.

DIFFUSE CORTICAL NECROSIS

Diffuse cortical necrosis (DCN) develops as a result of diffuse or patchy infarction of the cortices of the kidney secondary to ischemia. Often multifactorial and can progress to acute renal failure (ARF), especially in the third trimester of pregnancy.

PRESENTATION

Signs and symptoms of the systemic process (sepsis, disseminated intravascular coagulation [DIC], obstetric complications) resulting in cortical necrosis. Anuria, evidence of ARF, flank pain, and fever.

DIAGNOSIS

Based on the following findings:

- **Serum chemistry:** Azotemia, DIC (eg, low platelets, increased fibrin split products).
- **UA:** Proteinuria, hematuria, red blood cell casts, granular casts (derived from dead renal tubule cells).
- **Pathology:** Cortical necrosis, microthrombi of small vessels.

TREATMENT

Treat underlying condition.

PROGNOSIS

Reversible if treatment of underlying process is initiated early. Fatal if untreated.

RENAL PAPILLARY NECROSIS

Renal papillary necrosis results from an ischemic insult to the renal papillae.

PRESENTATION

Polyuria, rust-colored urine, ARF, flank pain.

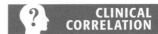

CLINICAL CORRELATION

Conditions associated with **DCN:**
- Abruptio placentae
- Eclampsia/preeclampsia
- Septic shock
- Hemolytic-uremic syndrome (in children)

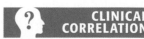

CLINICAL CORRELATION

Conditions associated with **renal papillary necrosis:**
- DM
- Acute pyelonephritis
- Chronic analgesic use, especially those containing phenacetin
- Sickle cell disease/trait

DIAGNOSIS

UA: Sediment, casts, blood, and necrotic renal papillae. Plain radiographs may show a ring of calcification (**nephrocalcinosis**), especially in disease resulting from analgesic use.

TREATMENT

No specific treatment. Treatment depends on underlying disease. Stop offending drugs if analgesic nephropathy is suspected.

RENAL FAILURE

Many conditions can lead to either ARF or chronic renal failure (CRF). Definitions of key terms pertinent to renal failure are provided in Table 8-20. The three main categories of renal failure are summarized in Table 8-21. Typical pathophysiologic mechanisms of renal failure are addressed in this section.

Acute Renal Failure

Abrupt-onset decrease in renal function as measured by GFR (not necessarily urine output). Leads to reduced ability to maintain serum electrolytes and excrete nitrogenous waste. ARF is classified as shown in Figure 8-36.

TREATMENT

- Maintain fluid and electrolyte balance and avoid nephrotoxic medications.
- Treat obstruction if indicated.
- **Dialysis** is indicated for severe uremia, hyperkalemia unresponsive to medication, metabolic acidosis, refractory fluid overload (usually presents as pulmonary edema), pericarditis, etc.

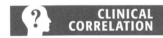

CLINICAL CORRELATION

Associated with **ATN:**
- Muddy brown casts
- Rhabdomyolysis
- Crush injury

Acute Tubular Necrosis

A disease state of the kidney clinically manifested as ARF and pathologically by destruction of tubular epithelial cells. Acute tubular necrosis (ATN) is an intrinsic renal disease and is the **most common cause of ARF**. It can be either ischemic or nephrotoxic in origin (Table 8-22).

TABLE 8-20. Renal Failure: Key Definitions

TERM	DEFINITION
Glomerular filtration rate (GFR)	The volume of filtrate that crosses the glomerular capillary membrane into Bowman capsule per unit time. Normal is 115–125 mL/min.
Azotemia	Elevated BUN and serum creatinine levels; may have causes other than renal dysfunction.
Uremia	Syndrome of biochemical derangement characterized by azotemia, acidosis, hyperkalemia, poor control of fluid volume, hypocalcemia, hyperphosphatemia, hypovitaminosis D, anemia, and hypertension.
Oliguria	Urine output < 500 mL/24 hours.
Anuria	Urine output < 100 mL/24 hours.
Polyuria	Urine output > 3 L/24 hours.

BUN, blood urea nitrogen.

TABLE 8-21.   Types of Renal Failure

VARIABLE	PRERENAL	RENAL	POSTRENAL
Urine osmolality (mOsm/kg)	> 500	< 350	< 350
Urine Na (mEq/L)	< 10	> 20	> 40
FE_{Na}	< 1%	> 2%	> 4%
BUN/Cr ratio	> 20	< 15	> 15

BUN, blood urea nitrogen; Cr, creatinine; FE_{Na}, fractional excretion of sodium.

PRESENTATION

Often asymptomatic; may have oliguria and azotemia. If left untreated, signs and symptoms of uremia and fluid overload develop.

DIAGNOSIS

Azotemia; $FE_{Na} > 1\%$ and **muddy brown casts** on microscopy (Figure 8-37).

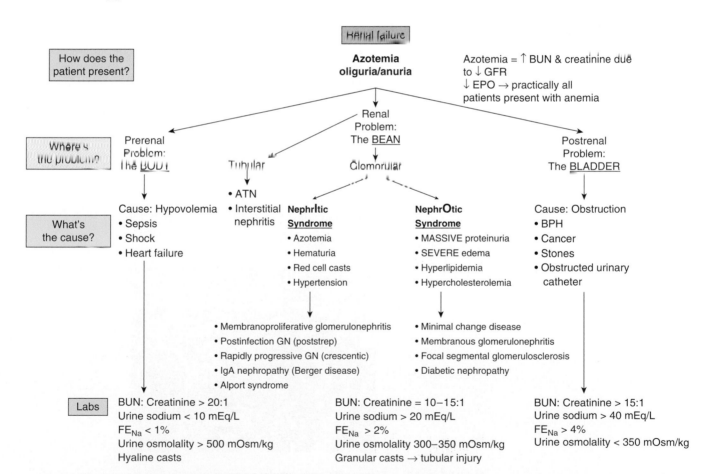

FIGURE 8-36.   Pathophysiology of renal failure.

TABLE 8-22. Common Causes of Acute Tubular Necrosis

Type	Etiology	Damage
Nephrotoxic	■ **Drugs:** NSAIDs, radiocontrast, cyclophosphamide, aminoglycosides, diuretics, and heavy metals (eg, lead, mercury). ■ **Disease:** Rhabdomyolysis, hemolysis, gout, pseudogout, and multiple myeloma.	■ PCT ■ Tubular basement membranes remain intact
Ischemic	■ Decreased blood flow to the kidney.	■ Straight segment of PCT ■ Medullary segment of TAL ■ Tubular basement membranes are disrupted

NSAIDs, nonsteroidal anti-inflammatory drugs; PCT, proximal convoluted tubule; TAL, thick ascending limb (of loop of Henle).

TREATMENT

Address the underlying disease, and remove the offending agent (medication, contrast medium, etc.). When rhabdomyolysis or crush injury is the insulting factor, large volumes of IV fluid are required to maintain adequate perfusion. Look for and treat electrolyte abnormalities.

Chronic Renal Failure

Also called chronic kidney disease (CKD), this disease is characterized by a substantial decrease in renal function, usually less than 20% of normal GFR, developing over a long period of time (usually > 6 months). CKD can be asymptomatic for many years, followed by increasing uremia and associated symptoms as GFR drops below 60 mL/min. Causes of CKD, all of which are chronic disease processes, are shown in Table 8-23.

TREATMENT

- Dietary management of protein and electrolytes.
- Dialysis (indicated when GFR ≤ 20 mL/min).
- Renal transplantation (cadaveric or living donor) when GFR < 20 mL/min.

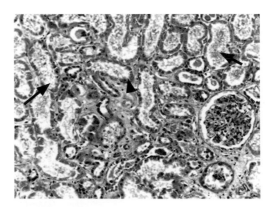

FIGURE 8-37. **Kidney with acute tubular necrosis.** Note the loss of nuclei (*arrowhead*), dilation of tubules, interstitial edema, sloughing of epithelium (*arrows*), and glomerular congestion. (Courtesy of Uniformed Services University of the Health Sciences.)

TABLE 8-23.   Causes of Chronic Renal Failure

	CAUSE
Prerenal	▪ Renal artery stenosis
	▪ Embolism (both kidneys)
Parenchymal	▪ DM
	▪ SLE
	▪ Hypertension
	▪ Amyloidosis
	▪ Chronic glomerulonephritis
	▪ Chronic tubulointerstitial nephritis
	▪ Adult polycystic kidney disease
	▪ Renal cancer
Postrenal	▪ Chronic urinary tract obstruction

DM, diabetes mellitus; SLE, systemic lupus erythematosus.

Consequences of Renal Failure

Renal failure results in multiple systemic consequences (Table 8-24). The primary effects of ARF are electrolyte imbalances and disruption of the kidneys' control of excretion. ARF typically manifests itself as uremic syndrome, hyperkalemia, and metabolic acidosis. CKD has more gradual effects on multiple systems, and the dysregulation of sodium and water can lead to **congestive heart failure (CHF)** and **pulmonary edema.**

CYSTIC KIDNEY DISEASE

Autosomal Dominant Polycystic Kidney Disease (ADPCKD)

PRESENTATION

An autosomal dominant disorder caused by mutations in PKD1 or PKD2. It is characterized by multiple cysts in both kidneys that destroy the intervening parenchyma. Patients usually present in their 40s with flank pain, intermittent hematuria, a palpable abdominal/flank mass, hypertension, and a positive family history of kidney disease.

DIAGNOSIS

A positive family history and bilateral kidney cysts detected by ultrasound. Liver cysts may also be present.

TREATMENT

Largely supportive, including antihypertensives, diuretics, and a low-salt diet. UTIs should be promptly treated with antibiotics. Treatment of ESRD includes dialysis and renal transplantation.

PROGNOSIS

CRF begins at age 40–60 and is the most common cause of death. Complications include refractory hypertension and urinary infection. There is an association with **saccular aneurysms** affecting the circle of Willis, leading to a high incidence of **subarachnoid hemorrhage.**

TABLE 8-24. **Consequences of Renal Failure**

Uremic syndrome	▪ Occurs as BUN rises; lethargy, seizures, myoclonus, asterixis, pericardial friction rub. ▪ Urea typically travels from the liver to the kidney, where it is excreted. The failing kidney cannot excrete urea and therefore the gut enzyme urease converts the extra urea into ammonia, causing **hyperammonemia.** ▪ Urinalysis: Isosthenuria (specific gravity of urine becomes fixed around 1.010, regardless of the fluid intake because the kidney cannot concentrate or dilute the urine), proteinuria, abnormal sediment with tubular casts.
Hyperkalemia	▪ When GFR significantly decreases, the kidney cannot excrete dietary K^+. ▪ Hyperkalemia → look for **peaked T waves on ECG, which can lead to ventricular fibrillation.**
Metabolic acidosis	▪ GFR < 50% impairs renal production of HCO_3^- so H^+ cannot be excreted. This causes an **elevated AG metabolic acidosis.**
Sodium and water retention	▪ **Early CKD** causes **decreased urine concentration,** which causes easy dehydration and sodium wasting. ▪ **Late CKD** causes **volume overload** as the kidney is no longer able to excrete sodium. This can lead to **pulmonary edema.**
Renal osteodystrophy	▪ Following hydroxylation in the liver by 25-hydroxylase, 25-hydroxycholecalciferol (25-(OH)-D_3) is then converted to its biologically active form, 1,25-dihydroxycholecalciferol (1,25-(OH)$_2$-D_3), in the kidney by 1α-hydroxylase. ▪ CKD causes loss of **1-α hydroxylase** activity in the kidney, thereby causing decreased vitamin D activation and increased bone turnover.
Anemia	▪ Failure of **EPO production** causes decreased hematocrit.
Hypertension	▪ Benign hypertension causes hyaline arteriolosclerosis. Malignant hypertension causes hyperplastic arteriolosclerosis, fibrinoid necrosis of the arterioles and small arteries, and intravascular thrombosis. ▪ Long-standing damage and scarring of the kidney from reflux nephropathy causes hypertension as one of the first indications of renal disease. ▪ Can be caused by APKD.
Fanconi syndrome	▪ Damage to proximal tubules compromises reabsorption of glucose, amino acids, phosphate, and bicarbonate.

AG, anion gap; APKD, adult polycystic kidney disease; CKD, chronic kidney disease; ECG, electrocardiogram; EPO, erythropoietin; GFR, glomerular filtration rate.

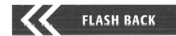
FLASH BACK

Expired tetracyclines can cause **Fanconi syndrome,** as can tenofovir and ifosfamide.

Autosomal Recessive (Childhood) Polycystic Kidney Disease (ARPCKD)

PRESENTATION

Rare, autosomal recessive, developmental disease due to mutations in PKHD1. Neonates present with enlarged kidneys at birth. Maternal oligohydramnios leads to Potter facies and pulmonary hypoplasia in newborns.

DIAGNOSIS

Ultrasound reveals enlarged kidneys. Disease can be diagnosed after 24 weeks in gestation in severe cases. Neither parent has renal cysts, which distinguishes ARPCKD from ADPCKD.

TREATMENT

No specific treatment. Mechanical ventilation, dialysis and blood pressure management may improve survival.

PROGNOSIS

Fifty percent of affected neonates die, and one-third of those who survive develop ESRD in 10 years. Patients who survive develop cysts in the liver and ultimately develop congenital hepatic cirrhosis.

INHERITED RENAL SYNDROMES

Liddle Syndrome

An autosomal dominant disorder characterized by severe hypertension due to gain of function mutation in the collecting duct epithelial sodium channel (ENaC). Excess sodium reabsorption increases ECF volume and causes hypertension.

PRESENTATION

Children are frequently asymptomatic. Adults can present with weakness, fatigue, and palpitations. Findings include **hypokalemia** and **metabolic alkalosis** with **hypertension**. Presentation is similar to hyperaldosteronism, but is independent of mineralocorticoids.

DIAGNOSIS

Persistent hypertension in the setting of low renin and low aldosterone. Genetic testing is available.

TREATMENT

ENaC antagonists, such as amiloride or triamterene.

PROGNOSIS

Excellent with blood pressure–lowering drugs and ENaC antagonists.

Bartter Syndrome

Rare autosomal recessive disorder due to mutations in any of the transporters of the thick ascending limb of Henle. Symptoms similar to those seen in patients taking loop diuretics.

PRESENTATION

Generally presents early in life with growth and mental retardation. Electrolyte abnormalities include **hypochloremic metabolic alkalosis, hypokalemia,** and **hypercalciuria. Hypomagnesemia** present in many but not all cases. **No hypertension.** Prenatal Bartter syndrome can present with **polyhydramnios.**

DIAGNOSIS

High renin, high aldosterone. Rule out vomiting and diuretic abuse. Genetic tests available.

TREATMENT

Potassium supplements and spironolactone to increase serum potassium. NSAIDs to reduce RBF and potassium wasting.

PROGNOSIS

With early treatment, prognosis is good and improves growth and intellectual development in affected children. In contrast, sustained hypokalemia and hyperreninemia can cause tubulointerstitial nephritis and result in ESRD.

Gitelman Syndrome

Rare autosomal recessive disorder due to defects in the thiazide-sensitive Na^+–Cl^- cotransporter in the distal tubule. Symptoms are similar to those seen in patients using thiazide diuretics. It is a more benign condition than Bartter syndrome and is often not diagnosed until late childhood or early adulthood.

PRESENTATION

Cramps and severe fatigue. Electrolyte abnormalities include **hypochloremic metabolic alkalosis, hypokalemia,** and **hypocalciuria.** Hypomagnesemia in many but not all cases. **No hypertension.**

DIAGNOSIS

High renin, high aldosterone. Rule out vomiting and diuretic abuse. Genetic tests available.

TREATMENT

Potassium supplements and spironolactone to increase serum potassium. NSAIDs to reduce RBF and potassium wasting.

PROGNOSIS

Prognosis for normal growth and intellectual development is excellent.

TUMORS OF THE RENAL SYSTEM

As with other neoplasms, tumors of the renal system can be malignant or benign, primary or secondary (metastatic). In this section, we address the most common malignancies of the kidneys.

Renal Cell Carcinoma

Renal cell carcinoma is the most common *primary* tumor of the kidney in the adult population, accounting for ~80% of kidney tumors (affecting men more than women, at an average age of 60–70 years). It arises from the tubular epithelium and can be sporadic (most common) or hereditary. Risk factors include smoking, exposure to cadmium, petroleum, gasoline, asbestos, and lead, and acquired cystic disease from chronic dialysis. Three common forms exist:

- Clear-cell carcinomas (80%) have **clear** or **granular cytoplasm** (Figure 8-38). Both familial and sporadic forms are commonly associated with an underlying genetic defect in the **VHL gene** (a tumor suppressor gene on **chromosome 3**).
- Papillary renal cell carcinomas (15%) have a **papillary growth pattern** and affect the proximal tubules. Familial and sporadic forms exist, with the underlying genetic defect being in the **MET gene** (a proto-oncogene on **chromosome 7**). Familial forms frequently exhibit **trisomy of chromosome 7.**
- Chromophobe renal carcinomas (< 5%) affect the cortical collecting ducts, stain darkly, and are characterized by **loss of an entire chromosome,** frequently chromosomes 1, 2, 6, 10, 13, 17, and 21.

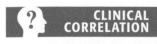
CLINICAL CORRELATION

Renal cell carcinoma can be associated with **von Hippel-Lindau disease (VHL).**

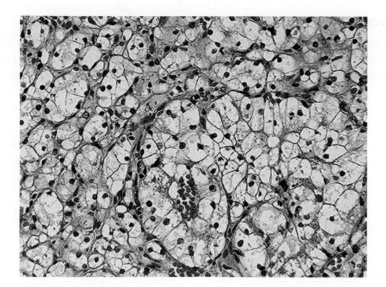

FIGURE 8-38. **Clear-cell carcinoma.** Histologically, the clear-cell variant is the most common type. The tumor has an alveolar architecture created by a prominent network of thin-walled vascular septae demarcating collections of tumor cells. Tumor cells have abundant clear cytoplasm. The nuclei are round and fairly uniform in appearance in low-grade tumors (as seen here) or may be highly pleomorphic and vesicular with prominent nucleoli in high-grade tumors. (Reproduced with permission from USMLERx.com.)

PRESENTATION

The classic **triad of clinical symptoms** includes:

- Painless hematuria (microscopic or macroscopic).
- Palpable flank mass.
- Flank pain.

But most patients will present without the full triad.

The cancer may spread hematogenously via the renal vein and interior vena cava (IVC) to the bones or lungs, causing bone pain or a lung mass, respectively. Invasion of the left renal vein can cause left-sided varicocele due to blockage of left spermatic vein drainage.

DIAGNOSIS

Ultrasound examination of the kidneys shows the presence of a mass. CT can provide precise information on the size and location of the tumor, as well as detect enlarged lymph nodes and metastases. The most common appearance of clear-cell renal carcinoma is an upper pole mass with cysts and hemorrhage.

TREATMENT

Standard treatment involves **radical nephrectomy** with removal of local lymph nodes.

- Partial nephrectomy/nephron-sparing surgery is commonly performed in cases of **VHL.**
- Additional treatments have included **interleukin-2** in metastatic disease.

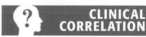

CLINICAL CORRELATION

Paraneoplastic syndromes associated with **renal cell carcinoma:**

- Hypercalcemia due to high levels of PTH-related protein.
- Polycythemia from excess EPO production.

KEY FACT

Schistosomiasis is associated with *squamous* cell carcinoma of the bladder, not transitional cell carcinoma.

MNEMONIC

Associated with problems in your Pee SAC:
Phenacetin
Smoking and **S**chistosomiasis
Aniline dyes (**A**romatic amines)
Cyclophosphamide

KEY FACT

Wilms tumor is associated with loss of *WT1* on chromosome 11 via a **two-hit mechanism.** Mutation of one copy of *WT1* in the germline followed by mutation of the second copy of *WT1* in the kidneys predisposes to tumor development.

CLINICAL CORRELATION

Syndromes associated with **Wilms tumor** include:
- **WAGR complex: W**ilms tumor, **A**niridia, **G**enitourinary malformation, and mental-motor **R**etardation.
- **Denys-Drash syndrome:** Gonadal dysgenesis, renal abnormalities (eg, mesangial renal sclerosis), and Wilms tumor.
- **Beckwith-Wiedemann syndrome:** Enlarged organs, hemihypertrophy of extremities, and Wilms tumor.

PROGNOSIS

Renal cell carcinoma usually metastasizes late and may recur years after the tumor has been removed. The prognosis is poor if the tumor has extended through the renal capsule or into the renal vein, with a 5-year survival rate of 10–15%. The best prognosis is with the chromophobe subtype.

Transitional Cell Carcinomas

Transitional cell carcinomas are twice as common as renal cell carcinomas and affect men more than women, frequently between the ages of 50 and 70 years. They arise in the urinary tract outside of the kidney, predominantly in the bladder, originating from transitional epithelium.

Bladder tumors are more common in people with exposures to β-naphthylamine, cigarette smoking, cyclophosphamide, and phenacetin (analgesic).

PRESENTATION

Painless hematuria with the risk factors mentioned and in the appropriate age range. Other presentations depend on the location of the tumor. If a ureter is involved or outflow of the ureters is blocked, there may be an obstructive presentation with flank pain, suprapubic fullness and pain, increased urinary frequency, and hydronephrosis.

DIAGNOSIS

Cystoscopy reveals the lesion within the bladder, and **urine cytology** shows malignant cells. **Pelvic CT** may help with level of invasion.

TREATMENT

Superficial tumors may be treated with transurethral resection and/or injection of chemotherapeutic agents, such as bacillus Calmette Guérin (BCG), into the bladder. More invasive tumors may require cystectomy with radiation or chemotherapy (or both).

PROGNOSIS

Tend to recur following treatment, but most low-grade recurrences can be treated with repeat conservative excision.

Wilms Tumor (Nephroblastoma)

Wilms tumor is the **most common** primary tumor of the kidney in early childhood (**between the ages of 2 and 5 years),** and is due to **loss of *WT1*** (a tumor suppressor gene on chromosome 11). **Nephrogenic rests** are precursor lesions associated with bilateral Wilms tumors.

PRESENTATION

Large, palpable abdominal mass that may extend into the pelvis. Hypertension results due to excessive renin secretion. Hemihypertrophy may be present. Tumors this size can also cause intestinal obstruction. Other presenting symptoms include abdominal pain, fever, and hematuria.

DIAGNOSIS

Abdominal ultrasound shows an intrarenal mass and any invasion into the IVC. **CT scan** (chest, abdomen, and pelvis) can evaluate for metastatic disease.

- Grossly, these tumors are **tan-gray with areas of hemorrhage and necrosis.**
- Histologically, there is a variable mix of blastemal, stromal, and epithelial cell types.

TREATMENT

Nephrectomy with chemotherapy (vincristine, actinomycin D, and doxorubicin if lung metastases are found). Abdominal radiation may also be used in selected patients.

PROGNOSIS

The aforementioned therapy offers excellent 5-year survival rates (> 90%).

ELECTROLYTE ABNORMALITIES

Electrolyte abnormalities (see Table 8-25) can be diagnosed with a standard laboratory chemistry panel and are frequently the manifestation of some underlying pathology. The common electrolyte abnormalities are discussed in the following sections.

Hypernatremia

Serum sodium level > 145 mEq/L.

TABLE 8-25.   Electrolyte Abnormalities

	PRESENTATION	CAUSES
Hypernatremia	Excessive thirst, **doughy skin,** and mental status changes.	Hypertonic saline, diuretics, diabetic ketoacidosis, and central or nephrogenic DI.
Hyponatremia	Headaches, nausea, muscle cramps, depressed reflexes, and disorientation.	Skin or GI losses, **SIADH,** water intoxication, and liver or heart failure; beware of **CPM** during correction.
Hyperkalemia	Palpitations, muscle weakness; peaked T waves, widened QRS interval, flattened P waves, ventricular fibrillation.	Lab error (hemolysis), renal failure, crush injury.
Hypokalemia	Fatigue, muscle weakness, hyporeflexia; flattened T waves, U waves, ST-segment depression.	Insulin, diuretics, vomiting, hyperaldosteronemia, hypomagnesemia.
Hypercalcemia	"Renal stones, abdominal groans, painful bones, and psychiatric moans." QT-segment shortening.	Malignancy, hyperparathyroidism, granulomatous disease.
Hypocalcemia	Muscle cramps, depression, tetany, convulsions; QT-segment prolongation; Chvostek and Trousseau signs.	DiGeorge syndrome (in children), hypoparathyroidism (following parathyroidectomy), furosemide, and vitamin D deficiency.
Hypomagnesemia	Often asymptomatic; anorexia, nausea, vomiting, lethargy.	Dietary deficiency; difficult to correct hypocalcemia or hypokalemia in the setting of hypomagnesemia.

CPM, central pontine myelinolysis; DI, diabetes insipidus; SIADH, syndrome of inappropriate secretion of antidiuretic hormone.

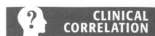

CLINICAL CORRELATION

Neurologic symptoms associated with **hypernatremia:** irritability, delirium, and coma.

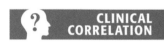

CLINICAL CORRELATION

Central pontine myelinolysis (CPM) develops as a result of severe damage to the myelin sheath of neurons in the pons. Most often caused by rapid correction of **chronic hyponatremia.** If the osmolarity of the external environment is suddenly increased, the neurons rapidly shrink, which causes myelinolysis.

Symptoms of CPM include sudden para- or quadriparesis, dysphagia, dysarthria, double vision, and loss of consciousness.

PRESENTATION

Excessive thirst, doughy skin, and mental status changes (confusion, seizures, and muscle twitching).

CAUSES

Most commonly, hypernatremia is due to a loss of free water versus a gain of sodium without adequate rehydration (due to impairment of the thirst mechanism or lack of access to water).

Specific causes include iatrogenic from hypertonic saline, medications (diuretics, lithium, or sodium-containing drugs), hyperglycemia in the setting of diabetic ketoacidosis, and central or nephrogenic diabetic insipidus.

TREATMENT

Treatment includes correction of the underlying cause and IV hydration with normal saline or lactated Ringer's solution. The amount of IV fluid to give is determined by the following formula:

$$\text{Free water deficit} = \text{Total body water} \times [(\text{Plasma Na}/140) - 1]$$

PROGNOSIS

Patients who becomes acutely hypernatremic have a worse prognosis than those in a chronic hypernatremic state.

Hyponatremia

Serum sodium level < 136 mEq/L.

PRESENTATION

The symptoms are largely manifested neurologically: headaches, nausea, muscle cramps, depressed reflexes, and disorientation.

CAUSES

To identify the cause of hyponatremia, it is essential to identify **serum osmolality.** Figure 8-39 offers an approach to identifying the cause of hyponatremia. Low serum sodium and low serum osmolality are most frequently encountered.

TREATMENT

Treatment of hyponatremia depends on the underlying cause, but if the patient is symptomatic, the administration of IV hypertonic saline (3% saline) may be indicated. Care must be taken to slowly correct the sodium level because of the risk that central pontine myelinolysis (CPM) may develop.

Hyperkalemia

Serum potassium > 5.0 mEq/L, making the resting membrane potential **less** negative and hence the cell **more** excitable.

PRESENTATION

Clinically, the patient may experience palpitations or muscle weakness. Potassium causes the heart to be more excitable (possibly leading to **ventricular**

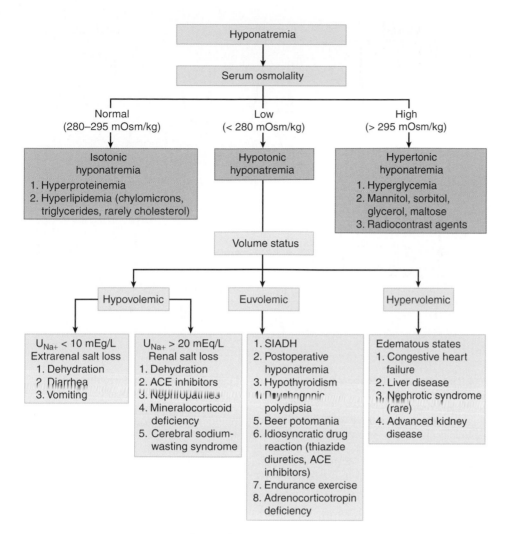

FIGURE 8-39. **Evaulation of hyponatremia using serum osmolality and extracellular fluid volume status.** (Reproduced with permission from Kasper DL, et al, eds. *Harrison's Principles of Internal Medicine*, 17th ed. Copyright 2008 © by The McGraw-Hill Companies, Inc.)

fibrillation) and the effects on the heart should be investigated with an **electrocardiogram (ECG)** (Figure 8-40A):

- Peaked T waves
- Widening of the QRS complex
- Flattening of the P wave

CAUSES

Most common underlying pathology includes renal failure or trauma due to extensive crush injury with release of potassium from muscle cells. Also common in diabetes patients as insulin facilitates potassium entry into cells.

TREATMENT

Treatment focuses on removing potassium from the body and stabilizing the myocardium (monitor the serum K^+ levels and ECG findings during treatment). The systematic approach to treating hyperkalemia includes:

- **Calcium gluconate** first to stabilize the myocardium.
- **Insulin** with concurrent glucose infusion (insulin ↑ cellular K^+ uptake).

KEY FACT

Lab error due to hemolysis of RBCs in the preparation of the specimen may provide false-positive results for hyperkalemia.

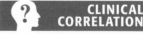
CLINICAL CORRELATION

Crush injury can cause renal failure, generalized edema, metabolic acidosis, ↑ nonprotein nitrogens normally excreted by the kidneys (eg, urea, creatinine, uric acid), and ↑ plasma ions normally excreted by the kidneys (eg, Na^+, K^+, H^+, etc.). The cause of death is usually **hyperkalemia → ventricular fibrillation.**

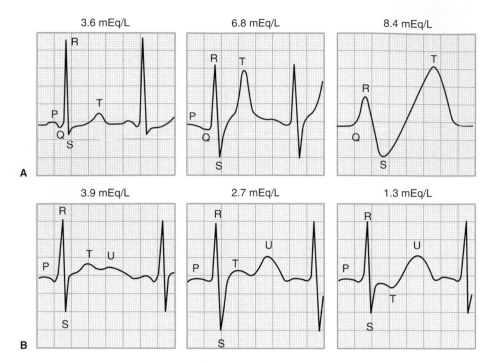

FIGURE 8-40. **Electrocardiographic effects of hyperkalemia (A) and hypokalemia (B).**
(A) Electrocardiographic changes characteristically progress from symmetrically peaked T waves, often with a shortened QT interval, to widening of the QRS complex, prolongation of the PR interval, loss of the P wave, loss of R-wave amplitude, and ST-segment depression (occasionally elevation)—to an ECG that resembles a sine wave—before final progression into ventricular fibrillation or asystole. (B) Note progressive flattening of the T wave, an increasingly prominent U wave, and ST-segment depression. (Modified with permission from Morgan GE, Mikhail MS, Murray MJ. *Clinical Anesthesiology*, 4th ed. New York: McGraw-Hill, 2006.)

- **β-Agonists** (drive K^+ into cells).
- **Sodium polystyrene sulfonate** (causes excretion of K^+ from the GI tract).
- Dialysis.

Hypokalemia

Serum $K^+ < 3.6$ mEq/L, making the resting membrane potential **more** negative and hence cell are **less** excitable.

PRESENTATION

Patients present with general, nonspecific symptoms of fatigue, muscle weakness, intestinal ileus, and/or hyporeflexia.

Classic ECG findings (Figure 8-40B) include:

- Flattened T waves.
- Presence of U waves.
- ST-segment depression.

CAUSES

Insulin, alkalosis, diuretics (loop or thiazide), vomiting (eg, eating disorders), increased aldosterone levels, and hypomagnesemia.

TREATMENT

Treat the underlying cause. Low-serum K^+ is treated with administration of IV or PO K^+. During treatment, monitor the ECG and plasma levels of K^+.

Hypercalcemia

Serum Ca^{2+} level > 10.2 mg/dL, increasing the threshold potential and thus cells are **less** excitable (acidosis has a similar effect).

PRESENTATION

Many patients are asymptomatic. Levels over 12.0 mg/dL may produce ECG changes (**shortened QT interval;** Figure 8-41), and more dramatic symptoms, such as renal **stones** (nephrolithiasis), abdominal **groans** (nausea, vomiting, constipation), psychiatric **moans** (delirium, psychosis), and painful **bones** (osteitis fibrosa cystica).

CAUSES

The most common cause in the inpatient setting is **malignancy** (metastases to bone or ectopic production of PTH-related protein), but the most common cause in the outpatient setting is primary **hyperparathyroidism** (adenoma > hyperplasia > carcinoma). Other common causes include hyperthyroidism, thiazide diuretic use, granulomatous disease (sarcoidosis), renal failure, and **milk-alkali syndrome.**

TREATMENT

Treat the underlying cause. If patients is symptomatic, hydrate with **IV normal saline** and give **furosemide** with consideration given to the addition of **bisphosphonates to inhibit bone resorption by osteoclasts.** In severe refractory cases, hemodialysis may be indicated.

Hypocalcemia

Serum calcium level < 8.5 mg/dL, decreasing the threshold potential and thus cells are **more** excitable (alkalosis has a similar effect).

PRESENTATION

Frequently asymptomatic. More severe symptoms occur at very low serum levels: muscle cramps, depression, **tetany,** and convulsions. **QT segment prolongation** is seen on ECG (see Figure 8-41).

?   **CLINICAL CORRELATION**

Renal stones, abdominal groans, painful bones, and psychiatric moans are classic findings for **hypercalcemia.**

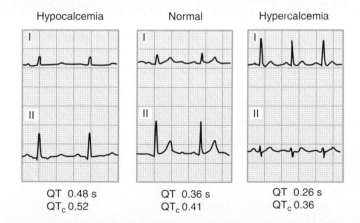

Hypocalcemia	Normal	Hypercalcemia
QT 0.48 s	QT 0.36 s	QT 0.26 s
QT$_c$ 0.52	QT$_c$ 0.41	QT$_c$ 0.36

FIGURE 8-41.   Electrocardiographic effects of hypocalcemia and hypercalcemia. Prolongation of the QT interval (ST-segment portion) is typical of hypocalcemia. Hypercalcemia may cause abbreviation of the ST segment and shortening of the QT interval. QT$_c$ is the QT interval corrected for heart rate. (Modified with permission from Kasper DL, Braunwald E, Fauci AS, et al, eds. *Harrison's Principles of Internal Medicine,* 16th ed. New York: McGraw-Hill, 2005: 1319.)

- **Chvostek sign:** Tapping the facial nerve results in twitching of facial muscles.
- **Trousseau sign:** Carpopedal spasm resulting from inflation of a BP cuff on the forearm.

CAUSES

In newborns and infants, consider **DiGeorge syndrome.** Hypoparathyroidism (secondary to treatment of hyperparathyroidism), pseudohypoparathyroidism, vitamin D deficiency, osteomalacia, rickets, and diuretics (furosemide).

TREATMENT

If the patient is symptomatic, calcium can be replaced via **IV calcium gluconate** while monitoring ECG. Less severe cases can be treated with **PO calcium** and **vitamin D.**

Hypomagnesemia

Serum Mg^{2+} level < 1.5 mEq/L.

PRESENTATION

Anorexia, nausea, vomiting, lethargy, and personality changes. Also look for hypocalcemia and hypokalemia in the setting of low Mg^{2+} levels because low magnesium decreases PTH release and increases efflux of intracellular K^+, which is then excreted.

CAUSES

Dietary deficiency complicated by poor absorption.

TREATMENT

Low Mg^{2+} is treated with magnesium replacement, usually magnesium sulfate.

Pharmacology

DIURETICS

Diuretics (Figure 8-42) are drugs that act to **increase urine volume** by altering ion transport in the nephron. A generally safe class, diuretics are **first-line drugs** in the treatment of **hypertension** and **edematous states** such as **CHF, nephrosis,** and **cirrhosis.**

Common side effects of diuretics (Table 8-26) are:

- Volume depletion.
- Hypokalemia (loop diuretics and thiazides).
- Hyponatremia (thiazides).
- Hyperglycemia (thiazides; opposite action on pancreatic β-cells as sulfonylurea drugs).
- Metabolic acidosis (acetazolamide).
- Specific side effects are discussed with each of the following drug classes.

There are **five main classes** of diuretics:

- Osmotic agents: Mannitol and urea (mainly in patients with SIADH).
- Carbonic anhydrase inhibitors: Acetazolamide.
- Loop agents: Furosemide, bumetanide, and ethacrynic acid.

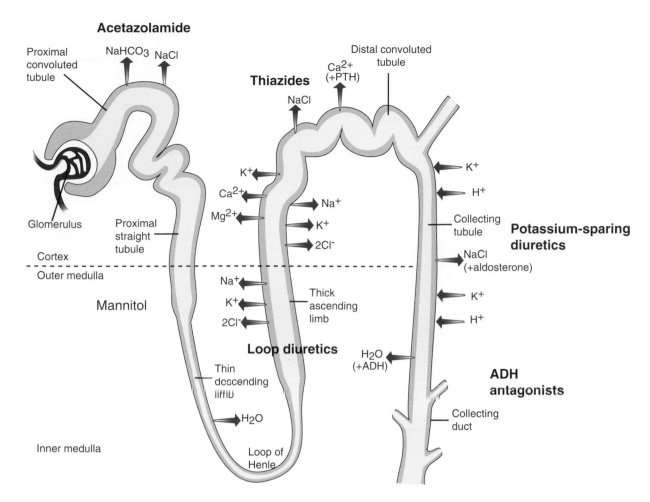

FIGURE 8-42. **Overview of diuretic sites of action.** (Modified with permission from Katzung BG. *Basic and Clinical Pharmacology*, 7th ed. Stamford, CT: Appleton and Lange, 1997, 743.)

- Thiazides: Hydrochlorothiazide (HCTZ) and metolazone.
- Potassium-sparing agents: Spironolactone, eplerenone, triamterene, and amiloride.

Osmotic Agents (Mannitol and Urea)

MECHANISM

Mannitol is filtered into the tubular lumen but not reabsorbed, increasing osmotic pressure in the lumen and retaining water in the urine.

USES

Reduction of intraocular or intracranial pressure, increases excretion of water more than sodium, urinary excretion of metabolic toxins.

SIDE EFFECTS

- Dehydration without adequate water intake.
- Increased ECF volume, leading to **pulmonary edema.**

Carbonic Anhydrase Inhibitors (Acetazolamide)

MECHANISM

Blocks carbonic anhydrase, primarily in the proximal tubule, preventing reabsorption of sodium bicarbonate and leading to diuresis.

TABLE 8-26. **Common Electrolyte Changes Seen With Diuretic Use**

CLASS	DRUGS	MECHANISM OF ACTION	ELECTROLYTE CHANGES
Carbonic anhydrase inhibitors	Acetazolamide	Inhibits carbonic anhydrase in PCT, blocks Na^+/H^+ exchange.	• Hyperchloremic metabolic acidosis ($\uparrow Cl^-$, $\uparrow H^+$) • Hypokalemia ($\downarrow K^+$)
Osmotic agents	Mannitol, urea	Increases tubular fluid osmolarity in entire tubule.	• Hypernatremia ($\uparrow Na^+$)
Loop agents	Furosemide, bumetanide, ethacrynic acid	Inhibits $Na^+-K^+-2Cl^-$ transporter in thick ascending limb of loop of Henle.	• Hypokalemia ($\downarrow K^+$) • Hyponatremia ($\downarrow Na^+$) • Hyperuricemia ($\uparrow urea$) • Hypocalcemia ($\downarrow Ca^{2+}$) • Hypomagnesemia ($\downarrow Mg^{2+}$) • Metabolic alkalosis ($\downarrow H^+$)
Thiazide diuretics	HCTZ, metolazone	Blocks Na^+-Cl^- cotransport in DCT.	• Hyperglycemia ($\uparrow glucose$) • Hyperlipidemia ($\uparrow lipids$) • Hyperuricemia ($\uparrow urea$) • Hypercalcemia ($\uparrow Ca^{2+}$) • Hypokalemia ($\downarrow K^+$) • Hyponatremia ($\downarrow Na^+$) • Metabolic alkalosis ($\downarrow H^+$)
Potassium-sparing agents	Spironolactone, eplerenone, amiloride, triamterene	• Spironolactone and eplerenone are competitive aldosterone receptor antagonists in the collecting tubule. • Other agents block Na^+ channels (ENaC) in the collecting tubule.	• Metabolic acidosis ($\uparrow H^+$) • Hyperkalemia ($\uparrow K^+$)

DCT, distal convoluted tubule; ENaC, epithelial sodium channel; HCTZ, hydrochlorothiazide; PCT, proximal convoluted tubule.

KEY FACT

Since it contains the sulfa group ($R-SO_2-NH_2$), acetazolamide is contraindicated in patients allergic to sulfonamides.

USES

Glaucoma (decreases production of aqueous humor), acute mountain sickness (stimulates ventilation via metabolic acidosis), elimination of acidic toxins (alkalinizes urine, leading to increased excretion of weak acids), and corrects alkalosis.

SIDE EFFECTS

- Renal stones (increases urine concentration of Ca^{2+} and phosphates).
- Potassium wasting (increased HCO_3^- in tubules attracts K^+).
- Hyperchloremic metabolic acidosis.

Loop Agents (Furosemide, Bumetanide, and Ethacrynic Acid)

MECHANISM

Inhibit $Na^+-K^+-2Cl^-$ transporter in thick ascending limb. Decreases positive luminal potential, leading to increased excretion of calcium and magnesium.

USES

Treatment of acute pulmonary or other edema, hypercalcemia, hyperkalemia, hypertension, and ARF.

SIDE EFFECTS

- Hypokalemic metabolic alkalosis.
- Ototoxicity.
- Hyperuricemia.
- Hypomagnesemia.
- Severe dehydration.
- Allergic reactions (all loop diuretics are sulfonamide derivatives except ethacrynic acid).

Thiazide Diuretics (Hydrochlorothiazide [HCTZ] and Metolazone)

MECHANISM

Inhibit Na^+–Cl^- cotransporter in DCT.

USES

First-line agent for treatment of hypertension, CHF, nephrosis, hypercalciuria, and nephrogenic DI (thiazides reduce ECF volume $\rightarrow$ activates RAAS $\rightarrow \uparrow$ proximal reabsorption of NaCl and $H_2O \rightarrow \downarrow$ delivery of fluid to distal nephron $\rightarrow \downarrow$ urine output).

SIDE EFFECTS

- Dehydration
- Hypokalemia
- Hypercalcemia
- Hyperglycemia
- Hyperlipidemia
- Hyperuricemia
- Hyponatremia
- Allergic reactions (sulfonamide derivatives)

Potassium-Sparing Agents (Spironolactone, Eplerenone, Amiloride, and Triamterene)

MECHANISM

Spironolactone and eplerenone directly antagonize the mineralocorticoid receptor (target of aldosterone), thereby reducing Na^+ reuptake in the late DCT and collecting duct. Both drugs prevent the aldosterone-mediated increase in apical membrane permeability to K^+ (ROMK channels) and therefore are considered "potassium-sparing."

Amiloride and triamterene directly inhibit ENaCs in the late DCT and collecting duct, which also reduces Na^+ reabsorption. This renders the charge in the lumen more positive, which is unfavorable for K^+ secretion. Hence, these ENaC antagonists are also considered "potassium-sparing."

USES

- **Spironolactone and eplerenone:** Primary hyperaldosteronism (Conn syndrome) and edematous states caused by secondary hyperaldosteronism (cirrhosis, nephrotic syndrome, and cardiac failure). Antiandrogen activity can be useful for treatment of polycystic ovary syndrome (PCOS) and hirsutism.
- **Amiloride and triamterene:** Counteract K^+ loss caused by other diuretics, adjunct therapy to other diuretics to treat edema or hypertension.

CLINICAL CORRELATION

Ethacrynic acid may be used in patients allergic to sulfonamides.

CLINICAL CORRELATION

Thiazides have added benefit in hypercalciuric patients.

KEY FACT

Spironolactone is a synthetic 17-lactone steroid with **antiandrogen activity;** binds and blocks the androgen receptor, resulting in **gynecomastia.**
Eplerenone is more specific for the mineralocorticoid receptor and hence does **not** have antiandrogen side effects.

SIDE EFFECTS

Hyperkalemia, hyperchloremic metabolic acidosis, gynecomastia (spironolactone), impotence (males), abnormal menses (females).

ANTIDIURETIC HORMONE (ADH) (VASOPRESSIN AND DESMOPRESSIN)

MECHANISM

Upregulates selective water channels (aquaporin 2) in apical membrane of collecting ducts.

USES

Central DI, enuresis.

SIDE EFFECTS

- Vasoconstriction
- Headache
- Nausea

ANTIDIURETIC HORMONE ANTAGONISTS

Demeclocycline

MECHANISM

Nonselectively inhibits action of ADH in collecting ducts by decreasing cAMP levels. Member of tetracycline family of antibiotics.

USES

SIADH, decrease intravascular fluid volume in heart or liver failure.

SIDE EFFECTS

- Nephrogenic DI
- Renal failure

Tolvaptan

MECHANISM

Competitively inhibits arginine vasopressin receptor 2, thus promoting excretion of free water.

USES

SIADH, decreases intravascular fluid volume in heart or liver failure.

SIDE EFFECTS

- GI upset
- Renal failure

ANGIOTENSIN-CONVERTING ENZYME INHIBITORS

Lisinopril, Enalapril, Captopril, and Ramipril

MECHANISM

Inhibit angiotensin-converting enzyme (ACE), which catalyzes conversion of angiotensin I to angiotensin II, thereby interrupting the renin–angiotensin–

aldosterone axis. Also **increases** levels of **bradykinin** (a potent vasodilator) because ACE normally degrades bradykinin. In the kidney, ACE inhibitors decrease efferent arteriolar resistance, improving glomerular blood flow and reducing GFR.

USES

Treatment of mild to moderate hypertension. Proven renal protective function in diabetics (decreases hyperfiltration and proteinuria and improves renal function in diabetic nephropathy).

SIDE EFFECTS

- Dry cough (due to increased levels of bradykinin).
- Teratogenic (do **not** give to pregnant women).
- Hypotension.
- Acute renal failure (patients with **bilateral renal artery stenosis**).
- Hyperkalemia.
- Angioedema (due to increased levels of bradykinin).

> **KEY FACT**
>
> **ACE inhibitors** reduce mortality in type 2 diabetes by hindering the development of **diabetic nephropathy.**

TABLE 8-27. Common Renal Manifestations of Adverse Drug Reactions and Toxins

DRUG CLASS	COMMON DRUGS	TOXIC RENAL ACTION(S)
Antihypertensives	ACE inhibitors, ARBs.	Fetal renal toxicity (teratogenic)
Antibiotics	Aminoglycosides (eg, gentamycin, neomycin), penicillins (esp. methicillin), β-lactams, sulfonamides (eg, sulfamethoxazole), trimethoprim, rifampin.	Range from mild renal impairment to ATN or AIN.
Antivirals	Acyclovir, ganciclovir, foscarnet.	Transient renal dysfunction.
Antifungals	Ampholericin B, polymyxin.	Dose-related nephrotoxicity (direct acute tubular injury).
Anti-inflammatory	NSAIDs (eg, ibuprofen, indomethacin, naproxen), COX-2 inhibitors (eg, rofecoxib).	■ AIN, renal papillary necrosis, direct tubular injury due to ischemia. ■ Inhibition of COX isoenzymes inhibits renal PGI_2 production, leading to altered excretion of Na^+, edema, and hypertension.
Immunosuppressive drugs	Cyclosporine, tacrolimus (FK506).	Dose-related nephrotoxicity (direct acute tubular injury).
Chemotherapy drugs	Cisplatin, cyclophosphamide.	Dose-related nephrotoxicity, hemorrhagic cystitis.
Radiocontrast dyes	Iodinated contrast agents.	CIARF, usually in patients with underlying renal disease (eg, diabetics).
Endogenous toxins	Myoglobin (rhabdomyolysis), hemoglobin (hemolysis).	ATN, oliguria.
Other exogenous toxins	Ethylene glycol. Heavy metals (eg, arsenic, lead).	Renal failure at high doses. ATN, oliguria.

ACE, angiotensin-converting enzyme; AIN, acute interstitial nephritis; ARBs, angiotensin receptor blockers; ATN, acute tubular necrosis; CIARF, contrast-induced acute renal failure; COX, cyclooxygenase; PGI_2, prostaglandin I_2.

ANGIOTENSIN RECEPTOR BLOCKERS

Losartan, Candesartan, Irbesartan, and Valsartan

MECHANISM

Block vasoconstriction and aldosterone-producing effects of angiotensin II at receptor sites in vascular smooth muscle and adrenal glands, thereby interrupting the renin–angiotensin–aldosterone axis. **Unlike ACE inhibitors,** angiotensin receptor blockers (ARBs) **do not affect bradykinin,** and thus are rarely associated with the persistent dry cough and/or angioedema that limit ACE inhibitor therapy.

USES

Treatment of mild to moderate hypertension. Alternative drug therapy for patients who cannot tolerate ACE inhibitors.

SIDE EFFECTS

- Hypotension.
- Teratogenic (do **not** give to pregnant women).
- Acute renal failure.
- Hyperkalemia.

NEPHROTOXIC DRUGS

The kidneys are critical organs for removal of most drugs from the body. Table 8-27 lists commonly used drugs and frequently encountered toxins that impair renal function.

CHAPTER 9

Reproductive

KEY FACT

Most disorders of sexual differentiation involve discordance between the gonadal sex and external genital appearance.

CLINICAL CORRELATION

The presence or absence of a Y chromosome determines the genetic sex, even in errors of sex chromosome nondisjunction. For example, individuals with Klinefelter syndrome (47,XXY) are considered to be genetically male and those with Turner syndrome (45,XO) are female.

KEY FACT

Steroid and peptide hormones secreted by the gonads lead to differentiation of the internal and external sexual structures and imprinting of the brain.

KEY FACT

The physiologic effects of testosterone, Müllerian-inhibiting factor (MIF), and dihydrotestosterone (DHT) are critical for the development of the male phenotype.

Embryology

REPRODUCTIVE DEVELOPMENT

Determination of Sex

According to the World Health Organization, human sex is defined as the biological and physiological characteristics that define men and women. Gender, on the other hand, is the social constructed role, behavior, and activity that society considers appropriate for a man or a woman. Human sex can be defined by three criteria:

- Genetic sex: Presence or absence of a Y chromosome.
- Gonadal sex: Presence of testes or ovaries.
- Phenotypic sex: Appearance of the external genitalia.

GENOTYPIC SEX

Genetic, or karyotypic, sex is determined at the time of conception. Under normal conditions, the oocyte provides an X chromosome, and the sperm cell carries either an X or Y chromosome. Thus, at fertilization, either an XX female or XY male is created. The **sex-determining region (SRY) gene** on the Y chromosome encodes the **testis-determining factor (TDF)**, a transcription factor whose targets induce a male phenotype. In the absence of SRY, a female phenotype develops. Notably, the genes from both X chromosomes are needed for female development, but can be overridden by SRY (ie, XXY). Additionally, sexual phenotype is affected by hormonal expression (Table 9-1). The **female phenotype is the default,** but the male phenotype requires expression of testosterone by the interstitial Leydig cells and Müllerian-inhibiting factor (MIF) by Sertoli cells.

Early Development

The SRY gene is not activated until the seventh week of embryonic development, so reproductive organs undergo an initial common stage of development beginning in the fifth week, known as the **indifferent stage.**

GONADS

Primordial germ cells, the precursor cells to the gametes, migrate out to the yolk sac wall during gastrulation. Between the fourth and sixth weeks, they return to the embryo through the GI tract, surrounding peritoneum, and dorsal mesentery while undergoing mitotic divisions (Figure 9-1). The cells

TABLE 9-1. **Hormones in Sexual Differentiation**

HORMONE	TIMING	INTERNAL STRUCTURES	EXTERNAL GENITALIA
Testosterone	8th week	Stimulates development of the vas deferens, seminal vesicles, and epididymis.	
MIF	8th week	Inhibits development of the uterus, fallopian tubes, cervix, and upper vagina.	
DHT	9th–12th weeks	Stimulates development of the prostate.	Stimulates development of the penis and scrotum.

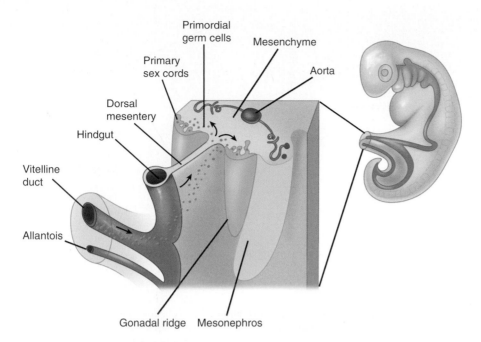

FIGURE 9-1.   Primordial germ cell migration and gonadal ridge formation. The primordial germ cells (*blue specs*) migrate from the wall of the yolk sac to the gonadal ridge, where they settle into the primary sex cords.

invade the gonadal ridge (a mass of mesodermal tissue at the back of the abdominal cavity), proliferate, and become embedded medial to the developing mesonephros. Three primary cell types (mesenchymal cells, mesothelial cells, and primordial germ cells) develop in the gonadal ridge (Table 9-2).

GENITAL DUCTS

The **mesonephric (Wolffian)** and **paramesonephric (Müllerian)** ducts are mesodermal derivatives that form the male and female genital duct systems, respectively (Figure 9-2).

The mesonephric ducts are derived from intermediate mesoderm. They form as longitudinal solid cords of tissue dorsolateral to the mesonephric tubules in the thoracic region. The solid cords grow caudally and fuse with the ventrolateral walls of the cloaca, the urogenital sinus. Subsequently, each cord detaches from everything except the urogenital sinus and canalizes, forming a lumen. During the sixth to tenth weeks, each duct **drains urine from the mesonephros,** a temporary kidney.

FLASH BACK

If embryologic terms are giving you trouble, remember that meso = middle, para = alongside, caudal = hind part, cranial = head part.

TABLE 9-2.   Gonadal Ridge Cell Types

CELL TYPE	FATE
Mesenchymal cells	Gonadal ridge medulla: Male = Leydig cells; Female = ovarian support stroma.
Mesothelial cells	Gonadal ridge and primary sex cord cortex: Male = seminiferous tubules; Female = ovarian follicles.
Primordial germ cells	Enter primary sex cords as future gametes: Male = spermatogonia; Female = oogonia.

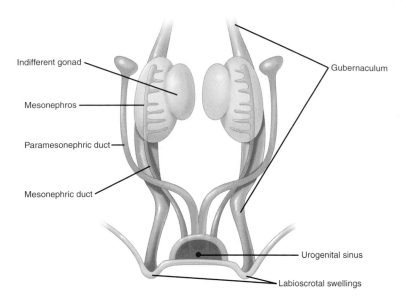

FIGURE 9-2. **Indifferent genital duct formation.** Once it becomes hollow, the mesonephric duct drains urine for the mesonephros. The paramesonephric duct forms lateral to the mesonephric duct and fuses at the midline. This fused tip becomes the uterus.

The paramesonephric duct forms lateral to the mesonephric duct via an invagination of celomic epithelium on the cranial aspect of the mesonephros. The invaginated portion of the paramesonephric duct forms the ostium at the future fimbriated end (infundibulum) of the uterine tube, which opens into the celomic cavity, the future peritoneal cavity. The duct then grows caudally and crosses over the mesonephric duct. At the midline it fuses with the duct growing from the other side, forming a canal that will **become the uterus** (see Figures 9-2 and 9-3). The fused tip then presses on the urogenital sinus, forming a small protrusion.

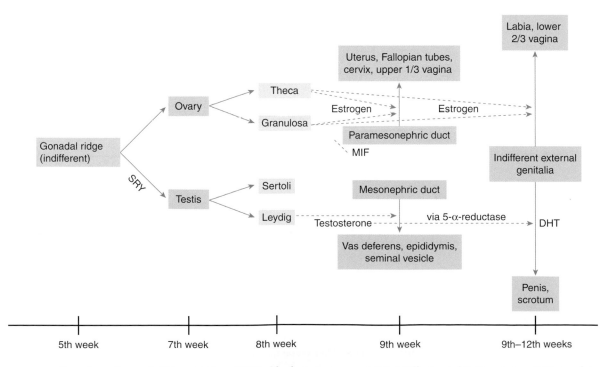

FIGURE 9-3. **Overview of sexual differentiation.** DHT, dihydrotestosterone; MIF, Müllerian-inhibiting factor; SRY, sex-determining region.

EXTERNAL GENITALIA

Around the fourth week, **five mesenchymal swellings** covered with ectoderm form around the cloacal membrane: one **genital tubercle,** two **urogenital folds,** and two **labioscrotal folds** (Figure 9-4). The cloacal membrane divides in half and ruptures, forming the urogenital orifice and anus. A ligament, the **gubernaculum,** forms between the indifferent gonads and the labioscrotal swellings (see Figure 9-2). This ligament guides the testes into the scrotum and forms the round ligament of the uterus and several ligaments of the ovary.

Differentiation

GONADS

At the seventh week of gestation, if a Y chromosome is present, the *SRY* gene leads to the development of testes; absence of *SRY* leads to formation of ovaries. Determination of the gonadal sex (ie, formation of either testes or ovaries) leads to differentiation of the germ cells. In male development, Leydig and Sertoli cells develop by week 8, producing testosterone and MIF, respectively.

For the male, the testes remain high in the abdomen until about the 30th week (seventh month) of gestation, when, under the influence of MIF and androgens (testosterone and dihydrotestosterone [DHT]), they undergo transabdominal and transinguinal descent, respectively.

GENITAL DUCTS

Testosterone stimulates differentiation of the Wolffian duct, producing the epididymis, vas deferens, and seminal vesicle. Meanwhile, MIF reduces aromatase biosynthesis, thereby reducing conversion of androgens to estrogens and suppressing development of the Müllerian duct. In females, the lack of these factors allows the Müllerian duct to develop into the Fallopian tubes, uterus, cervix, and upper part of the vagina, whereas the Wolffian duct degenerates. An overview of these pathways is illustrated in Figure 9-3.

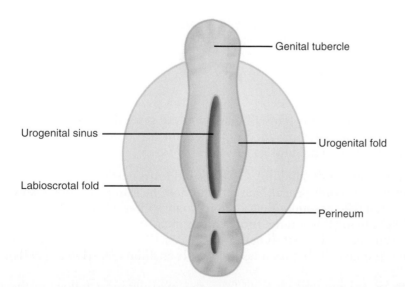

FIGURE 9-4.   Indifferent external genitalia development. The indifferent external genitalia consist of five mesenchymal swellings: one genital tubercle, two urogenital folds, and two labioscrotal folds.

EXTERNAL GENITALIA

Male and female external genitalia can be differentiated by the 9th week of fetal life and are fully developed by the 12th week.

Masculinization (virilization) or feminization of the external genitalia also depends on the presence or absence of male hormones. Whereas testosterone mainly affects the internal structures, **DHT** affects the development of the prostate, penis, and scrotum. In the female, lack of testes—and thereby vastly reduced levels of androgens—leads to development of the lower vagina and labia. Fetal estradiol has little effect on sexual differentiation, though estrogens from either the mother or exogenous sources can contribute to femininization of the genitalia in either gender. The roles of these hormones in determining gonadal and phenotypic sex are summarized in Table 9-1.

Disorders of Sex Development

GONADAL AGENESIS

If primordial germ cells do not form or migrate, gonads do not develop, and the duct systems and external genitalia differentiate along a female path until birth.

TRUE HERMAPHRODITISM

In ovotesticular disorder of sex development, which is very rare, there is one ovary, one testis, and external genitalia of both genders.

PSEUDOHERMAPHRODITISM

This condition is characterized by gonads and karyotype of one gender, combined with secondary sex characteristics of the other gender.

- Male pseudohermaphroditism (eg, complete androgen insensitivity syndrome):
    - XY, undervirilized male/female phenotype.
    - By definition, testes are present.
- Female pseudohermaphroditism:
    - XX, overvirilized female/male phenotype.
    - By definition, ovaries are present.

Male Development

TESTES

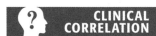 When the *SRY* gene is transcribed during the seventh week of development, its transcription factor product TDF acts on the indifferent gonads (Figure 9-5). They differentiate into:

- Primary sex cords (middle): Coiled, solid **testis cords.**
- Primary sex cords (ends): Stay straight, join near hilum = **rete testes.**
- Rete testes + mesonephric tubule remnants: **efferent ductules.**
- Mesenchyme thickening: **tunica albuginea.**
- Mesothelial cells: **Sertoli cells.**
- Mesothelial cells between testis cords: Interstitial cells (**Leydig cells**).

The testes enlarge and separate from the mesonephros, following the lower gubernacula to reach the scrotum via the inguinal canal (Figure 9-6). At the same time, the upper gubernacula degenerate to allow the testes to descend.

CLINICAL CORRELATION

5α-Reductase type 2 deficiency, one of the milder forms of 46,XY disorder of sex development, leads to deficiency of DHT and thereby to ambiguous external genitalia until puberty, when the external genitalia become more masculine. It is believed that the increase of levels of testosterone at the beginning of puberty produces sufficient levels of DHT either by the action of 5α-reductase type 1 (present in the adult liver, nongenital skin, and some brain areas) or through the expression of low levels of 5α-reductase type 2 in the testes.

CLINICAL CORRELATION

Direct inguinal hernias are acquired hernias that occur when bowel protrudes through a weak point of the abdominal wall: the superficial inguinal ring of the inguinal canal. **Indirect inguinal hernias** are congenital hernias and occur when bowel protrudes through the deep inguinal ring due to **patent processus vaginalis,** an incomplete closure of the inguinal canal. A **hydrocele** is a collection of serous fluid that can accumulate in the tunica vaginalis as a result of patent processus vaginalis.

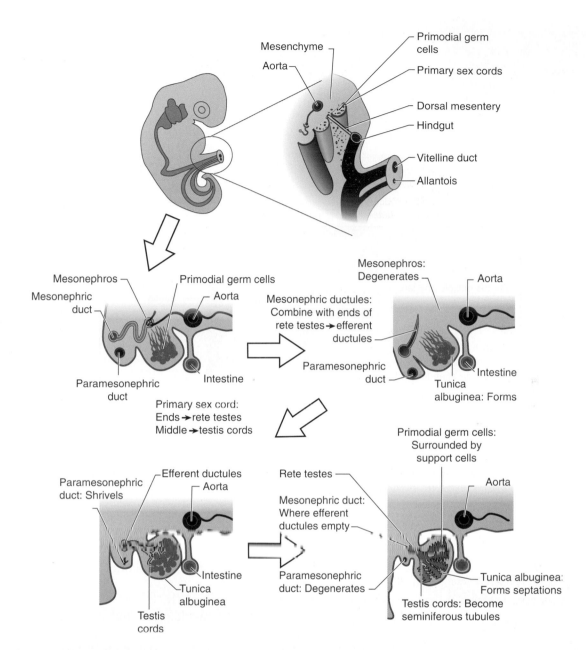

FIGURE 9-5. **Testis development.** As the testes develop, the testis cords, rete testes, and efferent ductules form, while the paramesonephric duct degenerates. As these structures mature, the tunica albuginea separates the testis cords whose mesothelial cells differentiate into Sertoli and Leydig support cells.

As the testes travel, the layers of the abdominal wall travel ahead, forming the layers of the scrotal wall and spermatic cord (see Figure 9-6). A thin fold of peritoneum, the **processus vaginalis,** also descends, but its connection to the abdomen is lost between the future deep ring of the inguinal canal and the upper pole of the testis. However, it remains in the scrotum as the **tunica vaginalis,** which covers the spermatic cord and testes. In a vast majority of cases, the testes finish their descent and are present in the scrotum at birth.

INTERNAL GENITALIA

Around the eighth week after fertilization, Sertoli cells secrete MIF, which induces **regression of the paramesonephric (Müllerian) ducts.** Leydig cells begin to secrete androgens that stimulate **differentiation of the mesonephric**

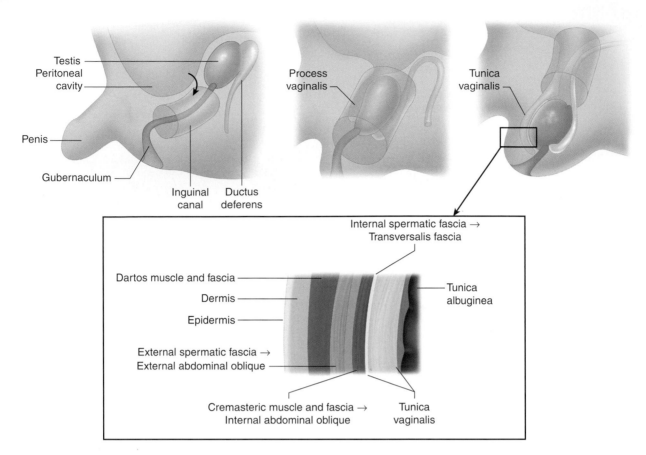

FIGURE 9-6. **Male testicular descent.** As the testes descend through the inguinal canal, portions of the abdominal wall precede them, forming the layers of the scrotal wall and sheath of the spermatic cord.

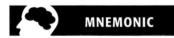

MNEMONIC

Mesonephric duct derivatives (SEED):
Seminal vesicles
Epididymis
Ejaculatory duct
Ductus deferens

(Wolffian) ducts. The mesonephric ducts form several structures (Figure 9-7).

- Seminal vesicles: Gland that is lateral to the ductus deferens and ends in the prostatic ejaculatory duct.
- Epididymis: Coiled ducts, form caudally.
- Ejaculatory duct: Connects ductus deferens and seminal vesicle ducts to the prostatic urethra.
- Ductus deferens: Thick smooth muscle coat, ends in prostatic ejaculatory duct.

Another important structure, the **prostate,** forms as an endodermal outgrowth from the urogenital sinus. There are two zones of glandular tissue surrounded by mesenchyme. The outer zone of prostatic glands constitutes the **posterior lobe.** The inner zone of mucus glands, which constitute the **median lobe,** also contains mesoderm from the mesonephric duct and Müllerian duct remnants. Additionally, the urogenital sinus forms the prostatic urethra.

EXTERNAL GENITALIA

Testosterone secreted by Leydig cells also induces changes in the external genitalia (Figure 9-8).

- Phallus enlarges to become the glans (distal end).
- Urogenital folds fuse to form the ventral shaft of the penis.
- Labioscrotal swelling develops into the scrotum.

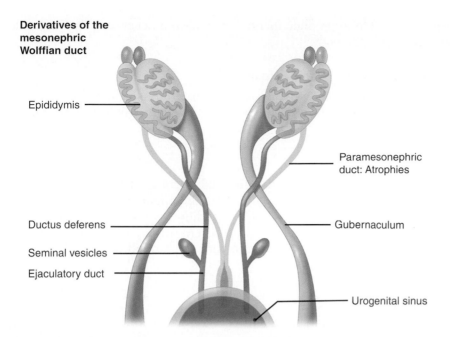

Derivatives of the mesonephric Wolffian duct

Epididymis

Paramesonephric duct: Atrophies

Ductus deferens

Gubernaculum

Seminal vesicles

Ejaculatory duct

Urogenital sinus

FIGURE 9-7.   Male internal genitalia development. The mesonephric (Wolffian) duct differentiates to form the epididymis, ductus deferens, seminal vesicle, and ejaculatory duct, whereas the paramesonephric (Müllerian) duct atrophies.

The fusion of the urogenital folds encloses the endodermally derived urethra. The fusion process leaves a line called the **scrotal/penile raphe.** All structures are covered in ectoderm, but the ectoderm over the glans breaks down to form the **foreskin,** or **prepuce.**

Male Congenital Malformations

CRYPTORCHIDISM

Failure of the testes to descend can occur secondary to abnormalities in either androgen production or shortening of the gubernaculum. Undescended testes typically migrate to the scrotum within 3–6 months after birth. If this does not occur, the child is said to have cryptorchidism, and surgical intervention is necessary either to lower them (orchidopexy) or remove them. Undescended

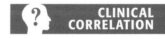

CLINICAL CORRELATION

A man with a past history of **cryptorchidism** has an increased risk of testicular cancer, testicular torsion, inguinal hernia, and lessened fertility.

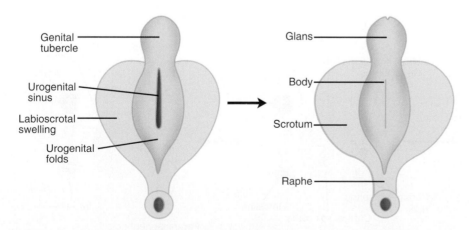

Genital tubercle

Glans

Urogenital sinus

Body

Labioscrotal swelling

Scrotum

Urogenital folds

Raphe

FIGURE 9-8.   Male external genitalia development. During development of the male external genitalia the phallus enlarges and the urogenital and labioscrotal folds fuse at the midline. This results in formation of the penile glans, penile body, and scrotum, respectively.

Hypospadias

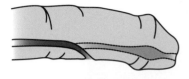

Epispadias

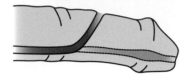

FIGURE 9-9. Penile urethral abnormalities. In hypospadias, an abnormal opening of the urethra occurs on the inferior side of the penis. In epispadias, an abnormal opening of the urethra occurs on the superior side of the penis.

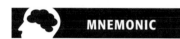

MNEMONIC

Hypospadias and epispadias defect locations:

Hypospadias: Urethra opens on the inferior side of the penis (**hypo** = below).
Epispadias: Urethra opens on the superior side of the penis (**epi** = on top of).

testes are unable to produce mature spermatozoa because of the higher temperature inside the body.

CONGENITAL (INDIRECT) INGUINAL HERNIA

Incomplete closure of the processus vaginalis/inguinal canal creates a passage from the abdominal canal to the scrotum through which the intestines can herniate.

HYPOSPADIAS

This condition is marked by an abnormal opening of the penile urethra on the inferior side of the penis (Figure 9-9). The opening is secondary to failure of the urogenital folds to close. This condition is the most common penile abnormality and must be corrected to prevent urinary tract infections (UTIs). Hypospadias occurs in 10% of patients with cryptorchidism.

EPISPADIAS

This condition is marked by an abnormal opening of the penile urethra on the superior side of the penis. This opening occurs due to malpositioning of the genital tubercle. This condition is associated with **exstrophy of the bladder,** a condition in which the bladder is exposed, inside out, and protrudes through the abdominal wall. Epispadias is less common than hypospadias.

Female Development

OVARIES

In the absence of the *SRY* gene, the indifferent gonads follow a female pattern of differentiation (Figure 9-10). They differentiate to form:

- Primary sex cords: Degenerate.
- Cortical sex cords: Break up into a single layer of mesothelial follicular cells surrounding each germ cell (**primordial follicles**).
- Primordial germ cells: Differentiate to **oogonia** and undergo mitosis to increase their numbers.
- Mesenchyme: Connective tissue stroma for follicular support.

Before birth, the oogonia enter meiosis I prophase, and no further division is possible. The ovaries separate from the mesonephros and become sus-

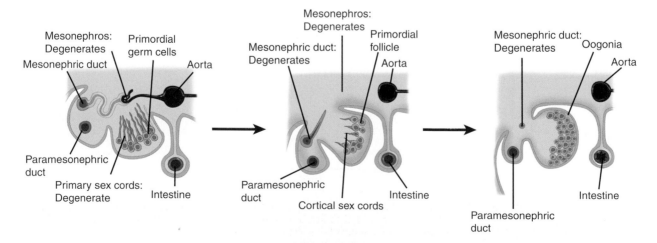

FIGURE 9-10. Ovarian development. As the ovaries develop, the mesonephros and primary sex cords degenerate. The primordial germ cells migrate into the cortical sex cords and form primordial follicles. These follicles then differentiate into oogonia.

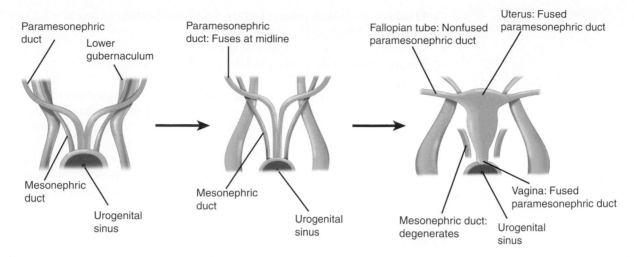

FIGURE 9-11. **Female internal genitalia development.** The lower portion of the paramesonephric duct fuses at the midline, forming the uterus and upper vagina. The upper portion of the paramesonephric duct does not fuse and forms the oviduct (Fallopian tube).

pended in the pelvic mesentery. The peritoneal covering of the ovary is lost. After puberty, the ova are extruded into the peritoneal cavity and gathered into the ostium of the infundibulum by the fimbriae.

INTERNAL GENITALIA

The female internal genitalia develop due to the **absence of testosterone** and **MIF.** Without these substances, the mesonephric (Wolffian) duct regresses and the paramesonephric (Müllerian) duct begins to differentiate. The paramesonephric ducts partially fuse at the midline to form several structures (Figure 9-11).

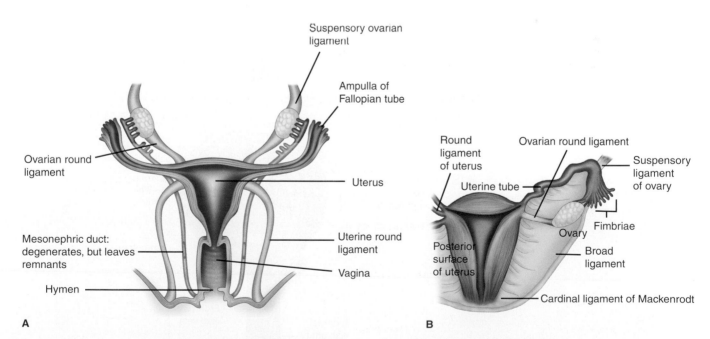

FIGURE 9-12. **Female ligament development.** The gubernaculum is separated into three segments that form the suspensory ovarian ligament, ovarian round ligament, and uterine round ligament. The broad ligament covers the entire uterus and forms as the developing uterus descends through the pelvis, pulling epithelium and mesenchyme from the lining of the body cavity.

- **Oviduct** (Fallopian tubes): Upper, nonfused portion of ducts.
- **Fimbriae:** Elongations of oviducts.
- **Uterus:** Lower, fused portion of ducts.
- **Vagina** (upper two-thirds): Lower, fused portion of ducts.

The uterus develops a layer of **myometrium** from the surrounding mesenchyme and a layer of peritoneal covering, the **perimetrium** (serosa). The lower third of the vagina is formed from two outgrowths of the urogenital sinus wall, the **sinovaginal bulbs.** The ascending sinovaginal bulbs fuse with the descending paramesonephric system, creating the vaginal plate. The vaginal plate canalizes with only the thin covering of the hymen remaining. The greater (**Bartholin glands**) and the lesser vestibular glands (**Skene glands**) are endodermal outgrowths of the urogenital sinus.

LIGAMENTS

Several peroneal ligaments are formed from the gubernaculum attached to the indifferent gonads (Figures 9-12 and 9-13). The gubernaculum is initially separated into an upper and lower portion. As the Müllerian ducts fuse in the midline, the lower ligament is further separated, creating a total of three segments: **suspensory ovarian ligament** (attaches ovary to pelvic wall, carries

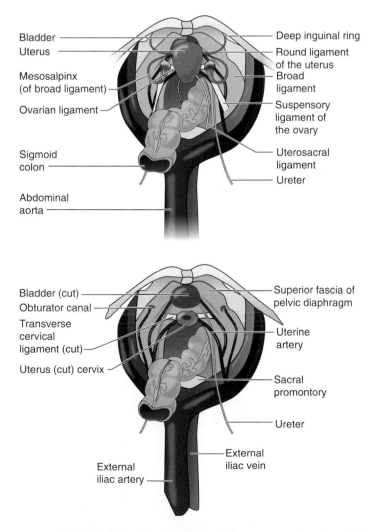

FIGURE 9-13. **Superior view of the ligaments of the uterus and ovaries in situ.** The bottom image, with the peritoneum and uterus removed, more clearly shows the course of the ureter, uterine vessels, and transverse cervical ligaments (cardinal ligaments).

TABLE 9-3. Female Peroneal Ligaments

LIGAMENT	CONNECTS	STRUCTURES CONTAINED
Suspensory ovarian ligaments	Ovaries to lateral pelvic wall	Ovarian vessels
Ovarian round ligaments	Ovary to uterus	
Uterine round ligament	Uterus to labia majora via inguinal canal	Sampson artery
Broad ligament	Uterus, Fallopian tubes, and ovaries to lateral pelvic wall	Uterus, round ligament of uterus, Fallopian tubes, ovaries, ovarian ligaments
Cardinal ligament of Mackenrodt	Cervix to lateral pelvic wall	Uterine vessels
Uterosacral ligaments	Cervix to sacrum	

ovarian vessels), **ovarian round ligament** (attaches ovary to lateral surface of uterus), and **uterine round ligament** (attaches uterus to labia majora via the inguinal canal; supplied by the Sampson artery).

The **broad ligament,** which covers the entire uterus, develops when the paramesonephric ducts descend through the pelvis, pulling a fold of celomic, or body cavity, epithelium and mesenchyme with them (see Figures 9-12 and 9-13). The broad ligament consists of three parts: mesovarium (covers ovaries), mesosalpinx (covers oviducts), and mesometrium (covers uterus). The **cardinal ligament of Mackenrodt** attaches the cervix to the lateral pelvic wall at the ischial spine and contains the uterine vessels (see Figures 9-12 and 9-13).

The female peroneal ligaments are summarized in Table 9-3.

EXTERNAL GENITALIA

Under the influence of estrogen (Figure 9-14):

- The genital tubercle becomes the glans, which then becomes the clitoris.
- Urogenital folds partially fuse to become labia minora.
- Labioscrotal swellings partially fuse to become labia majora.

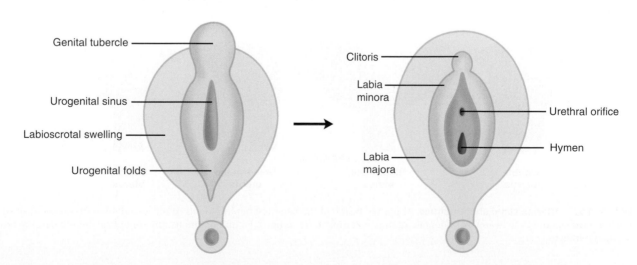

FIGURE 9-14. Female external genitalia development. The genital tubercle develops into the clitoris, and the urogenital and labioscrotal folds develop into the labia minora and labia majora, respectively.

The skin covering the clitoris does not break down as in male development, so there is no foreskin equivalent.

Breast Development

Mammary glands develop from **apocrine sweat glands** in the mesenchymal layer just beneath the skin. Embryologically, breast development is identical in males and females.

? CLINICAL CORRELATION

If portions of the mammary ridge do not regress, **accessory nipples** form. This is the most common congenital abnormality of breast development.

- Week 4: The **mammary ridge,** a line of thickened ectoderm, develops from the inguinal region to the axilla.
- Weeks 4–6: The mammary ridge regresses except in the pectoral region.
- Week 6: Single mammary buds form as downgrowths of the mammary ridge.
- Weeks 6–birth:
    - Placental hormones (eg, lactogen) cause lactiferous duct branching.
    - The surrounding mesenchyme develops into fat and connective tissue.
    - The nipple is formed by depression of the skin before birth.
- Postnatal: The skin surrounding the nipple pit grows, raising the nipple.
- Puberty: If estrogen is present, female mammary glands develop.

Female Congenital Malformations

UTERINE CANAL ABNORMALITIES

The paramesonephric ducts first fuse to form a **Y**-shaped tubular structure, which develops into the uterus and upper vagina. Once this **Y**-shaped structure is formed, fusion occurs followed by resorption/canalization of the intervening septum. Combinations of failed fusion and resorption can cause several different anomalies, including a double uterus, a bicornuate or septate uterus, or a unicornuate uterus (Figure 9-15).

ATRESIA OF THE UTERINE CANAL

This condition occurs when there is narrowing or complete occlusion of the paramesonephric ducts (uterine atresia) or of just the sinovaginal bulbs (vaginal atresia).

OVARIAN HYPOPLASIA

This underdevelopment of the ovary is seen in patients with Turner syndrome (XO). Primordial germ cells migrate toward the undifferentiated gonad, but

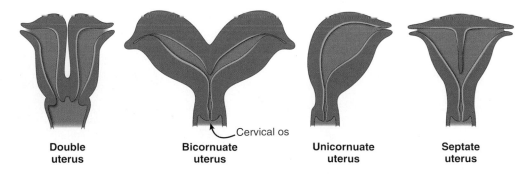

| Double uterus | Bicornuate uterus | Unicornuate uterus | Septate uterus |

Cervical os

FIGURE 9-15. **Uterine canal abnormalities.** Abnormal fusion of the paramesonephric ducts results in a double uterus (no fusion), a bicornuate uterus (incomplete fusion), or a septate uterus (incomplete resorption). Failure of one paramesonephric duct to develop results in unicornuate uterus.

TABLE 9-4.   Derivatives of Embryonic Urogenital Structures

	MALE	FEMALE
Mesonephric duct	Ureter, renal pelvis, calyces, collecting tubules, ductus (vas) deferens, duct of epididymis, ejaculatory duct, seminal vesicle.	Ureter, renal pelvis, calyces, collecting tubules.
Paramesonephric duct		Uterus, Fallopian tubes, cervix, upper two-thirds of vagina.
Urogenital sinus	Urinary bladder, urethra, prostate gland, bulbourethral glands.	Urinary bladder, urethra, lower third of vagina, urethral and paraurethral glands, greater vestibular glands.
Gubernaculum	"Scrotal ligament."	Ovarian ligaments, round ligament of the uterus.

follicles do not form. The vulnerable germ cells degenerate and the gonads do not produce hormones after birth, leaving the genitalia in an infantile state.

REVIEW: MALE AND FEMALE GENITAL HOMOLOGS

Table 9-4 and Figure 9-16 review the internal and external structural homologs between the reproductive systems of both sexes.

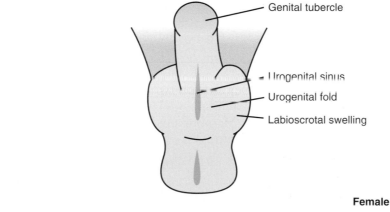

FIGURE 9-16.   Male and female genital homologs.

Anatomy

LOWER ABDOMEN AND PERINEUM

From superficial to deep, the abdominal wall consists of:

- Skin
- Subcutaneous fat (Camper fascia)
- Scarpa fascia
- External oblique muscle
- Internal oblique muscle
- Transversus abdominis muscle
- Transversalis fascia
- Preperitoneal fat
- Peritoneum

The aponeuroses of the abdominal muscles form the rectus sheath. Above the arcuate line, the sheath has anterior and posterior portions that wrap around the rectus abdominis. Below the arcuate line, however, the rectus sheath only travels anterior to the rectus abdominis. In other words, the posterior rectus sheath disappears (Figure 9-17).

The inguinal (Poupart) ligament is derived from the inferior border of the external oblique muscle aponeurosis. This ligament serves as the inferolateral border of the Hesselbach triangle and as the superiomedial border of the femoral triangle (Figure 9-18).

The pelvic region contains four named fasciae:

- Camper fascia: Fatty layer of the superficial fascia of the lower abdomen.
- Scarpa fascia: Membranous layer of the superficial fascia of the lower abdomen (deep to Camper fascia).
- Buck fascia: Membranous layer of the deep fascia of the penis.
- Colles fascia: Membranous layer of the superficial fascia of the urogenital region (perineum).

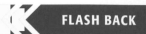

FLASH BACK

Protrusion of peritoneum through the femoral canal results in a **femoral hernia.**

KEY FACT

Scarpa and Colles fasciae are contiguous.

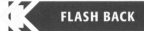

FLASH BACK

The **inguinal (Hesselbach) triangle** is the area defined by the **rectus abdominis muscle** medially, the **inguinal ligament** inferiorly, and the **inferior epigastric vessels** superiorly and laterally. It is in this region that **direct inguinal hernias** protrude through the abdominal wall.

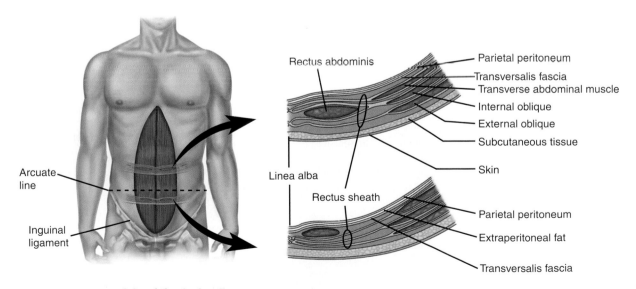

FIGURE 9-17. **Layers of the abdominal wall.**

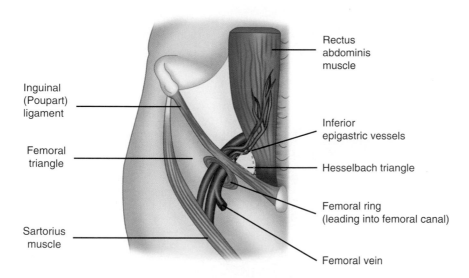

FIGURE 9-18. **Anatomic borders formed by the inguinal ligament.**

Of these, only the Buck fascia is unique to men.

Venous drainage of the gonads differs by side, not sex. The right gonadal vein drains directly into the **inferior vena cava (IVC)**, and the left drains first into the **left renal vein**, which then connects to the IVC.

Lymphatic fluid from the testes and ovaries drains to the **para-aortic lymph nodes,** regardless of the side of the body.

MALE REPRODUCTIVE SYSTEM

Reproductive structures in the male are located both within and outside the pelvis, as shown in Figure 9-19.

The pelvic fasciae are illustrated in Figures 9-19 and 9-20.

Between the testis and inguinal canal, the vas deferens runs within the **spermatic cord.** Cremasteric muscle fibers, the testicular artery, the pampiniform venous plexus, and the genital branch of the genitofemoral nerve are also found within this structure. The ilioinguinal nerve (a branch of the first lumbar nerve) runs atop the spermatic cord.

In the scrotum, the **tunica dartos,** a thin muscular layer superficial to Colles fascia, allows the scrotal skin to become tense. It also forms the scrotal septum, which keeps the spermatic cords from getting tangled. The **gubernaculum** (sometimes called the "scrotal ligament") further limits movement of the testes by tethering them to the inferior aspect of the scrotum. The left testis often hangs lower than the right.

In conjunction with the **cremaster muscle,** which covers each testis, the tunica dartos allows the testes and scrotum to be drawn up closer to the body in cold environments.

The layers of the scrotum are reviewed in Figure 9-21 and Table 9-5.

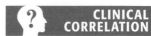

CLINICAL CORRELATION

Germ cell tumors (from testes or ovaries) spread first to the para-aortic lymph nodes.

MNEMONIC

The pathway sperm take to exit the body—

SEVEn UP
Seminiferous tubules (site of
   Spermatogenesis)
Epididymis
Vas deferens
Ejaculatory ducts
Urethra
Penis

KEY FACT

The superficial vein of the penis is the only subcutaneous penile structure not ensheathed by the Buck fascia.

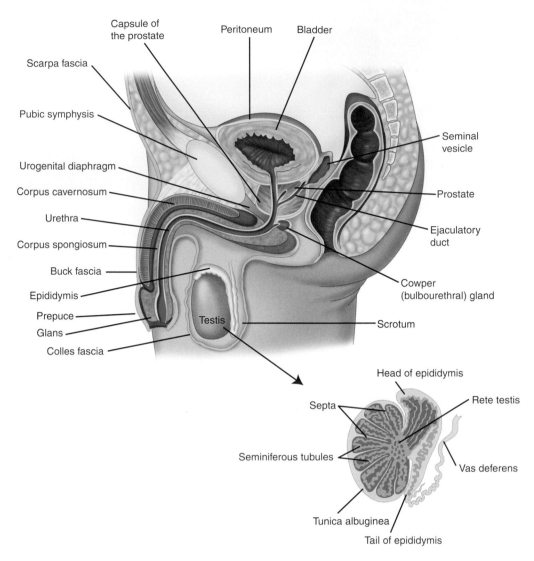

FIGURE 9-19. Lateral view of the male reproductive system.

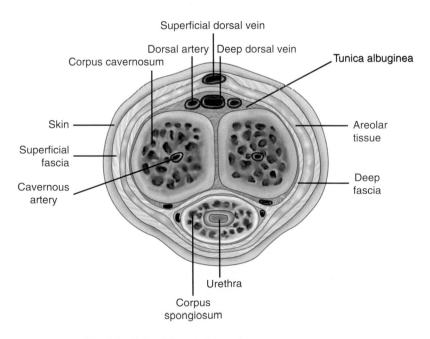

FIGURE 9-20. Cross-section of the penis.

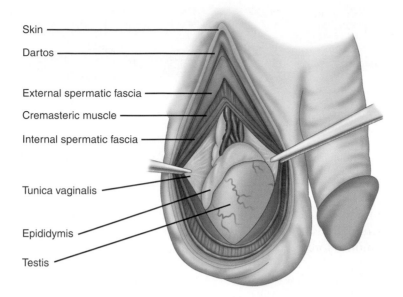

Skin
Dartos
External spermatic fascia
Cremasteric muscle
Internal spermatic fascia
Tunica vaginalis
Epididymis
Testis

FIGURE 9-21. **Layers of tissue within the scrotum.** (Modified with permission from Brunicardi FC, Andersen DK, Billiar TR, et al. *Schwartz's Principles of Surgery*, 8th ed. New York: McGraw-Hill, 2005: 1522.)

The penis is formed from three bodies of erectile tissue. During erection, this tissue stiffens because it is filled with blood from deep arteries of the penis and the arteries of the bulb of the penis. An erection is maintained because the expansion of erectile tissue compresses the dorsal veins of the penis, which keeps blood in the penis. The two dorsal erectile bodies are called corpus cavernosum, and the ventral body is called the corpus spongiosum. The urethra passes through the corpus spongiosum on the ventral side of the penis. At the distal end of the penis, the corpus spongiosum expands to form the glans penis (see Figures 9-19 and 9-20).

Sperm Cells

A sperm cell (Figure 9-22) is composed of a head, which includes the nucleus and acrosome; a middle piece; and a tail. The front part of the head contains the **acrosome,** a structure derived from the Golgi apparatus that contains enzymes to digest the extracellular matrix (ECM) and zona pellucida of the egg. The postacrosomal region contains a haploid nucleus. The sperm cell membrane in this region also contains receptors for the egg. The spiral midpiece consists of fused mitochondria that use fructose to generate adeno-

? CLINICAL CORRELATION

Mitochondria from the sperm are not included in the conceptus; thus, mitochondrially inherited disorders (eg, Leber hereditary optic neuropathy, Leigh syndrome, and mitochondrial encephalomyopathy with lactic acidosis and stroke-like episodes [MELAS]) are transmitted maternally.

TABLE 9-5. **Spermatic Cord Derivatives of Abdominal Layers**

ABDOMINAL STRUCTURE	DERIVATIVE IN SPERMATIC CORD
External oblique muscle aponeurosis	External spermatic fascia
Internal oblique muscle	Cremaster muscle
Transversalis fascia	Internal spermatic fascia
Extraperitoneal fatty tissue	Areolar tissue
Peritoneum	Processus vaginalis

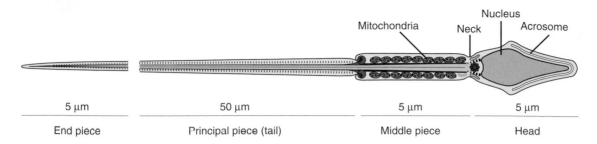

FIGURE 9-22. **Sperm anatomy.** (Modified with permission from Junqueira LC, Carneiro J. *Basic Histology*, 10th ed. New York: McGraw-Hill, 2003.)

KEY FACT

The prostatic tissue itself is strongly influenced by DHT. Normal, age-related increases in estradiol may lead to increased density of DHT receptors and subsequent growth of the prostate (benign prostatic hypertrophy, BPH).

sine triphosphate (ATP) to move the **9+2 axoneme** in the proximal portion of the tail (called the flagellum). The sliding of the microtubules generates the whip-like motive force characteristic of sperm cells.

Prostate

About the size and shape of a walnut, the prostate stores and secretes a clear, alkaline fluid found in semen. Located at a major anatomic hub with the seminal vesicles and vas deferens, this fluid from the prostate is mixed with seminal fluid and spermatozoa. The ejaculatory ducts, which are located in the middle lobe and lined with transitional epithelium, are found posterior to the urethra. Smooth muscle within the prostate helps expel semen during ejaculation.

Though the gross anatomy of the prostate can be described by lobes, the more common approach is by pathologic zones (Figure 9-23). Table 9-6 lists the approximate equivalencies between the two classification systems.

The stroma, which accounts for 5% of the weight of the prostate, contains no glands—only muscle and fibrous tissue.

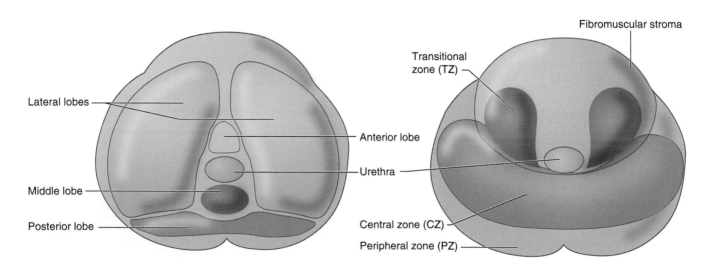

FIGURE 9-23. **Prostatic lobes (*left*) and prostatic zones (*right*).**

TABLE 9-6. Anatomic Lobes and Pathologic Zones of the Prostate

ANATOMIC LOBE	PATHOLOGIC ZONE
Anterior lobe (isthmus)	Transitional zone (TZ)
Posterior lobe	Peripheral zone (PZ)
Middle lobe (median lobe)	Central zone (CZ)
Lateral lobe	All zones

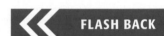

CLINICAL CORRELATION

BPH involves hyperplasia of cells in the periurethral zone (lateral and middle lobes), resulting in urinary symptoms. **Prostatic adenocarcinoma** affects the androgen-sensitive cells of the peripheral zone (posterior lobe), allowing easy metastasis to the spine via the Batson plexus.

FEMALE REPRODUCTIVE SYSTEM

The female reproductive organs and accessory structures are illustrated in Figure 9-24. In situ, the uterus is usually anteverted (tilted forward), with its anteroinferior face resting against the bladder. As such, it is the posterior side of the uterus that is visualized when looking down at the pelvic floor.

Once released by the ovary, ova are caught by the fimbriae of the Fallopian (uterine) tube and travel toward the uterus. The Fallopian tubes, also known as the **oviducts** or **salpinges,** contain four sections: the infundibulum, ampulla, isthmus, and interstitium. The infundibulum contains fimbriae and the ampulla is the usual site of fertilization.

The pelvic fasciae are labeled in Figure 9-25. As in the male, the female urogenital diaphragm is bordered by superior and inferior fascia. Colles fascia is continuous with the posterior aspect of the inferior fascia.

FLASH BACK

The ureters pass under (inferior to) the uterine arteries—"water under the bridge."

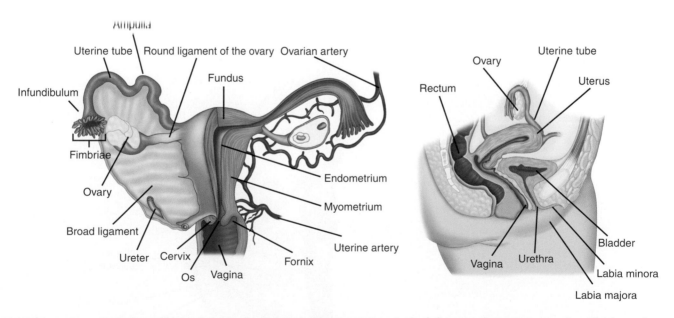

FIGURE 9-24. **Posterior and lateral views of female reproductive system.** In the left image, the ureter runs perpendicular to the plane of the page (the broad ligament).

Rectus sheath
Endopelvic fascia
Peritoneum
Tela subcutanea
Scarpa deep fascia
Camper superficial fascia
Pubic symphysis
Rectum
Uterus
Bladder
Fascia of levator ani
Urogenital diaphragm
Fascia of bulbocavernosus and ischiocavernosus muscles
Fascia diaphragmatis urogenitalis inferior (Colles fascia)

FIGURE 9-25. **Lateral view of the female perineum illustrating the pelvic fascia.** (Modified with permission from Benson RC. *Handbook of Obstetrics & Gynecology*, 8th ed. South Norwalk, CT: Appleton & Lange. Copyright © 1983 by The McGraw-Hill Companies, Inc.)

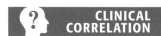

CLINICAL CORRELATION

Breast cancer in situ: Ductal carcinoma in situ (DCIS) tends to occur unilaterally, whereas lobular carcinoma in situ (LCIS) has a greater chance of affecting both breasts.

The Breasts

Breast tissue, a composite of connective tissue (collagen and elastin), adipose tissue, and glands, changes over time and secondary to hormonal influences. At puberty, the breasts increase in size and softness as the mammary glands develop and more fat is deposited. After the birth of a child, the number of glands roughly doubles, allowing for the secretion of milk. Overproduction of estrogen, either during menstruation or at the beginning of menopause, can

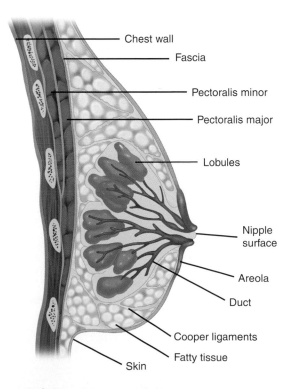

Chest wall
Fascia
Pectoralis minor
Pectoralis major
Lobules
Nipple surface
Areola
Duct
Cooper ligaments
Fatty tissue
Skin

FIGURE 9-26. **Lateral view of the female breast.**

TABLE 9-7.   Principal Nerves and Vessels of the Breast

Nerves	Anterior and lateral cutaneous branches of thoracic intercostal nerves T3–T5.
Arteries	Internal thoracic (internal mammary) artery, lateral thoracic artery, thoracodorsal artery, thoracoacromial artery.
Veins	Axillary vein, internal thoracic vein.

make the breast tissue more tender. The consistency of the breast tissue itself also varies during this period. With time, the **Cooper ligaments**—the suspensory ligaments of the breast—weaken.

A normal breast (Figure 9-26) possesses a nipple surrounded by the **areola,** a pigmented section of skin containing sebaceous glands. The mammary glands within the breast tissue connect to the nipple via lactiferous ducts. The breast itself sits atop the pectoralis major muscle, spanning from approximately the second to the sixth rib, though a thin layer of mammary tissue reaches several ribs above and below. The "tail of Spence" extends diagonally from the superior lateral quadrant to the axilla.

The majority of the lymph from the breast drains to the ipsilateral axillary lymph nodes. The parasternal, abdominal, and contralateral axillary lymph nodes may also be involved.

The nipples in both men and women are highly sensitive and highly vascular. Table 9-7 and Figure 9-27 review, respectively, the important nerves and vessels in the breast.

 KEY FACT

The dermatome at the level of the nipple is T4 in males.

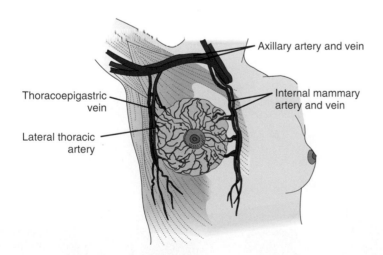

FIGURE 9-27.   Selected vessels in the female breast. (Modified with permission from DeCherney AH, Nathan L. *Current Obstetric & Gynecologic Diagnosis & Treatment*, 10th ed. New York: McGraw-Hill, 2007: 1033.)

TABLE 9-8. Overview of Gametogenesis in Males and Females

CHROMOSOMES	CELL TYPE (SINGULAR FORM)	CHROMATIDS
Diploid (46)	Spermatogonium/oogonium	2N
	Primary spermatocyte/primary oocyte	4N
Haploid (23)	Secondary spermatocyte/secondary oocyte	2N
	Spermatid/ootid	N
	Spermatozoon/ovum	

Physiology

GAMETOGENESIS

Human sexual reproduction depends on many factors, but formation of healthy gametes is probably the most important. Though the synchronicity and location of spermatogenesis and oogenesis differ, the cells go through

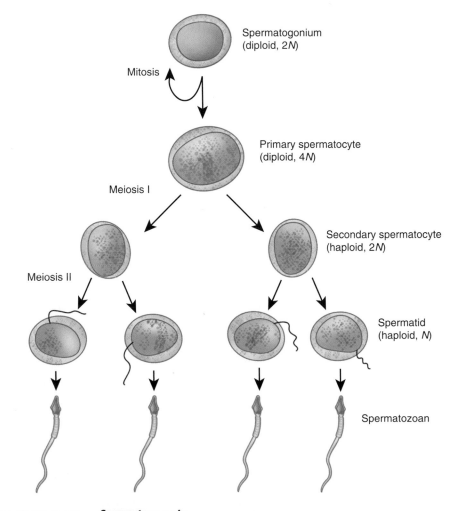

FIGURE 9-28. **Spermatogenesis.**

nearly analogous stages (as suggested by their suffixes). Table 9-8 reviews these stages.

SPERMATOGENESIS

Spermatogenesis, which occurs in the seminiferous tubules of the testes, is a simple stepwise process of mitosis and two rounds of meiosis (Figure 9-28). It is important to note two things: (1) Some spermatogonia undergo mitosis (replication) but do not advance further, thus maintaining a constant supply of cells for spermatogenesis, and (2) dividing sperm cells remain connected by threads of cytoplasm so they develop at the same time (Figure 9-29). Upon release from Sertoli cells, mature but nonmotile spermatozoa move from the lumen of the seminiferous tubules to the epididymis, where they become motile. However, it is muscle contraction in the male reproductive tract rather than flagellar movement that moves the sperm cells prior to ejaculation.

Sertoli cells are supportive "nurse" cells that make numerous contributions to developing sperm cells, including:

- The **blood-testis barrier,** which blocks penetration by cytotoxic agents.
- Secretion of substances that aid in meiosis.

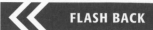

FLASH BACK

Ploidy = number of homologous sets of chromosomes:
- Diploid (46 chromosomes)
- Haploid (23 chromosomes): parent
- Chromatid = one-half of a replicated chromosome

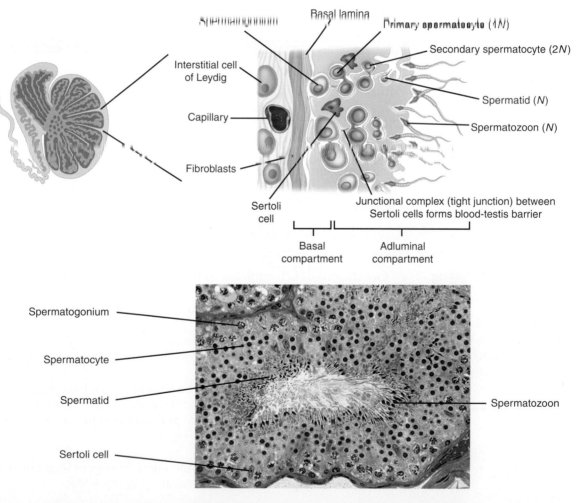

FIGURE 9-29. **Cells of the seminiferous tubules.** (Reproduced with permission from USMLERx.com.)

- Phagocytosis of residual cytoplasm during the final stage of spermatogenesis when spermatids become spermatozoa.
- Secretion of other factors, including androgen-binding protein (ABP), inhibin, giant-cell line–derived neutrophilic factor (GDNF), and estradiol.

Leydig cells are interstitial cells that produce testosterone, which diffuses into the seminiferous tubules. A very high local concentration of testosterone in the seminiferous tubules is required for spermatogenesis, and this is partly achieved by Sertoli cell–produced ABP, which traps androgens in the seminiferous tubules.

Leydig cells are stimulated by luteinizing hormone (LH), and Sertoli cells are stimulated by follicle-stimulating hormone (FSH); both hormones are secreted by the anterior pituitary.

Via standard feedback inhibition, inhibin secreted by Sertoli cells and testosterone secreted by Leydig cells inhibit the hypothalamus and anterior pituitary from secreting gonadotropin-releasing hormone (GnRH) and LH/FSH, respectively (Figure 9-30).

Spermatogenesis begins at puberty and continues until death, although the quantity and quality of the sperm cells wane somewhat in the later years as plasma testosterone levels fall.

OOGENESIS

The female sex cell, the ovum, is a spherical structure produced within **mature Graafian follicles** in the ovary. The outermost layer, the **corona radiata,** is two to three cells thick and is derived from the granulosa cells on the inner portion of the ovarian follicle. Deep to the corona radiata is the **zona pellucida (striata),** a glycoprotein layer that binds to invading sperm cells and allows the acrosome reaction to occur. Deeper still is the **perivitelline space,** which contains both the mature oocyte and, after fertilization, the second polar body. The mature oocyte possesses a cell membrane, copious cytoplasm, and a haploid nucleus.

Oogenesis occurs in the follicle without the aid of centrosomes. It is analogous to spermatogenesis, although the timing is different:

- Oocytogenesis is completed in the perinatal period, thus providing a newborn female with all the oocytes she will ever have ($\sim 7 \times 10^6$).
- Primary oocytes are arrested in **prophase I until ovulation.** This period is called dictyate or dictyotene.
- After ovulation, the oocyte continues through meiosis I, forming the first polar body and a secondary oocyte that is arrested in **metaphase II until fertilization.**
- Within minutes of fertilization, the secondary oocyte completes meiosis II and produces an ootid and second polar body. The ootid quickly becomes an ovum, a cell with both paternal and maternal pronuclei. When the pronuclei fuse, the ovum becomes a zygote.

Also in contrast to spermatogenesis, the effort in oogenesis is concentrated on one cell. The two **polar bodies** degenerate (Figure 9-31).

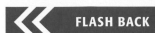

FLASH BACK

Steroid hormones are not stored in cells; their level in the bloodstream depends on their rate of synthesis.

KEY FACT

Upon fertilization, meiosis II is completed, allowing the secondary oocyte (2*N*) to become an ootid/ovum (*N*) and avoid multiploidy.

FLASH BACK

Breast budding **(thelarche)** and growth of pubic hair are the first signs of a girl's entry into puberty. Physicians monitor these changes using Tanner staging.

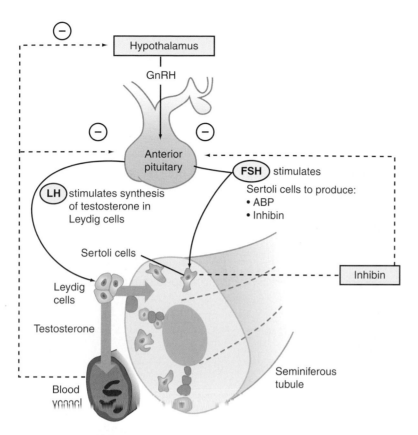

PRODUCTS	FUNCTIONS OF PRODUCTION
Androgen-binding protein (ABP)	Ensures that testosterone concentration in seminiferous tubule is high.
Inhibin	Inhibits FSH.
Testosterone	Differentiates male genitalia. Has anabolic effects on protein metabolism, maintains gametogenesis, maintains libido, inhibits GnRH.

FSH ⟶ Sertoli cells ⟶ Sperm production

LH ⟶ Leydig cells ⟶ Testosterone

FIGURE 9-30. **Hormonal regulation of spermatogenesis.** FSH, follicle-stimulating hormone; GnRH, gonadotropin-releasing hormone; LH, luteinizing hormone.

Until ovulation (and possible subsequent fertilization) occurs, maturation of the oocyte takes place within an ovarian follicle (Figure 9-32).

MENSTRUAL CYCLE AND OVULATION

Menarche, or a woman's first menstrual period, occurs, on average, at 12.5 years of age in American girls. It precedes regular ovulation by several months to a year.

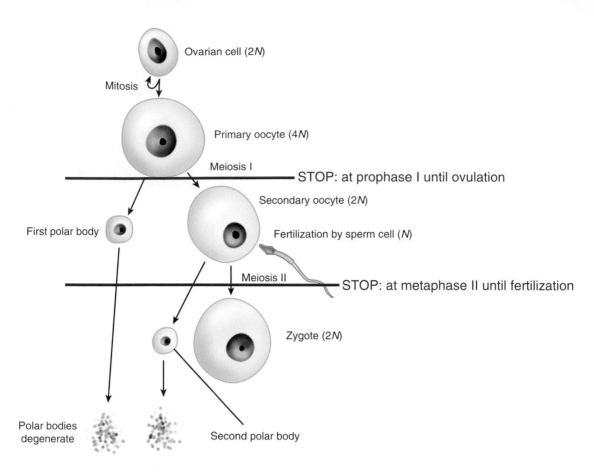

FIGURE 9-31. **Oogenesis and fertilization.**

 KEY FACT

Form follows function: Granulosa cells line the interior of the follicle, and theca cells form the outer border.

 KEY FACT

In the follicular phase, estrogens inhibit gonadotropin release (negative feedback on the pituitary), but then have a brief midcycle stimulatory action that induces the LH surge critical for ovulation.

 MNEMONIC

Progesterone **P**repares for and maintains **P**regnancy.

Granulosa cells, the female analog of Sertoli cells, respond to FSH and encourage growth of 15–20 follicles. LH-responsive theca cells stimulate growth of the corpus luteum and produce androgens, which can be converted to estrogen by the granulosa cells.

Estrogen encourages growth of the endometrium and generally provides negative feedback to the anterior pituitary to inhibit the release of FSH and LH (Figure 9-33). High levels of estrogen, which is the case at the end of the follicular phase, actually stimulate gonadotropin release, leading to a midcycle gonadotropin surge.

Approximately 1 week before ovulation, one of the developing follicles becomes dominant and increases its expression of FSH receptors above the other developing follicles (more sensitive to FSH). This follicle secretes inhibin, blocking the production of FSH from the anterior pituitary and thus causing the other follicles to undergo atresia. In anticipation of a preovulatory rise in estrogen levels from the dominant follicle, granulosa cells express both FSH and LH receptors, and theca cells increase their expression of LH receptors. An LH surge results in ovulation.

During ovulation, the wall of the ovary at the location of the dominant follicle degrades and ruptures, releasing the oocyte into the peritoneal space, where it can be captured by the fimbriae at the end of the Fallopian tube. The granulosa cells surrounding the ruptured follicle are filled with cholesterol esters and become the corpus luteum ("yellow body").

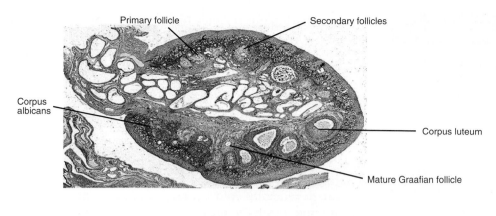

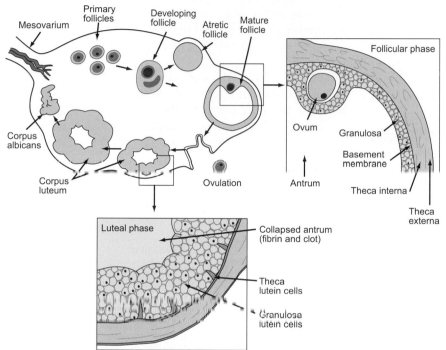

FIGURE 9-32. **Follicular development in situ.** (Reproduced with permission from USMLERx.com.)

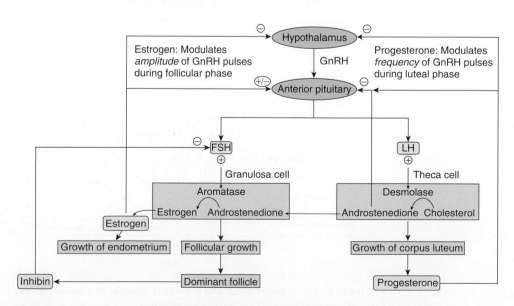

FIGURE 9-33. **Female hormonal axis (follicular phase).** FSH, follicle-stimulating hormone; GnRH, gonadotropin-releasing hormone; LH, luteinizing hormone.

CLINICAL CORRELATION

hCG is used to detect pregnancy because it appears in the urine approximately 8 days after successful fertilization.

CLINICAL CORRELATION

Insulin stimulates the ovaries to produce estrogen. Consequently, type 2 diabetics with insulin resistance and hyperinsulinemia may have a greater risk of breast cancer and endometrial carcinoma.

FLASH BACK

A female fetus has high levels of FSH and LH during the second trimester, owing to development of the genitalia.

The corpus luteum secretes high levels of progesterone and lower levels of estrogen. Progesterone transforms the proliferating endometrium into secretory endometrium to prepare the uterus for implantation. It also thickens the cervical mucus, rendering it impenetrable to sperm.

If fertilization and implantation occur, the extraembryonic trophoblasts produce **human chorionic gonadotropin (hCG)**. This hormone acts like LH and causes the corpus luteum to continue secreting high levels of progesterone, stimulating further development of the endometrium.

If fertilization and implantation do not occur (Figure 9-34), the corpus luteum degenerates into a mass of scar tissue called the **corpus albicans** ("white body") after approximately 14 days. Consequently, estrogen and progesterone levels drop, and the functional portion of the endometrium is shed via menstruation. The whole process of follicular recruitment through menstruation takes approximately 28 days.

Figure 9-35 shows the variation of FSH and LH levels with age. These two hormones normally stimulate production of estrogen, but after menopause, there are no more ovarian follicles, so estrogen, progesterone, and inhibin levels drop despite continuing high levels of FSH and LH. A woman's lifetime estrogen exposure is an important risk factor for the development of breast cancer and endometrial cancer. Increased estrogen exposure is associated with early menarche, late menopause, nulliparity, and not breast-feeding.

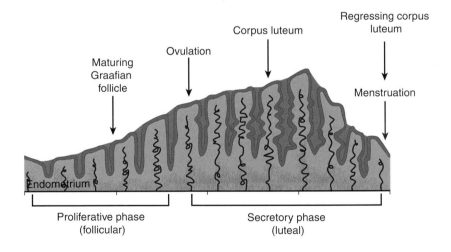

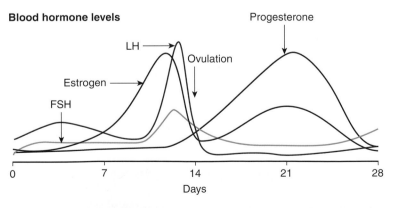

FIGURE 9-34. **Endometrial and hormonal changes in a menstrual cycle.** FSH, follicle-stimulating hormone; LH, luteinizing hormone.

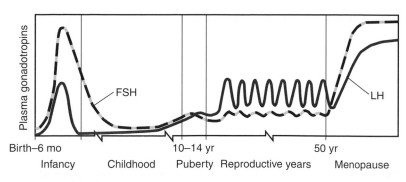

FIGURE 9-35. **Plasma gonadotropin levels throughout a woman's lifetime.** FSH, follicle-stimulating hormone; LH, luteinizing hormone. (Modified with permission from Kasper DL, Braunwald E, Fauci AS, et al. *Harrison's Principles of Internal Medicine*, 16th ed. New York: McGraw-Hill, 2005.)

GONADAL STEROIDS

Steroid hormones, which are derived from cholesterol (Figure 9-36), can be organized into five groups: mineralocorticoids, glucocorticoids, androgens, estrogens, and progestagens. The latter three groups are vital for normal genital development and, later, fertility. Their functions are reviewed in Table 9-9. Dehydroepiandrosterone (DHEA), a weak androgen, and androstenedione are both produced in the adrenal gland (zona reticularis) and the gonads. By comparison, the stronger androgens and estrogens (eg, testosterone, DHT, and estradiol) are primarily produced in the gonads.

SEXUAL RESPONSE

The trajectory of sexual response in both men and women consists of four phases: desire, excitation (parasympathetic), orgasm (sympathetic), and resolution. Men experience increased blood flow into and decreased venous return

KEY FACT

Testosterone and androstenedione are converted to estradiol and estrone, respectively, in adipose tissue by the enzyme **aromatase.**

CLINICAL CORRELATION

Like hyperinsulinemia, obesity can increase the risk of breast cancer. Adipocytes allow peripheral conversion of androgens to estrogens.

KEY FACT

Progesterone is the only naturally occurring human progestogen. Progestins are synthetic progestagens used for hormonal contraception because they inhibit ovulation by blocking the LH surge.

MNEMONIC

PRiSM
Progestagens cause **R**elaxation of **S**mooth **M**uscle, which accounts for the observed vasodilation and decreased myometrial excitability and GI motility.

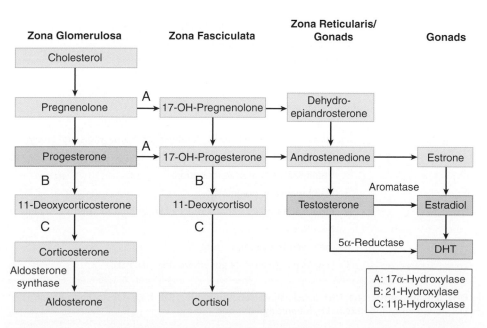

FIGURE 9-36. **Organization of steroid hormone synthesis.** Dihydrotestosterone (DHT) is produced by peripheral conversion. Estradiol can be made directly in the gonads or by peripheral conversion as well.

TABLE 9-9. Androgens, Estrogens, and Progestagens

ANDROGENS

Source	Testis (DHT and testosterone), adrenal glands (androstenedione).
Biological potency	DHT > testosterone > androstenedione.
Targets	Skin, prostate, seminal vesicles, epididymis, liver, muscle, brain.
Function	1. Differentiation of the Wolffian duct system into internal gonadal structures.
	2. Secondary sexual characteristics and growth spurt during puberty.
	3. Required for normal spermatogenesis.
	4. Anabolic effects (increased muscle size, increased RBC production).
	5. Increased libido.

ESTROGENS

Source	Ovary (estradiol), placenta (estriol), adipose (estrone, estradiol).
Biological potency	Estradiol > estrone > estriol.
Function	1. Growth of follicles.
	2. Endometrial proliferation.
	3. Development of genitalia.
	4. Stromal development of the breast.
	5. Female fat distribution.
	6. Hepatic synthesis of carrier proteins.
	7. Feedback inhibition of FSH.
	8. LH surge (estrogen feedback on LH and FSH secretion switches from negative to positive just before the LH surge).
	9. Increased myometrial excitability.
	10. Increased HDL, decreased LDL.

PROGESTAGENS

Source	Corpus luteum, placenta.
Function	1. Stimulation of endometrial glandular secretions and spiral artery development.
	2. Uterine smooth muscle relaxation.
	3. Maintenance of pregnancy.
	4. Production of thick cervical mucus, which inhibits sperm entry into the uterus.
	5. Increased body temperature.
	6. Negative regulation of gonadotropins (LH, FSH).

DHT, dihydrotestosterone; FSH, follicle-stimulating hormone; HDL, high-density lipoprotein; LDL, low-density lipoprotein; LH, luteinizing hormone.

out of the cavernous spaces of the penis, yielding an **erection.** Women, too, experience similar changes in blood flow to the clitoris and vestibular bulbs. This process is all mediated by the pelvic splanchnic nerves (parasympathetics, S2–S4).

In men, orgasm consists of two substeps: **seminal emission** and **antegrade ejaculation.** The sympathetic nervous system (T10–L2) controls closure of the bladder neck, contraction of the seminal vesicle, and deposition of semen in the posterior urethra. The somatic and visceral pudendal nerves (S2–S4) then stimulate rhythmic contraction of the ischiocavernosus and bulbocavernosus muscles, allowing ejaculation. Continued sympathetic stimulation ends the erection (**detumescence**) by inducing vasoconstriction of the arteries.

The components of semen primarily derive from five organs: seminal vesicle, prostate, testes, bulbourethral (Cowper) gland, and epididymis. The seminal vesicle secretes fructose, ascorbic acid, prostaglandins, phosphorylcholine, and flavins (60% of semen volume). The prostate secretes zinc, citric acid, phospholipids, acid phosphatase, and profibrolysin (20% of semen volume). The testes produce sperm (15% of semen volume). The bulbourethral gland secretes thick, alkaline mucus to help neutralize the acidity of the vagina (< 5% of semen volume). The epididymis secretes carnitine and acetyl carnitine (< 5% of semen volume).

In women, orgasm involves "tenting" of the vagina (relaxation of the vaginal muscularis) and contractions of the pelvic diaphragm and uterus. Detumescence of the clitoral and vestibular erectile tissue is slower, which allows women to experience multiple orgasms.

KEY FACT

The parasympathetics stimulate the release of nitric oxide (NO), which increases cyclic guanosine monophosphate (cGMP) in vascular smooth muscle and closes Ca^{2+} channels. The arterial smooth muscle relaxes, and the erectile tissue fills with blood.

MNEMONIC

Point (**P**arasympathetic) and **S**hoot (**S**ympathetic)

FERTILIZATION

Successful fertilization depends on four sequential steps:

- Gamete delivery.
- Binding of the sperm to the egg.
- Activation of the egg.
- Fusion of the sperm and egg.

Ovulation occurs within 24–48 hours of the midcycle surge of LH. Usually, only one egg is released, entering the Fallopian tube via ciliary action. The egg can survive only 24 hours in the female tract, so fertilization must occur around the time of ovulation.

By comparison, sperm can survive in the female tract for up to 5 days. In their journey to the Fallopian tubes, they are aided by estrogen-induced watery uterine mucus and peristaltic uterine contractions. Before being able to fertilize the egg, sperm must be **capacitated** in the female tract—a set of changes that alter membrane fluidity, membrane potential, and even movement of the tail.

Fertilization takes place in the Fallopian tube (ampulla). Capacitated sperm penetrate the corona radiata and bind to the zona pellucida. This species-specific interaction triggers the acrosome reaction and allows the entire sperm cell to burrow deeper into the egg.

The unfertilized egg is metabolically quiescent. After fusing with the sperm cell, the egg undergoes a signal transduction cascade that stimulates the egg to

KEY FACT

Fertilization of a single egg with multiple sperm would result in aneuploidy, **not** multiple, viable zygotes.

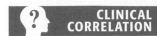

CLINICAL CORRELATION

Ectopic pregnancies occur when the zygote implants somewhere other than the uterus. Implantation in the Fallopian tube can lead to tubal rupture.

complete meiosis II (formation of the second polar body and a haploid ovum) and release cortical granules to prevent polyspermy (Figure 9-37). Sperm already bound to the zona pellucida are removed, and new ones are prevented from binding.

The egg's cytoplasm causes the sperm nucleus to decondense and form the male pronucleus. The mitochondria and tail disintegrate, but the sperm cell contributes a centriole for cell division. The male and female centrioles organize an aster, allowing the two pronuclei to slowly come together over the course of 12 hours. During this time, DNA replication occurs. Thus, when the male and female pronuclei finally fuse, the zygote can undergo mitosis to form two diploid cells.

While undergoing cell division, the zygote travels down the oviduct to the uterus, where it implants 5 days after fertilization.

At best, the probability of fertilization following intercourse is 35%, and only two-thirds of fertilized eggs develop successfully. Thus, the probability of a successful pregnancy is about 25%.

PREGNANCY

Designed to optimize the welfare of the fetus, numerous metabolic and physical changes occur in the mother's body during pregnancy.

Osmoregulation

Pregnancy is a state of chronic volume overload and has many features similar to those of congestive heart failure, including edema and polyuria. The fetus, placenta, and amniotic fluid contribute about half of the 6- to 8-L increase in the woman's total body water. As Figure 9-38 illustrates, increased glomerular filtration rate (GFR), progesterone, prostaglandins, and atrial natriuretic peptide (ANP) favor Na^+ excretion, whereas increased aldosterone, estrogen, deoxycorticosterone, and body position favor Na^+ retention. Despite net Na^+ retention, serum concentrations (and plasma osmolality) actually decrease due to dilution. Similarly, hemodilution causes **physiologic anemia** and a compensatory increase in cardiac output.

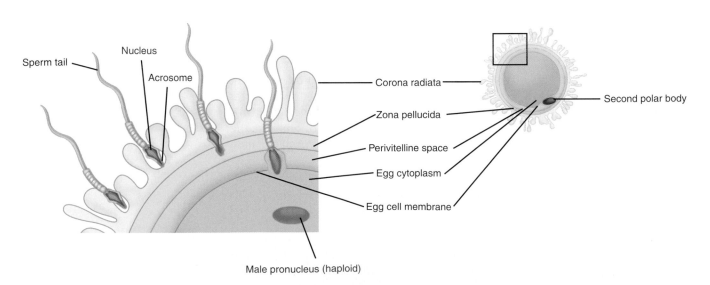

FIGURE 9-37. **Penetration of a sperm cell into the ovum.** The second polar body only appears after fertilization takes place.

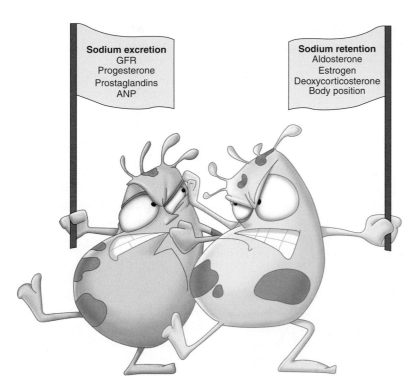

FIGURE 9-18. **Factors for Na⁺ retention and excretion.** ANP, atrial natriuretic peptide; GFR, glomerular filtration rate.

Urinary System

Positioning of the fetus can lead to decreased bladder capacity and increased urinary frequency and incontinence. An additional effect of progesterone-mediated smooth muscle relaxation is dilation of the ureters. Secondary to fluid overload, the renal pelves/calyces also dilate, literally opening the kidneys up to infection. Volume overload dilutes the serum levels of blood urea nitrogen (BUN), creatinine, and uric acid, and increases the effective renal plasma flow and GFR. The renal tubular absorptive capacity is surpassed, which may result in **glucosuria** (but not proteinuria). Similarly, small amounts of blood may also appear in the urine.

Cardiovascular System

Increased heart rate (HR) and stroke volume (SV) result in a 30–50% increase in cardiac output (CO). Nonetheless, blood pressure (BP) actually decreases secondary to progesterone acting on smooth muscle to decrease systemic vascular resistance (SVR). By the third trimester, BP returns to baseline. A low-grade systolic flow murmur and mild left ventricular hypertrophy are other normal physiologic changes seen during pregnancy.

Though the mother's blood volume increases about 50%, plasma expands at a faster rate than RBC mass, hastening the development of physiologic anemia. Platelet count may also progressively decline (gestational thrombocytopenia). Nonetheless, due to increased fibrinogen, decreased protein S, and increased venous stasis in the legs, the mother is actually in a **hypercoagulable state.**

Respiratory System

Pregnancy results in elevation of the diaphragm, which decreases the residual volume. The total lung capacity (TLC) decreases only slightly, however.

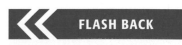

FLASH BACK

$CO = SV \times HR$
$BP = CO \times SVR$

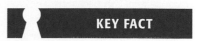

KEY FACT

The mother's respiratory rate (RR) generally remains unchanged; she takes deeper breaths at a normal frequency.

FLASH FORWARD

$MV = (TV - DV) \times RR$
where DV = dead volume, MV = minute ventilation, TV = tidal volume, and RR = respiratory rate

FLASH BACK

Do not confuse thyroglobulin (TGB) with thyroxine-binding globulin (TBG).

CLINICAL CORRELATION

Insufficient thyroid hormone levels during pregnancy, resulting from either a poorly functioning thyroid gland or low dietary iodine, can lead to severe neurologic and muscular problems in the fetus **(cretinism).**

KEY FACT

Only IgG can cross the placenta via the neonatal Fc (FcRn) receptors.

CLINICAL CORRELATION

Whereas some autoimmune diseases may improve during pregnancy, others may worsen or cause fetal complications. For example, though lupus flares are uncommon in pregnancy, systemic lupus erythematosus (SLE) increases the risk of preeclampsia, preterm birth, and fetal death.

The net effect is decreased residual volume but increased inspiratory capacity. Notably, on spirometry testing, forced vital capacity (FVC) and forced expiratory volume in 1 second (FEV_1), are unchanged.

These changes have no effect on respiratory muscle function itself. The tidal volume (TV) actually increases to allow for increased minute ventilation (MV) and chronic hyperventilation. Hyperventilation leads to decreased CO_2 partial pressure, which causes chronic (mild) respiratory alkalosis and compensatory metabolic acidosis, facilitating fetal off-loading of acidic wastes and CO_2.

On the negative side, estrogen can induce hyperemia and edema in the upper respiratory tract, which can lead to nasal stuffiness and epistaxis. Decreased pulmonary vascular resistance (PVR) and oncotic pressure can also lead to pulmonary edema.

Digestive System

Most changes to the digestive system are side effects of hemodilution, estrogen, and progesterone. Albumin and total protein levels appear decreased due to volume overload. Nonetheless, the body's new set point favors Na^+ and water absorption in the large intestine. Progesterone reduces small-bowel motility, leading to constipation. Estrogen increases 3-hydroxy-3-methylglutaryl coenzyme A (HMG-CoA) reductase activity, and progesterone delays gallbladder emptying, thus promoting supersaturation of bile with cholesterol and the formation of gallstones. Smooth muscle relaxation of the lower esophageal sphincter leads to gastroesophageal reflux disease (GERD) and nausea. Lastly, portal hypertension, spider angiomas, and palmar erythema due to high estrogen levels can mimic liver disease.

Endocrine System

Human placental lactogen (hPL) induces maternal insulin resistance to ensure continued transport of nutrients from mother to fetus. This leads to fasting hypoglycemia and postprandial hyperglycemia in the mother, in other words, glucose intolerance. With the body's response to insulin numbed, pancreatic β-cell hypertrophy results in **hyperinsulinemia** and an increased risk of gestational diabetes.

Triglycerides (TGs), high- and low-density lipoproteins (HDLs and LDLs), and total cholesterol levels all increase during pregnancy, as they are necessary precursors for steroidogenesis in the maternal adrenal glands. Progesterone, a cortisol antagonist, prevents Cushing-like effects that might otherwise be caused by increased adrenal function and delayed plasma clearance of cortisol.

Effects on the pituitary and thyroid are more subtle. Despite negative feedback by estradiol and progesterone (which decrease FSH and LH), the pituitary gland enlarges and increases its secretion of prolactin. Although hCG mimics the activity of thyroid-stimulating hormone (TSH) in the first trimester (potentially abnormal thyroid function tests), the mother remains euthyroid throughout the pregnancy. Estrogen causes an increase in hepatic synthesis of thyroxine-binding globulin (TBG), but free triiodothyronine (T_3) and thyroxine (T_4) levels remain relatively normal.

Immune System

Changes to immune function during pregnancy are complex. Estrogen and cortisol cause a progressive rise in WBC count—mostly polymorphonuclear leukocytes. This preference for granulocytes over lymphocytes and monocytes favors innate immunity over adaptive immunity. Progesterone, on the other hand, reduces the immune response, ostensibly to prevent rejection of the "foreign" fetus. The pregnant uterus is also an immune-privileged site, utilizing a number of sophisticated mechanisms to promote tolerance of the fetus.

Skin and Bones

To maintain her center of gravity, a pregnant woman experiences increased inward curvature of the spine (spinal lordosis). In anticipation of the birthing process, the woman's pubic symphysis also widens. **Relaxin,** the peptide hormone responsible for this process, causes relaxation of other ligaments as well.

Increased levels of active vitamin D [1,25-$(OH)_2$] increase intestinal absorption of Ca^{2+} so it can be transported across the placenta. Calcitonin keeps Ca^{2+} resorption from becoming overactive to protect the maternal skeleton. Parathyroid hormone (PTH) levels, on the other hand, are not particularly high because increased intestinal absorption keeps Ca^{2+} levels from falling too low. Despite all of these changes, the maternal serum ionized Ca^{2+} and phosphate levels remain normal.

Some of the most obvious changes during pregnancy occur in the skin. Estrogen-induced angiogenesis accounts for facial flushing, and estrogen also plays a role in the tearing of collagen that leads to stretch marks. Hyperinsulinemia may contribute to **linea nigra** (a hyperpigmented band down the midline) and hirsutism.

Table 9-10 reviews the key physiologic changes during pregnancy in these organ systems.

Other important aspects of pregnancy are related to the health of the fetus.

Prenatal Testing

Standard prenatal screening tests include routine blood work, urinalysis, and ultrasound examinations. Other tests may be offered based on the mother's risk factors, such as age, race, and comorbidities.

Maternal serum α-fetoprotein (AFP) was one of the first screening tests developed. High levels suggest an open neural tube defect such as cephalocele or spina bifida, whereas low levels suggest Down syndrome. The **quad test,** which makes use of multiple markers (AFP, estriol, hCG, and inhibin-A) is even more accurate (low false-positive rate).

Chorionic villus sampling (CVS) and amniocentesis are two common means of testing for chromosomal abnormalities. They are compared in Table 9-11.

The Placenta

Trophoblasts, cells forming the outer layer of the blastocyst, are the first cells to differentiate from the fertilized egg. They go on to develop into two layers:

CLINICAL CORRELATION

If blood tests show an Rh-negative mother is carrying an Rh-positive fetus, she should be given anti–Rh factor (RHOgam) injections late in the pregnancy to prevent development of maternal anti–Rh factor antibodies. Maternal anti–Rh factor antibodies do not affect the first Rh-positive fetus, but would put any future such pregnancies in jeopardy.

CLINICAL CORRELATION

hCG is also elevated in women with **hydatidiform moles** or **choriocarcinoma.**

CLINICAL CORRELATION

Failure of the placenta to properly implant in the uterine wall prevents dilation of the spiral endometrial arteries, resulting in insufficient blood flow to the fetus and **preeclampsia** (hypertension, edema, and proteinuria) in the mother.

CLINICAL CORRELATION

Though ABO blood type incompatibility occurs in approximately 20% of pregnancies, only a minority of these cases result in hemolytic anemia. This is because, unlike Rh incompatibility, which generates IgG antibodies that readily cross the placenta, ABO incompatibility generates IgM antibodies that do not. Thus, fetal hemolysis is uncommon in ABO incompatibility. Nonetheless, ABO blood type incompatibility is the most common cause of neonatal jaundice in the developed world.

TABLE 9-10. Maternal Adaptations to Pregnancy

System	Parameter	Pattern	
Renal	Renal flow	Increases 25–50%	
	Glomular filtration rate	Increases early, then plateaus	
Cardiovascular	Heart rate	Gradually increases 20%	
	Blood pressure	Gradually decreases 10% by 34 weeks, then increases to prepregnancy values	
	Stroke volume	Increases to maximum at 19 weeks, then plateaus	
	Cardiac output	Rises rapidly by 20%, then gradually increases an additional 10% by 28 weeks	
	Peripheral venous distention	Progressive increase to term	
	Peripheral vascular resistance	Progressive decrease to term	
Pulmonary	Respiratory rate	Unchanged	
	Tidal volume	Increases by 30–40%	
	Expiratory reserve	Gradual decrease	
	Vital capacity	Unchanged	
	Respiratory minute volume	Increases by 40%	
Blood	Volume	Increases by 50% in second trimester	
	Hematocrit	Decreases slightly	
	Fibrinogen	Increases	
	Electrolytes	Unchanged	
Gastrointestinal	Sphincter tone	Decreases	
	Gastric emptying time	Increases	
Weight	Uterine weight	Increases from about 60–70 g to about 900–1200 g	
	Body weight	Average 11-kg (25-lb) increase	

(Modified with permission from Gardner DG, Shoback D. *Greenspan's Basic and Clinical Endocrinology,* 8th ed, New York: McGraw-Hill, 2007: 648.)

TABLE 9-11. Diagnostic Testing for Chromosomal Abnormalities

	CVS	AMNIOCENTESIS
What is it?	Biopsy of rapidly dividing cells in the placenta.	Amniotic fluid retrieval of amniocytes.
When can it be done?	Early pregnancy (10–12 wk).	Midpregnancy (15–19 wk).
Risk of pregnancy loss?	1%	0.5%

CVS, chorionic villus sampling.

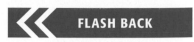

FLASH BACK

Oxygenated blood flows into the IVC → RA → foramen ovale → LA → LV → aorta → head.
Deoxygenated blood flows into the SVC → RV.
Mixed blood flows from the RV → pulmonary artery → ductus arteriosus → aorta → lower body.

KEY FACT

After birth, inspiration increases P_{O_2} and causes release of bradykinin, two factors that close the ductus arteriosus. Indomethacin, a nonsteroidal anti-inflammatory drug, can also be used to close the shunt in hypoxic newborns.

the inner cytotrophoblasts and outer syncytiotrophoblasts. The latter cells secrete hCG and attach to the uterine wall (endometrial stroma).

In the second trimester, the placenta takes over production of estrogen and progesterone, causing the corpus luteum to degrade into a corpus albicans.

The placenta is illustrated in Figure 9-39. Each gram of placenta can support 7 g of fetal tissue.

Fetal Circulation

The fetal circulatory system is different from that of the adult. It must both make use of the maternal blood supply via the placenta and avoid overperfusing the lungs while no gas exchange is occurring there. The three fetal shunts that allow this to occur are described in Table 9-12 (see also Figure 1-6).

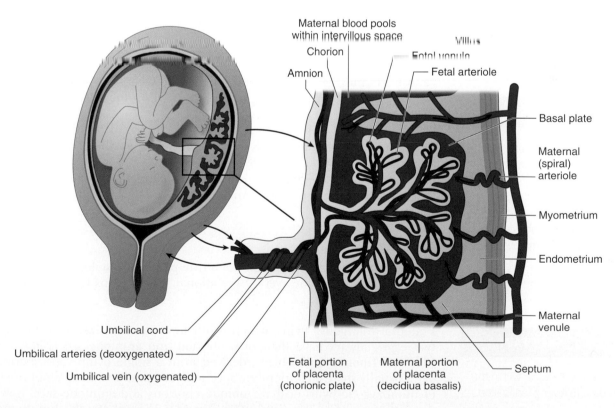

FIGURE 9-39. The mature placenta in cross-section. (Modified with permission from Morgan GE, Mikhail MS, Murry MJ. *Clinical Anesthesiology*, 4th ed. New York: McGraw-Hill, 2006: 880.)

There is no direct contact between maternal and fetal blood.

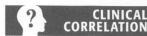

CLINICAL CORRELATION

Maintaining a patent ductus arteriosus (PDA) with prostaglandins may actually be necessary in anatomic abnormalities such as **coarctation of the aorta, transposition of the great arteries,** and **tetralogy of Fallot.**

KEY FACT

Monozygotic twins are always of the same sex (except in cases of meiotic nondisjunction, eg, XO). Dizygotic twins can be the same or different sex.

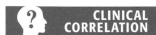

CLINICAL CORRELATION

Chorionicity in monozygotic twins can usually be determined by ultrasound. Some dichorionic, diamniotic gestations, however, feature a fused placenta, which falsely gives the appearance of a monochorionic, diamniotic pregnancy.

KEY FACT

Twinning can only occur within the first 15 days following fertilization.

TABLE 9-12. **Shunts in the Fetal Circulation**

SHUNT	LOCATION	FUNCTION	FLOW	OXYGENATION
Ductus arteriosus	Between the aorta and pulmonary trunk (artery).	Decreases pulmonary blood flow.	High PVR, low pulmonary blood flow.	Mixed blood.
Foramen ovale	Between the RA and LA.	Decreases pulmonary blood flow.	High PVR, low pulmonary blood flow.	Mixed blood.
Ductus venosus	Connects umbilical vein to the IVC (bypasses liver).	Import maternal blood.	Regulated by a sphincter.	Oxygen-rich blood.

IVC, inferior vena cava; LA, left atrium; PVR, pulmonary vascular resistance; RA, right atrium.

Furthermore, fetal hemoglobin (HbF) is more concentrated in fetal blood and has a greater affinity for O_2 than does maternal HbA. In other words, at any given oxygen partial pressure (Po_2), HbF has a greater O_2 saturation than HbA. This is the case because the γ-subunit of HbF has a weaker positive charge than the adult β-subunit, so 2,3-bisphosphoglycerate (2,3-BPG) has less of an effect on lowering its O_2 affinity.

For an adult, these circulatory modifications are unnecessary. Thus, three key changes allow for the transition from fetal to normal adult circulation:

- PVR decreases.
- SVR increases.
- The fetal shunts close so the pulmonary and systemic circulations operate in parallel.

At birth, the sphincter in the ductus venosus constricts and closes the ductus venosus; cutting off the placental blood supply causes portal blood to enter the hepatic sinusoids, resulting in a drop in BP in the IVC and right atrium (RA). Inspiration by the newborn increases Po_2 and causes release of bradykinin, which induces vasoconstriction and closure of the ductus arteriosus. Accompanied by reduced PVR from lung expansion, this results in increased pulmonary blood flow. The left atrial (LA) pressure rises and the RA pressure decreases, closing the foramen ovale, and thus functionally setting up the normal adult systemic circulation. Anatomic closure occurs with the formation of fibrous tissue.

Twinning

Multiple fetal gestation, though not a true pathologic state, is a natural cause of premature birth. The average gestational age for twins is 35 weeks, and for triplets it is 33 weeks.

Fraternal (dizygotic) twins, which result from two fertilized ova (two sperm, two eggs), always have their own chorion and amniotic sac (Figure 9-40). Identical (monozygotic) twins, derived from a single ovum (one sperm, one egg), usually share a chorion but have separate amniotic sacs. About one-third of monozygotic twins do have unique chorions and amniotic sacs, however, depending on when the ovum splits. Figure 9-41 illustrates this timeline.

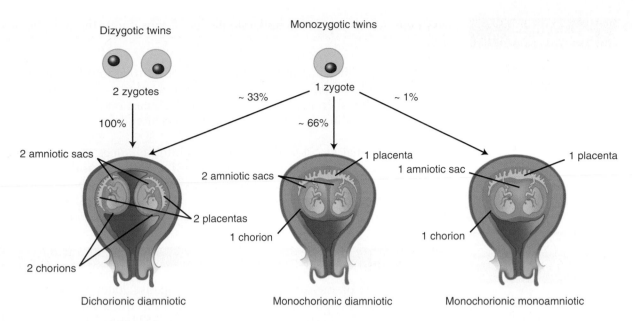

FIGURE 9-40. **Development of dizygotic and monozygotic twins.**

Breast-Feeding

During pregnancy, estrogen and progesterone levels are high. These hormones ready the breasts for milk production. However, estrogen antagonizes **prolactin,** preventing lactation. After expulsion of the placenta, estrogen and progesterone levels drop, removing the blockade of prolactin. The suckling of an infant on the breast stimulates prolactin secretion from the anterior pituitary and subsequent milk production. The posterior pituitary secretes

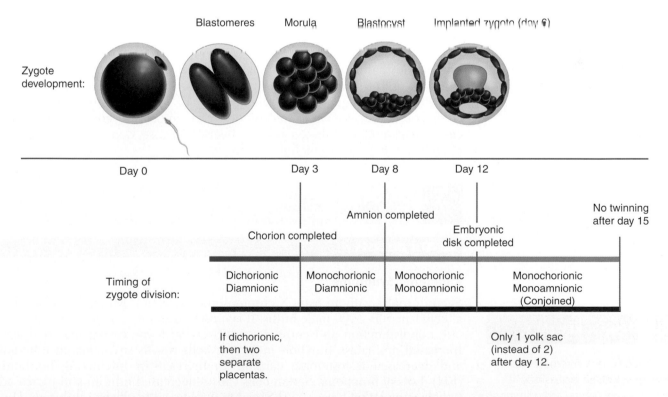

FIGURE 9-41. **Chorionicity in monozygotic twins.** Division of the zygote between days 12 and 15 results in conjoined twins.

CLINICAL CORRELATION

Having monozygotic twins is based on chance (1:250 pregnancies), whereas the likelihood of having dizygotic twins can be influenced by anything that increases fertility (eg, fertility drugs or increased FSH at either end of the reproductive lifetime). Thus, dizygotic twins may run in families, but monozygotic twins do not.

KEY FACT

Breast milk contains antimicrobial, immunomodulating, and anti-inflammatory agents not found in formula.

KEY FACT

Hormonal changes in menopause lead to reduced estrogen, higher FSH, higher LH (no surges), and higher GnRH.

MNEMONIC

Menopause creates HAVOC:
Hot flashes
Atrophy of the
Vagina
Osteoporosis
Coronary artery disease

KEY FACT

Each additional X chromosome correlates with an increasingly abnormal phenotype and with more severe mental retardation.

oxytocin, which expels the milk into the lactiferous ducts (the milk "letdown" reflex).

Breast milk is a dynamic fluid that changes both throughout the day and over the course of lactation. For example, though the volume decreases over a single feeding, the fat content increases. Similarly, breast milk is particularly rich in immunoglobulins (IgA) within the first 5 days after delivery.

It is believed that breast-feeding reduces a child's chances of acquiring acute infections (eg, respiratory syncytial virus, GI infections, and otitis media), chronic illnesses (eg, leukemia, irritable bowel disease, and obesity), and allergies. Similarly, breast-feeding seems to reduce the mother's risk of ovarian and premenopausal breast cancer, as well as that of osteoporosis and anemia.

MENOPAUSE

The cessation of menstruation, called menopause, occurs around age 52 and results from depletion of functional follicles in the ovaries. This leads to low serum levels of estradiol, elevated levels of FSH and LH, and secondary amenorrhea. Figure 9-35 shows the variation of FSH and LH levels with age. Recall that these two hormones normally stimulate production of estrogen, but after menopause, estrogen and inhibin levels drop due to ovarian failure. Lack of feedback inhibition generates very high levels of FSH and LH. A woman's lifetime estrogen exposure is an important risk factor for the development of breast and endometrial cancers. Increased estrogen exposure is associated with early menarche, late menopause, nulliparity, and not breast-feeding.

Some women experience symptoms such as palpitations, joint pain, decreased libido, vaginal dryness, and poor sleep (leading to forgetfulness and irritability) during menopause. Estrogen hormone replacement therapy (HRT) counteracts many of these symptoms, positively affecting the CNS to improve cognition and reducing depression. Estrogen therapy also preserves bone mass and inhibits hot flashes. However, unbalanced oral estrogen therapy increases a woman's risk of thromboembolic phenomena, stroke, and endometrial cancer. Similarly, estrogen-progesterone therapy (EPT), which reduces the risk of colorectal cancer, increases the risk of breast cancer and coronary heart disease. Development of these negative effects, of course, depends on the length of HRT and the age at which it is given.

Pathology—Male

GENETIC DISEASES

Klinefelter Syndrome

Seen in males with an extra X chromosome (47,XXY), Klinefelter syndrome affects 1 in 500–1000 male births. It is most commonly due to maternal meiotic nondisjunction and correlates positively with increasing maternal age. Increased aromatase function in Leydig cells results in increased estradiol and decreased testosterone, causing an increase in luteinizing hormone (LH). Loss of functional Sertoli cells causes decreased inhibin and increased follicle-stimulating hormone (FSH) due to reduced feedback inhibition. Histologically, there is hyalinization of the seminiferous tubules and prominent Leydig cells.

PRESENTATION

- Hypogonadism (very small [size of an almond], firm testes due to fibrosis and hyalinization) and infertility due to azoospermia.
- Tall, eunuchoid body shape with disproportionately long extremities.
- Female secondary sex characteristics at puberty such as **gynecomastia** and **female hair distribution** due to decreased testosterone:estradiol ratio.
- Elevated urinary gonadotropins result from lack of feedback inhibition.
- May present with developmental delay.

DIAGNOSIS

Klinefelter syndrome is suggested by classic phenotypic findings, including gynecomastia, tall stature, and small, firm testes.

- Hormonal findings include abnormally low testosterone and mildly elevated estrogen and gonadotropin levels (FSH and LH).
- Confirmed by demonstrating a 47,XXY karyotype with one of the X chromosomes inactivated in each cell (Barr body).

TREATMENT

- Most individuals receive lifelong testosterone therapy to induce puberty and maintain male secondary sex characteristics.
- Men with Klinefelter disease typically have azoosperima (no sperm in semen ejaculate). Many men with Klinefelter can achieve a pregnancy with their own gametes by advanced fertility techniques, such as testicular biopsy to retrieve sperm from the testes, and intracytoplasmic sperm injection (ICSI), whereby one sperm is directly injected into each egg that has been retrieved from a woman's ovaries during an in vitro fertilization (IVF) cycle.

XYY Syndrome

- Phenotypically normal male.
- Results from paternal nondisjunction at meiosis I, resulting in a sperm with an extra Y chromosome.
- XYY occurs 1 in 1000 male births.
- Increased risk of learning disabilities (speech and language skills) and behavioral problems.
- Reports of increased proportion of XYY males in prisons and mental hospitals are now known to be incorrect.
- Often are several centimeters taller than parents and siblings and have severe cystic acne.

Male Pseudohermaphrodite

Genetic male (46,XY) with ambiguous or female external genitalia (eg, vagina with blind pouch). Testes are present. However, there is effective testosterone deficiency, possibly due to any of the following causes:

- Defective testicular differentiation.
- Impaired secretion/production of testosterone.
- Failure of conversion of testosterone to dihydrotestosterone (DHT) (**5α-reductase deficiency**).
- Defect of androgen receptors (most common is **androgen insensitivity syndrome**).

KEY FACT

PSEUDOhermaphrodite is named after the **GONAD** present (eg, if testes are present, the subject is a **MALE** pseudohermaphrodite).

FLASH BACK

Formation of gonads (testes or ovaries) is genetically determined, whereas formation of male external genitalia is determined by the presence of functional testes and androgen receptors; in the absence of functioning testes or androgen receptors, development is female.

True Hermaphrodite

- Presence of both ovaries and testes in the same individual, which may be due to XX/XY mosaicism or abnormal crossover of a region of the Y chromosome containing the *SRY* region with the X chromosome in an XX individual.
- The external genitalia may be normal male, ambiguous (most common), or normal female.
- Cryptorchidism and hypospadias are common.
- The gonads are most often ovotestes, followed by ovaries, and, least commonly, testes.
- The development of the genital ducts follows that of the ipsilateral gonad.
- Germ cell tumors, inguinal hernias, and obstructed genital tracts frequently occur in true hermaphrodites.

5α-Reductase Type 2 Deficiency

- 5α-Reductase catalyzes the conversion of testosterone to dihydrotestosterone (DHT), a potent androgen required for the development of male external genitalia and secondary sexual characteristics.
- Males born with this enzyme deficiency have functional testes in addition to female or ambiguous **external genitalia.**
- Since functioning testes produce testosterone and Müllerian-inhibiting factor (MIF), **internal genitalia** develop in a male pattern.
- Increased testosterone production at puberty is able to generate sufficient levels of DHT either via 5α-reductase type 1 activity in the liver, skin, and brain or low-level expression of 5α-reductase type 2 in the testes. This causes masculinization and increased growth of external genitalia.

Androgen Insensitivity

- Mutations of androgen receptors render them nonfunctional. Testes are normal and produce testosterone, MIF, and other substances.
- Males with androgen insensitivity present with failure of development of male internal and external genitalia.
- Presence of MIF prevents the development of the paramesonephric ducts into the uterus, cervix, Fallopian tubes, and upper two-thirds of the vagina.
- **Complete** androgen insensitivity results in normal female external genitalia, whereas **incomplete** androgen insensitivity results in ambiguous external genitalia.

PENILE DISEASES

Phimosis

Extremely tight foreskin that is too small to be retracted over the glans penis. Although physiologic until 3 years of age, after that time it is considered pathologic. Often occurs in uncircumcised males that experience chronic infections and inflammation of the glans penis (**balanitis**), sometimes due to poor hygiene of the area. Circumcision can be used as a treatment after the initial infection is treated with broad-spectrum antibiotics.

Peyronie Disease

A dense, subcutaneous fibrous plaque forms on the tunica albuginea on the dorsal side of the penis, which causes the penis to curve laterally when erect. It mainly affects older men; however, the cause is unknown. If the curvature of the penis interferes with normal sexual intercourse, surgical correction is

KEY FACT

Mosaicism is the presence of two or more genetically distinct populations of cells in one individual.

KEY FACT

Phimosis is prone to infection, commonly due to *Candida.*

recommended. If erectile dysfunction or infertility occurs, then a penile implant should be considered.

Priapism

An erection that is persistent in the absence of sexual stimulation or desire and is often very painful. Can be a result of sickle cell disease, spinal cord injury, antidepressants (eg, trazodone), antipsychotics (eg, chlorpromazine), and penile trauma.

KEY FACT

Trazodone is an antidepressant that can cause **priapism.**

Balanitis

Inflammation of the glans penis. It is called **balanoposthitis** when the foreskin and prepuce are also inflamed. Balanitis is commonly seen in unhygienic uncircumcised men. The collection of smegma, which is carcinogenic, and the lack of aeration causes irritation and inflammation, accounting for the increased rates of penile cancer seen in uncircumcised males. Balanitis can be complicated by phimosis and meatal stenosis leading to urinary retention. Treatment includes cleaning of the area and antibiotics.

Bowen Disease

Intraepithelial neoplasia on the shaft of the penis/scrotum. It is associated with high-risk human papillomavirus (HPV) infection (eg, HPV-16). It presents as a gray, solitary, crusty plaque typically on the penis or scrotum. It is a precancerous lesion and has a **10% chance of progression to squamous cell carcinoma.**

Erythroplasia of Queyrat

Intraepithelial neoplasia on the shaft of penis/scrotum similar to Bowen disease. However, it presents as red, velvety plaques that typically involve the glans. Also associated with high-risk HPV and is a precursor to squamous cell carcinoma.

Bowenoid Papulosis

Small, multiple, red-, brown-, or flesh-colored patches on the skin of the penis. It is a premalignant condition with a 2–3% chance of progression to cancer. Bowenoid papulosis has a close link to high-risk HPV and is described as being between genital warts and Bowen disease of the penis in severity. Many cases of Bowenoid papulosis spontaneously regress, but close follow-up is required as it has malignant potential.

Cancer

Squamous cell carcinoma of the penis. Penile cancer is rare in the United States, representing < 1% of cancers in males. Penile cancer is frequently seen in an uncircumcised, unhygienic individual and is closely linked with genital warts and high-risk HPV.

FLASH FORWARD

High-risk HPV infection is also associated with cervical, oral, and anal cancer.

DISEASES OF THE TESTES

Congenital Abnormalities

CRYPTORCHIDISM

- A failure of one or both testes to descend into the scrotal sac.
- Most often unilateral, though sometimes occurs bilaterally.

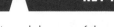
KEY FACT

Normal descent of the testes:
- Transabdominal phase (mediated by MIF)
- Inguinoscrotal phase (mediated by androgens, hCG)

- The undescended testis can frequently be palpated as a mass in the inguinal canal.
- Usually spontaneously descends by 3 months of age.
- A **greatly increased risk of germ cell tumors,** usually seminomas and embryonal carcinomas, is associated with cryptorchidism, even after surgical intervention, and in both the normal testis and cryptorchid testis.
- **Complications:** Ipsilateral inguinal hernia, testicular torsion, trauma, and infertility.
- **Treatment:** Orchiopexy decreases the risk of cancer if done prior to 10 years of age. It helps to fix the testes, prevent torsion, and increase fertility, and aids in detection of cancer because the external position of the testis facilitates examination and diagnostics.

Infectious Diseases

ORCHITIS

- An inflammation of the testes usually caused by the mumps virus (family Paramyxoviridae, genus *Rubulavirus*) and usually affects only one testis.
- If the condition is **bilateral (uncommon),** it **may lead to sterility** resulting from atrophy of the seminiferous tubules. In the case of sterility, levels of testosterone are decreased, but levels of FSH and LH are increased.

EPIDIDYMITIS

An infection of the epididymis that can be caused by a variety of bacteria.

- < 35 years old: *Chlamydia trachomatis* and *Neisseria gonorrhoeae*.
- > 35 years old: *Escherichia coli* and *Pseudomonas aeruginosa*.
- A tuberculous infection can start in the epididymis and travel to the seminal vesicles, prostate, and testicles.
- Patients often suffer from pain and swelling in the scrotum, tenderness, and a positive **Prehn sign** (a marked decrease in pain in association with elevation of the scrotum).

KEY FACT

Epididymitis is more common in men 19–40 years of age, and **orchitis** is more common in boys (< 10 years).

Other Abnormalities

TORSION

A twisting of the spermatic cord that compromises blood supply to the testes, potentially resulting in testicular infarction and gangrene (Figure 9-42).

- Most often caused by violent trauma to the testes or cryptorchidism.
- **Surgical correction** within 6 hours of occurrence usually results in full recovery of the testis.

VARICOCELE

Dilated and tortuous veins located in the pampiniform plexus of the spermatic cord that most often appears as a **"bag of worms"** on examination.

- The left testis is more likely to have a varicocele because its pampiniform plexus drains into the left renal vein before the inferior vena cava (IVC), causing increased pressure in the venous plexus.
- Any type of **obstruction of the left renal vein,** such as in renal cell carcinoma, can cause a varicocele.
- Varicocele is the most common cause of treatable male **subfertility.**

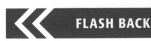
FLASH BACK

Right testicular vein → IVC
Left testicular vein → left renal vein → IVC

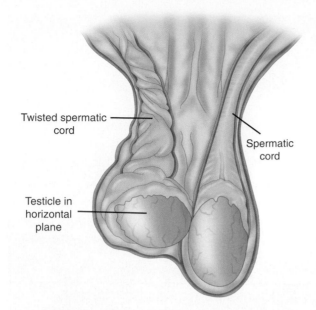

FIGURE 9-42. **Testicular torsion.** Note the unilateral pulling of the testis into the horizontal plane due to the twisting of the spermatic cord.

HYDROCELE

A collection of serous fluid that distends the tunica vaginalis. Most commonly caused by a **persistent processus vaginalis** that enables communication between the scrotum and the peritoneal cavity. Also can be due to infection or lymphatic blockage as a result of a tumor.

- The most frequent cause of **enlargement of the scrotum** in young boys.
- Can be distinguished from tumors by transillumination (Figure 9-43). Hydroceles transilluminate, tumors do not.

HEMATOCELE

A collection of blood in the tunica vaginalis. Hematocele often results from testicular trauma and presents with pain, tenderness, and absent transillumination. They sometimes result from tapping a hydrocele during examination. If a hematocele is not drained, a clotted hematocele is formed, which requires orchidectomy.

SPERMATOCELE

A retention cyst distended with fluid containing spermatozoa in the epididymis or rete testis. Spermatocele is often present in the head of the epididymis and behind the upper pole of the testis. Small ones can be ignored; larger ones should be aspirated or excised through a scrotal incision.

NEOPLASMS

Germ Cell Tumors

SEMINOMA

Most common germ cell tumor of the testes. Large, soft, well-demarcated, gray-white tumor that bulges from the cut surface of the affected testis. A

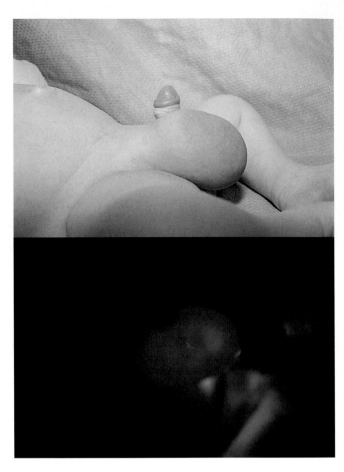

FIGURE 9-43. **Hydrocele and transillumination.** Note the translucent appearance when a light is shone through the testis filled with serous fluid. (Courtesy of Michael J. Nowicki, MD.)

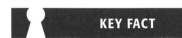

KEY FACT

Cryptorchidism results in an increased risk of **seminomas.**

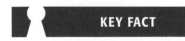

KEY FACT

Testicular tumors metastasize first to the periaortic lymph nodes.

seminoma is confined beneath an intact tunica albuginea. Microscopically, large cells with distinct cell borders, pale nuclei, and prominent nucleoli ("fried egg" appearance) as well as a lymphocytic infiltrate are seen. **Semi-noma** is associated with an increase in **hCG** and **placental-like alkaline phosphatase (PLAP).** It mainly affects males between the ages of 15 and 35 years old. Seminoma metastasizes via the lymphatics and is radiosensitive with an excellent prognosis (Figure 9-44 and Table 9-13).

YOLK SAC TUMOR

Large, may be well demarcated. Microscopically, cells appear as cuboidal to columnar epithelium forming sheets, glands, papillae, and microcysts, and are often associated with **hyaline globules. Schiller-Duval bodies,** which are structures resembling primitive glomeruli, are a distinctive feature of yolk sac tumors. This is the most common primary testicular neoplasm in children < 3 years. α-Fetoprotein (AFP) can be demonstrated within the cytoplasm of these neoplastic cells.

EMBRYONAL CARCINOMA

Ill-defined invasive mass containing foci of hemorrhage and necrosis. Metastases are common. Histologically, the cells are large and primitive looking, with basophilic cytoplasm, indistinct cell borders, and large nuclei with prominent nucleoli. The cells may be arranged in undifferentiated, solid sheets or glandular structures. Embryonal carcinoma is associated with **an increase in hCG.**

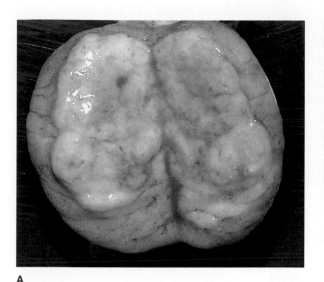
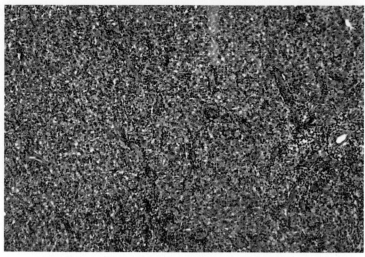

A **B**

FIGURE 9-44. **Testicular seminoma.** (A) Gross specimen shows well-defined borders with involvement of most of the parenchyma. (B) Histologic section shows infiltration of lymphocytes into the parenchyma. (Reproduced with permission from USMLERx.com.)

CHORIOCARCINOMA

Grossly, primary tumor is small and nonpalpable. Microscopically, choriocarcinoma is composed of sheets of small cuboidal cells irregularly intermingled with or capped by large, eosinophilic syncytial cells containing multiple dark, pleomorphic nuclei; these represent **cytotrophoblastic and syncytiotrophoblastic differentiation,** respectively. **hCG is elevated.** Choriocarcinoma metastasizes hematogenously.

TERATOMAS

Firm masses that contain cysts and recognizable areas of cartilage and other tissue types. Originating from germ cells, they neoplastically differentiate into

TABLE 9-13. **Characteristics, Tumor Markers, and Prognosis of Germ Cell Testicular Tumors**

MALIGNANCY	CHARACTERISTICS	TUMOR MARKERS	PROGNOSIS
Seminoma	Large, well-demarcated mass.	Increased hCG, PLAP	Excellent
Yolk sac tumor	Schiller-Duval bodies.	Increased AFP	Good
Embryonal carcinoma	Ill-defined masses with foci of necrosis and hemorrhage.	Increased hCG	Poor
Choriocarcinoma	Trophoblastic tissue.	Increased hCG	Poor
Teratoma	Derivatives from multiple germ layers (ectoderm, endoderm, mesoderm).	Increased AFP and/or hCG	Good

AFP, α-fetoprotein; hCG, human chorionic gonadotropin; PLAP, placental-like alkaline phosphatase.

ectoderm, endoderm, and mesoderm. Histologically, there are three major variants: mature, immature with or without malignant transformation, and mixed.

- **Mature:** Fully differentiated tissues from multiple germ cell layers (eg, neural tissue, cartilage, adipose, bone, and epithelium) in a random array.
- **Immature:** Immature somatic elements reminiscent of those in developing fetal tissue.
- **With malignant transformation:** Characterized by the development of frank malignancy in preexisting teratomatous elements, usually in the form of a squamous cell carcinoma or adenocarcinoma. Usually occurs in adults.
- **Mixed:** Combinations of any of the germ cell tumors above may occur in mixed tumors, the most common being a combination of teratoma, embryonal carcinoma, and yolk sac tumors. **hCG and AFP are elevated.**

Interstitial (Nongerm) Cell Tumors

LEYDIG CELL TUMOR

Arises from Leydig cells that contain rod-shaped **Reinke crystals,** and is usually benign in nature. Golden-brown mass consisting of large, uniform cells with indistinct cell borders. It produces androgens or estrogens, leading to gynecomastia in men and precocious puberty in boys. Treatment is orchidectomy.

SERTOLI CELL TUMOR

Arises from Sertoli cells. Grossly, it is a gray-white to yellow mass. Microscopically, it shows cord-like structures resembling seminiferous tubules. Secretes a small amount of androgens or estrogens that is typically insufficient to induce gynecomastia, loss of libido, and aspermia. It is usually a benign condition, and orchidectomy is curative.

MALIGNANT LYMPHOMA

Originates as a diffuse large-cell lymphoma and causes secondary involvement of both testes. It is the most common testicular cancer in elderly men. Prognosis is poor.

PROSTATE DISEASES

Prostatitis

Inflammation of the prostate gland.

PRESENTATION

- Dysuria, urinary frequency, malaise, lower back pain.
- Poorly localized pelvic pain.
- May be acute or chronic.
  - **Acute:** Caused by *E coli* and other gram-negative rods. Neutrophilic infiltrate, congestion, and edema. Microabscesses may form. The prostate is often **tender and boggy.** Leukocytosis and fever are also seen. In patients < 35 years of age, the pathogens *C trachomatis* and *N gonorrhoeae* are most likely. In patients older than 35 years of age, *E coli*, *P aeruginosa*, and *Klebsiella pneumoniae* are most likely.

- **Chronic:** Tissue destruction, **increased fibroblasts,** and inflammatory cells characteristic of chronic infections. Can be caused by recurrent UTIs or STDs. There are two types of chronic prostatitis:
  - **Bacterial:** Same organisms responsible for acute prostatitis.
  - **Abacterial:** The most common form of chronic prostatitis. Leukocytes are found in prostatic secretions but there are no bacteriologic findings. There is no history of recurrent UTI. However, *C trachomatis* and *Ureaplasma urealyticum* have also been implicated.

TREATMENT

For bacterial prostatitis, antibiotic treatment with trimethoprim/sulfamethoxazole or ciprofloxacin is effective. For abacterial prostatitis, no therapies have been shown to be effective. Nonsteroidal anti-inflammatory drugs (NSAIDs) can be used as an adjunctive therapy.

Benign Prostatic Hyperplasia (BPH)

Benign enlargement of the prostate gland due to cellular proliferation (**hyperplasia**), usually at the periurethral central zone (Figure 9-45).

- It is commonly seen in males > 50 years of age.
- Family history (first-degree relative) is a risk factor.
- With age, estrogen levels tend to increase, in turn inducing surface expression of androgen receptors in the central zone of the prostate. Therefore, despite the generally lower androgen levels in older men, their prostate hypertrophies because of increased **sensitivity** to DHT.

PRESENTATION

Patient presents with urgency, frequency, nocturia, dribbling of urine, poor stream, sensation of incomplete voiding, incontinence, urinary retention and often UTI. This may lead to distention and hypertrophy of the bladder due to incomplete emptying and straining during urination.

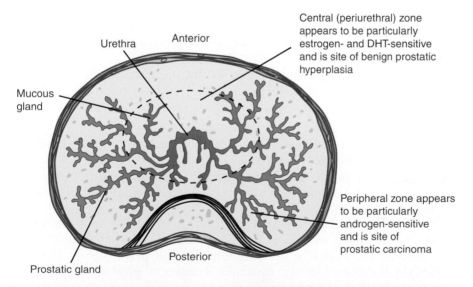

FIGURE 9-45. Transverse section of prostate showing location of benign prostatic hypertrophy (BPH) and prostatic carcinoma. The central portion of the prostate is sensitive to estrogen and dihydrotestosterone and is the site for BPH, whereas the peripheral zone is sensitive to androgen and is the site for prostatic carcinoma. DHT = dihydrotestosterone.

FLASH FORWARD

Prazosin, doxazosin, and terazosin relax the bladder neck and prostate by blocking α-adrenergic receptors located in smooth muscle. They are used to treat urinary retention in BPH.

FLASH FORWARD

The 5α-reductase inhibitor finasteride inhibits conversion of testosterone to DHT. DHT normally causes increased proliferation of smooth muscle in the central zone of the prostate.

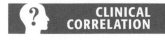

CLINICAL CORRELATION

PSA is often used to monitor tumor burden and recurrences. Digital rectal exams do **not** increase the false-positive rate of PSA.

DIAGNOSIS

- Firm, smooth, and uniform enlargement of the prostate on digital rectal examination.
- Sonogram shows a diffusely enlarged prostate.
- Prostate-specific antigen (PSA) level is checked to rule out prostate cancer. PSA can be elevated in BPH, but is typically <10 ng/mL.

TREATMENT

Medical treatment includes nonselective α-blockers (doxazosin, prazosin, and terazosin), selective α-blockers (tamsulosin), and 5α-reductase inhibitors (finasteride). Surgical management involves transurethral resection of the prostate (TURP) or prostatectomy.

Adenocarcinoma of the Prostate

- Arises mostly from the peripheral zone (70%) of the prostate (see Figure 9-45).
- It occurs in 20–30% of men > 50 years of age and in 90% of men > 70 years of age.
- Most are very slow growing and never present in the man's lifetime.
- With advancing age, the androgen level declines. When the androgen level declines, regressive changes occur, mainly in the peripheral zone, and prostatic carcinoma arises in these settings.

PRESENTATION

- Appears as a hard, irregular mass during digital rectal examination.
- Since the peripheral zone is typically involved, urinary symptoms are a late manifestation of the disease.

SPREAD

- Spreads via hematogenous or lymphatic channels and by direct invasion.
- Spreads to the **lungs** hematogenously and via the vertebral venous plexus to **pelvic bones and lumbosacral spine.**
- Lymphatic spread occurs to presacral, internal iliac, para-aortic, and supraclavicular nodes, whereas direct spread may invade the bladder, ureter, seminal vesicles, and other pelvic structures.
- The rectum is rarely involved due to the presence of the rectovesical fascia.

DIAGNOSIS

- On digital rectal examination, the prostate appears to be **stony hard with obliteration of the median sulcus.**
- PSA (glycoprotein produced by normal and abnormal ductal epithelium) > 10 ng/mL is suggestive, and > 35 ng/mL is diagnostic of advanced cancer.
- **Alkaline phosphatase** is elevated either due to hepatic or bone metastasis.
- Radiologic findings in case of metastasis include characteristic sclerotic, osteoblastic metastases in lumbar vertebrae and pelvic bones. However, osteolytic metastases are also common. Transrectal prostatic biopsy always confirms the diagnosis when in doubt.

TREATMENT

Radical prostatectomy can be done as a curative treatment for early disease, but palliative treatment is the only option for advanced disease. The palliative treatment involves deprivation of androgens via bilateral orchidectomy or by giving antiandrogens such as flutamide. Other treatment options include radiation and gonadotropin-releasing hormone (GnRH) agonists administered in a continuous fashion (suppresses anterior pituitary secretion of FSH and LH).

Pathology—Female

GENETIC DISEASES

Turner Syndrome

Primary hypogonadism in phenotypic females resulting from partial or complete monosomy (45,X). Short stature is related to loss of regions on the short arm of the X chromosome. Loss of regions of the long arm of the X chromosome is associated with amenorrhea and premature loss of ovarian follicles but not with short stature. If there is any Y chromosome mosaicism, there is increased risk for gonadoblastoma (germ cell tumor) and gonadal extirpation is required. Patients typically have either primary ovarian failure (primary amenorrhea) or premature ovarian failure (premature menopause).

PRESENTATION

- Newborns may have webbed neck (**cystic hygroma**), edema of the hands and feet, coarctation of the aorta, characteristic triangular facies, pulmonary stenosis, and bicuspid aortic valve.
- Affected girls often fail to develop secondary sex characteristics.
- The genitalia may remain infantile with little pubic hair.
- Patients generally a short stature with a "shield chest" with widely spaced nipples, **streak ovaries,** and amenorrhea.
- Short stature and primary amenorrhea in adult patients should prompt strong suspicion of Turner syndrome.

DIAGNOSIS

Karyotyping (no Barr body), high FSH:LH ratio due to decreased estrogen.

TREATMENT

Teenage patients need counseling regarding stigmata of their condition and treatment with hormone therapy. Estrogen is given for development of secondary sexual characteristics, normal menstruation, and osteoporosis prevention. Growth hormone may be given to increase the height of affected patients.

PROGNOSIS

Patients with 45,X (most common) or 45,X mosaicism have a low fertility rate. Those who become pregnant have increased rates of spontaneous abortion (30%), stillbirths (6–10%), and maternal death (2%).

Female Pseudohermaphrodite

- Genetic females (XX) with virilized or ambiguous external genitalia due to excessive and inappropriate exposure to androgens during the 8th to 13th weeks of gestation.
- Commonly seen in **congenital adrenal hyperplasia.**

Müllerian Agenesis

Characterized by the congenital absence of the vagina with variable uterine development. It is the second most common cause of primary amenorrhea.

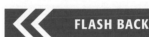

Indifferent gonads develop into ovaries without the genetic signal *SRY* (sex-determining region of the Y chromosome) to turn into testes. If no germ cells are present in the indifferent gonad, it will fail to develop and become a streak gonad.

Turner syndrome is the most common cause of primary amenorrhea.

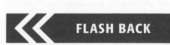

Fused lower ends of the Müllerian (paramesonephric) ducts form the uterus, Fallopian tubes, cervix, and upper two-thirds of the vagina.

KEY FACT

The stratified squamous epithelium of the anus and vagina are derived from the cloaca and have somatic innervation from the pudendal nerve. The structures superior have columnar epithelium and visceral innervation.

The incidence rate is 1 in 4000–5000 live female births. Affected individuals have normal ovaries and normal secondary sexual characteristics. The exact cause is unknown.

PRESENTATION

- Primary amenorrhea in the presence of normal secondary sexual characteristics.
- The vagina may be absent or shortened.
- The labia majora, labia minora, and clitoris are normal.
- Ectopic kidneys are common. Other patients may present with voiding difficulties, recurrent UTIs, and urinary incontinence.

DIAGNOSIS

- Ultrasound or MRI can often be diagnostic.
- Laparoscopy is performed if there is an unclear diagnosis or pain from functioning obstructed Müllerian remnants, possibly with a higher rate of endometriosis.
- After administration of IV contrast medium and subsequent excretion by the kidneys, a pyelogram is performed to assess for frequently associated urinary tract abnormalities.

KEY FACT

Renal abnormalities are found in 20–30% of women with Müllerian duct abnormalities.

TREATMENT

- Progressive dilation or reconstructive surgery on the foreshortened vagina can be performed to make the vagina more functional, and this may establish sexual functioning. Sometimes intercourse itself can serve this same purpose.
- Rudimentary uterine horns may need to be excised to prevent pain if they have functioning endometrium.

VAGINAL DISEASES

Vaginismus

The involuntary contraction of the muscles of the pelvic floor, which causes pain and prevents vaginal penetration, including sexual intercourse and insertion of a speculum in gynecologic examinations. The exact cause is unknown, but it is important to investigate both physiologic and psychological causes. Treatment should be individualized based on the patient's condition.

Condyloma Acuminata (Genital Warts)

Occurs on the female genitalia, perineum, perianal area, and rectum. Genital warts result from HPV infection acquired during sexual intercourse. Genital warts appear as soft, tan, cauliflower-like warts. Histologically, genital warts have epidermal hyperplasia with cytoplasmic vacuolization (**koilocytosis**) (Figure 9-46).

KEY FACT

Koilocytes are cells infected with HPV. They appear to have vacuolated cytoplasm.

Neoplasms

SQUAMOUS CELL CARCINOMA

Most common form of vaginal cancer with a mean age of presentation of 60 years. Squamous cell carcinoma may present with painless vaginal bleeding and discharge, commonly after intercourse. Commonly, it is an extension of a cervical squamous carcinoma with the primary lesion associated with high-risk HPV (eg, types 16, 18).

FLASH FORWARD

HPV types 16 and 18 cause 70% of cervical cancers. HPV expresses E6 and E7 oncoproteins that interact with p53 and Rb, respectively, leading to malignant transformation.

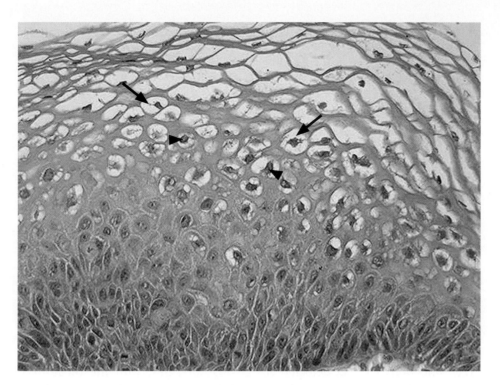

FIGURE 9-46. **Koilocytosis caused by human papillomavirus.** Cytoplasmic vacuolization (*arrows*) is found around pyknotic nuclei (*arrowheads*). (Reproduced with permission from USMLERx.com.)

CLEAR CELL ADENOCARCINOMA

Correlated with girls in their late teens whose mothers took **diethylstilbestrol** (DES), an estrogen once believed to prevent miscarriage, during pregnancy. In one-third of the at-risk population, small glandular or microcystic inclusions appear in the vaginal mucosa (vaginal adenosis). Microscopically, malignant cells appear with clear cytoplasm.

SARCOMA BOTRYOIDES (EMBRYONAL RHABDOMYOSARCOMA)

Rare (except on examinations). Encountered in children < 5 years who present with vaginal bleeding and soft polypoid grape-like masses that protrude from the vagina. Histologically, sarcoma botryoides appears as a small, round, blue-cell tumor with skeletal muscle differentiation. It also expresses muscle-specific proteins including **desmin.**

> **KEY FACT**

The most common cancer of the vagina is squamous cell carcinoma, followed by adenocarcinoma. Malignant melanoma is the third most common cause of vaginal cancer.

The most common cancer of the vulva is also squamous cell carcinoma. However, melanoma ranks second for vulvar cancer.

CERVICAL DISEASES

Cervical Dysplasia

Abnormal organization of cells in cervical epithelium starting from the basal layer. It has a tendency to progress from mild to severe dysplasia, and finally to invasive carcinoma. Ninety percent of cervical intraepithelial neoplasia (CIN) is associated with HPV infection. On biopsy, CIN is histologically classified as:

- CIN I (mild dysplasia): Involves the basal third of the epithelium.
- CIN II (moderate dysplasia): Involves the basal two-thirds of the epithelium.
- CIN III (severe dysplasia): Involves more than two-thirds of the epithelium.
- Carcinoma in situ: Involves the entire thickness of the epithelium.

KEY FACT

CIN is the histologic classification derived from biopsy, whereas ASCUS, LGSIL, or HGSIL is the cytologic classification derived from Pap smear examinations.

FLASH BACK

Carcinoma in situ (biopsy) is a preinvasive neoplasm with an intact basement membrane. Dysplasia (cytology) does not necessarily progress to cancer.

According to the Bethesda system for cytologic Papanicolaou (Pap) smear examinations, atypical squamous cells are classified into those of undetermined significance (ASCUS), low-grade squamous intraepithelial lesion (LGSIL), and high-grade squamous intraepithelial lesion (HGSIL).

Invasive Carcinoma

Early cervical cancer is often asymptomatic. Risk factors for development are related to infection with oncogenic HPV, including **early age at first intercourse, multiple partners, cigarette smoking,** and **high-risk HPV infection** (most important risk factor). Progression from CIN III to invasive carcinoma requires approximately 10 years (Figure 9-47). Cervical cancer can invade directly into the uterus, vagina, peritoneal cavity, bladder, or rectum, and by lymphatic or hematogenous dissemination.

PRESENTATION

Postcoital vaginal bleeding, abnormal vaginal bleeding, or a mucinous discharge. In late-stage disease, the patient may present with foul-smelling vaginal discharge, weight loss, or obstructive uropathy.

High-Risk HPV (Types 16, 18, 31, 33, 35, and 39)

HPV infections can be detected in 85–90% of cases, with the most common types being 16 and 18. High-risk HPVs integrate into the host's DNA and express the proteins E6 and E7, which inactivate p53 and Rb respectively, allowing uncontrolled cellular proliferation.

DIAGNOSIS

Pap smear is a screening test that looks for abnormal cervical cells while the patient is asymptomatic. Increased detection of abnormal cells with Pap smears has reduced the number of cervical cancer cases in developed countries. Women with abnormal cytology should undergo colposcopy. Rectal

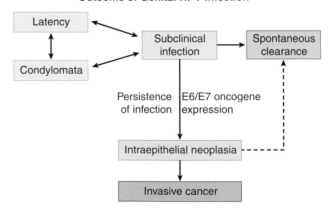

FIGURE 9-47. The potential outcomes of genital human papillomavirus (HPV) infection. Subclinical infection and spontaneous resolution are the most common outcomes. Progression to invasive cancer usually develops over a period of approximately 10 years. (Reproduced with permission from Shorge JO, Schaffer JL, Halvorson LM, et al. *Williams Gynecology.* New York: McGraw-Hill, 2008: Figure 29-4.)

examinations may reveal nodularity when carcinoma invades into the parametrium. Biopsy alone is sufficient for diagnosis.

PREVENTION

Vaccination against HPV-16 and -18 reduces the risk of developing cervical neoplasia and cervical cancer.

TREATMENT

Cervical conization, simple hysterectomy, radical hysterectomy, or radiation therapy and chemotherapy, depending on the stage.

PROGNOSIS

Five-year survival is > 80% with early-stage disease. Five-year survival is < 10% with late-stage disease.

KEY FACT

The most common form of cervical cancer is squamous cell carcinoma. The second most common form is adenocarcinoma.

UTERINE DISEASES

Clues to uterine pathology include lower abdominal pain, changes in the menstrual cycle (more or less frequent, heavier or lighter), or a range of constitutional symptoms (fever, chills, and unintentional weight loss). To determine the specific underlying cause, pay attention to the age of the patient and the characteristics of the menstrual cycle with regard to symptoms.

Pelvic Inflammatory Disease

Pelvic inflammatory disease (PID) is infection and inflammation of the upper genital tract. Causative organisms include:

- *Neisseria gonorrhoeae.*
- *Chlamydia trachomatis.*
- *Gardnerella vaginalis*
- *Anaerobic bacteria.*
- Less commonly *Haemophilus influenzae*, enteric gram-negative rods, and streptococci.
- In regions where tuberculosis is endemic, PID is commonly caused by *Mycobacterium tuberculosis.*

PID commonly occurs in young, sexually active, nulliparous women. Progestin-containing oral contraceptive pills and barrier methods may have a protective effect against PID. Risk factors include smoking, douching, and nonwhite race.

PRESENTATION

Patients present with lower abdominal pain, fever with chills, and purulent cervical discharge. On examination, cervical motion tenderness (**chandelier sign**) and adnexal tenderness may be noted. However, many patients with PID may exhibit subtle signs and symptoms, making it difficult to diagnose. Because the sequelae are grave, PID criteria are defined broadly with low sensitivity in order to catch all cases.

TREATMENT

Azithromycin and ceftriaxone are used to cover *C trachomatis* and *N gonorrhoeae*, respectively.

KEY FACT

PID with right upper quadrant tenderness suggests associated perihepatitis (infection of the liver capsule) from bacterial transmigration across the peritoneum. This condition is known as **Fitz-Hugh-Curtis syndrome.**

COMPLICATIONS

Even with treatment, 25% of patients with acute PID develop recurrent PID, chronic pelvic pain, dyspareunia, **ectopic pregnancy,** or **infertility.** May also progress to Fitz-Hugh-Curtis syndrome.

Endometritis

Infection of the endometrium. Frequently preceded by parturition or miscarriage and is related to retained products of conception. Presents with fever and abdominal pain in the postpartum period. Chronic endometritis can occur in association with chronic gonorrheal disease, miliary tuberculosis, intrauterine devices, or spontaneously. Histologically, there is irregular proliferation of the glands with chronic inflammatory cells present.

Endometriosis

Presence of functional endometrial tissue outside the uterus. The most common sites of implantation are the pelvic viscera (ovaries are most common, rectosigmoid pouch of Douglas is second most common) and the peritoneum (Figure 9-48). Other sites of implantation include laparotomy scars, lungs, pleura, diaphragm, kidneys, nasal mucosa, spinal canal, stomach, and breast. Endometriosis is believed to occur in 6–8% of women of reproductive age in the United States.

PATHOPHYSIOLOGY

The exact cause of endometriosis is unknown; however, several theories have been proposed to explain its occurrence, including the retrograde menstrual flow theory, celomic metaplasia, and multifactorial genetic predisposition.

- **Regurgitant flow theory (retrograde menstruation, or Sampson's theory):** Menstrual regurgitation occurs in 80–90% of women during normal menstruation. The endometrial cells get implanted elsewhere and function as if they were in the uterine cavity.
- **Celomic metaplasia:** Conversion of one normal cell type to another (eg, hemoptysis and epistaxis concurrent with each menstrual period suggest upper respiratory endometriosis).

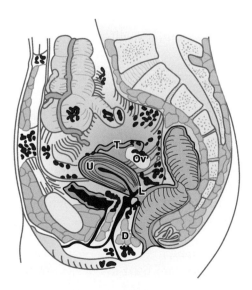

FIGURE 9-48. Common locations of endometriosis. The most common sites of endometrial implants are the uterus (U), uterine tubes (T), ovaries (Ov), uterine ligaments (L), and the rectosigmoid pouch of Douglas (D).

- **Induction theory:** Some believe that under the influence of immunologic and hormonal factors, undifferentiated peritoneal cells get transformed into endometrial cells.
- **Genetic factors:** A relative risk of 7 has been shown in women who have first-degree relatives affected with endometriosis. Twin studies support the role of genetic influences.

PRESENTATION

There are a variety of manifestations, ranging from no complaints to the following:

- Cyclic bleeding with **dysmenorrhea** (severe menstrual pain).
- Subfertility or infertility.
- Dyspareunia.
- Chronic pelvic pain.
- Pain on defecation.
- Pain on urination.
- GI symptoms like nausea, vomiting, bloating, distention, and altered bowel habits.

The physical examination may be normal in the majority of women. However, the following findings may be present:

- Pelvic tenderness.
- Adnexal tenderness.
- Tenderness and nodularity over the uterosacral ligaments or in the posterior cul-de-sac.
- Unilateral ovarian enlargement.
- Retroverted uterus.

DIAGNOSIS

- A transvaginal sonogram has excellent specificity and sensitivity in detecting ovarian endometriotic cysts.
- Laparoscopic findings of endometriosis with histologic confirmation remain the gold standard for the diagnosis of endometriosis.
- Laparoscopic findings include typical lesions that appear to be like **powder burns,** or red implants, serous or clear vesicles, white plaques, yellow-brown discoloration of the peritoneum, and scarring. The pathologic diagnosis requires the presence of two or more of the following: endometrial glands, endometrial stroma, and hemosiderin-laden macrophages.

TREATMENT

- Progestins and progestin dominant, estrogen-progestin contraceptives stop proliferation of endometrial cells by shutting down the hypothalamic-pituitary-ovarian axis, resulting in endometrial atrophy.
- Danazol is useful in endometriosis because of its antigonadotropin activity. Danazol directly acts on the pituitary to decrease the level of gonadotropins.
- A GnRH analog given in a continuous fashion (vs. pulsatile) also acts by decreasing the levels of LH and FSH, thereby decreasing the estrogen level.
- The goal of **surgical management** is to preserve fertility and decrease symptomatology. The least expensive and least invasive procedures should be the preferred choices.

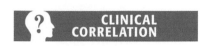

CLINICAL CORRELATION

Suspect **endometriosis** in women with new-onset cyclic dysmenorrhea.

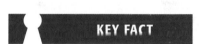

KEY FACT

Endometrioma is a pseudocyst formed by accumulation of menstrual debris from shedding and bleeding of a small endometrial implant over the ovarian cortex. These are also called **chocolate cysts** because of the color of the fluid.

Adenomyosis

Presence of endometrial glands and stroma in the myometrium of the uterus. The proliferating stratum basalis is nonfunctional, and it may occur focally or diffusely.

PRESENTATION

- Menorrhagia and dysmenorrhea.
- Asymptomatic in one-third of cases.
- Pelvic examination may reveal an enlarged soft, bulky uterus, a uterine mass, or uterine tenderness.

DIAGNOSIS

- Transvaginal sonography is the initial imaging technique of choice.
- MRI is the most accurate diagnostic test for adenomyosis.

TREATMENT

Hysterectomy is the only definitive treatment.

COMPLICATION

Anemia due to menorrhagia.

Neoplasms

ENDOMETRIAL HYPERPLASIA

Proliferation of endometrial glands and stroma in a greater-than-normal gland:stroma ratio. **Endometrial hyperplasia usually occurs due to prolonged unopposed action of estrogen on endometrial tissue.** Causes include early menarche, late menopause, nulliparity, polycystic ovary syndrome (PCOS), and any other condition associated with anovulation (unopposed estrogen), granulosa cell tumor (secretes estrogen), tamoxifen (an endometrial estrogen-receptor agonist, despite being a breast estrogen-receptor antagonist), or unopposed estrogen therapy without concomitant use of a progestin.

The different types of endometrial hyperplasia are described in Table 9-14.

TABLE 9-14. Types of Endometrial Hyperplasia, Cytologic Features, and Progression to Endometrial Carcinoma

TYPE	CYTOLOGIC FEATURES	PROGRESSION TO ENDOMETRIAL CANCER (%)
Simple	Cystic hyperplasia without atypia.	1
Complex	Adenomatous hyperplasia without atypia.	3–5
Simple with atypia	Cystic hyperplasia with atypia.	8–10
Complex with atypia	Adenomatous hyperplasia with atypia.	29

PRESENTATION

Patients with endometrial hyperplasia present with abnormal uterine bleeding, such as menorrhagia, metrorrhagia, or postmenopausal bleeding. Amenorrhea may also be a presenting symptom, especially in anovulatory patients.

DIAGNOSIS

The diagnosis is based on histologic examination of specimens obtained either from dilatation and curettage (D&C) or endometrial biopsy in an office setting.

TREATMENT

Progesterone therapy is quite effective for hyperplasia without atypia. However, complex hyperplasia with atypia may require hysterectomy because 25% of patients with atypical hyperplasia detected on endometrial biopsy or curettage specimens are found to have well-differentiated endometrial carcinoma. Women who have not completed childbearing can be treated with progestins and followed closely to preserve fertility.

> **KEY FACT**
>
> Any factor that causes the endometrium to undergo unopposed estrogen exposure increases the risk of **endometrial carcinoma.**

LEIOMYOMA

A benign tumor arising from smooth muscle and connective tissue of the uterus. **Most common of all tumors in females.** Leiomyomas are clonal and arise from a single myometrial cell. Leiomyomas occur in 20–50% of women of reproductive age and may be:

- **Intramural:** Tumors embedded within the myometrium.
- **Submucosal:** Tumors directly beneath the endometrium (Figure 9-49).
- **Subserosal:** Tumors directly beneath the serosa.

Sometimes leiomyomas are found in the peritoneal cavity, broad ligament, and cervix. The exact cause is unknown. Grossly, leiomyomas are sharply circumscribed, firm, gray-white masses with a **characteristic whorled cut surface.** Microscopically, the cells appear to have uniform size and shape with scarce mitotic figures. Malignant transformation is very rare.

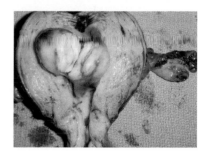

FIGURE 9-49. Submucosal leiomyoma. (Courtesy of Dr. Paban Sharma, Patan Hospital, Kathmandu, Nepal.)

PRESENTATION

Peak incidence is 20–40 years of age. The clinical features of leiomyoma depend on the location, size, and number of tumors. Symptoms include the following:

- Menorrhagia, which may lead to iron deficiency anemia.
- Pain symptoms such as dysmenorrhea, dyspareunia, or pelvic pressure. Acute pain may result from torsion of a pedunculated fibroid.
- Pressure symptoms such as frequency, urgency, incontinence, constipation, or venous stasis of the lower extremities.
- Recurrent abortions in the first trimester.
- Ascites.
- Polycythemia.

DIAGNOSIS

Pelvic examination may reveal an asymmetrically enlarged uterus or an adnexal or pelvic mass. Sonography shows a concentric, solid hypoechoic mass. The diagnosis is confirmed by histopathology, which shows uniform-sized cells with few mitotic figures.

KEY FACT

Red degeneration is a form of coagulative necrosis in a hemorrhagic, meaty, cut surface.

TREATMENT

- **Medical:** Continuous administration of GnRH agonists decreases the levels of FSH, LH, and estrogen. Long-term use of GnRH agonists is limited by their side effects (eg, hot flashes).
- **Surgical:** Hysterectomy or myomectomy.

COMPLICATIONS

Calcification, ossification, mucinous or cystic degeneration, and **red degeneration**; anemia and venous stasis in the lower extremities are common complications of leiomyoma. Leiomyomas are estrogen-sensitive and therefore may enlarge during pregnancy.

ENDOMETRIAL CARCINOMA

Cancer arising from the endometrium of the uterus. It is the **most common gynecologic malignancy,** and 2–3% of women develop endometrial carcinoma in their lifetime. Seventy-five percent of endometrial cancer occurs in women > 50 years of age. It ranks as the fourth most common malignancy in women after breast, lung, and colon cancers. The most common risk factors for endometrial carcinoma include:

- Nulliparity
- Late menopause
- Early menarche
- Obesity
- Diabetes mellitus
- Estrogen replacement therapy
- Atypical endometrial hyperplasia
- Tamoxifen therapy for breast cancer

Endometrial carcinoma can arise in two different pathologic settings:

- **Endometrioid:** Carcinomas frequently arise on a backdrop of endometrial hyperplasia. These tumors are termed endometrioid because they appear similar to normal endometrial glands. They originate in the mucosa and may infiltrate the myometrium and enter the vascular spaces, with metastases to regional lymph nodes.
- **Papillary serous and clear cell:** Poorly differentiated cancers that do not arise from endometrial hyperplasia and are much more aggressive tumors. Not associated with unopposed estrogen exposure.

KEY FACT

There is no appropriate screening test for endometrial carcinoma.

Most patients present at their perimenopausal or postmenopausal period with complaints of vaginal bleeding or discharge. The peak age of incidence is in the sixth and seventh decades of life.

DIAGNOSIS

Endometrial aspiration biopsy is the best initial investigation of choice.

TREATMENT

Total abdominal hysterectomy plus bilateral salpingo-oophorectomy with peritoneal sampling is routinely done.

CLINICAL CORRELATION

Postmenopausal vaginal bleeding is endometrial carcinoma until proven otherwise.

LEIOMYOSARCOMA

- Arises from mesenchymal cells of the myometrium, *not* from preexisting leiomyomas.
- Appears similar to leiomyomas but diagnostic features include **pleomorphic spindle cells with relatively frequent mitoses.**

- Older females are affected, and pathology reveals at least 10 mitotic figures per high-power field, atypia, and necrosis.
- Treat with surgical resection.

KEY FACT

Leiomyosarcoma does not arise from leiomyoma.

OVARIAN DISEASES

Polycystic Ovary Syndrome

Characterized by chronic anovulation, hirsutism, obesity, and enlarged polycystic ovaries. The most important features of PCOS are anovulation and signs of hyperandrogenism. Ovaries are enlarged with multiple small cysts and the cortex is thickened.

PATHOGENESIS

Most women with PCOS have elevated LH secretion, which stimulates the ovarian theca and stroma to secrete excessive quantities of androgens, including androstenedione and testosterone. In addition, many women with PCOS are insulin resistant with chronic hyperinsulinemia. Although the women are insulin resistant, the ovaries are stimulated by the insulin to secrete excess quantities of androgens. The elevated ovarian androgens are associated with poor follicle growth. Follicle growth is stunted, with follicles achieving a maximal size of 2–9 mm in diameter. These follicles are too small to trigger an LH surge, and anovulation results (Figure 9-50).

PRESENTATION

Patients with PCOS present with hirsutism, obesity, chronic anovulation, insulin resistance, infertility, and anemia. Symptoms typically begin around menarche. They are also at increased risk for endometrial hyperplasia and carcinoma due to prolonged unopposed estrogen exposure.

DIAGNOSIS

There are three major diagnostic criteria (two of three should be met for diagnosis):

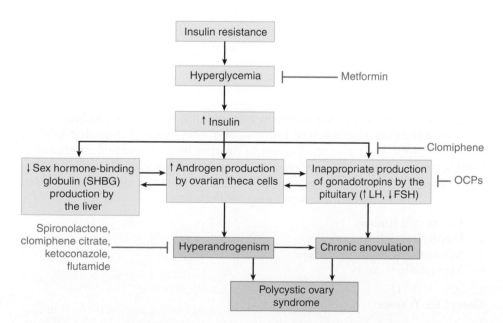

FIGURE 9-50. **Pathophysiologic pathways in polycystic ovary syndrome.**

- Any form of hyperandrogenism: clinical (eg, acne, hirsutism) or endocrine (high levels of androgens).
- Oligomenorrhea or amenorrhea indicating ovarian dysfunction.
- Sonogram showing enlarged ovaries, with multiple (> 12) small cysts (2–9 mm in diameter) in a "string of pearls" configuration.
- Other endocrinopathies must be ruled out, such as hypothyroidism, hyperprolactinemia, or late-onset congenital adrenal hyperplasia.
- Laboratory studies show increased LH production (leading cause of anovulation) and hyperandrogenism due to inappropriate increased synthesis of androgens by theca cells.

TREATMENT

Weight loss, oral contraceptive pills (OCPs), GnRH agonists, metformin, ketoconazole, spironolactone, clomiphene citrate, and pergonal (menotropins) have been used with varying degrees of success.

Follicular Cyst

When the LH surge does not occur and the Graafian follicle does not extrude the ovum, it grows and results in a follicular cyst that does not usually require treatment. It goes away on its own after two or three menstrual cycles. Sometimes an OCP can be used.

Corpus Luteum Cyst

Hemorrhage into a persistent corpus luteum. Normally after the LH surge, the ovum is extruded. The follicle then turns into a corpus luteum. However, the corpus luteum can sometimes accumulate fluid, thus becoming a corpus luteum cyst. It can grow up to 6 cm in diameter and has a potential to rupture, which consequently can cause ovarian torsion. Corpus luteum cysts are also called *hemorrhagic cysts*. The cysts usually regress spontaneously. There is an association of corpus luteum cysts with the use of ovulation-inducing medication such as clomiphene citrate.

Theca Lutein Cyst

Lined with theca interna cells, theca lutein cysts are usually bilateral and often regress spontaneously. They may grow to a large size and rupture. The cysts are associated with molar pregnancy, choriocarcinoma, twin pregnancy, Rh isoimmunization, and ovulation-inducing agents such as clomiphene citrate.

Neoplasms

Asymptomatic until growing tumor becomes large enough to produce symptoms of abdominal distention or fullness, or a dragging sensation due to mass effect. A tumor mass also predisposes to ovarian torsion, causing intermittent intense and sharp pain. Constitutional symptoms of fever, chills, and unintentional weight loss may also be present. Ovarian neoplasms are broadly divided into the following categories, depending on their origin:

- **Germ cell tumors**
- **Epithelial cell tumors**
- **Sex cord/stromal cell tumors**
- **Metastatic tumors**

GERM CELL TUMORS

Derived from primordial germ cells of ovaries and constitute 20% of all ovarian tumors. They are similar to testicular germ cell tumors (see previous discussion).

KEY FACT

Hemorrhagic (corpus luteum) cysts are a common gynecologic cause of ovarian torsion and acute abdomen in a young female.

PRESENTATION

Can occur at any age, but peak incidence is in the early 20s.

- About one-third of germ cell tumors diagnosed in children and adolescents are malignant, but most diagnosed in adults are benign (primarily mature cystic teratomas).
- Often present at early stages, unlike epithelial ovarian tumors, which are slow growing and often present at late stages.
- Pelvic pain.
- Menstrual irregularities.
- Rapidly growing pelvic mass with pressure symptoms on the bladder and rectum.
- Adnexal mass, ascites, and pleural effusion may be present.

DIAGNOSIS

- **Sonogram** may reveal adnexal mass measuring > 2 cm with cystic or solid components.
- Karyotyping may be necessary because germ cell tumors tend to occur in dysgenetic gonads (can be seen in 46,XY females).

TYPES

- Dysgerminoma
- Endodermal sinus tumor
- Embryonal carcinoma
- Choriocarcinoma
- Teratomas

DYSGERMINOMA

The most common malignant germ cell tumor in females. Analogous to seminoma of the testes. Associated with elevated **placental-like alkaline phosphatase (PLAP)**, **lactate dehydrogenase (LDH)**, and **human chorionic gonadotropin (hCG)** (Table 9-15).

- Typically unilateral; bilateral in **10–15% of cases.**
- The capsule appears thin, and the cut surface is spongy and gray-brown in color (Figure 9-51). Histologically, dysgerminomas exhibit large, round cells with clear cytoplasm and large nuclei with prominent nucleoli.

TABLE 9-15. Germ Cell Tumors, Tumor Markers, and Characteristic Features

GERM CELL TUMORS	TUMOR MARKERS	CHARACTERISTIC FEATURES
Dysgerminoma	PLAP, LDH, and hCG	Large round cells with clear cytoplasm.
Endodermal sinus tumor	AFP	Blood vessels with cancer cells resembling primitive glomeruli (Schiller-Duval bodies).
Embryonal carcinoma	hCG and AFP	Large cells, basophilic cytoplasm with indistinct borders.
Choriocarcinoma	hCG	Syncytiotrophoblast and cytotrophoblast.
Teratoma	AFP and hCG	Differentiated somatic cells from endoderm, ectoderm, and mesoderm.

AFP, α-fetoprotein; hCG, human chorionic gonadotropin; LDH, lactate dehydrogenase; PLAP, placental-like alkaline phosphatase.

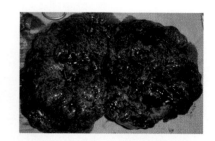

FIGURE 9-51. Dysgerminoma of ovary. (Courtesy of Dr. Paban Sharma, Patan Hospital, Kathmandu, Nepal.)

- Increased risk in Turner syndrome and pseudohermaphrodites (46,XY females).
- Highly sensitive to radiation and chemotherapy.

ENDODERMAL SINUS TUMOR

Also known as yolk sac tumor both in males and females.

- Second most common germ cell tumor of the ovary; occurs in those < 30 years of age.
- Associated with **elevated AFP** levels (see Table 9-15).
- Shows glandular and papillary structures.
- Papillary structures resemble primitive glomeruli (**Schiller-Duval bodies**).
- Radioresistant but chemosensitive.

EMBRYONAL CARCINOMA

- **hCG** and **AFP** are usually **elevated.**
- Appears as an ill-defined invasive mass containing foci of hemorrhage and necrosis.
- The cells are large and primitive looking, with basophilic cytoplasm, indistinct cell borders, and large nuclei with prominent nucleoli.
- May secrete estrogens, leading to precocious puberty.
- Responds to combination chemotherapy.

KEY FACT

hCG is a product of the trophoblast.

CHORIOCARCINOMA

Grossly, primary tumors are small, nonpalpable lesions. Microscopically, **cytotrophoblasts** and **syncytiotrophoblasts** are seen.

- **hCG** is elevated (see Table 9-15).
- Increased frequency of theca-lutein cysts.
- Responds well to chemotherapy; therefore, good prognosis.

KEY FACT

AFP is a product of yolk sac cells.

TERATOMA

Differentiated neoplastic germ cells along somatic cell lines. They contain differentiated somatic cells from multiple germ layers (ectoderm, mesoderm, and endoderm). Teratomas are firm masses that on cut surface often contain cysts and recognizable areas of cartilage. AFP and hCG are associated tumor markers. Histologically, there are three major variants:

- **Mature dermoid cyst:** "Dermoid" because this tumor has hair and keratin (Figure 9-52). Most frequent benign ovarian tumor.
  - **Benign.**
  - **Bilateral in 10–15%** (Figure 9-53).
  - **Most common during reproductive years.**
  - Cyst lined by epidermis and adnexal structure.
  - Contains **well-differentiated** bone, cartilage, hair, muscle, and/or thyroid follicles.
- **Immature dermoid cyst:**
  - **Malignant.**
  - Common in younger age groups.
  - Solid tumor (Figure 9-54) with areas of hemorrhage and necrosis.
  - Contains **poorly differentiated** elements of bone, cartilage, hair, muscle, and/or thyroid tissues.
  - Immature areas are always immature neuroepithelium.
- **Specialized teratoma:** Primarily monodermal in origin. An example is **struma ovarii,** which contains mostly mature thyroid tissues. Sometimes can cause **hyperthyroidism** (rare).

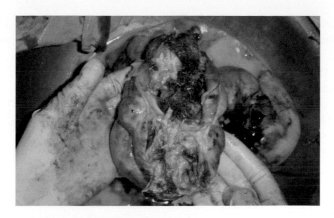

FIGURE 9-52. **Cut section of mature dermoid cyst showing hairs.** (Courtesy of Dr. Paban Sharma, Patan Hospital, Kathmandu, Nepal.)

EPITHELIAL CELL TUMORS

Arises from the epithelial lining of the ovary. It usually appears at the fifth or sixth decade of life and accounts for 90% of all ovarian cancer. CA-125 is a surface-derived ovarian cancer marker that is used to follow tumor burden during treatment and to detect recurrence; however, it is not diagnostic of ovarian cancer because it can be elevated in other conditions. Risk factors include low parity, infertility, early menarche, and late menopause. Genetic predisposition, such as **BRCA-1** and **Lynch syndrome (hereditary nonpolyposis colon cancer [HNPCC])**, is the most significant risk factor. The use of oral contraceptive pills has been documented to help prevent ovarian cancer.

Types include:

- Serous
- Mucinous
- Brenner
- Endometrioid

SEROUS

- **Serous cystadenoma:**
  - Benign.
  - Filled with pale yellow serous fluid.

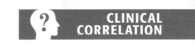

CLINICAL CORRELATION

CA-125 is used to assess treatment efficacy and detect recurrence but is never diagnostic!

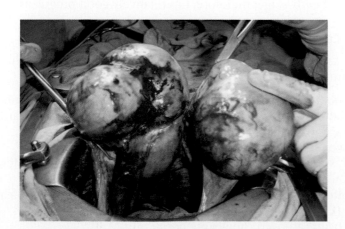

FIGURE 9-53. **Intraoperative image showing bilateral mature dermoid cysts.** (Courtesy of Dr. Paban Sharma, Patan Hospital, Kathmandu, Nepal.)

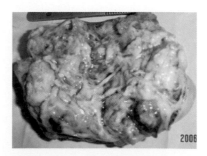

FIGURE 9-54. **Immature dermoid cyst.** (Courtesy of Dr. Paban Sharma, Patan Hospital, Kathmandu, Nepal.)

MNEMONIC

PSaMMoma bodies are round collections of calcium seen in:
- **P**apillary carcinoma of the thyroid
- **S**erous cystadenocarcinoma
- **M**eningioma
- **M**esothelioma

- Bilateral in 10–25% of cases.
- Treatment is either unilateral salpingo-oophorectomy or ovarian cystectomy.
- **Serous cystadenocarcinoma:**
  - Malignant.
  - Characterized by ingrowths of papillary and glandular structures with stromal invasion.
  - **Psammoma bodies** are present in 80% of cases.
  - **Poorly differentiated** cancer may present as solid sheets of cells.

MUCINOUS

- **Mucinous cystadenoma:**
  - Benign.
  - Filled with sticky mucin; tends to be **multiloculated.**
  - Bilateral in < 5% of cases.
  - Can present very large.
  - Treatment is either unilateral salpingo-oophorectomy or ovarian cystectomy.
- **Mucinous adenocarcinoma:**
  - Malignant.
  - Characterized by multiple loculi lined with mucin-secreting epithelium and stromal invasion.
  - Bilateral in 8–10% of cases.
  - **Pseudomyxoma peritonei** is a potential complication and involves tumor production of mucus in the abdominal cavity. If not treated, mucin will accumulate to such an extent that vital structures in the abdomen are compressed.

BRENNER TUMOR

- Usually benign.
- Characterized by **transitional (bladder) epithelium** with stromal invasion.

ENDOMETRIOID CARCINOMA

- Characterized by similar adenomatous pattern seen in endometrial carcinoma of the uterus.
- Endometrioid carcinoma of the ovary correlates with concurrent lesions in the endometrium.
- Often present with abdominal distention, pelvic or abdominal pain, and **abnormal vaginal bleeding.**
- Presents at early stage; therefore, has relatively good prognosis.

GRANULOSA CELL TUMOR

Estrogen-secreting tumor. Granulosa cells secrete estrogen, which can be used as a tumor marker.

- In prepubertal girls, often associated with pseudoprecocious puberty.
- In reproductive age group, associated with menstrual irregularities, endometrial carcinoma (5%), and endometrial hyperplasia (50%).
- Some secrete inhibin, which can be used as a tumor marker.
- Grossly, smooth with lobulated surfaces; size can range from few millimeters to 20 cm.
- Cells often arrange themselves around a central cavity like a primordial follicle (**Call-Exner bodies**).
- Coffee bean (grooved) nuclei are common.
- Bilateral in < 2% of cases.

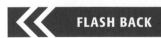

FLASH BACK

Granulosa cells convert androstenedione and testosterone into estrone and estradiol, respectively, via aromatase.

SERTOLI-LEYDIG CELL TUMOR

Androgen-producing tumor and may contain **Reinke crystals.**

- Occur between 30 and 40 years of age.
- Because of the type of hormone produced, commonly presents with signs of virilization such as amenorrhea, breast atrophy, acne, hirsutism, deepening of the voice, and receding hairline.
- Elevated testosterone and androstenedione with normal dehydroepiandrosterone sulfate (DHEA-S).
- Bilateral in < 1% of cases.

METASTATIC TUMORS

- **Krukenberg tumor:** Metastatic tumor to ovaries commonly from the stomach and less commonly from other sites such as the colon, breast, or biliary tract.
- Occurs in ovarian stroma.
- Cells are typically mucin-filled, with **"signet ring" appearance.**
- Usually bilateral (evidence for hemometastasis).

PREGNANCY COMPLICATIONS

Placental Disorders

ABRUPTIO PLACENTAE

Separation of normally implanted placenta due to hemorrhage in the decidua basalis of the endometrium before the delivery of the fetus. Severe abruptions have a 25% rate of perinatal mortality.

PRESENTATION

Vaginal bleeding, tender uterus, fetal distress, hypertonus, and/or stillbirth. Sometimes, the bleeding may be severe, leading to shock, and it can also lead to disseminated intravascular coagulation (DIC). The bleeding is often painful.

DIAGNOSIS

Mainly clinical. A retroplacental clot on ultrasound is specific for abruption.

TREATMENT

Prompt delivery of the fetus via cesarean section. Vaginal delivery is preferred if the fetus is deceased and the mother is stable.

PLACENTA ACCRETA

Defect in the decidua basalis leading to abnormal implantation of the placenta. When the Nitabuch membrane is deficient, the trophoblastic tissue attaches directly to the myometrium. Incomplete separation of the placenta during delivery leads to profuse hemorrhage.

PRESENTATION

Profuse placental hemorrhage during delivery.

DIAGNOSIS

Sonography may help diagnosis in the antepartum period.

KEY FACT

Abruption: Painful
Previa: Painless

MNEMONIC

Abrupt (**A**bruptio) **D**etachment causes **D**eath.

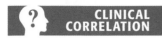

Do not perform vaginal examination in any woman who is > 20 weeks pregnant with vaginal bleeding. The digital examination may rupture the previa.

TREATMENT

Hysterectomy.

PLACENTA PREVIA

Implantation of the placenta over or near the internal cervical os. The incidence of placenta previa is 1 in 300 deliveries in the United States.

PRESENTATION

Painless vaginal bleeding at the end of the second trimester or later. The uterus is soft and nontender.

DIAGNOSIS

Sonography is the initial investigation of choice for localization of the placenta.

TREATMENT

The choice of treatment depends on gestational age, maternal and fetal conditions, and the amount of bleeding.

EXPECTANT MANAGEMENT

If fetal lung maturity is not achieved, the pregnancy may be prolonged using tocolytics and dexamethasone.

DELIVERY

Cesarean section.

COMPLICATIONS

- **Maternal:** Hemorrhage, shock, and death.
- **Fetal:** Prematurity and perinatal mortality.

Ectopic Pregnancy

Implantation of blastocysts outside the uterine cavity. The most common location for ectopic pregnancy is the **ampulla of the Fallopian tube.** The rate of ectopic pregnancy is 2% of all pregnancies in the United States, with African Americans at increased risk. Risk factors include **previous tubal or abdominal surgery, previous ectopic pregnancy, IUD use, PID,** infertility, and current smoking. A pregnancy in a patient with an IUD is more likely to be ectopic because the chances of an intrauterine pregnancy are greatly reduced.

PRESENTATION

Patient classically presents with amenorrhea, abdominal pain, vaginal bleeding, fainting, or dizziness. On examination, abdominal tenderness and cervical motion tenderness may be present, and an adnexal mass can be palpated.

DIAGNOSIS

Urine pregnancy test, sonogram, and measurement of β-hCG are extremely sensitive diagnostic tests. Transvaginal sonography is more sensitive for a gestational sac.

TREATMENT

- **Medical:** Methotrexate (MTX) is the drug of choice for medical management. MTX is a folate antagonist that is able to kill rapidly dividing trophoblastic cells.
- **Surgical:** Laparoscopic salpingostomy or salpingectomy. A laparotomy approach can be used in unstable patients.

Amniotic Fluid Disorders

Amniotic fluid is produced by the fetus, aids in normal growth and development, and helps protect the fetus. Too much (polyhydramnios) or too little (oligohydramnios) amniotic fluid can lead to abnormalities in the developing fetus.

POLYHYDRAMNIOS

- May result from inability to swallow amniotic fluid.
- Associated with fetal intestinal atresia, esophageal/duodenal atresia, anencephaly, maternal diabetes, neural tube defects, and multiple gestations.
- Amniotic fluid index (AFI) > 24 cm or amniotic fluid volume > 1.5–2 L.

OLIGOHYDRAMNIOS

- Associated with ruptured membranes, **Potter syndrome,** placental insufficiency, and agenesis of posterior urethral valves (in males) and resultant inability to excrete urine.
- AFI < 5 cm or amniotic fluid volume < 0.5 L.

Hypertensive Disorders

PREECLAMPSIA

Defined as new onset **hypertension** and **proteinuria** after 20 weeks of gestation. It has an incidence of 23.6 per 1000 deliveries in the United States. Placental dysfunction causes release of excess soluble fms-like tyrosine kinase-1 (sFlt-1), which binds growth factors vascular endothelial growth factor (VEFG) and **placental growth factor** (PGF), rendering them unavailable. This leads to vascular endothelial damage, vasoconstriction, hypertension, renal glomerular endothelial cell damage, and coagulation abnormalities. Intense vasospasm is induced by the release of various mediators like endothelin and thromboxane A_2. The degree of preeclampsia depends on the level of trophoblastic invasion by the placenta.

The criteria for preeclampsia:

- Systolic blood pressure (BP) > 140 mm Hg or diastolic BP > 90 mm Hg after 20 weeks of gestation, on two readings taken 6 hours apart while the patient is on bed rest.
- Proteinuria: 0.3 g or more per 24 hours.
- With or without edema (caused by loss of albumin in the urine).

SEVERE PREECLAMPSIA

Preeclampsia is considered severe if there is severe end-organ dysfunction as manifested by one or more of the following criteria:

- Systolic BP > 160 mm Hg or diastolic BP > 110 mm Hg after 20 weeks of gestation measured on two readings taken 6 hours apart while the patient is on bed rest.

FLASH BACK

MTX inhibits dihydrofolate reductase, resulting in a decrease in deoxythymidine monophosphate, purine nucleotides, and amino acids and a consequent decrease in DNA and protein synthesis.

KEY FACT

The fetus drinks and pees amniotic fluid. If it can't drink, **polyhydramnios** results; if it can't pee, **oligohydramnios** results.

FLASH BACK

Prostacyclins and nitric oxide (potent) are vasodilators, and endothelin (potent), thromboxane A_2, and angiotensin II are vasoconstrictors.

KEY FACT

When symptoms of preeclampsia are present at < 20 week's gestation, suspect an underlying disorder such as lupus or a gestational trophoblastic neoplasm.

- Proteinuria: > 5 g per 24 hours or > 3 g on two random samples collected 4 hours apart.
- Oliguria (< 500 mL/24 h).
- Severe headache.
- Cerebral or visual disturbances.
- Pulmonary edema or cyanosis.
- Epigastric or right upper quadrant tenderness.
- Elevated liver enzymes.
- Low platelets (<100,000/mm^3).
- Intrauterine growth restriction.
- Death resulting from **cerebral hemorrhage** and **acute respiratory distress syndrome (ARDS).**

ECLAMPSIA

New-onset grand mal seizure in the setting of preeclampsia.

PRESENTATION

High BP with proteinuria or signs of severe preeclampsia with convulsive seizures, as discussed earlier. May lead to DIC.

TREATMENT

Delivery of the fetus is the definitive cure for preeclampsia. During labor and delivery, **magnesium sulfate** may prevent severe preeclampsia and eclampsia. Hydralazine and labetalol can be used to lower the BP. Vaginal delivery should be attempted whenever possible, weighing possible risks and benefits.

GESTATIONAL HYPERTENSION

Elevated BP without proteinuria after 20 weeks of gestation and followed by disappearance within 12 weeks of delivery.

PREECLAMPSIA SUPERIMPOSED ON CHRONIC HYPERTENSION

Sudden new-onset proteinuria, acute increase in hypertension, and/or development of HELLP syndrome.

HELLP SYNDROME

- **H**emolysis, **E**levated **L**iver enzymes, and **L**ow **P**latelets in a pregnant woman.
- Mortality rate of 7–35%.
- Can occur during antepartum period and up to 1 week postpartum with or without superimposed preeclampsia or eclampsia.
- A positive feedback loop of endothelial damage and platelet activation, leading to release of thromboxane A$_2$ and serotonin, causing vasoconstriction and platelet aggregation.

PRESENTATION

- May present with vague complaints of malaise, epigastric pain, nausea and vomiting, and headache.
- The diagnosis is often delayed in the absence of superimposed eclampsia.
- Physical examination may reveal epigastric or right hypochondriac tenderness, edema, and hypertension with or without proteinuria.

DIAGNOSIS

- Hemolytic anemia (microangiopathic).
- Elevated liver enzymes and low platelets.

KEY FACT

Eclamptic seizures may occur as long as 48 hours after delivery.

CLINICAL CORRELATION

Complete blood count and liver function tests should be done in any pregnant woman in the third trimester presenting with malaise. Suspect HELLP syndrome in a pregnant woman with a low platelet count.

TREATMENT

The best treatment for HELLP syndrome is termination of the pregnancy. **Corticosteroids** should be given to all patients with HELLP syndrome. Severe HELLP syndrome requires immediate delivery.

Sheehan Syndrome

Necrosis of the pituitary gland due to postpartum hemorrhage. During pregnancy, the pituitary gland enlarges, and sudden massive obstetrical bleeding or hypovolemia may cause hypoxia, leading to pituitary necrosis. The anterior pituitary is more often involved than the posterior pituitary.

PRESENTATION

- Difficulty in lactation or failure to lactate (lack of prolactin) is the most common initial presentation.
- Other features include oligomenorrhea or amenorrhea.
- If diagnosis is missed at an earlier stage, may present with features of panhypopituitarism, such as hypothyroidism, secondary adrenal insufficiency, or adrenal crisis.

DIAGNOSIS

- Diagnosis made by features of hypopituitarism seen in a patient with a history of postpartum hemorrhage.
- Decreased levels of pituitary hormones, such as adrenocorticotropic hormone (ACTH), thyroid-stimulating hormone (TSH), FSH, LH, and growth hormone (GH), followed by a decreased level of target hormones, such as thyroxine, cortisol, estrogen, and progesterone.

TREATMENT

Replacement of target hormones, such as hydrocortisone, thyroxine, estrogen, and progesterone.

Amniotic Embolism

- Embolism of amniotic fluid during labor and delivery.
- High mortality rate of 80–90%.
- Exact mechanism is unknown, but inflammatory cytokines and mediators are probably involved.

PRESENTATION

- Sudden-onset dyspnea, tachypnea, and cyanosis during or after labor and delivery.
- May also present with cardiovascular collapse, hypoxemia, seizures, DIC, and bleeding.

DIAGNOSIS

- Arterial blood gas (ABG) shows severe hypoxemia.
- Prolonged bleeding times, clotting times, hypofibrinogenemia, and increased fibrin degradation products can occur in the setting of DIC.
- Electrocardiogram (ECG) may reveal sinus tachycardia, right ventricular strain pattern, and nonspecific ST segment changes.

TREATMENT

Supportive.

Erythroblastosis Fetalis

- Alloimmunization because of previous maternal exposure to foreign fetal RBCs leads to destruction of fetal RBCs by maternal antibodies directed against them.
- There are several types of RBC alloimmunization, but the most common is Rh incompatibility (especially RhD).
- An Rh-negative mother is sensitized with Rh-positive fetal RBCs and produces antibodies.
- During a subsequent pregnancy, Rh-specific IgG crosses the placenta into the fetus and coats Rh-positive fetal RBCs, causing hemolysis, hydrops, and hemolytic disease of the newborn.

PRESENTATION

- Anemia, hepatosplenomegaly, and jaundice.
- May present with edema, ascites, and pericardial/pleural effusion.
- Respiratory distress due to deficiency of surfactant and pulmonary hypoplasia.

DIAGNOSIS

Blood typing, Rh factor, and antibody screening of all pregnant patients, with paternal testing if maternal antibodies are found.

TREATMENT

- Rh immunoglobulin (RhoGAM) consisting of IgG anti-RhD antibodies (passive immunization) is given to the mother at 28 weeks of gestation, and again within 72 hours after delivery as prophylaxis.
- This solution of immunoglobulins bind and lead to the destruction of fetal RhD-positive red blood cells that have passed from the fetal circulation into the mother's circulation, and hence do not allow for the mother to mount an immune response to RhD antigens.
- RhoGAM is also routinely given to the Rh-negative mothers after abortion, D&C, amniocentesis, chorionic villus sampling, abruptio placentae, placenta previa, and ectopic pregnancy, or after any bleeding during pregnancy.

KEY FACT

Passive immunization: Transfer of active presynthesized antibodies.
Active immunization: Transfer of an immunogen that stimulates the host's humoral immune system.

GESTATIONAL NEOPLASMS

Hydatidiform Mole

Benign tumors of the chorionic villus resulting from abnormal fertilization of an ovum and characterized by abnormal proliferation of trophoblastic cells. The incidence is 7–10 times higher in Southeast Asian countries than in the Western world. Occurs in 1 of 1500 live births in the United States. Increased maternal age is only a risk factor for complete mole and *not* incomplete mole.

Hydatidiform moles are classified into two different types:

- **Complete mole:** Results from fertilization of an empty ovum by two sperms or a haploid sperm that divides its nuclear material and forms **diploid chromosomes** (**46,XX** or **46,XY**). Therefore, the **complete** mole is **completely** paternal in origin. Fetal parts are **completely** absent, and the placenta is **completely** neoplastic (Table 9-16).
- **Partial mole:** Results from fertilization of a normal ovum by two sperm cells or duplication of one sperm. It has **triploid chromosomes** (**69,XXY, 69,XXX,** or **69,XYY**). Partial mole is both maternal and paternal in origin

TABLE 9-16. **Classification of Hydatidiform Moles**

	COMPLETE MOLE	INCOMPLETE MOLE
Karyotype	46,XX (most common) or 46,XY	69,XXY or 69,XXX or 69,XXY
Components	Empty egg + 1 duplicated sperm or empty egg + 2 sperm	1 egg + 1 duplicated sperm or 1 egg + 2 sperm
Fetal parts	No	Yes
Histologic features	▪ Generalized swelling of chorionic villi ▪ Diffuse trophoblastic hyperplasia ▪ Marked trophoblastic atypia	▪ Focal swelling of chorionic villi ▪ Focal trophoblastic hyperplasia ▪ Mild trophoblastic atypia
hCG levels	Excessively elevated	Sometimes elevated
Progress to choriocarcinoma	2%	Rare
Risk of complications	15–20% malignant trophoblastic disease	Low risk of malignancy (< 5%)

and **partially** consists of identifiable fetal parts (see Table 9-16). Not all placental villi are neoplastic.

PRESENTATION

- **Complete mole:** First-trimester vaginal bleeding is the most common presentation. Additional features include excessive elevations in hCG, theca lutein cysts > 5 cm in diameter, excessive uterine size, hyperemesis gravidarum, **symptoms of preeclampsia in the first trimester,** and hyperthyroidism.
- **Partial mole:** Vaginal bleeding or the features of missed or incomplete abortion are the most common presentations of partial mole. The uterus is usually small for date.

DIAGNOSIS

- **Complete mole:** hCG is excessively elevated. Sonography is sensitive and specific, revealing a "snowstorm" pattern. "Honeycombed" uterus, appearance like a cluster of grapes on imaging, and swollen villi without fetal RBCs are other important features (Figure 9-55).
- **Partial mole:** hCG is rarely elevated above levels that are normal for pregnancy. Sonography shows focal cystic changes in the placenta and a ratio of transverse to anteroposterior diameter > 1.5.

TREATMENT

- **Suction curettage** is the method of choice for evacuation of the uterine cavity. It should be followed by curettage with a sharp curette to confirm complete evacuation of the products of conception.
- **Follow-up:** Postevacuation molar pregnancy should be followed up with weekly hCG measurements until three consecutive tests are negative.

 KEY FACT

The amount of hCG is directly proportional to the volume of trophoblasts.

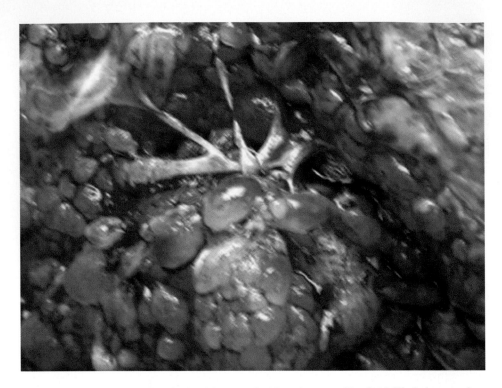

FIGURE 9-55. **Complete hydatidiform mole.** Note the grape-like fluid-filled clusters of chorionic villi. (Reproduced with permission from Shorge JO, Schaffer JL, Halvorson LM, et al. *Williams Gynecology.* New York: McGraw-Hill, 2008: Figure 37-3.)

PROGNOSIS

With complete mole, there is a 15–20% chance of development of postmolar gestation trophoblastic neoplasia (invasive mole and choriocarcinoma). With partial mole, the risk is only 2–4%.

Choriocarcinoma

Aggressive, malignant tumors composed of cytotrophoblasts and syncytiotrophoblasts arising from gestational chorionic epithelium. They usually follow evacuation of a mole with 2% of complete moles becoming choriocarcinoma.

PRESENTATION

- Recurrent vaginal bleeding after evacuation of a mole or following delivery, ectopic pregnancy, or abortion. hCG levels continue to rise after evacuation. Histologically, the cancer appears as hemorrhagic, necrotic masses within the uterus. **Chorionic villi are not present.**
- Metastases spread hematogenously and seed the lung (50%), vagina (35%), liver, and brain. Chemotherapy (methotrexate) is often curative.

BREAST DISEASES

Benign Breast Disease

The female breast progresses through normal anatomic changes during pre-, peri-, and postmenopausal years. Differentiating normal from pathologic anatomic changes is important in clinical practice and in answering test questions. Keys to identifying the underlying disease process are the patient's age, history, changes related to the menstrual cycle, nipple discharge, and findings on ultrasound, mammogram, or biopsy (Table 9-17).

TABLE 9-17.   Classification of Benign and Malignant Breast Diseases

BENIGN BREAST DISEASES	BREAST CARCINOMA
■ Fibrocystic changes	Carcinoma in situ
■ Intraductal papilloma	■ Ductal
■ Fibroadenoma	■ Lobular
■ Phyllodes tumor (benign or malignant)	Invasive carcinoma
■ Traumatic fat necrosis	■ Ductal
■ Acute mastitis	■ Medullary
	■ Tubular
	■ Mucinous (colloid)
	■ Papillary
	■ Inflammatory
	■ Lobular

FIBROCYSTIC CHANGE

Fibrocystic changes are common, benign changes involving the tissues of the breast that manifest as palpable lumps. They are the consequence of an exaggeration and distortion of the cyclic breast changes that occur normally in the menstrual cycle. Fibrocystic changes are divided into two categories: nonproliferative and proliferative.

■ **Nonproliferative (cysts and fibrosis):** The most common fibrocystic change, it is characterized by an increase in fibrous stroma associated with dilation of ducts and formation of cysts of various sizes without epithelial cell hyperplasia. The secretions within the cysts can calcify and appear radiodense on mammograms. Types of nonproliferative change include blue dome cysts (filled with serous, turbid fluid), and apocrine metaplasia (cysts lined by large, polygonal cells that have abundant granular, eosinophilic cytoplasm with small, round deeply chromatic nuclei).

■ **Proliferative (hyperplasia and sclerosing adenosis):** The terms *epithelial hyperplasia* and *proliferative fibrocystic change* encompass a range of lesions within the ductules, terminal ducts, and sometimes lobules of the ducts. Atypical hyperplasia is associated with the development of carcinoma and is estrogen sensitive.

INTRADUCTAL PAPILLOMA

A neoplastic papillary growth (double-layered epithelial cells overlying a myoepithelial layer) within a lactiferous duct or sinus. Presentation includes **serous or bloody nipple discharge,** subareolar tumors, or, rarely, nipple retraction. There may be a single papillary growth or multiple growths (more likely to be subsequently associated with carcinoma).

FIBROADENOMA

Most common benign tumor of the female breast, and the most common tumor in women < 25 years of age. It is thought to be caused by an increase in estrogen activity. Grossly, fibroadenomas are firm, with a uniform tan-white color on cut section, punctuated by softer yellow-pink specks. Clinically, they present as a **solitary, discrete, movable mass** in a young woman and rarely become malignant.

KEY FACT

Intraductal papilloma is the most common cause of bloody nipple discharge in women < 50.

Phyllodes Tumor

Arises from the intralobular stroma and rarely from preexisting fibroadenoma. Most grow to a massive size, distending the breast. On gross section, they exhibit leaf-like clefts and slits (**phyllon** is Greek for leaf). Only about 15% are malignant, and < 20% metastasize. **There is no ductal invasion and, therefore, no bleeding.**

Acute Mastitis

Inflammation of the breast tissue caused by infection. Bacteria are the most common pathogen; fungi are rare. Staphylococcal infections can lead to abscess formation. Treatment includes antibiotics (cephalosporins, dicloxacillin) and continuation of breast feeding (if caused by milk engorgement).

Traumatic Fat Necrosis

An uncommon and innocuous lesion significant only because it produces a mass, usually after some antecedent trauma to the breast. The lesion consists of a central focus of necrotic fat cells surrounded by polymorphonuclear neutrophils; it later becomes enclosed by fibrous tissue, and then scars. **The necrotic fat is phagocytosed by macrophages, which then become lipid-laden.** Can progress and cause skin retraction.

Breast Cancer

In the United States, approximately 210,000 new cases of invasive breast cancer will be diagnosed in females and 1970 new cases in males each year. Risk factors include family history, early menarche, late menopause, late first pregnancy (after 30 years), nulliparity, never having breast-fed, previous history of breast cancer, and family history of first-degree relative with breast cancer at a young age. Women having mutations in *BRCA1* and *BRCA2* genes have a 60–80% chance of developing breast cancer in their lifetimes. *BRCA1* and *BRCA2* gene mutations are transmitted in an autosomal dominant fashion. Treatment of breast cancer is specialized based on the location of the primary lesion, lymph node involvement, and the expression of hormone receptors or the HER2 protein.

- **Estrogen/progesterone receptors:** It is believed that estrogen and progesterone receptors normally present in breast epithelium, and often present in breast cancer cells, may interact with various growth promoters to create an autocrine mechanism of tumor development. Assessment of these receptors' expression is critical as there are targeted therapies such as tamoxifen (a breast estrogen receptor antagonist) and aromatase inhibitors.
- *ERBB2:* The *ERBB2* (formerly *HER2/neu*) protooncogene has been found to be amplified in up to 30% of sporadic breast cancers. It is a member of the epidermal growth factor receptor family and is associated with a poor prognosis. The importance of evaluating *ERBB2* expression is to predict responsiveness to the monoclonal antibody trastuzumab, which targets the *ERBB2* receptor. It is one of the first antitumor antibody therapies based on specific genetic abnormalities.
- **Sentinel node biopsy:** This has been introduced as an alternative, less morbid procedure to replace a full axillary nodal dissection. The first one to two draining nodes are identified with a dye or radiolabel. A negative sentinel node is highly predictive of no metastatic cancer in the remaining nodes. However, the significance of finding micrometastases is unknown.

KEY FACT

Staphylococcus causes localized abscess, but *Streptococcus* causes disseminated infection throughout the breast.

KEY FACT

Tamoxifen acts as an estrogen receptor antagonist in breast tissue and an agonist in endometrium and bone tissue. **Raloxifene** acts as an estrogen receptor antagonist in breast tissue and an agonist in bone tissue. It has no effect on the endometrium.

PRESENTATION

The initial chief complaint may be a palpable breast mass. Others may present with abnormal mammographic findings such as irregular masses and calcifications. The key to identifying the underlying pathology involves breast examination and tissue biopsy of the mass.

Classification of Breast Cancer

CARCINOMA IN SITU

- **Ductal carcinoma in situ (DCIS):** Usually arises from the major ducts. Nonpalpable. Commonly contain microcalcifications. One-third of cases eventually invade. Treated with lumpectomy.
- **Lobular carcinoma in situ (LCIS):** Involves the terminal duct lobular unit. Nonpalpable. Signet ring cells are common. Usually estrogen and progesterone receptor-positive. One-third of cases eventually invade. Fifty percent to 75% increased incidence of cancer in the opposite breast.

FRANK CARCINOMA

DUCTAL

Term used for all nonlobular carcinomas that cannot be subclassified into one of the specialized types listed here; they account for most breast cancers (70–80%). It is usually associated with DCIS. Invasion of lymphovascular spaces or nerves may be seen. Roughly two-thirds express estrogen-progestin receptors and about one-third overexpress ERBB2. Types of frank ductal carcinoma include the following (Table 9-18):

- **Medullary:** 1–5% of all breast cancers. Associated with *BRCA1* mutations. Occur at younger age. Bulky, soft tumor with large cells and infiltrate of leukocytes. Although they lack estrogen and progesterone receptors, they have a better prognosis.
- **Tubular:** Presents as irregular mammographic densities. The carcinoma consists of well-formed tubules with low-grade nuclei. Affects young

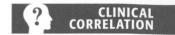

CLINICAL CORRELATION

The most common site for breast cancer is the upper outer quadrant, including the axilla, because lymphatics drain into this area.

TABLE 9-18. Characteristics of Different Subtypes of Invasive Ductal Carcinoma

TYPE	AGE	PATHOLOGIC FINDINGS	PROGNOSIS
Medullary	Young	- Sheet-like growth with absent ducts or alveolar pattern. - Estrogen/progesterone receptor absent.	Better
Tubular	Young	- Well-formed tubules with low-grade nuclei. - Estrogen/progesterone receptor present.	Better
Mucinous	Elderly	- Neoplastic cells surrounded by mucin. - Estrogen/progesterone receptor present.	Better
Papillary	Elderly	- Papillary architecture with fibrovascular cores. - Estrogen/progesterone receptor present.	Better
Inflammatory	Young	- Swollen, erythematous base with invasion to dermal lymphatics and dimpling of the skin (peau d'orange). - Estrogen/progesterone receptor present in < 50%.	Poor

females. Metastases are rare, prognosis is good, and hormone receptors are normally expressed.

- **Mucinous (colloid):** Cancer cells produce mucus and grow into a jelly-like tumor; associated with a better prognosis. Usually affect the elderly.
- **Papillary:** Papillary architecture and fibrovascular cores. Often expresses progesterone and estrogen receptors.
- **Inflammatory:** Presents as an enlarged, swollen, erythematous breast, usually without a palpable mass. The blockage of numerous dermal lymphatic spaces by carcinoma results in dimpling like an orange peel—"peau d'orange". Most of these have distant metastases and an extremely poor prognosis.

LOBULAR

Often bilateral but less common than infiltrating ductal carcinoma. The cells invade individually into stroma and are often aligned in strands or chains. Lobular carcinomas, more often than ductal carcinomas, metastasize to cerebrospinal fluid and elsewhere. Nearly all of these tumors express hormone receptors.

PAGET DISEASE OF THE NIPPLE

Caused by the extension of DCIS into the lactiferous ducts and the skin of the nipple. Clinically, there is a unilateral crusting exudate over the nipple and areolar skin (Figure 9-56). Paget cells have an abundant clear cytoplasm. Palpable mass in only 50% of cases.

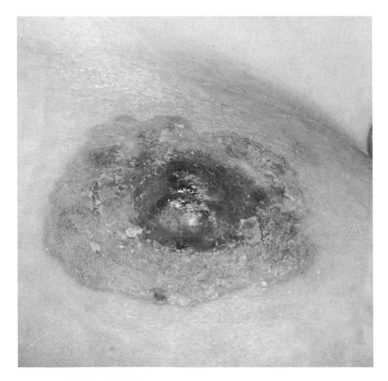

FIGURE 9-56. **Paget disease of the nipple.** Scaly and erythematous plaque involving the nipple and areola. (Reproduced with permission from Wolff K, Goldmith LA, Katz SI, et al. *Fitzpatrick's Dermatology in General Medicine,* 7th ed. New York: McGraw-Hill, 2008: Figure 121-1.)

SEXUALLY TRANSMITTED INFECTIONS AND OTHER GENITAL INFECTIONS

Sexually transmitted infections (STIs) are a significant cause of morbidity with short- and long-term consequences. Table 9-19 summarizes the common STIs and other genital infections.

TABLE 9-19. Sexually Transmitted Infections and Other Genital Infections

DISEASE (PATHOGEN)	PRESENTATION	DIAGNOSIS	TREATMENT
Syphilis (*Treponema pallidum*)	**Primary:** Small papule that turns into a painless ulcer (chancre) with well-defined borders. **Secondary:** Lymphadenopathy, rash on the palms and soles of the feet, condylomata lata, meningitis, hepatitis. **Tertiary:** Thoracic aneurysm, tabes dorsalis, gummas, Argyll Robertson pupils. **Congenital:** Stillbirth, hepatomegaly, snuffles, rash, bone abnormalities (eg, saber shins, mulberry molars, saddle nose, Hutchinson triad [notched central incisors, interstitial keratitis, 8th nerve palsy]).	■ Darkfield microscopy. ■ VDRL/RPR (nonspecific): Measure cardiolipin antibody; titers fall after treatment. ■ FTA-Abs (specific): Remains positive after treatment.	Penicillin G, azithromycin, ceftriaxone, or erythromycin.
Gonorrhea (*Neisseria gonorrhoeae*)	■ Attaches to the mucosal epithelium of the urethra via pili. May ascend to infect the prostate, epididymis, and testes in men or cause PID in women. ■ Purulent urethral discharge. ■ Swelling around the meatus. ■ Pain with urination.	Culture of discharge shows gram-negative diplococci.	Ceftriaxone (also treat for *C trachomatis* with azithromycin or doxycycline).
Nongonococcal urethritis (*Chlamydia trachomatis*, serotypes D-K or *Ureaplasma urealyticum*)	■ Most common STI. ■ Purulent urethral discharge. ■ Pain with urination. ■ May ascend to infect the prostate, epididymis, and testes in men or cause PID in women.	■ Gram-negative intracellular organism. ■ Serologic testing. ■ **Reiter syndrome:** Uveitis, arthritis, urethritis ("can't see, can't pee, can't climb a tree").	Azithromycin or doxycycline (also treat for *N gonorrhoeae* with ceftriaxone).
Lymphogranuloma venereum (*C trachomatis*, serotypes L1-L3)	■ Ulcerative genital lesion. ■ Regional lymphadenopathy (buboes): Granulomatous inflammatory reaction with irregularly shaped foci of necrosis and neutrophilic infiltrate; potential formation of draining sinuses. ■ Proctitis, rectal strictures.	■ Gram-negative intracellular organism. ■ Serologic testing.	Tetracycline, doxycycline, erythromycin, or cotrimoxazole.
Chancroid (*Haemophilus ducreyi*)	■ Tender, erythematous papule that ulcerates. ■ Lesions are painful. ■ Base of ulcer covered by yellow-gray exudate.	Based on clinical criteria. Very difficult to culture.	Azithromycin, ceftriaxone, or erythromycin.

(continues)

TABLE 9-19.   Sexually Transmitted Infections and Other Genital Infections (continued)

DISEASE/PATHOGEN	PRESENTATION	DIAGNOSIS	TREATMENT
Granuloma inguinale (donovanosis, caused by *Klebsiella granulomatis*)	■ Sharply demarcated ulcer with beefy-red granulation tissue. ■ Lymph nodes are spared. ■ Lesion is painless.	Based on clinical criteria. Very difficult to culture.	Erythromycin, tetracycline, ampicillin, or TMP-SMX.
Condylomata acuminata (HPV types 6 and 11)	■ Squamous cell proliferation (genital warts). ■ Small sessile lesions to large papillary lesions.	**Koilocytosis:** Hyperchromatic nuclei surrounded by a perinuclear halo.	Chemical destruction (podophyllin, trichloroacetic acid, or 5-FU/epinephrine gel) or surgical excision.
Genital herpes (HSV types 1 and 2)	■ Usually caused by HSV-2. ■ Prodrome of burning and tingling. ■ Active lesions are painful vesicles.	Microscopy: **Cowdry type A inclusion bodies** (viral inclusions that appear as light purple intranuclear structures surrounded by a clear halo).	Acyclovir, famciclovir.
Bacterial vaginosis (*Gardnerella vaginalis*)	■ **Fishy-smelling** discharge after unprotected intercourse. ■ No inflammatory signs on examination.	■ Microscopy: **Clue cells** (epithelial cells covered with adherent *Gardnerella vaginalis*; Figure 9-57). ■ pH > 4.5 (abnormal).	Metronidazole or clindamycin.
Trichomoniasis (*Trichomonas vaginalis*)	■ Purulent, thin, greenish frothy vaginal discharge associated with pruritus, dysuria, and dyspareunia. ■ Erythema of the vulva and vagina. ■ Punctate hemorrhages on the vagina and cervix ("strawberry cervix").	■ Microscopy: Motile trichomonads and leukocytes. ■ **Whiff test** (addition of KOH to vaginal discharge generates fishy amine-like odor) may be positive.	Metronidazole.
Candidiasis (*Candida albicans*)	■ Thin to homogeneously thick vaginal discharge. ■ Vaginal soreness, pruritus, dyspareunia, and vulvar burning. ■ Curdy white patches on the vulva and vagina. ■ May have had recent antibiotic use, pregnancy, or diabetes as these conditions decrease lactobacilli and allow overgrowth of fungi.	■ pH < 4.5 (normal). ■ Mycelia on KOH preparation.	Topical azoles or oral fluconazole.

FTA-Abs, fluorescent treponemal antibody absorption; 5-FU, 5-flurouracil; HPV, human papillomavirus; HSV, herpes simplex virus; PID, pelvic inflammatory disease; STI, sexually transmitted infection; TMP/SMX, trimethoprim-sulfamethoxazole; VDRL/RPR, Venereal Disease Research Laboratory, rapid plasma reagin.

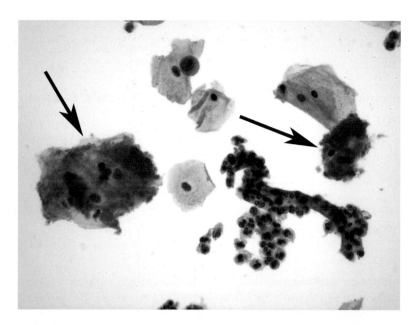

FIGURE 9-57. **Clue cells.** Clue cells can be seen on Pap smears of patients with bacterial vaginosis caused by overgrowth of *Gardnerella*. The image shows the organisms coating squamous cells forming a purple, velvety coat (*arrows*). (Reproduced with permission from USMLERx.com.)

The pH of the normal vagina is < 4.5 and is maintained by the production of lactic acid. Estrogen-stimulated vaginal epithelial cells are rich in glycogen, which is broken down into glucose. The vaginal cells and lactobacilli convert glucose into lactic acid. Frequent sexual intercourse or the use of douches cause the vaginal pH to be alkaline, which predisposes to bacterial vaginosis (Figure 9-57).

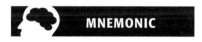

MNEMONIC

Haemophilus "do cry" (*ducreyi*) is extremely painful.

Pharmacology

DRUGS THAT MODULATE THE GONADOTROPIN AXIS

Gonadotropin-Releasing Hormone Agonists (Leuprolide, Buserelin, Nafarelin)

MECHANISM

Influences anterior pituitary secretion of FSH and LH (see Figure 9-33). Synthetic GnRH is termed **gonadorelin,** which is no longer available as a pharmacologic agent in the United States. Secretion of GnRH is controlled by neural input from other parts of the brain and, through negative feedback, by sex steroids.

USES

Intermittent GnRH administration stimulates FSH and LH release, which can be used for infertility treatment. Continuous GnRH and long-acting GnRH agonist analogs suppress FSH and LH release, which can be used to induce hypogonadism and treat prostate cancer, uterine fibroids, endometriosis, polycystic ovary syndrome, and precocious puberty.

SIDE EFFECTS

Headache, light-headedness, nausea, and hypoestrogenic state (eg, hot flashes, vaginal dryness, bone density loss).

Gonadotropin-Releasing Hormone Antagonists (Ganirelix, Cetrorelix)

MECHANISM

Binds to the pituitary GnRH receptor and inhibits gonadotropin secretion and reduces estrogen synthesis.

USES

Suppression of premature LH surges in IVF cycles. Also used for endometriosis, menorrhagia, and gynecomastia.

SIDE EFFECTS

GI disturbances, weight gain, fluid retention, dizziness, muscle cramps, headache, and virilizing effect in females.

Gonadotropin-Modulating Agents (Leuprolide, Goserelin)

MECHANISM

Acts as an agonist when used in pulsatile fashion but acts as an antagonist when used continuously. Leuprolide and goserelin are synthetic peptide analogs of GnRH. These analogs are more potent than the natural hormone.

USES

Infertility (used in pulsatile fashion). Prostate cancer and uterine fibroids (continuous; use with flutamide).

SIDE EFFECTS

Antiandrogen, nausea, vomiting.

DRUGS THAT MODULATE THE MALE REPRODUCTIVE SYSTEM

Testosterone

MECHANISM

Modifies gene transcription upon conversion to DHT in target cells. Testosterone negatively regulates LH production in anterior pituitary cells.

USES

Replacement therapy in testicular failure, anemia, and as an anabolic agent.

SIDE EFFECTS

Eventual decrease of gonadotropin release, with resultant infertility and salt and water retention; edema.

Cyproterone

MECHANISM

Competitive antagonist of androgen receptor. Inhibits androgen activity in peripheral tissues.

USES

No current approved uses in the United States. May be effective in hirsutism, prostate cancer, BPH, hypersexuality, and priapism.

SIDE EFFECTS

Breast swelling, decreased libido, inability to generate or keep an erection, excess milk flow from the breast.

Flutamide

MECHANISM

Antiandrogen that competitively antagonizes the testosterone receptor.

USES

Prostate cancer, hirsutism in women.

SIDE EFFECTS

Hot flashes, diarrhea, nausea, gynecomastia, impotence, hepatitis, decreased libido, decreased volume of ejaculate, breast tenderness or enlargement.

Finasteride

MECHANISM

Antiandrogen that acts as a 5α-reductase inhibitor. Decreases conversion of testosterone to DHT.

USES

BPH; male pattern baldness.

SIDE EFFECTS

Breast enlargement/tenderness, lip swelling, testicular pain, GI distress (diarrhea, abdominal pain), loss of libido, erectile dysfunction. Women who are or may be pregnant must not use or come into contact with finasteride because it may cause hypospadias in a male fetus.

Sildenafil, Vardenafil, Tadalafil

MECHANISM

Inhibits cGMP phosphodiesterase (PDE5), causing increased cGMP levels. Increased cGMP levels vasodilates vascular smooth muscle in the corpus cavernosum and increases blood flow for penile erection.

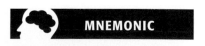

MNEMONIC

Sildena**fil,** vardena**fil,** and tadala**fil** all **fill** the penis.

USES

Erectile dysfunction.

SIDE EFFECTS

Headache, flushing, dyspepsia, alterations in blue-green color vision, risk of life-threatening hypotension in patients taking nitrates.

DRUGS THAT MODULATE THE FEMALE REPRODUCTIVE SYSTEM

Estrogens

MECHANISM

Stimulates endometrial growth, reduces LDL, raises HDL.

TYPES

- Natural: Premarin-conjugated estrogens.
- Steroidal: Ethinyl estradiol and mestranol.
- Nonsteroidal: Diethylstilbestrol (DES).

USES

Hormone replacement therapy (HRT) in patients without breast cancer history; osteoporosis; birth control.

SIDE EFFECTS

Nausea, weight gain, breast tenderness, thrombosis (predisposes to hypercoagulable state), endometrial hyperplasia, migraine, increased risk of endometrial cancer; DES increases the risk of clear cell vaginal adenocarcinoma in offspring.

Clomiphene

MECHANISM

Estrogen receptor antagonist in hypothalamus → reduced negative feedback → increased GnRH → increased FSH, LH → increased ovulation.

USES

Fertility.

SIDE EFFECTS

Abdominal pain, breast tenderness, multiple births, hot flashes, ovarian enlargement, visual disturbances.

Tamoxifen

MECHANISM

Partial estrogen receptor agonist/antagonist (selective estrogen receptor modulator [SERM]) → agonist in endometrial tissue and bone, but antagonist in breast tissue. Upregulates transforming growth factor-β (TGF-β).

USES

HRT in patients with family history of breast cancer, estrogen-sensitive breast cancer, progesterone-resistant endometrial and ovarian cancers, melanoma, osteoporosis.

SIDE EFFECTS

Thrombosis, endometrial cancer, endometriosis, hair/nail thinning, hot flashes.

Raloxifene

MECHANISM

Another SERM similar in action to tamoxifen, except that it has antagonistic activity in the endometrium.

USES

Estrogen receptor-positive breast cancer; safe to use in patients with history of endometrial cancer. Osteoporosis.

SIDE EFFECTS

Hot flashes, sudden sweating/warmth, increased vaginal discharge, joint/muscle pain, weight gain, increased thromboembolism risk.

Progestins (Medroxyprogesterone, Norethindrone)

MECHANISM

Progesterone stimulates endometrial glandular secretions and spiral artery development for maintenance of pregnancy. Suppresses ovulation.

USES

Used with estrogens for birth control; stimulates appetite in cachectic patients. Norplant is a time-release strip implanted subcutaneously; slowly releases levonorgestrel into the body and provides contraception for up to 5 years.

SIDE EFFECTS

Increased BP, increased incidence of thromboembolism, weak androgenic effects, acne, hirsuitism, fluid retention, weight change, decreased HDL, increased LDL, depression, change in libido, breast discomfort, premenstrual symptoms, irregular menstrual cycles, and breakthrough bleeding.

Oral Contraceptives (Combined Progesterone and Estrogen)

MECHANISM

Inhibits secretion of LH and FSH via negative feedback, suppresses development of ovarian follicles, and inhibits secretion of LH, preventing ovulation.

USES

Contraception, reduction of endometrial/ovarian cancer risk and incidence of ectopic pregnancy.

SIDE EFFECTS

Increased risk of breast cancer in women receiving HRT and increased triglyceride levels. Increased risk for depression, weight gain, nausea, hypertension, and hypercoagulable state. Progesterone side effects include nausea, fluid retention, and weight gain.

Trastuzumab (Herceptin)

MECHANISM

Helps kill breast cancer cells that overexpress *ERBB2*, possibly through antibody-dependent cytotoxicity. Herceptin is a monoclonal antibody against *ERBB2* (*HER2/neu*).

USES

Metastatic breast cancer overexpressing *ERBB2*.

SIDE EFFECTS

Cardiotoxicity.

Mifepristone (RU-486)

MECHANISM

Competitively inhibits progestins at progesterone receptors.

USES

Pharmacologic alternative to surgical termination of pregnancy.

SIDE EFFECTS

Diarrhea, pain, heavy bleeding, GI effects, nausea, vomiting, anorexia, abdominal pain.

Oxytocin, Ergometrine

MECHANISM

Binds oxytocin receptor, which stimulates release of intracellular calcium stores and induces contraction of smooth muscle cells in the uterus and myoepithelial cells in the mammary gland.

USES

Uterine contractions (induction of labor, abortion). Oxytocin induces milk letdown and is also used for control of postpartum uterine hemorrhage.

SIDE EFFECTS

Normal doses have few reported side effects. Reported adverse reactions are maternal deaths due to hypertensive episodes, uterine rupture, water intoxication, and fetal deaths.

Ritodrine, Salmeterol

MECHANISM

β_2-Adrenergic agonists.

USES

Blockade of uterine contractions. These uterine relaxants are used in selected patients to prevent premature labor occurring between 22 and 33 weeks of gestation.

SIDE EFFECTS

Risks to the mother, such as pulmonary edema, tremor, and arrhythmia.

Ketoconazole, Spironolactone

MECHANISM

Inhibits steroid synthesis (ketoconazole and spironolactone), displaces estradiol and dihydrotestosterone from sex hormone–binding protein (spironolactone but not keotoconazole), and increases the estradiol-to-testosterone ratio.

USES

PCOS and hirsutism. Antiandrogen.

SIDE EFFECTS

Liver toxicity, which is rare but fatal. Other side effects include GI disturbances, pruritus, gynecomastia.

CHAPTER 10

Respiratory

Embryology

RESPIRATORY DEVELOPMENT

The respiratory system provides the means by which blood is oxygenated and cleared of carbon dioxide, sustaining aerobic energy production and playing a role in acid-base homeostasis. In preparation for a baby's first breath, the respiratory system develops in the fluid-filled womb, devoid of the air with which it is so intimately associated. This developmental process occurs in a **cranial-to-caudal** fashion. The upper respiratory tract (consisting of the larynx and trachea) develops first, followed by the lower respiratory tract (the bronchi and lungs). Lung development is further subdivided into pseudoglandular, canalicular, saccular, and alveolar stages, which are discussed in detail later in this section (Figure 10-1).

In the third to fourth week of gestation, the primordial respiratory system arises from the laryngotracheal groove on the ventral foregut (Figure 10-2). The groove deepens into an outpouching (diverticulum), which then elongates to form the laryngotracheal tube, partitioned off from the esophagus by the tracheoesophageal septum except for a thin opening at the junction with the pharynx. The proximal end of this tube becomes the larynx, the middle becomes the trachea, and the distal end forms the lung buds.

Larynx

The larynx is a musculocartilaginous structure in the anterior neck that functions to protect the airways, aid in respiration, and produce vocalization. Its location, just below the pharynx, marks the first division between the respiratory and digestive systems. It is suspended by muscle and ligaments to the hyoid bone superiorly and attached to the trachea inferiorly.

The laryngeal cartilage and musculature are derived from the **fourth and sixth pharyngeal arch** mesenchyme, with derivatives of the fourth arch inner-

> **KEY FACT**
>
> The larynx, trachea, and lung buds develop as an outpouching of the esophagus.

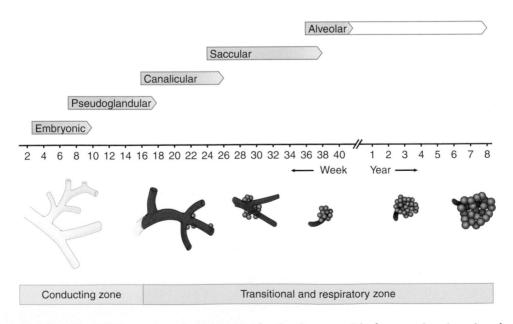

FIGURE 10-1. **Overview of respiratory system development.** After development of the larynx and trachea, the other conducting zones develop through branching. The transitional and respiratory zones develop after the conducting zone.

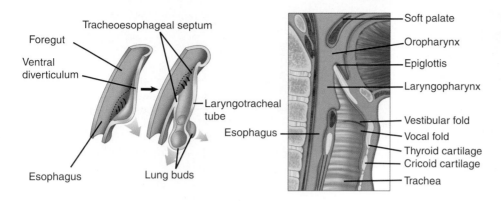

FIGURE 10-2. **Larynx and trachea development.** The larynx begins as a small herniation in the esophagus, known as the ventral diverticulum. As the diverticulum lengthens, lung buds form at its distal end. This will ultimately give rise to the trachea and lungs.

vated by the **superior laryngeal nerve (CN X)** and derivatives of the sixth arch innervated by the **recurrent laryngeal nerve (CN X).** As the pharyngeal arches develop, a primitive laryngeal orifice arises below the fourth arch. During week 5, swellings occur lateral to the orifice; these eventually become the arytenoid cartilages. Additionally, an anterior swelling develops that becomes the epiglottis. During week 6, continued growth in the region results in a **T**-shaped orifice (Figure 10-3). Epithelial tissue occluding the orifice breaks down during week 10, and surrounding epithelial folds differentiate into the false and true vocal folds.

Trachea

The trachea, or "windpipe," is a conducting airway that derives from the middle portion of the laryngotracheal tube. The epithelium and glands form from the tube endoderm, whereas cartilage, smooth muscle and connective tissue are derived from splanchnic mesoderm (the ventral part of the lateral mesoderm).

Bronchi

The lower laryngotracheal tube divides into bronchi, which further divide into bronchioles (Figure 10-4). The first division is asymmetrical, accompanied by movement of the **smaller left bud** to a **more lateral position** than the **larger right bud.** The second division of the bronchi is also asymmetrical, with three branches arising on the right and only two branches on the left, where the heart is also situated. In a fractal-like fashion, the tertiary bronchi continue to divide dichotomously until terminal bronchioles with distal alveoli are formed.

Lungs

At the end of the fourth week, the laryngotracheal diverticulum forms the lung buds as two lateral outpouchings. These two lung buds go on to develop the bronchi and bronchial tree between 2 and 7 months of gestation (the **pseudoglandular** and **canalicular** periods). The lungs mature relatively late compared with many of the other organs: the terminal sacs and eventually alveoli only begin to form in week 26 when the bronchial tree is completed, and surfactant production begins between weeks 25 and 28 with a rise in production over time (the **saccular** and **alveolar** periods). As a result, the developmental maturity of the lungs is one of the most critical determinants of survival in premature infants.

FLASH BACK

Humans have **six pharyngeal arches,** which develop from **neural crest tissue** surrounding their **aortic arches.**

1st (**M**'s)
- Muscles (muscles of **M**astication, anterior belly of the digastric, **M**ylohyoid, tensor tympani, tensor veli palatini)
- Skeletal (**M**axilla, **M**andible, **M**alleus, incus, **M**eckel cartilage)
- Nerves (CN V_2 and V_3)
- Arteries (**M**axillary artery, external carotid artery)

2nd (**S**'s)
- Muscles (muscles of facial expression, **S**tapedius, **S**tylohyoid, buccinator, platysma, posterior belly of the digastric)
- Skeletal (**S**tapes, **S**tyloid process, hyoid—lesser horn and upper part of body, Reichert cartilage)
- Nerve (CN VII)
- Artery (**S**tapedial artery)

3rd
- Muscle (stylopharyngeus)
- Skeletal (hyoid—greater horn and lower part of body, thymus)
- Nerve (CN IX)
- Artery (common carotid/internal carotid)

4th
- Muscles (cricothyroid muscle, all intrinsic muscles of soft palate)
- Skeletal (thyroid and epiglottic cartilages)
- Nerve (CN X—superior laryngeal nerve)
- Artery (right subclavian artery, aortic arch)

5th (only exists transiently during embryonic development; no adult structures)

6th
- Muscles (all intrinsic muscles of the larynx except the cricothyroid)
- Skeletal (cricoid, arytenoid, and corniculate cartilages)
- Nerve (CN X—recurrent laryngeal nerve)
- Arteries (pulmonary arteries, ductus arteriosus)

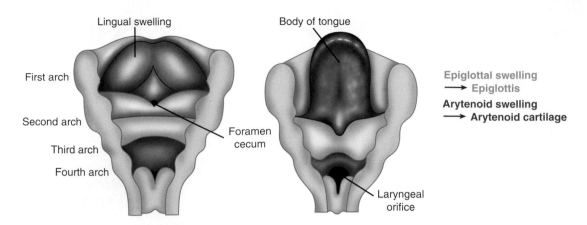

FIGURE 10-3. **Larynx development from pharyngeal arches.** The cartilage and musculature of the larynx are derived from the pharyngeal arches. An epiglottal swelling will give rise to the epiglottis, and an arytenoid swelling will give rise to the arytenoid cartilages.

PSEUDOGLANDULAR PERIOD (WEEKS 5–16)

During this period, **branching** continues and all major parts of the lung are formed with the exception of the gas-exchange elements—the respiratory bronchioles and the alveoli.

CANALICULAR PERIOD (WEEKS 16–26)

During the canalicular period, the **airways increase in diameter and lung vasculature** develops. **Primitive end-respiratory units,** consisting of a respiratory bronchiole, alveolar duct, and terminal sac, are formed during this period.

SACCULAR PERIOD (WEEK 26–BIRTH)

Terminal sacs develop, distinguished by their **thin epithelial lining.** Type I squamous epithelial cells form the gas-exchange surface, and type II secretory pneumocytes produce surfactant.

ALVEOLAR PERIOD (PRENATAL–CHILDHOOD)

Clusters of primitive alveoli form, allowing "breathing" in utero via aspiration and expulsion of amniotic fluid. The fluid in the lungs keeps the pulmonary

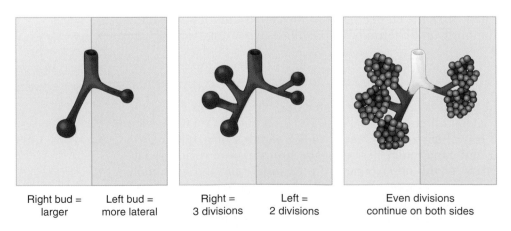

FIGURE 10-4. **Bronchiole divisions.** The initial two divisions of the trachea are asymmetrical. During the first division, the smaller left lung bud becomes more lateral. During the second division, the larger right lung bud divides three times, while the left bud divides only twice. All subsequent divisions on both sides result in two branches.

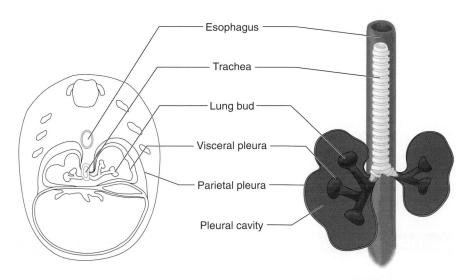

FIGURE 10-5. **Pleural cavity development.** The pleural cavity develops when the lung penetrates the body cavity. While some of the lining, the visceral pleura, becomes attached to the lung, the rest, the parietal pleura, remains attached to the body wall.

vascular resistance high throughout gestation. At birth, the lungs are half-filled with liquid that must be emptied through the mouth or absorbed into the blood and lymph. The replacement of fluid with air results in a dramatic fall in pulmonary vascular resistance at birth. The alveoli continue to mature after birth, growing in number only for the first 3 years and then increasing in both number and size for the next 5 years.

Pleural Cavities

The lungs invaginate to penetrate part of the intraembryonic coelom, or body cavity, as they grow and branch. This leaves a layer of **visceral pleura** from the splanchnic mesoderm covering the lung, and a layer of **parietal pleura** from the somatic mesoderm covering the body wall (Figure 10-5).

Diaphragm

The diaphragm develops more superiorly than its postnatal location but maintains its innervation from cervical roots C3, C4, and C5. It is formed from four embryologic structures that fuse by week 7 of gestation (Figure 10-6):

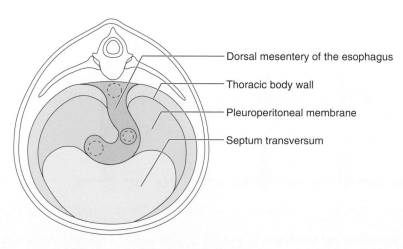

Dorsal mesentery of the esophagus

Thoracic body wall

Pleuroperitoneal membrane

Septum transversum

FIGURE 10-6. **Embryonic origins of the diaphragm.**

> **KEY FACT**
>
> To understand pleural cavity formation, imagine stepping on a partially inflated beach ball (the lining of the thoracic cavity) that is contained within a box (the thoracic cavity [ie, the chest wall and diaphragm]). As your foot (the growing lung) pushes down on the beach ball, two juxtaposed layers of the ball are now between your foot and the floor of the box. The surface of the ball that is in contact with your foot is the **visceral pleura,** and the surface in contact with the box is the **parietal pleura.** In between is the **pleural cavity,** which in reality is a **potential space** that contains < 10 mL of lubricating fluid.
> **Visceral = organ side**
> **Parietal = wall side**

MNEMONIC

C3, 4, 5 keep the diaphragm alive.

MNEMONIC

Several Parts Build a Diaphragm:
Septum transversum
Pleuroperitoneal folds
Body wall
Dorsal mesentery of the esophagus

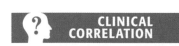

CLINICAL CORRELATION

The aspiration of amniotic fluid is essential for lung development, and fetal breathing movements are important for respiratory muscle development. **Pulmonary hypoplasia** may result from **oligohydramnios** (too little amniotic fluid which may be caused by renal malformation in **Potter syndrome.**

- The **septum transversum** is formed by mesodermal tissue that projects from the ventral body wall to partially separate the thoracic cavity and abdominal cavity. In the adult, the septum transversum forms the **central tendon** of the diaphragm.
- The **pleuroperitoneal folds** extend from the dorsolateral sides of the body wall to form the pleuroperitoneal membranes, which then fuse with the septum transversum.
- The **body wall** also extends from the dorsal and lateral sides (after the pleuroperitoneal folds have closed the thoracic cavity) to form the peripheral, muscular portion of the adult diaphragm.
- The **dorsal mesentery of the esophagus** forms the diaphragmatic portion that is dorsal to the esophagus and ventral to the aorta.

CONGENITAL MALFORMATIONS

Esophageal Atresia and Tracheoesophageal Fistula

The ventral laryngotracheal diverticulum is separated from the dorsal gut tube (the esophagus at this region) by the **tracheoesophageal septum** (mesoderm-derived tissue). Anomalies in the tracheoesophageal septum can lead to **esophageal atresia** (EA) and/or **tracheoesophageal fistula** (TEF) (see also Chapter 3).

The most common combination of findings is a proximal EA with the distal esophagus forming a fistula with the trachea. However, a multitude of other variants have been observed and are diagrammed in Figure 10-7.

An **esophageal closure** can form as a result of posterior deviation of the tracheoesophageal septum (see Figure 10-7). Embryos in whom there is an EA with no proximal TEF are unable to swallow amniotic fluid, leading to fluid accumulation and an enlarged uterus.

On the other hand, infants with a TEF have a conduit by which oral contents and/or acidic gastric contents may communicate with the lung, leading to the presentation of coughing during feedings. Chemical irritation of the airway mucosa by gastric contents is termed **aspiration pneumonitis.** Infection of the lungs by this process is called **aspiration pneumonia.** In addition, passage of air into the stomach causes gastric dilation, elevation of the diaphragm, and impaired breathing. Air may be seen in the stomach on a chest radiograph.

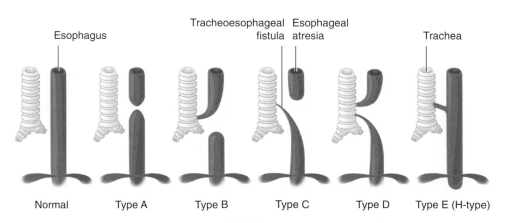

FIGURE 10-7. Congenital malformations of the trachea and esophagus. (1) Normal. (2) Type A (8%): esophageal atresia (EA) only. (3) Type B (1%): proximal tracheoesophageal fistula (TEF) and distal EA. (4) Type C (86%): proximal EA and distal TEF. (5) Type D (1%): proximal TEF and distal TEF. (6) Type H (4%): TEF only.

TEF and EA may be part of a larger pattern of congenital anomalies known by the acronym **VACTERL**, which includes **V**ertebral defects, **A**nal atresia or imperforate anus, **C**ardiac defects, **T**EF, **E**sophageal atresia, **R**enal agenesis/ obstruction, and **L**imb hypoplasia.

Laryngeal Atresia

Physical discontinuity of the larynx is thought to be a consequence of failed recanalization during development. Although rare, this condition is considered a medical emergency, because a neonate with laryngeal atresia will asphyxiate unless tracheostomy is performed.

Laryngomalacia

Laryngomalacia is a congenital weakness of the laryngeal cartilages that leads to collapse of the larynx during inspiration, audible as a "wet" inspiratory stridor. The condition is common in neonates and usually resolves spontaneously.

Congenital Diaphragmatic Hernia

A **congenital diaphragmatic hernia** (CDH) may result if the four embryonic components of the developing diaphragm fail to properly fuse. The newborn presents with respiratory distress, and a chest radiograph shows abdominal contents (loops of bowel) within the thoracic cavity (Figure 10-8). Additionally,

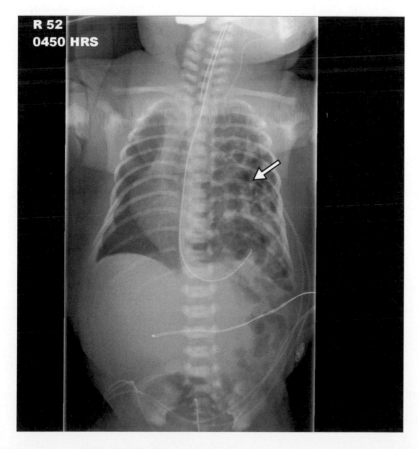

FIGURE 10-8. **Congenital diaphragmatic hernia.** Anteroposterior portable chest and abdomen film (babygram) shows numerous air-filled loops of bowel (indicated by the *arrow*) are seen in the left hemithorax in this neonate with a congenital diaphragmatic hernia. There is a shift of mediastinal structures to the right. An orogastric tube lies within the stomach. (Reproduced with permission from USMLERx.com.)

bowel sounds may be heard during chest auscultation. CDH is the most common cause of pulmonary hypoplasia, as explained in the following section.

Pulmonary Hypoplasia (Figure 10-9)

Failure of the lungs to develop fully may be primary or, more commonly, secondary to another defect, such as oligohydramnios or encroachment of the chest cavity by a CDH or tumor. The hypoplastic lung lacks respiratory exchange capacity and has overgrowth of smooth muscle elements, which leads to pulmonary hypertension. Unilateral hypoplasia is compatible with life. In rare cases, the lungs may fail to develop entirely, termed **pulmonary aplasia.**

Congenital Cysts

These saccular enlargements of the terminal bronchiole are usually solitary and can be associated with chronic infection secondary to poor drainage.

Respiratory Distress Syndrome (RDS)

During weeks 25–28, type II pneumocytes begin to produce surfactant, a phospholipoprotein fluid that facilitates alveolar opening by reducing surface tension. Due to the absence of surfactant, a fetus delivered prior to 25 weeks of gestation is not viable. A baby delivered prematurely during the period between the onset of surfactant secretion and term gestation has some degree of surfactant deficiency. As such, he or she is unable to fully inflate the lungs, leading to formation of hyaline membranes in the alveoli (Figure 10-10). Clinically, the infant exhibits superficial, rapid breathing (**tachypnea**) and **cyanosis.** The incidence of RDS is inversely related to gestational age at birth. Current treatments include antenatal maternal steroids (stimulates fetal surfactant production) and surfactant replacement.

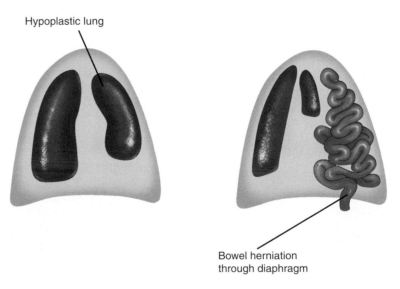

Hypoplastic lung

Bowel herniation through diaphragm

FIGURE 10-9. **Lung hypoplasia and congenital diaphragmatic hernia (CDH).** Failure of a lung to fully develop may occur as an isolated event (*left*) or as the result of another defect such as bowel herniation through a diaphragmatic hernia (*right*).

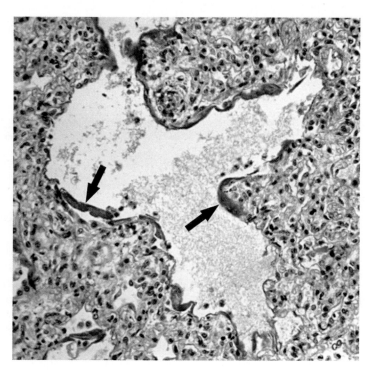

FIGURE 10-10. **Histologic features indicating surfactant deficiency in a premature infant.** Photomicrograph (original magnification, ×75; H&E stain) shows collapsed alveoli surrounding dilated alveolar ducts lined by smooth homogeneous hyaline membranes (*arrows*). (Reproduced with permission from the Armed Forces Institute of Pathology.)

Anatomy

The respiratory system consists of the nasal passages and mouth, pharynx, trachea, bronchi, bronchioles, lungs, and the muscles that control respiration, as shown in Figure 10-11.

KEY FACT

The conducting airways contain a surrounding smooth muscle layer that hypertrophies and undergoes spastic constrictions in **asthma,** an obstructive lung disease.

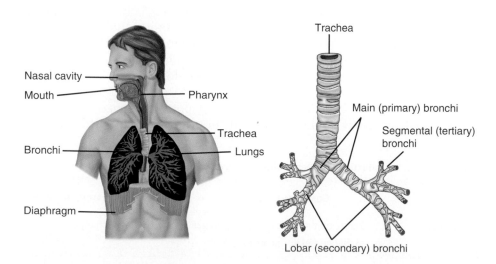

Nasal cavity
Mouth
Pharynx
Trachea
Bronchi
Lungs
Diaphragm

Trachea
Main (primary) bronchi
Segmental (tertiary) bronchi
Lobar (secondary) bronchi

FIGURE 10-11. **Gross anatomy of the respiratory system.** Overview (*left*) and conducting airways (*right*).

RALS:
Right pulmonary artery is **A**nterior,
Left pulmonary artery is **S**uperior to
the bronchi.

KEY FACT

An aspirated foreign object is more
likely to lodge in the right mainstem
bronchus than the left mainstem
bronchus due to the former's
smaller angle of entry and wider
diameter (see Figure 10-11).

KEY FACT

The visceral pleura lacks sensory
innervation; however, the parietal
pleura is innervated by branches of
the intercostal and phrenic nerves.
Thus, the parietal pleura is highly
sensitive to pain, but the visceral
pleura is not.

MNEMONIC

The **P**arietal pleura feels **P**ain.

FLASH BACK

A pleural effusion may be the result
of a **transudative** or **exudative**
process.
- **Transudate:** increased
  capillary pressure or decreased
  oncotic pressure secondary to
  congestive heart failure (CHF),
  cirrhosis, or nephrotic syndrome.
- **Exudate:** increased vascular
  permeability and inflammation
  secondary to lung infection,
  malignancy, or pulmonary
  embolism (PE).

AIRWAYS

The passages that transmit air from the environment to the lungs can be
divided into conducting airways and respiratory airways, as described in Table
10-1.

LUNGS

The right and left lungs are structurally distinct, as described in Table 10-2.

Blood Supply of the Lungs

- The right and left **pulmonary arteries** transport relatively deoxygenated
  blood from the right ventricle to the lungs.
- The **bronchial arteries** branch from the descending aorta to supply the
  bronchi and pulmonary connective tissues with nourishing, O_2-rich blood.
- Branches of the pulmonary and bronchial arteries enter the **bronchopulmonary segments** centrally alongside the **segmental (tertiary) bronchi.**
- The **bronchial veins** drain blood supplied by the bronchial arteries; the
  small bronchial veins unite to form a single vessel in each lung that empties into the **azygos vein** on the right and the **hemiazygos vein** on the left.
- The **pulmonary veins** transport oxygenated blood from the alveoli to the
  left atrium.

The relationship among the conducting airways, respiratory airways, and
blood supply to the alveoli is shown in Figure 10-12.

Pleura

The lungs are located within a bilayered pleural sac in the thoracic cavity.

- The **visceral pleura**, or **pulmonary pleura** adheres tightly to the outer surface of the lungs.
- The **parietal pleura** covers the inside of the thoracic cavity, including the
  diaphragm, chest wall, and the mediastinum.
- The **pleural reflections** are the angled boundaries between the parietal
  pleura lining one surface and the parietal pleura lining another. For example, the costal pleura is continuous with the diaphragmatic pleura, forming
  the costal line of pleural reflection at the boundary between the ribs and
  the diaphragm, also called the **costophrenic angle.**

Between the visceral and parietal pleura is a potential space, the **pleural
cavity,** which normally contains < 10 mL of circulating fluid. In some dis-

TABLE 10-1. Conducting and Respiratory Airways

	CONDUCTING AIRWAYS	**RESPIRATORY AIRWAYS**
Function	Warm, humidify, and filter air; no gas exchange (anatomic dead space)	Gas exchange
Structures	Nose/mouth, pharynx	Respiratory bronchioles
	Trachea	Alveolar ducts
	Bronchi	Alveoli
	Bronchioles	
	Terminal bronchioles	

TABLE 10-2.   Anatomy of the Right and Left Lungs

	RIGHT	**LEFT**
Lobes	Three (upper, middle, and lower)	Two (upper with lingula, and lower)
Main bronchus entry	Smaller angle (more continuous with trachea)	Sharper angle (greater deviation from trachea)
Main bronchus shape	Shorter and wider	Longer and narrower
Pulmonary artery entry	Anterior to right mainstem bronchus	Superior to left mainstem bronchus

ease states, fluid accumulates in the pleural cavity, forming a **pleural effu-sion.** When the patient is erect, the fluid fills the **costodiaphragmatic recess** located at the inferior part of the thoracic cavity. On a chest radiograph, the costophrenic angles are normally sharply demarcated and unoccupied by tis-sue or fluid, but pleural effusions blunt these angles, as seen in Figure 10-13.

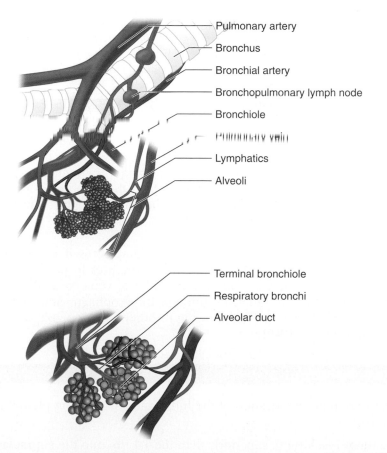

Pulmonary artery
Bronchus
Bronchial artery
Bronchopulmonary lymph node
Bronchiole
Pulmonary vein
Lymphatics
Alveoli

Terminal bronchiole
Respiratory bronchi
Alveolar duct

FIGURE 10-12.   Anatomy of the bronchopulmonary segments. Each lobe of the lung is subdivided into several functional bronchopulmonary segments, each supplied by its own artery and tertiary bronchus. The pulmonary and bronchial arteries approach the alveoli along-side the bronchi, and the pulmonary vein drains blood separately.

> **? CLINICAL CORRELATION**
>
> A pneumothorax occurs when air fills the pleural cavity due to compromise of one or both of the pleurae (often caused by trauma or ruptured air blebs). Positive pleural pressure resulting from air entering the thorax leads to collapse of the ipsilateral lung, as well as dissociation of the lung–chest wall system. These events may manifest as shortness of breath (dyspnea), particularly when the pneumothorax is large.

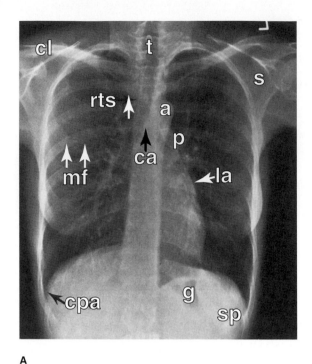

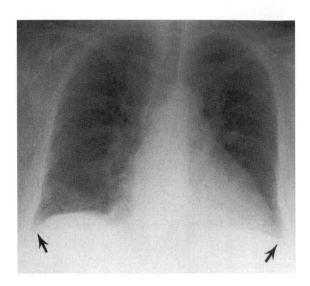

A   B

FIGURE 10-13. **Chest radiographs.** (A) Normal chest radiograph. (B) Chest radiograph showing respiratory fluid with meniscus in the left pleural space, compressing the adjacent lung. Note the sharp costodiaphragmatic (costophrenic) angles in the normal radiograph and blunting of the angles in a pleural effusion (*black arrows*). (Key a, aorta, ca, carina, cpa, costophrenic angle, cl, clavicle, g, gastric air bubble, la, left atrium, mf, minor fissure, p, main pulmonary artery, rts, right tracheal [or paratracheal] stripe, s, scapula, sp, spleen, and t, trachea.) (Reproduced with permission from USMLERx.com.)

FLASH BACK

The **right crus** of the diaphragm wraps around the esophagus to prevent the formation of a **hiatal hernia**, in which the stomach begins to slide into the thoracic cavity (refer to the Pathology section in Chapter 3 for details).

MNEMONIC

I 8 10 EGGs AAT 12 ("I ate ten eggs at twelve"):
Inferior vena cava: T8
Esopha**G**us, va**G**us nerve: T10
Aorta, **A**zygos vein, **T**horacic duct: T12

MNEMONIC

The intercostal **V**ein, **A**rtery, and **N**erve travel in a **VAN** inferior to the rib. The vein is most protected by the rib, and the nerve is least protected.

DIAPHRAGM

The thoracic diaphragm is a domed, musculotendinous structure that forms the inferior border of the thoracic cavity. During physiologic inspiration, the central part of the diaphragm descends, decreasing intrathoracic pressure and increasing lung volume. The peripheral parts of the diaphragm are fused to the thoracic wall and are thus immobile. The left and right crura (singular: crus) affix the diaphragm posteriorly to the vertebral column.

The diaphragm is a useful landmark in radiographs, as it has three openings at specific vertebral levels, which allow structures to penetrate: (1) the caval opening at T8, allowing through the inferior vena cava (IVC); (2) the esophageal hiatus at T10, allowing through the esophagus and vagus nerve; and (3) the aortic hiatus at T12, allowing through the aorta, azygos vein, and thoracic duct (Figure 10-14).

EXTERNAL ANATOMY

Landmarks outline the location of the lungs and surrounding pleural cavities (Figure 10-15).

- The lungs reach more superiorly than the 1st rib, into the **supraclavicular fossa.**
- At full exhalation, the lower lung borders extend to the 6th rib anteriorly, the 8th rib at the midaxillary line, and the 10th rib posteriorly. At full inspiration, the lungs reach about two ribs beyond the respective borders listed previously.
- The pleural reflection extends to the 8th rib anteriorly, descending to the level of the 10th rib at the midaxillary line, and to the 12th rib posteriorly.

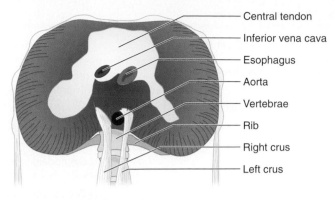

Central tendon
Inferior vena cava
Esophagus
Aorta
Vertebrae
Rib
Right crus
Left crus

Inferior view

FIGURE 10-14. **The diaphragm and penetrating structures.**

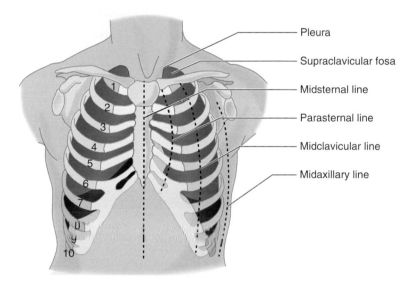

Pleura
Supraclavicular fosa
Midsternal line
Parasternal line
Midclavicular line
Midaxillary line

FIGURE 10-15. **External landmarks of the thoracic cavity.** Note the difference between the extent of the lungs at normal inflation (*pink*) and at full inspiration (*dark red*). The floating ribs (11 and 12) are not illustrated.

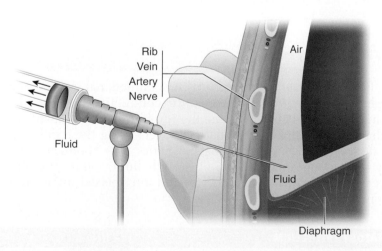

Rib
Vein
Artery
Nerve
Air
Fluid
Fluid
Diaphragm

FIGURE 10-16. **Thoracentesis.**

TABLE 10-3.   **Respiratory Muscles**

	QUIET RESPIRATION	FORCED RESPIRATION
Inspiration	**Diaphragm**	Diaphragm
	External intercostals	External intercostals
	Internal intercostals	Internal intercostals
	(interchondral part)	(interchondral part)
		Scalenes
		Sternocleidomastoids
Expiration	None (passive)	Rectus abdominis
		Internal/external obliques
		Transversus abdominis
		Transversus thoracis
		Internal intercostals
		(interosseous part)

These landmarks are important when performing thoracic procedures. A **thoracentesis** allows for sampling of pleural effusions by introducing a needle into the pleural space. The needle is typically inserted **above** the rib, because the intercostal vein, artery, and nerve travel along the inferior margin of each rib (Figure 10-16).

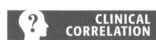

CLINICAL CORRELATION

A lesion of the phrenic nerve results in ipsilateral paralysis of the diaphragm. On a chest radiograph, this can be seen as elevation of the ipsilateral diaphragm.

MUSCLES OF RESPIRATION

The diaphragm is the primary muscle involved in respiration. It is innervated by the **phrenic nerve,** which is formed by branches of the C3, C4, and C5 nerve roots.

The diaphragm (and to a lesser extent, the external intercostals and scalenes) is involved in **quiet inspiration** (inspiration at rest), while **quiet expiration** is a passive activity. Multiple additional accessory muscles are involved in **forced respiration,** which occurs during heavy activity (Table 10-3).

Histology

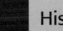

Within the lungs proper, there are two distinct functional regions, as suggested in the earlier gross anatomy discussion: the **conducting airways,** which partition, humidify, and filter the air, and the **respiratory airways,** which allow for gas exchange. Specialized epithelial cell layers along these different airways contribute to their distinct functional capacities. The conducting airways are lined by thick pseudostratified columnar epithelium, and the alveoli are lined by exceedingly thin type I pneumocytes and interspersed surfactant-secreting type II pneumocytes.

RESPIRATORY EPITHELIUM

The conducting portion of the respiratory tract is lined mostly by **ciliated pseudostratified columnar epithelium** ("respiratory epithelium") from the nasal cavity to the terminal bronchioles, where the lining transitions to ciliated simple cuboidal (respiratory bronchioles) and then simple squamous (alveolar ducts and alveoli) epithelium.

Cilia of the respiratory epithelium sweep mucus and foreign particles toward the mouth, thereby protecting the lower respiratory tract. **Goblet cells,** which secrete mucus, are interspersed in the respiratory epithelium from the nasopharynx to the primary bronchioles. These cells can be identified by their distinct shape and pale-staining cytoplasm.

Clara cells are located in the terminal bronchioles and secrete protein to help protect the airway lining from damage. Microscopically, Clara cells can be identified by secretory granules located in the apical cytoplasm. They lack cilia.

ALVEOLI

The alveoli are composed of multiple cell types critical for proper alveolar function. These cells are described in Table 10-4 and illustrated in Figure 10-17.

Pulmonary surfactant is a mixture of phospholipids (80%, primarily DPPC, which is a type of lecithin), surfactant-associated proteins (12%), and lipids (8%). Surfactant is secreted by type II alveolar cells in order to decrease alveolar surface tension and prevent alveolar collapse. Surfactant is stored in the whorled cytoplasmic **lamellar bodies** of type II alveolar cells.

Pulmonary capillary endothelial cells are joined by tight junctions to form a continuous endothelium without fenestrations. This configuration prevents fluid leakage but still permits gas exchange across the thin cell bodies.

OLFACTORY CELLS

In the nasal cavity, the **pseudostratified olfactory epithelium** is found in the superior conchae. Among other supportive cells in this epithelium, **olfactory cells** are bipolar neurons that generate action potentials in response to spe-

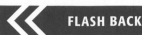

FLASH BACK

In **Kartagener syndrome** (immotile cilia syndrome), a defect in the protein dynein prevents cilia from moving properly. This results in impaired clearance of secretions and **frequent respiratory infections,** as well as **infertility** and **situs inversus** or **situs ambiguus (heterotaxy).**

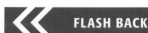

FLASH BACK

Alveolar macrophages, which phagocytize RBCs that leak into alveoli in CHF, are also called "heart failure cells." See Left-Sided Heart Failure in Chapter 1 for more details.

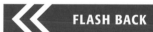

FLASH BACK

Increased capillary hydrostatic pressure within the lungs, as occurs in severe left ventricular systolic failure, can cause leakage of fluid into the lungs **(pulmonary edema).**

TABLE 10-4. Types of Alveolar Cells

	TYPE I CELLS	TYPE II CELLS	ENDOTHELIAL CELLS	MACROPHAGES
Prevalence	Cover 95% of alveolar surface area. Comprise 10% of cell population.	Cover 5% of alveolar surface area. Comprise 12% of the cell population.	40% of the cell population.	Variable
Structure	Flat and extremely thin (< 500 nm).	Cuboidal.	Thin, wrapped into cylinders to form capillaries.	Amorphous
Function(s)	Allow for gas exchange with the adjacent capillaries. Nonproliferative.	Secrete surfactant. Proliferate after lung damage. Are source of precursors for new alveolar cells (types I and II).	Allow for gas exchange with the alveolus.	Engulf debris ("dust cells")

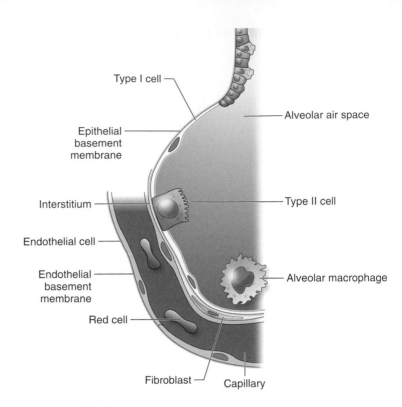

FIGURE 10-17. **Alveolar structure.**

KEY FACT

Ideal Gas Law

$PV = nRT$

where

P = absolute pressure (pascals)

V = volume (m³)

n = number of gas molecules (moles)

R = universal gas constant (8.314 J/[K * mol])

T = temperature (kelvins)

KEY FACT

Boyle's Law

Special case of the ideal gas law that states: For a fixed amount of an ideal gas kept at a constant temperature, the pressure and volume of the gas are inversely proportional.

$PV = k$, where k is a constant.

cific odor molecules. Each olfactory cell has a single dendrite containing a few nonmotile cilia that increase the surface area for olfactory receptors.

Physiology

The respiratory system is fundamentally a means for taking in air, facilitating exchange of the gases in the air with a liquid (the blood), and finally expelling air with a differing composition. As illustrated by the ideal gas law and Boyle's law, air and its component gases are characterized by their quantity, volume, and pressure. Likewise, respiratory physiology may be described as a series of **pressure-driven changes in the volume of gas in the lung** that enable the **regulation of oxygen, carbon dioxide, and pH in the blood.** This section introduces lung volumes and capacities and then discusses in detail (1) the movement of gas into and out of the lungs (**ventilation**) and (2) the regulation of O_2 and CO_2 transport (the **blood gases**).

LUNG VOLUMES AND CAPACITIES

Important lung volumes and capacities are defined in Table 10-5 and depicted graphically in Figure 10-18.

- FEV_1 is normally 70–80% of the FVC, or **FEV_1/FVC = 0.7–0.8.**
- In obstructive lung diseases, like **asthma** or **emphysema**, FEV_1 is decreased more than FVC, so **FEV_1/FVC < 0.7** (Figure 10-19 and Table 10-6).
- In restrictive lung diseases, like **pulmonary fibrosis**, FEV_1 is decreased to the same extent as, or less than, FVC, so **FEV_1/FVC ≥ 0.7.**

Measurement of Lung Volumes and Capacities

Some lung volumes and capacities can be measured simply by having a patient perform various breathing maneuvers into a spirometer. For example, having a patient take a maximal inspiration to TLC followed by a maximal expiration to RV generates a volume equivalent to the VC. However, since RV, FRC, and TLC cannot, by definition, be measured as expired volumes on spirometry, other methods are used. They include:

- **Dilution tests:** A known volume and concentration of an inert gas such as helium is inhaled at the end of a tidal expiration. This inert gas is diluted by the air already in the lungs, so the change in concentration of the gas that is expired can be used to calculate the FRC. Specifically, if X is the unknown lung volume of the patient, then

$$X = \frac{V_o \cdot (C_o - C)}{C}$$

where V_o and C_o are the original volume and concentration of helium in the spirometer, and C is the final concentration of the helium after equilibration with the patient's lungs.

TABLE 10-5. Lung Volumes and Capacities

Name	Description	Typical Value*
Volumes		
Tidal volume (TV or V_T)	Volume of air taken into the lungs during resting inspiration after a resting expiration.	0.5 L
Inspiratory reserve volume (IRV)	Maximal additional volume of air that can be inspired beyond tidal inspiration.	3.3 L
Expiratory reserve volume (ERV)	Maximal volume of air that can be expired beyond resting expiration	1.0 L
Residual volume (RV)	Volume of air in lungs that cannot be expired regardless of effort.	1.2 L
Capacities (Sums of 2 or more volumes)		
Inspiratory capacity (IC)	IC = IRV + TV	3.8 L
Functional residual capacity (FRC)	Volume of air remaining after tidal expiration. FRC = ERV + RV	2.2 L
Vital capacity (VC) Forced vital capacity (FVC)	The vital capacity is the maximum expiratory volume after a maximal inspiration. The forced vital capacity is the *measured* vital capacity when the patient exhales at a rapid pace after maximal inspiration. VC = IRV + TV + ERV = TLC − RV	4.8 L
Forced expiratory volume in 1 second (FEV$_1$)	After maximal inspiration, the *measured* volume of air that can be forced out quickly within 1 second.	3.8 L
Total lung capacity (TLC)	Total volume of air contained in the lungs after maximal inspiration.	6.0 L

*For 70-kg male.

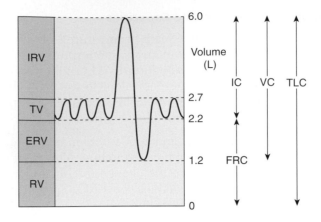

FIGURE 10-18. **Lung volumes and capacities.** A spirometry tracing showing all of the lung volumes and capacities. Values are typical for a 70-kg male. ERV, expiratory reserve volume; FRC, functional residual capacity; IC, inspiratory capacity; IRV, inspiratory reserve volume; RV, residual volume; TLC, total lung capacity; TV, tidal volume; VC, vital capacity.

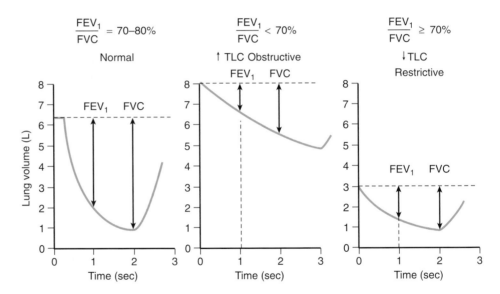

FIGURE 10-19. **Obstructive versus restrictive lung diseases.** Forced vital capacity (FVC) and forced expiratory volume in 1 second (FEV$_1$) in normal subjects and patients with lung disease. TLC, total lung capacity.

TABLE 10-6. **Lung Volumes in Restrictive Versus Obstructive Disease**

	RV	FRC	TLC	FVC	FEV$_1$	FEV$_1$/FVC
Obstructive	↑↑	↑	↑	↓	↓↓	↓
Restrictive	↓	↓	↓	↓↓	↓	↑ or normal

FEV$_1$ = forced expiratory volume in 1 second; FRC = functional residual capacity; FVC = forced vital capacity; RV = residual volume; TLC = total lung capacity.

- **Body plethysmography:** The patient sits in an airtight box that measures the pressure of the air within the box and, via a mouthpiece, the pressures at the airway opening. The FRC is computed by having the patient first exhale to FRC and then pant against a closed shutter, expanding and compressing the gas within the thorax. By measuring the changes in airway pressure and the pressure and volume changes in the box, Boyle's law (conservation of PV) may be applied to compute the volume of air contained in the thoracic cavity. In contrast to dilution tests, body plethysmography can detect air that is not in communication with the airways.

Anatomic Dead Space

The volume of air in the conducting airways that does not participate in gas exchange (ie, everything but the respiratory bronchioles, alveolar ducts, and alveoli). It is **normally ~150 mL** and should not change for a given individual under different respiratory conditions.

Physiologic Dead Space (Total Dead Space)

The total volume of inspired air that does not participate in gas exchange, comprised of the **anatomic dead space** and the **alveolar dead space**. The alveolar dead space represents the alveoli that are filled with air but not perfused by blood (V/Q mismatch, where V is ventilation rate and Q is blood flow; see Hypoxemia section under Blood Gases). Conceptually, dead space (or more specifically V_D/V_T) is proportional to the fraction of tidal volume that reaches areas that do not contribute expired CO_2 (no gas exchange due to absence of perfusion). Thus, in healthy lungs, the total dead space is essentially equal to the anatomic dead space, while diseased lungs may have elevated physiologic dead space. The Bohr equation computes the physiologic dead space:

$$V_D = V_T \frac{Pa_{CO_2} - Pe_{CO_2}}{Pa_{CO_2}}$$

where V_D is the physiologic dead space (mL); V_T is the tidal volume (mL); Pa_{CO_2} is the arterial partial pressure of carbon dioxide (mm Hg); and Pe_{CO_2} is the partial pressure of carbon dioxide in expired air (mm Hg).

VENTILATION

Alveolar Function

GAS EXCHANGE

The alveolus is exquisitely constructed to enable robust gas exchange, even during rigorous exercise. To accomplish this, the approximately spherical alveolar surface is criss-crossed by a network of narrow capillaries barely wider than a single red blood cell, or about 10 μm. Oxygen and carbon dioxide must diffuse across a trilaminar barrier: the endothelial cell wall, the basement membrane, and a type I pneumocyte; remarkably, the total thickness of this barrier is on the order of 500 nm in the healthy human lung. At normal respiratory rates, RBCs are fully saturated with oxygen after traversing just a quarter of the length of an alveolar capillary. The remaining length provides the capacity to accommodate the increased cardiac output during exertion.

SURFACE TENSION

The collapsing pressure of the alveoli is governed by Laplace's law:

$$P = (2T)/r$$

where P is collapsing pressure (the pressure required to hold the alveolus open); T is surface tension; and r is the alveolar radius.

When r is small, greater pressure is required to keep the alveolus open. Thus, alveoli are most likely to collapse on expiration, when their radii are at a minimum; this alveolar collapse is called **atelectasis. Surfactant** reduces the surface tension to protect small alveoli from collapsing.

SURFACTANT

As described in greater detail previously (see under Alveoli in the Histology section), surfactant is synthesized by **type II alveolar cells** and is made up primarily of **DPPC.**

KEY FACT

Decreased or dysfunctional surfactant in acute respiratory distress syndrome (ARDS) and the lack of surfactant in neonatal RDS contribute to decreased lung compliance and atelectasis.

- Surfactant lines alveoli and acts as a detergent, reducing surface tension. This helps prevent alveolar collapse.
- Surfactant production in the fetus may begin as early as week 24, and is usually present by week 35. A **lecithin (DPPC):sphingomyelin ratio > 2:1** indicates mature surfactant production.
- **Neonatal respiratory distress syndrome** can occur in premature infants due to their lack of surfactant production. These infants have **atelectasis, decreased compliance,** trouble with inspiration, and **hypoxemia** due to V/Q mismatch.

OTHER LUNG PRODUCTS

The lung produces many important substances besides surfactant, including:

- **Prostaglandins:** Various functions, including contraction or relaxation of vascular smooth muscle.
- **Histamine:** Promotion of vascular permeability and exudative processes.
- **Kallikrein:** Activates bradykinin.
- **Angiotensin-converting enzyme (ACE):** Converts angiotensin I to angiotensin II (see also Renin-Angiotensin-Aldosterone System in the Physiology section of Chapter 8); inactivates bradykinin.

KEY FACT

ACE inhibitors increase bradykinin levels, potentially causing cough and angioedema as side effects.

Ventilation Rate

MINUTE VENTILATION

The total amount of air inspired in 1 minute.

Minute ventilation = Tidal volume × Breaths/min

ALVEOLAR VENTILATION

The total amount of air that reaches the alveoli (air that participates in gas exchange) in 1 minute. It is different from minute ventilation due to dead space.

$$\text{Alveolar ventilation} = (V_T - V_D) \times \text{Breaths/min}$$
$$\dot{V}_A = \dot{V}_{CO_2}/F_{ACO_2} = 0.863\ \dot{V}_{CO_2}/P_{aCO_2}$$

where $\dot{V}_A$ is alveolar ventilation (L/min), $\dot{V}_{CO_2}$ is the rate of CO_2 production in the body (mL/min), F_{ACO_2} is the fraction of alveolar CO_2, P_{aCO_2} is the partial pressure of CO_2 in the arterial blood, and 0.863 is the temperature and pressure-adjusted conversion between F_{ACO_2} and P_{aCO_2}.

Increasing alveolar ventilation through increased depth (tidal volume) or rate of breathing results in a proportionate decrease in P_{aCO_2}.

INSPIRATION

An **active** process that always requires at least some muscle activity (see also Table 10-3).

- **Diaphragm:** The most important muscle in inspiration. When the diaphragm contracts, the volume of the thoracic cavity increases in the vertical dimension. This creates negative intrathoracic pressure, thus drawing air into the lungs.
- **External intercostals, interchondral part of internal intercostals, scalenes, and sternocleidomastoids:** Normally used only during **exercise,** but may be used for inspiration **at rest in patients with lung disease,** noted on physical exam as observable **increased work of breathing.** The actions of these muscles on the upper and lower ribs are different because the upper ribs are firmly attached to the sternum and relatively parallel to the horizontal plane, whereas the lower ribs descend as they curve around the body. As a result, movement of the upper ribs is often compared to a pump-handle, where the ribs and sternum move up and out as a unit and increase the anteroposterior (AP) diameter of the chest. In contrast, movement of the lower ribs is more like lifting bucket handles from either side of the thorax, resulting in an increased transverse diameter (Figure 10-20).

EXPIRATION

Expiration is normally a passive maneuver, secondary to the natural elastic recoil of the lung–chest wall system. The lung–chest wall system is minimally distended at FRC, so once the active muscle activity of inspiration is removed, the lungs recoil back to FRC.

Expiratory muscles are used during **exercise,** coughing, or when airway resistance is elevated in disease (eg, **asthma**). Such muscles include the interosseous part of the internal intercostals, rectus abdominis, transversus abdominis, and internal/external obliques.

Lung Compliance

Compliance (C) is a measure of the distensibility of an object; in other words, the volume change that results per unit of pressure applied. The more compliant the lung, the easier it is to inflate and deflate it. Compliance is the reciprocal of elastance and is therefore inversely proportional to the amount of elastic tissue.

$$\text{Compliance } (C) = \Delta \text{ Volume } (V) / \Delta \text{ Pressure } (P)$$

where C is in mL/cm H_2O, V is in mL, and P is in cm H_2O (1 cm H_2O = 0.74 mm Hg).

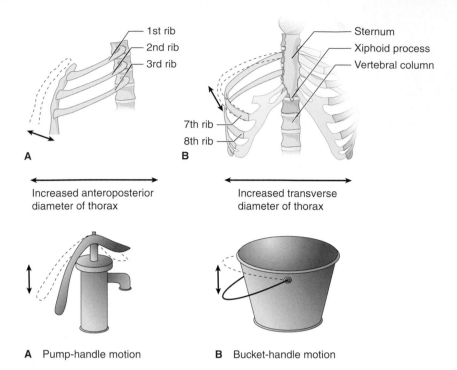

FIGURE 10-20. **Pump-handle versus bucket-handle movement.** (A) When accessory muscles lift the upper ribs, which are directly affixed to the sternum, the sternum lifts up and out as if it were a water pump, thereby increasing the anteroposterior diameter of the thorax. (B) When accessory muscles lift the lower ribs, which have a significant downward angle and indirect attachment to the sternum, they primarily lift up like the handle of a bucket, thereby increasing the transverse diameter of the thorax.

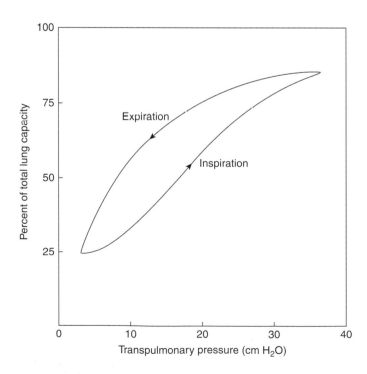

FIGURE 10-21. **Hysteresis curve.** Percent of total lung capacity versus transpulmonary pressure.

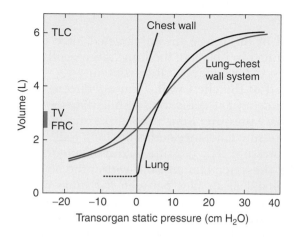

FIGURE 10-22. Lung–chest wall system. Pressure and volume tracings for the lung, chest wall, and the combined system. FRC, functional residual capacity; TLC, total lung capacity; TV, tidal volume.

When inspiration and expiration are plotted on a volume-versus-pressure graph (Figure 10-21), the slope of the curve is the compliance (note that this is a **static compliance** curve, meaning that the points correspond to measurements made after airflow is halted at different stages of inspiration or expiration). Notice that the compliance changes as a function of pressure and according to whether a person is breathing in or out (this path-dependence is termed *hysteresis*).

COMPLIANCE OF THE LUNG–CHEST WALL SYSTEM

Since the act of breathing involves both the lungs and the chest wall, the separate compliance curves for both must be summed in order to understand the mechanics of the respiratory cycle (Figure 10-22).

Mechanics of Breathing During the Respiratory Cycle

The respiratory cycle involves the repeating pattern of inspiration → expiration → rest. The volumes and key pressures during a prototypical tidal breath are graphed in Figure 10-23 and described in detail in the following sections.

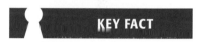

KEY FACT

In **emphysema,** there is destruction of elastic tissue, so **C** ↑.

In **fibrotic lung disease,** the lungs become stiffer, so **C** ↓.

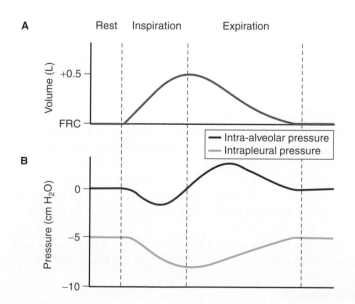

FIGURE 10-23. Spontaneous respiration. (A) Volume of the lung relative to functional residual capacity (FRC) during spontaneous respiration. (B) Intrapleural (*blue*) and intra-alveolar (*red*) pressures during spontaneous respiration.

FORCES DEFINED

- **Inward recoil of the lungs:** Inward-directed force created by the elastic tissue in the lungs. In isolation, the lungs always collapse to a minimal volume, regardless of how much air they contain.
- **Outward recoil of the chest wall:** Outward-directed force created by the chest wall's tendency to expand to its resting state (~70% of TLC).
- **Transpulmonary pressure:** Intra-alveolar pressure minus intrapleural pressure, ie, the pressure difference across the lung wall.
- **Intrapleural pressure:** The pressure within the pleural cavity.
- **Intra-alveolar pressure:** The pressure within the alveoli of the lungs; the major determinant of air flow between the lungs and the environment. Varies from negative during inspiration to positive during expiration.
- **Negative pressure:** When the intra-alveolar pressure is lower than the ambient pressure at the airway opening, air flows down the pressure gradient into the lungs.
- **Positive pressure:** When the intra-alveolar pressure is greater than the airway opening pressure, air flows down the pressure gradient out of the lungs.

AT REST

At rest, when the gas volume in the lungs is equal to FRC, the pressures created by the lungs (inward recoil) and the chest wall (outward recoil) are equal and opposite (see Figure 10-22). The lungs create positive pressure because they tend to collapse due to their elasticity. At the same time, the chest wall generates negative pressure because the ribcage and the rest of the thoracic wall to which the lungs are affixed resist deformation from their natural shape. These opposing forces cancel out, establishing a distending pressure (alveolar pressure) of 0 (see Figure 10-23). The respiratory muscles are not involved in this process.

$$\text{Intrapleural pressure} = -5 \text{ cm H}_2\text{O}$$
$$\text{Intra-alveolar pressure} = 0 \text{ cm H}_2\text{O}$$

In **emphysema,** the lungs have a decreased tendency to collapse due to a loss of elasticity (compliance ↑). As a result, the lung–chest wall system recalibrates to a new, **higher FRC** at which the forces balance. This is why patients with emphysema are **barrel-chested.**

In **lung fibrosis,** the lungs have an increased tendency to collapse (compliance ↓), so the system equilibrates to a new, **lower FRC** at which the forces balance.

DURING INSPIRATION

The muscles of inspiration contract, generating negative pressure. The intra-alveolar pressure is therefore negative. However, inspiration does not continue indefinitely because the pressure exerted by the chest wall becomes positive as it expands beyond its natural shape, thus opposing the muscles of inspiration. Approximate values for a young, healthy subject are given below; note that there can be significant variation based on age, weight, or health:

$$\text{Intrapleural pressure: Decreases from } -5 \text{ to } -8 \text{ cm H}_2\text{O}$$
$$\text{Intra-alveolar pressure} < 0 \text{ cm H}_2\text{O, so air flows into the lungs}$$

AT MAXIMUM INSPIRATION

At TLC, the positive inward pressures due to the distension of the chest wall and lungs have increased to the point where they exactly cancel out the negative outward pressure generated by the muscles of inspiration. Thus, the lungs are held at full capacity, neither expanding nor contracting.

$$\text{Intrapleural pressure} = -8 \text{ cm } H_2O$$
$$\text{Intra-alveolar pressure} = 0 \text{ cm } H_2O, \text{ so no air flows}$$

DURING EXPIRATION

The muscles of inspiration relax, removing their strong negative outward force and allowing the intra-alveolar pressure to become positive. This allows the lung–chest wall complex to return to its equilibrium at FRC.

$$\text{Intrapleural pressure: Increases from } -8 \text{ to } -5 \text{ cm } H_2O \text{ (may increase into positive range, depending on the patient)}$$
$$\text{Intra-alveolar pressure} > 0 \text{ cm } H_2O, \text{ so air flows out of the lungs}$$

AT MAXIMUM EXPIRATION

At RV, there is still some gas left in the lungs. That is, **we can never exhale enough to fully collapse the lungs.** At RV, the chest wall exerts such a strong negative outward pressure (due to its tendency to recoil outward to its resting shape) that the expiratory muscles are unable to create enough positive inward pressure to exhale any further.

$$\text{Intrapleural pressure} = -5 \text{ cm } H_2O$$
$$\text{Intra-alveolar pressure} = 0 \text{ cm } H_2O, \text{ so no air flows}$$

MECHANICAL VENTILATION

Mechanical ventilators allow physicians to manipulate the pressures and volumes that govern inspiration and expiration. A detailed explanation of mechanical ventilation is beyond the scope of this text, but a brief discussion of the most common modes of mechanical ventilation and how they work may be useful.

- **Assist control (AC):** The ventilator is set to deliver a minimum number of breaths at a set tidal volume and, in effect, breathes for the patient. It automatically delivers the preset volume if the patient initiates a breath. This mode fully supports a patient.
- **Synchronized intermittent mandatory ventilation (SIMV):** The ventilator delivers a specified tidal volume at a predetermined rate, which is defined by the time interval during which one breath must be delivered (eg, at least one breath every 6 seconds). The ventilator allows the patient to initiate the breath as long as the maximum time interval has not elapsed, but if no breath is initiated by the end of each time interval, it automatically delivers the specified tidal volume. On the other hand, if the patient takes an extra breath within the time interval, the ventilator does not deliver the full preset volume; rather, it allows the patient to determine the tidal volume.
- **Pressure support ventilation (PSV):** Each patient-initiated breath is supported by the ventilator, which provides a specified amount of positive pressure to the airway. The volume of each breath therefore varies.
- **Positive end-expiratory pressure (PEEP):** PEEP is an option that can be added to other forms of ventilation. With it, airway pressure at the end of expiration does not fall to 0, but is instead maintained at a fixed value (eg, 10 cm H_2O). This helps to maintain airway patency during expiration and is particularly useful in hypoxemic states such as acute respiratory distress

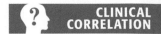

CLINICAL CORRELATION

Obstructive sleep apnea occurs when excess body weight, extra pharyngeal tissue, or abnormal anatomy (eg, severe scoliosis) blocks the upper airway passages when the patient is supine. This obstruction causes periods of hypoventilation and hypoxia, resulting in nocturnal awakenings, poor sleep, and daytime somnolence. Treatment includes continuous positive airway pressure (CPAP), which is the equivalent in spontaneous breathers of positive end-expiratory pressure (PEEP).

syndrome (ARDS). In a patient who is initiating all breaths, the equivalent of PEEP is continuous positive airway pressure (CPAP), which may be applied by mask or endotracheal tube in order to maintain airway patency. CPAP is commonly used in the treatment of obstructive sleep apnea.

- **High-frequency ventilation (HFV):** Delivers very small tidal volumes at high respiratory rates. Thought to decrease ventilator-induced injury in patients with acute lung injury or ARDS (see Interstitial Lung Diseases in the Pathology section of this chapter).

Airways

FLOW

Airflow is proportional to the pressure difference between the mouth (or nose) and the alveoli and is inversely proportional to the resistance of the airway.

$$\dot{V} = \Delta P / R$$

where $\dot{V}$ is the ventilation rate (airflow); ΔP is the pressure gradient; and R is resistance.

Note that the dot over the $\dot{V}$ in the ventilation rate indicates that it is the change in volume with respect to time (ie, dV/dt).

RESISTANCE

Governed by Poiseuille's law:

$$R = (8 \eta l)/(\pi r^4)$$

where R is resistance, η is the viscosity of the gas, l is the length of the airway, and r is the radius of the airway.

Since airway radius is the major determinant of resistance (r^4), the major source of airway resistance is the **medium-sized bronchi** (the smaller bronchi have greater numbers arranged in parallel, thus offering less net resistance than the medium-sized bronchi).

FACTORS THAT INFLUENCE PULMONARY RESISTANCE

- Contraction of bronchial smooth muscle:
  - **Sympathetic stimulation:** Airways dilate via β_2-adrenergic receptors, thus decreasing resistance. **Albuterol** is a common β_2 agonist and is used in an inhaled form by patients with asthma or chronic obstructive pulmonary disease (COPD).
  - **Parasympathetic stimulation:** Airways constrict via M_3-cholinergic receptors, thus increasing resistance. This is seen in **asthma** as part of the immune response. **Ipratropium** is a common anticholinergic drug used to counter this parasympathetic bronchoconstriction in asthma or COPD.
- **Secretions:** Increased and/or thickened airway secretions, which are a hallmark of COPD and cystic fibrosis (CF), lead to increased airway obstruction and resistance.
- **Lung volumes:**
  - **High lung volumes:** The lung tissue surrounding and attached to the airways expands, pulling the airways open, so resistance is decreased.
  - **Low lung volumes:** When the lung volume is low, there is less traction and increased resistance. Airways are more prone to collapse.

BLOOD GASES

Oxygen Transport

HEMOGLOBIN

- **Structure:** Hemoglobin is a globular protein made up of four subunits (two α-family chains and two β-family chains). Each subunit contains a **heme moiety,** which is a porphyrin ring containing a single iron atom at its core. The iron in hemoglobin is in the **ferrous (Fe^{2+})** state and can bind O_2. If the iron is in the **ferric (Fe^{3+})** state, it is called **methemoglobin** and is unable to bind O_2.
- **O_2 saturation (SpO_2):** The percentage of total oxygen-binding sites on hemoglobin that are actually occupied by oxygen, also called the saturation of peripheral oxygen.
- **O_2 content:** The total amount of O_2 in the blood, both dissolved and bound to hemoglobin. Measured in mL of O_2 per deciliter of blood. Depends on hemoglobin concentration, partial pressure of O_2 (PO_2), and the 50% percent hemoglobin capacity (P_{50}) of the hemoglobin. Calculated by the equation:
    - O_2 content = O_2 bound to hemoglobin + O_2 dissolved in blood
    - O_2 content (mL/dL blood) = (1.34 mL O_2/dL blood × [Hemoglobin] × SpO_2) = (0.0031 mL/mm Hg O_2 × PaO_2)
    - Using typical values of hemoglobin = 14 g/dL, SpO_2 = 1.00 (100%), and partial arterial pressure of oxygen (PaO_2) = 100 mm Hg, one finds that the vast majority (98.5%) of oxygen in the blood is bound to hemoglobin.
- **O_2 capacity:** The maximum amount of O_2 that can be bound to hemoglobin (in mL/dL blood), computed as 1.34 mL O_2/dL blood × [Hemoglobin]. This is approximately equal to the O_2 content of blood at 100% saturation.

OXYGEN-HEMOGLOBIN DISSOCIATION CURVE

The oxygen-hemoglobin dissociation curve describes how the oxygen saturation of hemoglobin varies with the PO_2 in the blood (Figure 10-24). Its sigmoidal **S**-like shape reflects positive cooperativity among the four subunits, such that the more oxygen molecules that are bound, the easier it is for an additional oxygen molecule to bind. Factors that decrease the affinity of hemoglobin for oxygen cause the curve to shift right, leading to greater oxygen unload-

KEY FACT

Methemoglobinemia may result from treatment with nitrites and is thus sometimes induced when amyl nitrite or sodium nitrite is given to treat cyanide poisoning. Methemoglobinemia is treated by administering **methylene blue,** which is converted in the body into a reducing agent that reduces the ferric iron (Fe^{3+}) in methemoglobin to ferrous iron (Fe^{2+}).

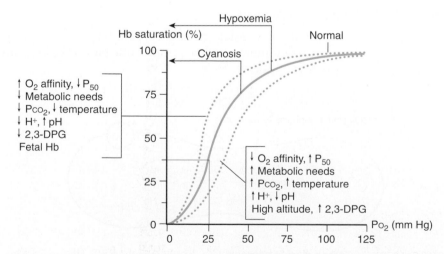

FIGURE 10-24. **Oxygen–hemoglobin dissociation curve.** The dashed lines indicate a right or left shift. 2,3 DPG, 2,3 diphosphoglycerate; Hb, hemoglobin; P_{50}, 50% hemoglobin capacity; PCO_2, partial pressure of carbon dioxide.

MNEMONIC

A rule of thumb for translating between P_{O_2} and Sp_{O_2} is the 40–50–60: 70–80–90 rule, where P_{O_2}s of 40, 50, and 60 mm Hg translate to 70%, 80%, and 90% saturation, respectively.

MNEMONIC

Factors that cause a right shift of the oxygen-hemoglobin dissociation curve—

CADET

↑ P_{CO_2}
Higher **A**ltitude
↑ 2,3-**D**PG
Exercise (buildup of lactic acid → ↓ pH)
↑ **T**emperature

KEY FACT

Carbon monoxide (CO) binds to hemoglobin with 240 times greater affinity than O_2 does, thus creating an allosteric change in the hemoglobin that prevents the unloading of O_2 from the three other binding sites. This causes a left shift of the curve and results in hypoxemia in CO poisoning. Treatment includes high-flow O_2 to competitively remove the CO from hemoglobin.

ing. On the other hand, a left shift causes more oxygen to become bound in the blood.

- Increases in P_{CO_2}, altitude, 2,3 diphosphoglycerate (2,3-DPG), or temperature, or a decrease in pH, will cause a rightward shift of the curve.
- Decreases in P_{CO_2}, altitude, 2,3-DPG, or temperature, or an increase in pH, will cause a leftward shift of the curve.
- During exercise, P_{CO_2} and temperature rise, and pH falls in the active muscle tissue. This promotes a right shift and greater O_2 unloading to the tissues.
- At high altitudes, 2,3-DPG synthesis is increased, facilitating O_2 unloading.
- Fetal hemoglobin ($\alpha_2\gamma_2$) does not bind 2,3-DPG as strongly as adult hemoglobin ($\alpha_2\beta_2$), shifting the curve to the left. This helps the fetus obtain O_2 from the mother's RBCs.

There are several important regions of the oxygen-hemoglobin dissociation curve worth remembering:

- At a P_{O_2} of > 70 mm Hg, hemoglobin is essentially 100% saturated. **Arterial blood** has a P_{O_2} of around 100 mm Hg.
- At a P_{O_2} of 40 mm Hg, hemoglobin is 70% saturated. **Venous blood** is at this level of oxygenation.
- At a P_{O_2} of 25 mm Hg, hemoglobin is 50% saturated. This is the P_{50} (50% saturation point) of hemoglobin.

Carbon Dioxide Transport

CO_2 is produced in the body's tissues and carried to the lungs via the venous blood. It is transported in three forms:

- HCO_3^- **(bicarbonate)**, formed by the combination of CO_2 and H_2O by the enzyme **carbonic anhydrase**. This is the **major mode** of carbon dioxide transport. This reaction reverses in the lungs, where HCO_3^- enters RBCs in exchange for Cl^-, and CO_2 is reformed by carbonic anhydrase and expired (Figure 10-25).
- Dissolved CO_2, which is free in the bloodstream.
- Carbaminohemoglobin, which is CO_2 bound to hemoglobin. In the lungs, the oxygenation of hemoglobin promotes the dissociation of CO_2 from hemoglobin. This is known as the **Haldane effect** (Figure 10-26).

Respiratory Acid-Base Disturbances

The lungs and kidneys are the major determinants of acid-base balance within the body. The kidneys can eliminate and reabsorb both base (HCO_3^-) and

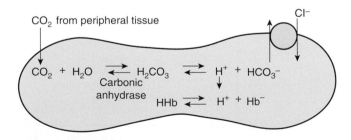

FIGURE 10-25. Carbon dioxide transport. CO_2 handling in the RBC. Hb^-, ionized hemoglobin; HHb, deionized hemoglobin. (Modified with permission from Ganong WF. *Review of Medical Physiology*, 22nd ed. New York: McGraw-Hill, 2005: 670.)

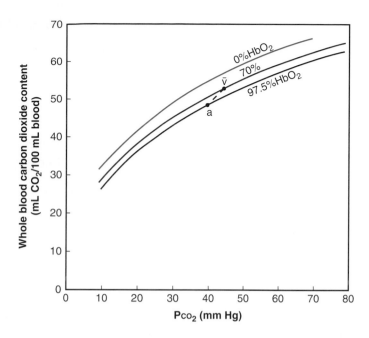

FIGURE 10-26. **Haldane effect.** As RBCs pass through the alveolar capillaries and the partial pressure of oxygen increases from 70% to almost 100%, the CO_2 dissociation curve shifts downward. This promotes the dissociation of CO_2 from the RBCs. $\bar{v}$, mean venous conditions; a, arterial conditions; HbO_2, oxygenated hemoglobin; Pco_2, partial pressure of carbon dioxide. (Modified with permission from Levitzky MG. *Pulmonary Physiology*, 7th ed. New York: McGraw-Hill, 2007: 157.)

acid (H^+ and fixed [nonvolatile] acids) in the urine, whereas the lungs remove volatile acid from the circulation in the form of exhaled CO_2.

- **Respiratory acidosis:** Caused by a **decrease in alveolar ventilation** (hypoventilation) and retention of CO_2 (**$Paco_2 > 40$ mm Hg**), leading to an increase in blood $[H^+]$ and $[HCO_3^-]$.
    - **Renal compensation:** Increased excretion of H^+ and NH_4^+ and increased reabsorption of HCO_3^-.
    - **Acute respiratory acidosis:** Renal compensation has not yet occurred (intracellular fluid buffering only). Each 10 mm Hg increase in $Paco_2$ leads to a 1 mEq/L rise in HCO_3^- and a 0.08 decrease in pH.
    - **Chronic respiratory acidosis:** Renal compensation has occurred. Each 10 mm Hg increase in $Paco_2$ leads to a 3.5 mEq/L rise in HCO_3^- and a 0.03 decrease in pH.
    - Causes of respiratory acidosis include opiates, sedatives, and anesthetics (due to inhibition of the medullary respiratory center), Guillain-Barré syndrome, amyotrophic lateral sclerosis (ALS), and multiple sclerosis (MS) (due to weakening of respiratory muscles), airway obstruction, ARDS, and COPD (due to decreased CO_2 exchange).
- **Respiratory alkalosis:** Caused by an **increase in alveolar ventilation** (hyperventilation) and a loss of CO_2 (**$Paco_2 < 40$ mm Hg**), leading to a decrease in blood $[H^+]$ and $[HCO_3^-]$.
    - **Renal compensation:** Decreased excretion of H^+ and NH_4^+, decreased reabsorption of HCO_3^-.
    - **Acute respiratory alkalosis:** Renal compensation has not yet occurred (intracellular fluid buffering only). Each 10 mm Hg decrease in $Paco_2$ leads to a 2 mEq/L decrease in HCO_3^- and a 0.08 rise in pH.
    - **Chronic respiratory alkalosis:** Renal compensation has occurred. Each 10 mm Hg decrease in $Paco_2$ leads to a 5 mEq/L decrease in HCO_3^- and a 0.03 rise in pH.

FLASH BACK

The kidneys play a vital role in acid-base disturbances. In the case of metabolic acidosis and alkalosis, the role of the respiratory system is to try to compensate for the skewed pH. Hyperventilation helps blow off excess carbonic acid and therefore compensates for metabolic acidosis. On the other hand, hypoventilation helps to retain carbonic acid and therefore compensates for metabolic alkalosis.

- Causes of respiratory alkalosis include pulmonary embolism (PE), high altitude (due to hypoxemia and increased ventilation rate), psychogenic hyperventilation, pregnancy, cirrhosis, and salicylate intoxication (due to direct stimulation of the medullary respiratory center).

The lungs play a compensatory role in the cases of metabolic acidosis and alkalosis, which are discussed in greater detail in Chapter 8.

- In **metabolic acidosis,** hyperventilation occurs to blow off excess CO_2 and thus carbonic acid, although this cannot completely compensate for the acidosis.
- Conversely, in **metabolic alkalosis,** hypoventilation occurs to retain CO_2 and thus carbonic acid, although this cannot completely compensate for the alkalosis.

Pulmonary Circulation

CHARACTERISTICS

The pulmonary vasculature has unique characteristics that set it apart from the rest of the vascular system. These properties relate directly to the physiologic function of the respiratory system.

- **Pressures** are much **lower** in the pulmonary circulation than in the systemic circulation (normal pulmonary arterial pressure = 25 mm Hg systolic and 10 mm Hg diastolic).
- **Resistance** is much **lower** than in the systemic circulation.
- Normal pulmonary vascular resistance (PVR) = 20–120 dynes $\cdot$ s $\cdot$ cm^{-5}. This is ~1/10 of systemic vascular resistance (SVR) (Table 10-7).
- PVR changes with lung volume. At high volumes, the **alveolar vessels** are compressed by stretched alveolar walls and contribute more to PVR. At low volumes, larger **extra-alveolar pulmonary vessels** are compressed due to decreased elastic traction and contribute more to resistance.
- Total PVR is at its minimum at FRC.

DISTRIBUTION OF PULMONARY BLOOD FLOW

When a person is supine, blood flow is nearly uniform throughout the entire lung. When standing, however, the lungs are divided into three zones based on blood flow and ventilation as affected by gravity, with zone 1 at the apices,

TABLE 10-7. Calculating Cardiac Output, Pulmonary Vascular Resistance, and Systemic Vascular Resistance

		CALCULATION	**NORMAL VALUE**
CO	SV × HR		5–6 L/min
PVR	[(MPAP – MLAP)/(CO)] × 80	**Note:** Units for pressure and CO should be mm Hg and L/min, respectively. The factor of 80 converts the units to dynes $\cdot$ s $\cdot$ cm^{-5}.	20–120 dynes $\cdot$ s $\cdot$ cm^{-5}
SVR	[(MAP – MRAP)/(CO)] × 80		770–1500 dynes $\cdot$ s $\cdot$ cm^{-5}

CO = cardiac output; MAP = mean arterial pressure; MLAP = mean left atrial pressure; MPAP = mean pulmonary artery pressure; MRAP = mean right atrial pressure; PVR = pulmonary vascular resistance; SVR = systemic vascular resistance.

zone 2 in the middle, and zone 3 at the bases. Both blood flow and ventilation are increased as one moves down the lung due to gravity, but blood flow increases to a greater degree than ventilation, resulting in a mismatch between ventilation ($\dot{V}$) and perfusion ($\dot{Q}$). This is known as $\dot{V}/\dot{Q}$ mismatch.

- **Zone 1 (apices):** Reduced perfusion.
    - Alveolar pressure > arterial pressure > venous pressure.
    - High alveolar pressures compress the capillaries and reduce blood flow.
    - $\dot{Q}$ is reduced relative to $\dot{V}$, therefore $\dot{V}/\dot{Q}$ is increased. In extreme cases. Zone 1 can approximate dead space ($\dot{Q} = 0$, so $\dot{V}/\dot{Q} = \infty$).
    - Po_2 is the highest and Pco_2 is the lowest in zone 1 due to having greater ventilation relative to blood flow; there is unspent (wasted) ventilation left over even after full oxygenation of the blood.
- **Zone 2 (middle):** Well-matched.
    - Arterial pressure > alveolar pressure > venous pressure.
    - Blood flow here is driven by the difference between arterial and alveolar pressures.
- **Zone 3 (bases):** Excess perfusion.
    - Arterial pressure > venous pressure > alveolar pressure.
    - Blood flow here is driven by the difference between arterial and venous pressures, as in the systemic circulation.
    - $\dot{Q}$ is increased relative to $\dot{V}$, so $\dot{V}/\dot{Q}$ is decreased. In extreme cases, zone 3 can approximate shunt ($\dot{Q} \gg \dot{V}$, so $\dot{V}/\dot{Q} \to 0$).
    - Po_2 is the lowest and Pco_2 is the highest in zone 3 due to decreased gas exchange and airway closure.

REGULATION OF PULMONARY BLOOD FLOW

- **Hypoxia:** In the lungs, hypoxia leads to **vasoconstriction.** This is in contrast to other organs, in which hypoxia leads to vasodilation. Hypoxic vasoconstriction allows blood to be redirected away from poorly ventilated regions and toward well-ventilated areas.
- Several other factors also affect pulmonary blood flow (Table 10-8).

Hypoxemia

Hypoxemia is defined as a below-normal O_2 content in the arterial blood (as opposed to **hypoxia,** which means low O_2 in tissues), usually indicated by a reduced Pao_2. In a normal individual, the blood leaving the lungs should have an O_2 tension (Pao_2) approximately equal to the O_2 tension within the alveoli (Pao_2).

$$Pao_2 = Fio_2(Pb - Ph_2o) - (Paco_2/R)$$

where Fio_2 is the fraction of inspired air that is O_2 (0.21 on room air, 1.00 for pure oxygen); Pb is the barometric pressure (760 torr at sea level, where 1 torr = 1 mm Hg = 133 Pa); Ph_2o is the vapor pressure of H_2O in the alveoli

KEY FACT

Pulmonary blood flow can be measured using radioactive isotopes. This method, called **$\dot{V}/\dot{Q}$ scanning,** can detect areas of decreased perfusion and is useful for evaluating for pulmonary embolism (PE) and assessing regional lung function. CT pulmonary angiograms can also be used to identify PEs.

TABLE 10-8. **Factors Regulating Pulmonary Blood Flow and PVR**

	LOW pH	HISTAMINE	PROSTAGLANDINS	NITRIC OXIDE	ENDOTHELIN	SYMPATHETIC TONE	PARASYMPATHETIC TONE
Vasoconstriction	X				X	X	
Vasodilation		X	X	X			X

(47 torr at 37°C); $Paco_2$ is the arterial CO_2 tension; and R is the respiratory quotient.

The respiratory quotient, R, which represents the number of molecules of CO_2 produced for every molecule of O_2 consumed, depends on diet. $R = 0.7$ for fat metabolism, 0.8 for protein metabolism, and 1.0 for carbohydrate metabolism. The typical Western diet is assumed to have an R of about 0.8.

For a patient breathing room air, this can be simplified to:

$$Pao_2 = 150 - 1.25(Paco_2)$$

Once Pao_2 is calculated, the actual Pao_2 can be measured via arterial blood gas testing. The difference between the Pao_2 and Pao_2 is the **alveolar-arterial O_2 gradient** (A-a gradient, or $AaDo_2$), and should be **< 15 torr**, although this value can increase with normal aging. A good rule of thumb is that the gradient should be less than the patient's age/4 + 4. For example, a 60-year-old should have an A-a gradient no greater than 19 torr. The A-a gradient is important for determining the cause(s) of hypoxemia, discussed in greater detail later and diagrammed in Figure 10-27. In particular, the A-a gradient is increased in the case of shunt, V/Q mismatch, and diffusion impairment, but it is unchanged in the case of pure hypoventilation or low Fio_2.

ETIOLOGY

There are five main causes of hypoxemia (Figure 10-27). They include:

1. **Hypoventilation:** Hypoventilation is relatively common in lung disease. It is characterized by a reduced Pao_2 and an **increased $Paco_2$**. Since alveolar ventilation is also reduced, there is **no increase in A-a gradient.**
2. **Decreased inspired O_2:** This occurs most commonly at high altitudes, where the P_B is decreased. This causes a reduction in Pao_2 due to the decrease in Pao_2. Thus, there is **no increase in A-a gradient.** There are several physiologic adaptations to high altitude (Table 10-9).
3. **Poor gas exchange (diffusion impairment):** Diffusion impairment occurs due to a failure of Po_2 in the pulmonary capillary blood to equilibrate with alveolar gas. This is a rare cause of hypoxemia because most abnormalities in diffusion are too mild to cause hypoxemia unless the patient is exercising. The **A-a gradient is increased.**
   - O_2 is normally a **perfusion-limited** gas. This means that O_2 equilibrates early along the length of the pulmonary capillary (within the first

KEY FACT

In the fetus, PVR is very high due to hypoxic vasoconstriction. This allows blood to be diverted away from the developing lungs via the ductus arteriosus. When the infant is born and begins to breathe, the PVR decreases due to the action of vasodilators while the ductus arteriosus closes up. This results in increased blood flow to the lungs.

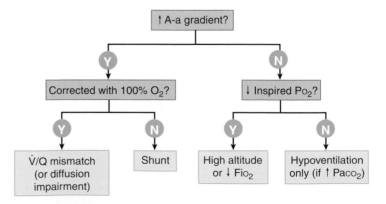

FIGURE 10-27. **Hypoxemia decision tree.** The different causes of hypoxemia can be distinguished as shown. Note, however, that combinations of different mechanisms are common.

TABLE 10-9.   Response to High Altitude

PARAMETER	RESPONSE
Pao_2	Decreased (hypoxemia)
Pao_2	Decreased (due to $\downarrow$ barometric pressure)
Ventilation rate	Increased (hyperventilation due to hypoxemia)
Arterial pH	Increased (respiratory alkalosis)
Hemoglobin concentration	Increased (polycythemia)
2,3-DPG concentration	Increased
Hemoglobin-O_2 curve	Right shift
PVR	Increased (hypoxic vasoconstriction)

2,3-DPG = 2-3-diphosphoglycerate; Pao_2 = partial alveolar pressure of oxygen; Pao_2 = partial arterial pressure of oxygen; PVR = pulmonary vascular resistance.

one-third). This leaves a lot of room for compensation in disease states; thus, a failure in O_2 diffusion is a very rare cause of hypoxemia.

- O_2 can become a **diffusion-limited** gas under certain circumstances, in which case it does not equilibrate by the end of the pulmonary capillary, resulting in the maintenance of a partial pressure gradient between the alveolus and the capillary. This can occur in **strenuous exercise** (due to increased cardiac output), **pulmonary fibrosis** (due to alveolar membrane thickening), and **emphysema** (due to decreased surface area for gas diffusion).
- Diffusion capacity can be measured using carbon monoxide, resulting in a DLCO (diffusion capacity of the lung for carbon monoxide) value. CO is used in place of oxygen because of the very high affinity of hemoglobin for CO. DLCO is a surrogate for the surface area available for gas exchange.
  - DLCO is decreased when useful surface area for gas exchange is lost, such as in emphysema, interstitial lung disease, and pulmonary vascular disease.
  - DLCO may be increased in the presence of intraparenchymal hemorrhage, increased blood volume due to CHF, or polycythemia (increased hematocrit).

4. **V̇/Q mismatch:** The V̇/Q ratio is the ratio of ventilation to pulmonary blood flow. Under normal circumstances, V̇/Q ≈ 0.8, although it varies with position in the lungs (see previous discussion of lung zones). When the V̇/Q ratio is altered, hypoxemia can result. There is also an **increased A-a gradient.**
  - **V̇/Q mismatch in airway obstruction:** If the airway is completely blocked and blood flow remains, then V̇ = 0, so V̇/Q = 0, and there is a **shunt.** Since there is no gas exchange, the values of Po_2 and Pco_2 for pulmonary capillary blood approach the values of mixed venous blood (Pao_2 = 40 mm Hg, $Paco_2$ = 46 mm Hg).
  - **V̇/Q mismatch in pulmonary embolism:** If blood flow is completely blocked, then Q = 0, so V̇/Q = ∞ and there is **complete dead space.** This results in increased CO_2 retention, although this is rarely seen since patients with PE often hyperventilate and may even become

hypocapnic as a result. Local bronchospasm due to the PE can also contribute to hypoxemia. If the blood flow is low but not zero, the values of Po_2 and Pco_2 for pulmonary capillary blood approach that of inspired air ($Pao_2 = 150$ mm Hg, $Paco_2 = 0$ mm Hg).

  - In most cases of $\dot{V}/\dot{Q}$ mismatch, there is neither true shunt nor complete dead space, but simply an **abnormal $\dot{V}/\dot{Q}$ ratio.** Blood from well-ventilated areas is already saturated at baseline, so no amount of effort from well-ventilated areas can compensate for the desaturated blood emerging from areas that are poorly ventilated. Giving the patient **100% O_2 increases the patient's Pao_2.**

5. **Shunt:** As mentioned previously, shunt is an extreme case of $\dot{V}/\dot{Q}$ mismatch that occurs when some blood reaches the systemic circulation without being oxygenated, reducing Pao_2. Since the Pao_2 is unaffected, the **A-a gradient is increased.**

  - **Right-to-left shunt:** Occurs when blood from the right side of the heart enters the systemic circulation without passing through the lungs. It is seen in **tetralogy of Fallot** (and other congenital heart conditions causing right-to-left shunts) and always causes a reduction in Pao_2.
  - **Left-to-right shunt:** More common than right-to-left shunt because pressures are higher on the left side of the heart. It is seen with several congenital abnormalities, including patent ductus arteriosus (PDA), atrial septal defect, and ventricular septal defect, as well as with traumatic injury. Left-to-right shunts **do not decrease Pao_2** since oxygenated blood is returning to the right side of the heart, raising the Po_2.
  - True shunt can be differentiated from $\dot{V}/\dot{Q}$ mismatch by giving the hypoxemic patient 100% O_2. This increases Pao_2 in the case of $\dot{V}/\dot{Q}$ mismatch but not in the case of a shunt, since in the latter, the blood never communicates with the alveolar gas, regardless of its composition. A patient with no shunt should achieve a Pao_2 of at least 400 torr on 100% oxygen.

CLINICAL CORRELATION

Over time, left-to-right shunts can cause pressures on the **right side** of the heart to become greater than those on the **left.** This leads to a reversal of the shunt to right-to-left, causing hypoxemia. This is called **Eisenmenger syndrome.**

Hypercapnia

Alveolar ventilation is the main determinant of $Paco_2$. Hypercapnia occurs when alveolar ventilation is reduced, which can happen in a number of ways:

  - Decreased total minute ventilation without a change in the V_D/V_T ratio.
  - Constant minute ventilation with increasing V_D/V_T. This can occur with decreased V_T (eg, a greater percentage of the V_T is taken up by dead space) and increased respiratory rate.
  - $\dot{V}/\dot{Q}$ mismatch. Well-perfused areas may be underventilated, whereas underperfused areas may be overventilated. When a large amount of ventilation is "wasted" on underperfused sections of lung, the effect is similar to increasing the dead space: less air is available to exchange gases with the blood, and CO_2 levels in the blood increase.

The response of the body to hypercapnia is often to increase alveolar ventilation by hyperventilating and blowing off more CO_2. Thus, CO_2 retention may not occur even if the preceding criteria are met as long as the body is able to compensate.

Control of Respiration

CENTRAL CONTROL OF RESPIRATION

  - **Medullary respiratory center:** Located in the reticular formation. Damage to or suppression of this region due to stroke, opioid overdose, or other causes can lead to respiratory failure and death.

- **Dorsal respiratory group:** Responsible for **inspiration** and determines the **rhythm of breathing** (normally 12–20 breaths/minute with an I:E [inspiration-to-expiration] ratio of 1:2). The dorsal respiratory group receives sensory input from peripheral chemoreceptors and lung mechanoreceptors via the vagus and glossopharyngeal nerves. Output travels via the phrenic nerve (C3–C5) and the intercostal nerves (T1–T11) to the diaphragm and the external intercostal muscles, respectively.
  - **Ventral respiratory group:** Responsible for **forced expiration;** not active during ordinary passive expiration. Also involved with increased inspiratory effort (eg, during exercise).
- Pons:
  - **Pneumotaxic center:** Located in the upper pons. **Inhibits inspiration,** helping to regulate inspiratory volume and rate.
  - **Apneustic center:** Located in the lower pons. **Stimulates inspiration.**
- **Cerebral cortex:** Exerts voluntary control over breathing.

CHEMORECEPTORS

- **Central chemoreceptors in the medulla:** Respond to the pH of the cerebrospinal fluid (CSF), with decreases in pH causing hyperventilation. CO_2 from arterial blood diffuses into the CSF and combines with H_2O to form H^+ and HCO_3^-.
- **Peripheral chemoreceptors in the carotid and aortic bodies:** Increased Pa_{CO_2} or decreased pH or Pa_{O_2} stimulate these chemoreceptors to increase respiratory rate. Pa_{O_2} must reach quite low levels (< 60 mm Hg) before breathing is stimulated.

OTHER RECEPTORS

- **Lung stretch receptors:** Mechanoreceptors located in the airway smooth muscle, these receptors are stimulated by distention of the lungs and produce reflex inspiratory time shortening and Hering-Breuer inflation and deflation reflexes. In the Hering-Breuer inflation reflex, excessive stretching of the lungs during a large inspiratory effort leads to inhibition of the dorsal respiratory group and the apneustic center to promote expiration. The deflation reflex acts during expiration to activate the inspiratory control areas.
- **Irritant receptors (nociceptors):** Located between airway epithelial cells and stimulated by noxious substances.
- **Juxtacapillary (J) receptors:** Located close to the capillaries in the alveolar walls. Increases in interstitial fluid, such as during pulmonary edema, PE, or pneumonia, stimulate these receptors, causing rapid, shallow breathing.
- **Joint and muscle receptors:** These are activated by limb movement and help to stimulate breathing early in exercise.

Pathology

There are five major categories of lung diseases: obstructive, restrictive, vascular, malignant, and infectious. Although the range of diseases affecting the lungs is large and perhaps daunting at first, the pathophysiologic processes underlying these diseases can be understood by considering the unique position the respiratory system occupies within the body.

In contrast to most organ systems, the respiratory system is constantly challenged with foreign matter. Particles from the environment are responsible for obstructive diseases such as COPD and asthma, malignancies such as lung squamous cell carcinoma and malignant mesothelioma, and, of course, a whole host of infectious diseases. The respiratory system is particularly susceptible to inflammation and infiltration because of the delicacy of the gas-exchange membrane.

At the same time, the lungs are the only organs aside from the heart that must bear responsibility for the entire cardiac output. This puts them at risk for vascular disease as well as hematogenous spread of malignancy.

Unfortunately, despite the diverse pathogeneses of respiratory illness, many of the classic symptoms of respiratory disease are particularly nonspecific: shortness of breath, chest pain, cough. Thus, working from a patient's initial presentation to the underlying disease process requires that the results of physical exam, history, and diagnostic testing be informed by an understanding of the physiology underlying ventilation and gas exchange. Treatment can then be chosen based on the conclusions of this comprehensive problem-solving process.

PATHOLOGY ON PHYSICAL EXAM

The physical exam of the respiratory system is essential for forming a differential diagnosis as well as for monitoring changes in a patient's respiratory status. This section defines common physical exam findings as a glossary for subsequent sections on respiratory disease, but discussion of physical exam techniques is beyond the scope of this text.

- **Inspection:**
  - The main goal of inspection is to identify respiratory distress, which appears as tachypnea, flaring of the nasal ala, retractions (accessory muscles causing the chest to "retract" inward), and abdominal breathing (using abdominal muscles to aid the diaphragm). Increased **work of breathing** not in the context of exercise is concerning.
  - Hyperinflated lungs can be a sign of COPD, in particular the "**barrel chest**" seen in emphysema.
- **Auscultation:**
  - **Physiologic breath sounds** can be divided by their origin: tracheal, bronchial, bronchovesicular, and vesicular (alveolar). Simply listening to the lungs of many healthy people is the best way to appreciate the broad range of normal breath sounds.
  - **Diminished breath sounds** unilaterally is suggestive of pneumothorax. Bilateral diminished sounds occur acutely when a patient is in respiratory distress (due to asthma, ARDS, etc.) as well as chronically in the case of emphysema (due to reduced lung tissue).
  - **Adventitious breath sounds** indicate pathology:
    - **Coarse breath sounds** (ie, a potpourri of sounds of different frequencies and intensities) are nonspecific but can indicate lower respiratory tract infections such as bronchiolitis and pneumonia. Care should be taken to distinguish coarse sounds originating in the lung versus transmitted upper airway noise that can be heard over the trachea and mouth.
    - **Crackles (rales)** are nonpitched sounds. **Fine crackles** resemble static, a burning fireplace, or Rice Krispies in a bowl of milk and may reflect the opening of collapsed alveoli in atelectasis. **Coarse crackles** resemble the sound produced by exhaling slowly underwater and are associated with airway opening and fluid in the lungs.

- **Wheezes** are high-pitched, polyphonic sounds that indicate obstruction of airways, usually heard in the setting of obstructive disease such as asthma or COPD. In children, sudden onset of wheezes is suggestive of foreign body aspiration. Diversity of pitch broadly correlates with the number of airways obstructed (think of the airways as a chorus of elementary school recorders or slide-whistles).
  - **Rhonchi** are low-pitched, monophonic sounds indicative of airway secretions and obstruction. They resemble the slurping sound produced when one sucks in air through a straw at the bottom of a drink.
  - **Stridor** is a high-pitched sound heard over the trachea, reflecting tracheal or laryngeal obstruction.
  - **Egophony** is an auditory phenomenon in which a patient asked to say "E" is heard through the stethoscope to be saying "A." This may be a sign of lung consolidation (eg, pneumonia).
- **Percussion:**
  - By serially percussing the lungs from top to bottom during inspiration and expiration, one can estimate the size of the lungs and assess for inflation status. The lungs normally sound resonant, like a drum.
  - **Dullness to percussion** may indicate lung consolidation (eg, pneumonia).
- **Palpation: Tactile fremitus** is elicited by asking the patient to utter a phrase rich in low-frequency vowel sounds (eg, "blue balloon" or "toy boat") while placing one's hands on the patient's back. Increased tactile fremitus is felt as a rumbling vibration and is associated with lung consolidation (eg, pneumonia).

OBSTRUCTIVE LUNG DISEASES

Obstructive lung diseases are a group of disorders whose distinguishing feature is **airflow obstruction.** The three major obstructive disorders are COPD (which includes emphysema and chronic bronchitis), asthma, and bronchiectasis. Airflow obstruction can originate at any point in the respiratory tree, from the bronchioles to the mainstem bronchi. All lead to a marked decrease in forced expiratory volume in 1 second (FEV_1), a normal or decreased forced vital capacity (FVC), and therefore a **decreased FEV_1: FVC ratio.** This is the hallmark of obstructive lung disease.

Emphysema

Destruction of alveolar walls leads to **loss of elastic recoil** within the lung and **dilation of the terminal air spaces.**

- Proteolytic enzymes (eg, **elastase**) digest elastin, the component responsible for elastic recoil in alveolar walls. Enzymes like α_1-antitrypsin prevent elastase from being active constitutively.
  - **Smoking:** Cigarette smoke attracts neutrophils and macrophages (which produce elastase) and inactivates α_1-antitrypsin.
  - **Hereditary α_1-antitrypsin deficiency:** This makes up a small subgroup of cases of emphysema (approximately 1%).
- The loss of elastic recoil in the lung parenchyma shifts the compliance curve of the lung upward and to the left (Figure 10-28), resulting in:
  - Decreased driving pressure for expiratory airflow, which leads to prolonged expiration time to maximally empty the lungs.
  - Loss of radial traction on the airways due to destruction of parenchymal tissue. This leads to airway collapse during expiration and air trapping.

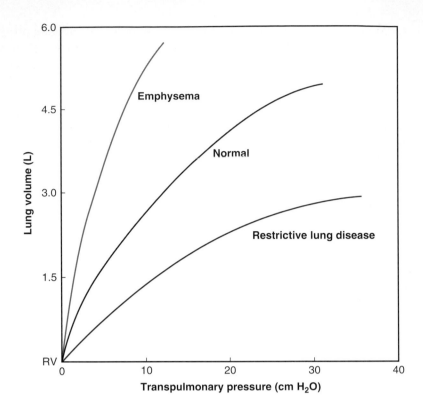

FIGURE 10-28.   Lung compliance in pulmonary disease. The lung compliance curve shifts up and to the left in emphysema and down and to the right in restrictive lung disease.

The prolonged expiratory phase seen in emphysema lengthens the overall duration of a single respiratory cycle. Because patients need to ventilate at a high enough rate to remain oxygenated despite the prolonged respiratory cycle, they often begin inhaling their next breath before all of the air from the previous breath is expired. This traps the nonventilated air in their lungs. Over the course of several breaths, they breathe at higher and higher volumes (**dynamic hyperinflation**).

PRESENTATION

■ Chronic dyspnea with or without cough. Dyspnea and desaturation are often worsened by exertion and can be exacerbated by respiratory tract infections, air pollutants, bronchospasm, or CHF.

■ **"Pink puffer"**: Pa_{O_2} is well preserved, so patients are not cyanotic ("pink"). Although ventilation and perfusion are both decreased, they are often well matched (alveoli and pulmonary capillaries are destroyed equally), so $\dot{V}/\dot{Q}$ mismatch is not severe. Patients require a high minute ventilation to maintain normal levels of P_{O_2} and P_{CO_2}, so they "puff," working hard to get air in. Although this is the classic presentation, many patients do not fit this description.

DIAGNOSIS

■ **Physical exam:**
  ■ Thin or cachectic.
  ■ Leaning forward on extended arms ("tripoding"), using accessory muscles of respiration.
  ■ Signs of hyperinflation: Resonance to percussion lower in the back than expected; diminished breath sounds bilaterally. There may be a

perceived increase in the AP diameter of the chest, although systematic studies have failed to verify this observation and it is more likely that the fixed size of the ribcage appears increased relative to the thin or cachectic abdomen.
  - Prolonged expiration and occasional wheezes on forced exhalation.
- **Chest film:** Hyperinflated lungs, flattened diaphragm. In classic emphysema (smoking related), paucity of vascular markings (arterial deficiency) in the upper lobes with or without bullae. These changes can be seen in the lower lobes in α_1-antitrypsin deficiency.
- **Pulmonary function testing:** Decreased FEV_1 and FEV_1:FVC ratio. FVC is often preserved. Air trapping leads to increased TLC, FRC, and RV.
- **Diffusing capacity:** Surface area for gas exchange is decreased, so D_{LCO} is reduced.
- **Arterial blood gas testing:** PaO_2 normal or slightly decreased; $PaCO_2$ variable but is often chronically increased in severe emphysema. During acute exacerbation, PaO_2 may drop and $PaCO_2$ may rise, with a corresponding drop in pH.
- **Pathology:** Two major subtypes of emphysema.
  - **Panacinar (panlobar) emphysema:** Characterized by dilation of the entire acinus (including the respiratory bronchioles, alveolar ducts, and alveolar sacs). Primarily affects the lower lobes. Associated with α_1-antitrypsin deficiency.
  - **Centriacinar (centrilobular) emphysema:** Characterized by dilation of the proximal part of the acinus (the respiratory bronchioles). The pattern of involvement is more irregular and is often localized to the upper parts of the lungs. Associated with smoking.

TREATMENT

Inhaled bronchodilators (β_2-agonists [albuterol, salmeterol] or anticholinergics [ipratropium, tiotropium]) can reduce airflow obstruction (see further discussion of these drugs in the following section on Asthma). IV or PO corticosteroids are used during acute exacerbations and are given long-term via inhaler for chronic disease. Supplemental O_2 is useful in patients with hypoxemia. Lung volume reduction surgery has been found to benefit a small subset of emphysema patients but may not be appropriate for the majority of them. Pulmonary rehabilitation is often helpful.

PROGNOSIS

Lifelong and chronic. Often coexists with, or may be complicated by, chronic bronchitis. Pneumothorax can occur due to rupture of a surface bleb or tear in the airways.

Chronic Bronchitis

Defined clinically as a **productive cough** occurring for at least 3 months per year over at least 2 consecutive years. Characterized by excessive mucus production in the airways. The mucus itself is typically more viscous than normal.

Smoking causes proliferation and hypertrophy of bronchial mucous glands. It also damages cilia lining the bronchial lumen, impeding mucus clearance. There is also an influx of inflammatory cells, leading to airway inflammation.

The increased mucus production and airway wall thickness decreases the cross-sectional area of the lumen, increasing resistance and inhibiting air flow. The obstruction to airflow in chronic bronchitis is in the terminal bronchioles, which is proximal to the obstruction in emphysema.

PRESENTATION

■ Chronic productive cough, dyspnea.

■ **"Blue bloater"**: Patients are often hypoxemic and cyanotic ("blue"), due to decreased ventilation in diseased airways with relative preservation of perfusion, resulting in significant $\dot{V}/\dot{Q}$ mismatch. They are also frequently obese and can have peripheral edema due to right ventricular failure ("bloater"). However, there is a great deal of overlap between chronic bronchitis and emphysema in many patients (COPD).

DIAGNOSIS

■ **Physical exam:**
  ■ Often obese and sometimes cyanotic. The fingertips, lips, and tongue in particular may appear purplish blue.
  ■ Clubbing of fingertips associated with hypoxemia.
  ■ Breath sounds characterized by wheezing and rhonchi.

■ **Chest film:** May show increased airway markings (appearing as a "dirty lung"), and there may be evidence of pulmonary hypertension and cor pulmonale.

■ **Pulmonary function testing:** Airflow obstruction results in decreased FEV_1 and FEV_1:FVC ratio. FVC is often preserved. In patients with dynamic hyperinflation, TLC, FRC, and RV may be increased.

■ **Diffusing capacity:** Typically normal.

■ **Arterial blood gas testing:** PaO_2 is often decreased, and $PaCO_2$ is increased. Bicarbonate is elevated by the kidneys in an attempt to compensate for the decreased pH.

■ **Pathology:** Increased number of goblet cells. The **Reid index,** which is the ratio of bronchial mucous gland depth to the total thickness of the bronchial wall, is abnormally high in chronic bronchitis.

TREATMENT

Bronchodilators and corticosteroids are used as in emphysema. Supplemental O_2 can prevent hypoxemia, reduce hypoxic vasoconstriction and polycythemia, thereby reducing the incidence of pulmonary hypertension. It is the only intervention that has been shown to reduce mortality. Chest physiotherapy (percussion, coughing, and postural changes) can loosen and clear airway secretions, and pulmonary rehabilitation is helpful.

PROGNOSIS

Increased risk of developing **pulmonary hypertension** secondary to hypoxemia and pulmonary vasoconstriction. May evolve to **cor pulmonale** (right ventricular dilation acutely and right ventricular hypertrophy chronically).

Asthma

Reversible obstructive disease characterized by hyperreactive and hyperresponsive airways that lead to exuberant bronchoconstriction on minimal irritation. Prevalence is approximately 9% in the United States, although there is variation between races and sexes. Extrinsic and intrinsic subtypes exist, although patients frequently have a combination of both.

■ **Extrinsic asthma:** Mediated by a **type I hypersensitivity** reaction involving IgE and mast cells (see also the section on Allergy at the end of this chapter). Often begins in childhood in patients with a family history of allergy. Common allergens include animal dander (especially cats), pollen, mold, and dust mites.

- **Intrinsic asthma:** Includes asthma associated with chronic bronchitis as well as asthma induced by exercise, cold/hot temperatures, pollutants such as cigarette smoke, medications (especially aspirin, see Key Fact), or stress.

In both types of asthma, airway inflammation leads to bronchial hyper-responsiveness. Implicated in this inflammation are eosinophils, lymphocytes, histamine, leukotrienes, and IgE (see Table 10-10 for specific mediators). As a result of airway smooth muscle contraction, mucosal edema, and secretions within the lumen, the airway narrows, thereby increasing resistance and reducing airflow, especially during expiration. Unlike COPD, the process in asthma is reversible, so between attacks, most asthmatics have relatively normal physiology.

PRESENTATION

Acute exacerbation manifests with wheezing, dyspnea, tachypnea, coughing, and chest tightness or chest pain.

DIAGNOSIS

- **Physical exam:** Tachypnea. Prolonged expiration and wheezing on auscultation.
- **Methacholine/histamine challenge:** Consists of inhalation of methacholine or histamine. Compared with a person with normal airways, an asthmatic experiences bronchoconstriction at a lower dose of the drug (hyperreactive), along with increased severity of bronchoconstriction (hyperresponsive).
- **Pulmonary function testing (PFTs):** During an acute attack, airflow obstruction results in decreased FEV_1 and FEV_1:FVC ratio (FVC is often

KEY FACT

Some asthmatics may be sensitive to aspirin, which inhibits cyclooxygenase and favors the production of leukotrienes from arachidonic acid. Leukotrienes play a role in airway inflammation and are potent bronchoconstrictors.

TABLE 10-10. **Epithelial-Derived Inflammatory Mediators in Asthma**

MEDIATOR	PHYSIOLOGIC EFFECT(S)
Endothelin-1	Bronchoconstriction
NO PGE$_2$ 15-HETE	Vasodilation
Cytokines: ■ GM-CSF ■ IL-8 ■ RANTES ■ Eotaxin	Inflammation
Growth factors: ■ EGF ■ IGF-1 ■ PDGF	Fibrosis Smooth muscle hyperplasia

EGF = epidermal growth factor; GM-CSF = granulocyte-macrophage colony-stimulating factor; IGF-1 = insulin-like growth factor-1; 15-HETE = 15-hydroxyeicosatetraenoic acid; IL-8 = interleukin-8; NO = nitric oxide; PDGF = platelet-derived growth factor; PGE$_2$ = prostaglandin E$_2$.

normal), and dynamic hyperinflation leads to a normal or increased TLC, and an increased FRC and RV. Between attacks, PFTs are often normal, although there may be small changes, such as decreased maximal mid-expiratory flow (appearing as a marked concavity on the exhalation curve termed **expiratory coving**) and increased RV (Figure 10-29).

- Patients with asthma can often monitor their own respiratory status with portable peak flow meters.
- **Arterial blood gas testing:** During an attack, PaO_2 is often reduced due to hypoxemia resulting from $\dot{V}/\dot{Q}$ mismatch. $PaCO_2$ is also reduced due to hyperventilation. $PaCO_2$ levels that normalize or become elevated during an asthma attack may indicate worsening airway obstruction or a tiring individual who can no longer maintain a high minute ventilation rate.
- **Pathology:** Edema and cellular infiltrates (eosinophils and lymphocytes) seen in the bronchial wall on bronchoscopy. Denuding of the epithelium, hypertrophy and hyperplasia of the smooth muscle layer, and enlargement of mucous glands with an increased number of goblet cells are also seen.
- **Differential diagnosis:** CHF ("cardiac asthma" or paroxysmal nocturnal dyspnea), foreign body aspiration, bronchiolitis, cystic fibrosis.

TREATMENT

- **Relievers:** Used to resolve acute symptoms.
  - **Short-acting β_2-agonists** (albuterol, terbutaline): Administered through metered-dose inhaler or nebulizer to promote bronchodilation and reduce airflow obstruction. Side effects are generally related to off-target agonism on β_1 (and to a much lesser extent, α) adrenergic receptors: hypertension, angina, vomiting, vertigo, central nervous system (CNS) stimulation, and drying/irritation of the oropharynx.
  - **Ipratropium:** Anticholinergic that competitively blocks acetylcholine from binding to muscarinic M_1, M_2, and M_3 receptors of smooth muscle cells, thereby preventing acetylcholine-mediated bronchoconstriction. Although useful in acute asthma exacerbation and COPD, long-term use has not been established as useful. Side effects are rare due to chemical modifications that impair systemic absorption, but there may

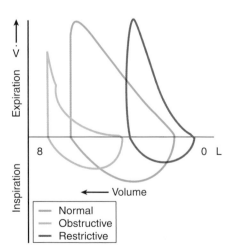

FIGURE 10-29. **Spirometry in obstructive and restrictive disease.** In obstructive disease, the patient's breathing cycles operate at higher-than-normal volumes, with the decreased FEV_1/FVC reflected in the marked concavity of the expiratory curve known as expiratory coving. In contrast, patients with restrictive diseases operate at lower volumes, and TLC is reduced. FVC, forced vital capacity; FEV_1, forced expiratory volume in 1 second; TLC, total lung capacity; $\dot{V}$, ventilation.

be off-target anticholinergic effects such as dry mouth, dry bronchial secretions, and urinary retention.

- ▪ **Oral and parenteral steroids** (prednisone, methylprednisolone): Reduce inflammatory response by decreasing the formation of cytokines, inactivating nuclear factor kappa light-chain enhancer of activated B cells (NF-κB), inhibiting generation of vasodilators, decreasing microvascular permeability, and reducing mediator release from eosinophils. Often given IV in severe acute exacerbations and may be taken PO (prednisone, methylprednisolone) for long-term control. Side effects of long-term steroid use include glaucoma, cataracts, weight gain (nuchal hump, moon-shaped facies), sore throat, seizures, mood changes (especially depression), confusion, muscle twitching, shaking, difficulty with sleep, increased osteoporosis, and bulging eyes.
- ▪ The management of a **severe asthma attack** consists of repeated administrations of albuterol (with or without ipratropium), 100% oxygen, and IV corticosteroids such as prednisone/prednisolone; if those therapies fail, **magnesium sulfate** or **epinephrine** is administered. Intubation is a last resort because of the difficulty of managing ventilation in the setting of severe obstruction.
- ▪ **Controllers:** Used long-term to prevent future exacerbations.
  - ▪ **Inhaled corticosteroids** (fluticasone, beclomethasone): Used to reduce inflammation in the long term, but onset is too slow for acute management.
  - ▪ **Long-acting β₂-agonists** (salmeterol): Similar to short-acting agonists, but have a longer half-life. May also be used as prophylaxis in COPD. Side effects include coughing, tremor, arrhythmia, chest pain, headache, and hives.
  - ▪ **Xanthines** (theophylline, theobromine, caffeine): These drugs increase cAMP in smooth muscle cells through inhibition of phosphodiesterase isoenzymes, leading to airway dilation. They may also have an anti-inflammatory effect. Rarely used due to drug interactions and a side effect profile including cardiotoxicity and neurotoxicity.
  - ▪ **Mast cell stabilizers** (cromolyn): Inhibit the release of inflammatory mediators from mast cells. Toxicity is rare due to poor absorption. Side effects may include throat irritation, cough, dry mouth, chest tightness, and wheezing.
  - ▪ **Leukotriene blockers** (zileuton, montelukast, zafirlukast): Zileuton inhibits 5-lipoxygenase, which reduces the conversion of arachidonic acid into leukotrienes. Montelukast and zafirlukast are cysteinyl leukotriene receptor 1 antagonists. Leukotriene inhibition helps to relax airways (Figure 10-30).
  - ▪ **Omalizumab:** Monoclonal antibody that binds circulating IgE, reducing airway inflammation. Rarely used due to cost. Table 10-11 summarizes these treatments.

PROGNOSIS

May improve with age or be a life-long condition. Avoidance of triggers can avert the worst symptoms. A severe attack that is refractory to bronchodilators **(status asthmaticus)** may require assisted ventilation and can result in death.

Bronchiectasis

An irreversible dilation of airways caused by inflammatory destruction of airway walls, leading to colonization by bacteria and pooling of secretions. The ability to fight off infection is compromised with chronic colonization. The bacteria and host may form a stable relationship that can be interrupted by

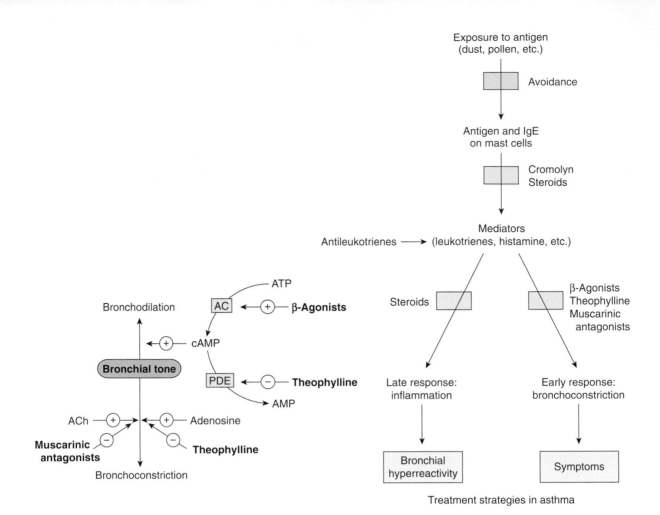

FIGURE 10-30. **Treatment of asthma.** Sites of action for β-agonists, muscarinic antagonists, theophylline, cromolyn, corticosteroids, and antileukotrienes. ACh, acetylcholine; PDE, phosphodiesterase. (Modified with permission from Katzung BG, Trevor AJ. *Pharmacology: Examination and Board Review*, 5th ed. Stamford, CT: Appleton & Lange, 1998: 159 and 161. Copyright © McGraw-Hill.)

acute exacerbations of the infection. Bronchiectasis has multiple causes, including:

- **Infection:** May be viral, bacterial, or fungal. Examples include tuberculosis, pertussis, and allergic bronchopulmonary aspergillosis.
- **Obstruction,** often by tumor.
- A defect in airway clearance of (or protection against) bacterial pathogens can also lead to bronchiectasis. An example is **Kartagener syndrome,** in which a genetic defect in dynein results in ciliary dysfunction and manifests as **sinusitis, bronchiectasis,** and **situs inversus.**
- Patients with **cystic fibrosis** develop bronchiectasis due to the production of thick secretions that are difficult to clear as well as chronic infection with multiple pathogens (Figure 10-31). The lungs of these patients are often colonized with *Pseudomonas aeruginosa*, *Staphylococcus aureus*, and *Haemophilus influenzae*; less common organisms include *Burkholderia cepacia*, which almost exclusively appears in patients with cystic fibrosus.

PRESENTATION

Cough; copious mucoid, mucopurulent, or purulent sputum production; dyspnea; rhinosinusitis; hemoptysis.

TABLE 10-11. Common Pharmacotherapeutics in the Treatment of Asthma

Drug Class	Specific Drug	Route of Administration
Nonspecific β-agonists	**Isoproterenol**—relaxes bronchial smooth muscle (β_2). Major adverse effect is tachycardia (β_1).	IV
Specific β_2-agonists	**Albuterol**—relaxes bronchial smooth muscle (β_2). Use during acute exacerbation. **Salmeterol**—long-acting agent for prophylaxis. Adverse effects are tremor and arrhythmia.	MDI or nebulizer
Methylxanthines	**Theophylline**—causes bronchodilation by inhibiting phosphodiesterase, thereby ↓ cAMP hydrolysis. Usage is limited because of narrow therapeutic index (cardiotoxicity, neurotoxicity).	PO
Muscarinic antagonists	**Ipratropium**—competitive block of muscarinic receptors, preventing bronchoconstriction.	MDI or nebulizer
Corticosteroids	**Fluticasone, beclomethasone, prednisone**—inhibit the synthesis of virtually all cytokines. Inactivate NF-κB, the transcription factor that induces the production of TNF-α, among other inflammatory agents. First-line therapy for chronic asthma.	MDI, nasal spray, or PO
Mast cell stabilizers	**Cromolyn, nedocromil**—prevents release of mediators from mast cells. Effective only for the prophylaxis of asthma. Not effective during an acute asthmatic attack. Toxicity is rare.	MDI or nebulizer
Antileukotrienes	**Zileuton**—5-lipoxygenase inhibitor. Blocks conversion of arachidonic acid to leukotrienes. **Zafirlukast, montelukast**—block CysLT1 leukotriene receptors. Especially good for aspirin-induced asthma.	PO

MDI = metered dose inhaler; NF-κB = nuclear factor kappa light-chain enhancer of activated B cells; TNF-α = tumor necrosis factor alpha.

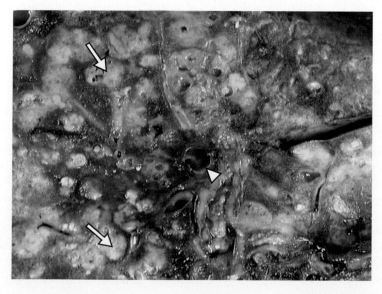

FIGURE 10-31. **Bronchiectasis.** Fibrotic lung parenchyma with numerous areas of pneumonia (*arrows*) and thick inspissated secretions in areas of bronchiectasis (*arrowhead*) in a patient with cystic fibrosis. (Reproduced with permission from USMLERx.com.)

DIAGNOSIS

- **Physical exam:**
  - Localized crackles or rhonchi may be heard. Some patients also present with wheezing.
  - Clubbing of the fingernails may also be seen in some patients.
- **Chest film:** Often nonspecific abnormal findings, including increased markings, crowded vessels, or "ring" shadows corresponding to the dilated airways.
- **CT:** Has become the preferred method both to diagnose bronchiectasis and to evaluate location and extent of disease.
- **PFT:** Often normal, but can also show obstructive pattern.
- **Arterial blood gas testing:** Usually normal, except in patients with very diffuse disease, who can exhibit hypoxemia and hypercapnia.
- **Pathology:** Marked dilation of the airways in one of three patterns: cylindrical, varicose, or saccular (Figure 10-31). Increased secretions are also seen. The arteries also enlarge and proliferate. New anastomoses may form, leading to hemoptysis.

TREATMENT

Inhaled bronchodilators (see section on Asthma Treatment) are useful in patients with coexisting airway obstruction. Antibiotics are given to treat both acute and chronic infections. Bronchopulmonary drainage with physical therapy helps to clear secretions from the dilated airways. In CF patients, DNase is used to break up thick secretions.

PROGNOSIS

In severe cases, cor pulmonale can develop. Colonization with *P aeruginosa* is frequent.

RESTRICTIVE LUNG DISEASES

Restrictive lung diseases are characterized by reduced expansion of the lungs and a **decrease in TLC. FEV_1 and FVC are both reduced,** but the **FEV_1:FVC ratio is normal or increased** (see Figure 10-29 for representative spirometry). The two main categories of restrictive lung diseases are **extrapulmonary disorders,** in which the defect is extrinsic to the lung parenchyma, and **interstitial lung disease,** in which the problem is within the lung parenchyma (Figure 10-32).

Extrapulmonary Restrictive Disease

Includes disorders of the chest wall and neuromuscular disease, leading to impaired ability to fully expand the lungs.

- **Neuromuscular diseases:** Lead to weakness of the respiratory muscles. Patients alter their pattern of breathing, taking more frequent, shallow breaths. This increases the $V_D:V_T$ ratio, reducing alveolar ventilation and increasing $Paco_2$. Ineffective cough can lead to recurrent respiratory infections, accumulation of secretions, and atelectasis. (See Chapter 6 for more detail on neuromuscular diseases.)
  - **Guillain-Barré syndrome:** Autoimmune demyelinating disorder primarily affecting peripheral motor fibers, causing ascending muscle weakness. Often postinfectious (eg, following *Clostridium jejuni* gastroenteritis).
  - **Myasthenia gravis:** Autoimmune disorder involving antinicotinic acetylcholine receptor (anti-nAChR) antibodies that cause muscle weakness.

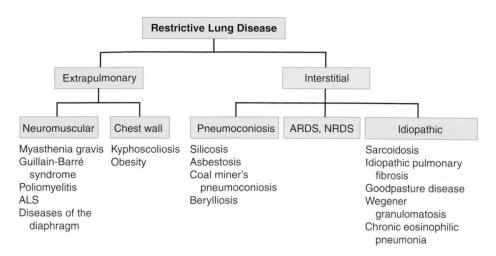

FIGURE 10-32. **Classification of restrictive lung diseases.** ALS, amyotrophic lateral sclerosis; ARDS, acute respiratory distress syndrome; NRDS, neonatal respiratory distress syndrome.

- **Poliomyelitis:** Picornavirus infection leading to ablation of anterior horn motor neurons and therefore symptoms of lower motor neuron (LMN) paralysis.
- **Postpolio syndrome:** Occurs decades after initial poliovirus infection, causing muscle weakness.
- **Amyotrophic lateral sclerosis (ALS):** Purely motor neuron disease leading to loss of spinal cord anterior horns and demyelination of lateral corticospinal tracts. Symptoms of both upper motor neuron (UMN) and LMN paralysis.
- **Diaphragmatic disease:** Can lead to dyspnea, hypoventilation and respiratory failure, although depending on severity, diaphragmatic disease may be asymptomatic in isolation due to compensatory recruitment of accessory muscles of respiration.
  - **Diaphragmatic fatigue:** Due to increased work of breathing, decreased energy supply to the diaphragm, and/or inefficient diaphragmatic contraction.
  - **Unilateral diaphragmatic paralysis:** Due to trauma or disease affecting the ipsilateral phrenic nerve, including impingement by tumor.
  - **Bilateral diaphragmatic paralysis:** Often due to a neuromuscular cause or bilateral phrenic nerve palsy.
- **Diseases affecting the chest wall:** Distortion of the chest wall or diaphragm leads to hypoventilation of lung regions, V/Q mismatch, and occasionally hypoxemia.
  - **Kyphoscoliosis:** Abnormal curvature of the spine in the lateral and anteroposterior directions. As a result, the rib cage becomes stiffer and more difficult to expand.
  - **Obesity:** Excess soft tissue makes the chest wall stiffer and less compliant, in addition to exerting pressure on the abdominal contents, forcing the diaphragm up to a higher resting position. One serious consequence of this is obesity-hypoventilation syndrome, also known as **Pickwickian syndrome,** which is characterized by a reduced central drive to breathe.

PRESENTATION

Most often dyspnea, especially with exertion.

DIAGNOSIS

- **Physical exam:**
  - **Neuromuscular disease:** Nonpulmonary manifestations of specific neuromuscular disease (see Chapter 6).
  - **Diaphragmatic disease:** Paradoxical movement of paralyzed regions of the diaphragm upward (and abdominal wall inward) during supine inspiration or during a sniff (can use a fluoroscopic sniff test to visualize).
  - Assess for kyphoscoliosis.
- **Chest film:** Assess for kyphoscoliosis, diaphragmatic paralysis.
- **Respiratory muscle forces** (maximal inspiratory [MIP] or expiratory [MEP] pressure): These measurements represent the maximum forces that a patient can generate against a closed mouthpiece. Assesses the strength of the respiratory muscles.
- **PFT:** Generally, decreased TLC, FRC, RV, FEV_1 and FVC, with a normal or increased FEV_1:FVC ratio. However, if neuromuscular disease becomes very severe, RV may increase due to inability to engage in active expiration.

TREATMENT

Supplemental O_2 or mechanical ventilation may be needed for patients with severe disease. The underlying disorder must be treated before irreversible pulmonary sequelae develop.

PROGNOSIS

Extrapulmonary restrictive diseases resulting in hypoxemia can lead to pulmonary hypertension and cor pulmonale. Progressive disease can lead to chronic respiratory acidosis.

Interstitial Lung Diseases

ACUTE RESPIRATORY DISTRESS SYNDROME AND ACUTE LUNG INJURY

ARDS and its precursor, acute lung injury (ALI), are characterized by acute-onset diffuse alveolar damage and leakage of fluid out of the pulmonary capillaries into the interstitium and alveolar spaces. ARDS and ALI are defined by four major criteria, all of which must be met:

1. Reduced arterial oxygen to inspired oxygen ratio:
   - In ALI, $200 < PaO_2/FIO_2 < 300$ mm Hg.
   - In ARDS, $PaO_2/FIO_2 < 200$ mm Hg.
   - A low ratio reflects poor oxygenation despite ample inspired oxygen; normal ratio is 500 mm Hg.
2. Acute onset.
3. Bilateral lung infiltrates (Figure 10-33).
4. Pulmonary capillary wedge pressure (PCWP) < 18 mm Hg (or normal left atrial pressures), to rule out left-sided CHF as a cause of the lung infiltrates.

Causes include pneumonia, inhalation of irritants, O_2 toxicity, heroin overdose, shock, sepsis, aspiration of gastric contents, trauma, uremia, acute pancreatitis, head trauma, multiple transfusions, disseminated intravascular coagulation (DIC), and fat or amniotic fluid embolism. In all of these cases, the initial injury in ARDS affects the type I pneumocytes and/or capillary endothelial cells, resulting in leakage of protein-rich fluid. Alveoli become flooded with fluid, reducing pulmonary compliance and preventing ventilation. This leads to hypoxemia in the forms of shunting and V̇/Q̇ mismatch, with the latter being exacerbated by altered distribution of pulmonary blood

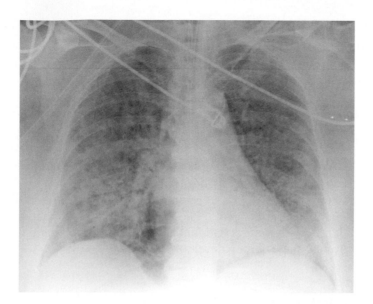

FIGURE 10-33.   **Chest film of a patient with acute respiratory distress syndrome.** Diffuse, bilateral interstitial and alveolar infiltrates are seen. (Reproduced with permission from Kasper DL, Braunwald E, et al. *Harrison's Principles of Internal Medicine*, 16th ed. New York: McGraw-Hill, 2005: 1593.)

flow due to increased PVR. Additionally, surfactant function and production is altered, resulting in alveolar collapse.

PRESENTATION

Dyspnea and tachypnea, usually in a critically ill patient.

DIAGNOSIS

- **Physical exam:** Crackles are often heard on auscultation.
- **Chest film:** Diffuse, symmetrical interstitial and alveolar edema (see Figure 10-33; note that this is criterion 3 from the previous diagnostic criteria). Air bronchograms—visualization of distal bronchioles due to the contrasting opacity of infiltrates around the airway—may be present.
- **PFT:** Not usually performed, but would see a restrictive pattern with a reduced D_{LCO}.
- **Arterial blood gas testing:** Hypoxemia and hypocapnia, with a large A-a gradient. Supplemental O_2 may not increase PaO_2 significantly due to shunt.
- **Differential diagnosis:** Cardiogenic pulmonary edema (ie, left heart failure), pneumonia, severe obstructive disease.

PATHOLOGY

Damage to type I alveolar epithelial cells, with regenerative hyperplasia of type II cells. Interstitial and alveolar fluid is present, with an inflammatory cell infiltrate. Areas of alveolar collapse. **Hyaline membranes** (composed of eosinophilic, acellular material), fibrosis, and changes in the pulmonary vasculature can also be seen (Figure 10-34).

TREATMENT

Treat the underlying cause of ARDS. Patients are typically intubated, mechanically ventilated using low-volume ventilation with PEEP, and treated in an ICU.

KEY FACT

Pulmonary edema is an intraalveolar accumulation of fluid. It can be caused by increased hydrostatic pressure (eg, left ventricular failure), increased capillary permeability (eg, ARDS), or several other mechanisms (eg, high altitude, neurologic injury, or opiate overdose).

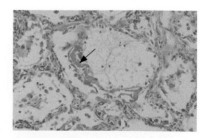

FIGURE 10-34.   **Alveolar damage in acute respiratory distress syndrome.** The alveoli are congested and edematous, and the classic hyaline membrane can be seen (*arrow*). (Courtesy of the Uniformed Services University of the Health Sciences.)

PROGNOSIS

High mortality (30–50%), largely due to the underlying cause rather than the pulmonary effects of ARDS. In patients who recover, long-term respiratory sequelae are often minor.

NEONATAL (INFANT) RESPIRATORY DISTRESS SYNDROME

Neonatal respiratory distress syndrome (RDS) is the most common cause of respiratory failure in newborns and the most common cause of death in premature infants. It results from a deficiency of surfactant in immature lungs, leading to atelectasis due to increased surface tension in the air-liquid interface, V/Q mismatch, and shunting. Predisposing factors include prematurity, maternal diabetes mellitus, and delivery by cesarean section. Incidence and mortality decrease dramatically with gestational age, with the most severe disease seen prior to the alveolar stage of lung development.

PRESENTATION

Dyspnea and tachypnea.

DIAGNOSIS

- **Physical exam:** Infants may appear cyanotic, and crackles can be heard on auscultation.
- Fetal pulmonary maturity can be assessed by measuring the **ratio of surfactant lecithin to sphingomyelin in the amniotic fluid.** A ratio of 2:1 or greater indicates lung maturity.
- **Chest film:** Low lung volumes, diffuse ground-glass appearance with air bronchograms.
- **Arterial blood gas testing:** Hypoxemia, hypocapnia, with a large A-a gradient. Hypoxemia that is refractory to supplemental O_2 due to shunting.
- **Pathology:** Lungs are heavier than normal, with alternating atelectatic areas and dilated alveoli. The pulmonary vessels are engorged, with leakage of fluid into the alveoli. Hyaline membranes are also seen (note that neonatal RDS was formerly called hyaline membrane disease).
- **Differential diagnosis:** Transient tachypnea of the newborn (TTN—self-resolving, relatively benign respiratory distress associated with pulmonary edema), bacterial pneumonia, congenital heart disease.

TREATMENT

Exogenous surfactant administration. Mechanical ventilation with PEEP. Inhaled nitric oxide. Antenatal maternal corticosteroid therapy to promote surfactant production.

PROGNOSIS

Mortality rates have improved dramatically with the use of exogenous surfactant but remain over 10%. Bronchopulmonary dysplasia may develop due to treatment with high-concentration O_2 and mechanical ventilation. Neonatal RDS may also be associated with patent ductus arteriosus (PDA), intraventricular hemorrhage, and necrotizing enterocolitis.

PNEUMOCONIOSIS

A group of interstitial lung diseases caused by the inhalation of inorganic and organic particulate matter. This produces varying degrees of pulmonary fibrosis, characterized by decreased compliance, reduced lung volumes, and

TABLE 10-12. **Common Inorganic Pneumoconioses**

NAME	INHALED SUBSTANCE	FEATURES
Silicosis	Silica dust (in quartz, sand, and many other minerals)	Seen in sandblasters, rock miners, quarry workers, and stone cutters.
Coal worker's pneumoconiosis (CWP)	Coal dust	Coal dust contains both carbon and silica. Progresses from anthracosis, a mild, asymptomatic form of carbon build-up commonly seen in city-dwelling residents and smokers.
Asbestosis	Asbestos, especially amphibole fibers	Seen in insulation, shipyard, and construction workers, as well as mechanics.
Berylliosis	Beryllium dust	Seen in workers who manufacture aerospace materials, nuclear weapons, and electronics.

destruction of the alveolar-capillary interface, leading to $\dot{V}/\dot{Q}$ mismatch and hypoxemia. Four common inorganic pneumoconioses are listed in Table 10-12.

PRESENTATION

Dyspnea, especially with exertion.

DIAGNOSIS

- **Physical exam:** Bibasilar crackles heard on auscultation. Clubbing may also be seen.
- **Chest film.** Nodular opacities seen in silicosis, coal worker's pneumoconiosis, and berylliosis. A more linear pattern is seen in asbestosis. Calcified pleural plaques are also seen in asbestosis.
- **PFT:** Decreased TLC, FRC, RV, FEV_1, and FVC, with a normal or increased FEV_1:FVC ratio. DLCO is also decreased.
- **Arterial blood gas testing:** Hypoxemia, often with normo- or hypocapnia.
- **Pathology** (Figures 10-35 [silicosis], 10-36 [coal worker's pneumoconiosis], and 10-37 [asbestosis]). In **berylliosis,** granulomas form due to the cellular immune reaction against the beryllium.

TREATMENT

Avoid further exposure. No curative treatment.

PROGNOSIS

- **Silicosis:** Associated with increased susceptibility to tuberculosis (TB).
- **Coal worker's pneumoconiosis (CWP):** Simple CWP is often inconsequential. If CWP is complicated by progressive massive fibrosis (PMF), it can lead to bronchiectasis, pulmonary hypertension, and death from respiratory failure or right-sided heart failure.
- **Asbestosis:** Predisposes to bronchogenic carcinoma and, less commonly, malignant mesothelioma of the pleura or peritoneum. Concomitant cigarette smoking multiplies the risk of developing cancer.
- **Berylliosis:** Can mimic sarcoidosis, with granulomas in multiple organ systems.

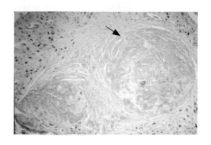

FIGURE 10-35. **Silicotic nodule.** Silica dust is engulfed by macrophages, initiating an inflammatory response. Concentric areas of cellular fibrosis are seen (*arrow*). (Courtesy of the Uniformed Services University of the Health Sciences.)

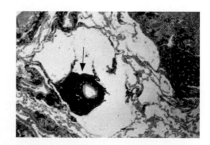

FIGURE 10-36. **Coal macule.** Black, nonfibrotic coal macule (*arrow*) seen in a patient with coal worker's pneumoconiosis. The macule is a collection of coal dust surrounded by little tissue reaction. Small areas of focal emphysema (surrounding the coal macule in this image) may also be seen. (Courtesy of the Uniformed Services University of the Health Sciences.)

KEY FACT

Pneumoconiosis associations:
Silicosis → lung nodules, "egg-shell" calcification in hilar nodes, tuberculosis
CWP → "dust cells" (alveolar macrophages with anthracotic pigment)
Asbestosis → bronchogenic carcinoma >> malignant mesothelioma
Berylliosis → granulomas mimicking sarcoidosis

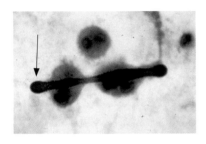

FIGURE 10-37. Ferruginous body. Prussian blue stain of a ferruginous body in a patient with asbestosis. The asbestos fibers are taken up by alveolar macrophages and coated with iron (which stains with Prussian blue) to form ferruginous bodies that cause diffuse interstitial fibrosis. Ferruginous bodies appear as yellow-brown rods with clubbed ends (*arrow*). Dense, hyalinized, fibrocalcific plaques on the parietal pleura are also seen in asbestosis (not shown). (Courtesy of the Uniformed Services University of the Health Sciences.)

SARCOIDOSIS

Inflammatory disease characterized by **noncaseating granulomas**, often involving multiple organ systems. The initial exposure that leads to granuloma formation is unknown.

PRESENTATION

More common in women and African Americans. Presents in young adulthood. Most often discovered incidentally on chest film. Can present with dyspnea or nonproductive cough. Less often, presents with extrapulmonary symptoms.

DIAGNOSIS

- **Chest film:** Bilateral hilar lymphadenopathy, diffuse reticular densities. Divided into four stages based on chest radiograph and CT findings:
  - **Stage 1:** Hilar lymphadenopathy.
  - **Stage 2:** Hilar lymphadenopathy and interstitial changes.
  - **Stage 3:** No lymphadenopathy, only interstitial changes.
  - **Stage 4:** Pulmonary fibrosis.
- Reduced sensitivity/anergy to skin test antigens.
- **Laboratory findings:** Hypercalcemia (due to increased 1-α-hydroxylase production by activated macrophages leading to increased 1,25-$(OH)_2$-vitamin D), hypercalciuria, hypergammaglobulinemia, increased ACE activity. Hypercalcemia/hypercalciuria may present as nephrolithiasis.
- **Biopsy** showing noncaseating granulomas in the lung with a negative microbiology work-up is highly suggestive. Granulomas are often seen in other organs as well. The granuloma consists of a core of macrophages surrounded by T lymphocytes, as illustrated in Figure 10-38.
- **Differential diagnosis:** TB, fungal infections (see Table 10-15), other infectious diseases, hematologic malignancy, rheumatologic disease.

TREATMENT

Many patients do not need treatment. Criteria for receiving treatment include impaired pulmonary function or worsening radiologic findings, systemic

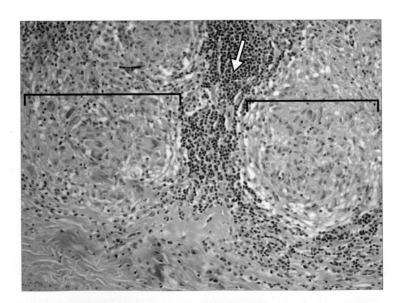

FIGURE 10-38. Photomicrograph from a patient with sarcoidosis. Granulomas consist of macrophages and multinucleated giant cells (*brackets*) surrounded by lymphocytes (*arrow*). (Reproduced with permission from USMLERx.com.)

symptoms that interfere with activities of daily living, ocular disease, heart disease, and hypercalcemia. Treatment consists of systemic corticosteroids or other immunosuppressive drugs.

PROGNOSIS

Natural history varies widely. In some patients, clinical and radiographic manifestations resolve spontaneously. In others, symptoms persist without progression. In a small minority, the disease progresses to widespread pulmonary fibrosis.

IDIOPATHIC PULMONARY FIBROSIS

Accounts for approximately 15% of cases of chronic interstitial lung disease. The pathogenesis of idiopathic pulmonary fibrosis (IPF) is believed to involve repeated cycles of cytokine release and inflammation initiated by an unknown factor.

PRESENTATION

Insidious onset, often between 40 and 70 years of age. Most commonly presents with progressive dyspnea. Two subtypes exist: **usual interstitial pneumonia (UIP)**, comprising most cases of idiopathic pulmonary fibrosis (IPF), and **nonspecific interstitial pneumonia (NSIP)**.

DIAGNOSIS

- **Physical exam:** Dry crackles or rales on auscultation, clubbing of fingernails.
- **Chest film and CT:** Diffuse, interstitial pattern bilaterally. Seen more at the bases and peripheral portions of the lung. **UIP** classically appears with *honeycombing*—a cavernous network of fibrosis within the lungs (Figure 10-39). In contrast, **NSIP** appears as *ground-glass opacities*.
- **Biopsy/pathology:** Provides definitive diagnosis; shows chronic inflammation and fibrosis of the alveolar walls as well as interstitial fibrosis; dilation

MNEMONIC

Causes of hypercalcemia—

CHIMPANZEES

Calcium excess intake (milk-alkali syndrome)
Hyperparathyroidism and hyperthyroidism
Iatrogenic (thiazides, etc.)
Multiple myeloma
Paget disease of bone
Addison disease
Neoplasms (parathyroid hormone-related protein—PTHrP, etc.)
Excess vitamin D
Excess vitamin A
Sarcoidosis
The **Z** can remind you that both hyperparathyroidism and Zollinger-Ellison syndrome can be seen in multiple endocrine neoplasia (MEN 1).

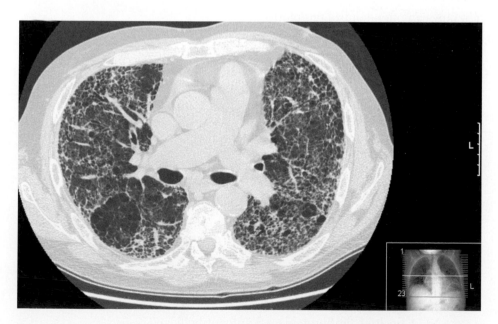

FIGURE 10-39.   CT of a patient with idiopathic pulmonary fibrosis. Image demonstrates bibasilar reticular abnormalities with traction bronchiectasis and honeycombing characteristic of usual interstitial pneumonia. (Courtesy of Wikipedia.)

of bronchioles proximal to fibrotic alveoli produces "honeycomb lung" appearance in UIP.

TREATMENT

Systemic corticosteroids and other immunosuppressive drugs are used but are not very effective. Lung transplantation may be an option for younger patients.

PROGNOSIS

Rapid disease progression with a mean survival of 2–5 years.

GOODPASTURE SYNDROME

Autoimmune disease targeting the lungs and kidney. Caused by type II hypersensitivity against the $\alpha 3$-chain of type IV collagen, located in the basement membranes of alveoli and glomeruli.

PRESENTATION

Pulmonary hemorrhage with concomitant nephritic syndrome (hematuria, etc.; see Chapter 8).

DIAGNOSIS

- **Anti–type IV collagen autoantibodies.**
- **Kidney biopsy:** Immunofluorescence demonstrates linear, ribbon-like deposition of IgG along the glomerular basement membrane. Lung biopsy may be necessary if renal biopsy is not possible.

TREATMENT

Plasmapheresis with or without immunosuppressive therapy to reduce the burden of autoantibodies.

PROGNOSIS

Therapy can often control symptoms.

WEGENER GRANULOMATOSIS

Wegener granulomatosis (also called antineutrophil cytoplasmic antibody [ANCA]–associated granulomatous vasculitis) is an autoimmune vasculitis affecting primarily the upper respiratory tract, lungs, and kidneys, but also affecting the joints, skin, eyes, or nervous system in certain cases. Characterized by vasculitis of small and medium blood vessels in affected organs, with granulomas surrounding these vessels.

PRESENTATION

Extremely varied. Cough, dyspnea, hemoptysis. Persistent rhinorrhea, bloody/purulent nasal discharge, nasal pain. Nonrespiratory symptoms include nephritic syndrome, eye and ear symptoms, arthritis, and cutaneous vasculitis.

DIAGNOSIS

- **CT:** One or several nodules ("coin lesions") and infiltrates, often with cavitation (Figure 10-40).
- **c-ANCA-positive** (antiproteinase 3 autoantibodies).
- **Biopsy:** Necrotizing granulomatous vasculitis.

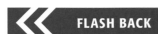

FLASH BACK

Both **Goodpasture syndrome** and **Wegener granulomatosis** are causes of **rapidly progressive glomerulonephritis,** which presents as a nephritic syndrome. Histology will reveal crescent-shaped proliferation of glomerular parietal cells and accumulation of fibrin in glomeruli.

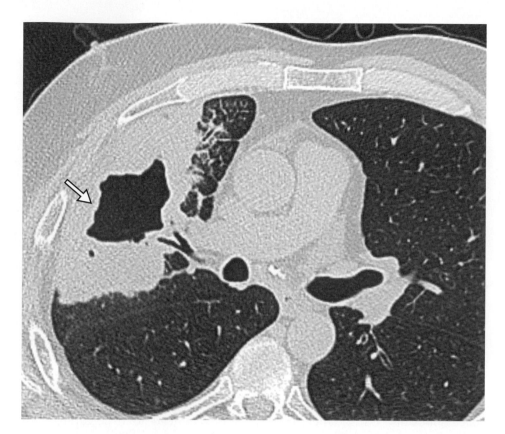

FIGURE 10-40.   CT of a patient with Wegener granulomatosis. This CT scan shows a large cavitary lesion in the right upper lobe (*arrow*) (surgically proven Wegener). (Reproduced with permission from USMLERx.com.)

TREATMENT

Prednisone used during initial therapy. Cytotoxic agents like cyclophosphamide are also used.

PROGNOSIS

Complete and long-term remission can often be achieved with proper treatment.

CHRONIC EOSINOPHILIC PNEUMONIA

PRESENTATION

Presents over weeks to months, with fever, weight loss, dyspnea, and nonproductive cough.

DIAGNOSIS

- **Chest film:** Peripheral pulmonary infiltrates and a pattern suggestive of alveolar filling.
- **Eosinophilia.**
- **Pathology:** Pulmonary interstitium and alveolar spaces infiltrated by eosinophils and macrophages.

TREATMENT

Administration of corticosteroids.

Prognosis

Clinical improvement can be seen within days to weeks after therapy (eg, prednisone) is initiated.

PULMONARY VASCULAR DISEASES

The pulmonary vasculature receives the entire cardiac output and is susceptible to a number of disease processes. The two major entities discussed here are pulmonary embolism (PE) and pulmonary hypertension.

Pulmonary Embolism

PE is often missed clinically and is seen in > 60% of autopsies. It occurs when a blood clot from a systemic vein lodges in one or more branches of the pulmonary artery. Most often, a PE arises from a deep vein thrombosis (DVT), but it can also result from embolization of tumor cells, fat, amniotic fluid, infectious vegetations, or foreign material. The **Virchow triad** (hypercoagulability, endothelial damage, and stasis of blood flow) predisposes to thrombus formation. Common predisposing factors include immobilization, cancer, multiple fractures, and use of oral contraceptive pills. Genetic causes of hypercoagulability (eg, **factor V Leiden**) can amplify the risk of thromboembolic events.

Decreased perfusion with continued ventilation causes an increase in dead space following a PE. One may expect this to lead to hypercapnia, but patients often hyperventilate and may be surprisingly hypocapnic. The release of inflammatory mediators can lead to bronchoconstriction, V/Q mismatch, and hypoxemia. Reduced forward output of the right ventricle can lead to hypotension, syncope, and/or shock.

Presentation

Tachycardia, tachypnea, dyspnea, hemoptysis, pleuritic chest pain. Syncope and hypoxemia may also be seen. Smaller PEs are often asymptomatic.

Diagnosis

- **Physical exam:**
  - Tachycardia and tachypnea.
  - Localized crackles or wheezes; however, the lung exam is often normal.
  - A pleural rub may be present. The pleural rub is produced by a fibrinous exudate that is released from the pleural surface overlying the region of ischemic lung tissue.
  - In the case of a massive PE, the sudden increase in vascular resistance can lead to right ventricular overload (acute cor pulmonale), in which case a right-sided S_4 and loud P_2 may be heard (see Heart Sounds, discussed in Chapter 1). Jugular venous distention (JVD) may also be observed.
  - Lower extremity tenderness, swelling, and a palpable clot within a vessel suggestive of a DVT may be seen.
- **Laboratory results and imaging:**
  - **CT angiography** can show the filling defect due to the thrombus (Figure 10-41). This is the preferred method of definitive diagnosis.
  - **V/Q scan** shows an area of ventilation without perfusion. Infrequently performed but can be done in the absence of CT.
  - **Chest film:** Usually nonspecific, including atelectasis and elevation of the hemidiaphragm. Dilation of the pulmonary artery, Hampton hump

---

FLASH BACK

The differential diagnosis for hypercoagulable states includes primary thrombotic disorders and acquired risk factors. Primary genetic disorders include factor V Leiden, prothrombin G20210A, antithrombin deficiency, protein C or S deficiency, and dysfibrogenemias. Secondary risk factors include antiphospholipid syndrome (APLS), immobility, pregnancy, oral contraceptive use, and obesity.

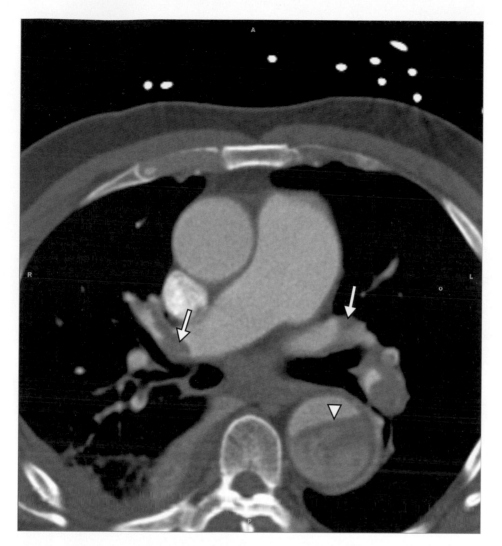

FIGURE 10-41. **CT of a patient with a pulmonary embolism.** Bilateral pulmonary emboli (*arrows*) appear as contrasting regions within the pulmonary vasculature. This axial CT also shows a type B aortic dissection (*arrowhead*), with the true lumen narrower than the false lumen. (Reproduced with permission from USMLERx.com.)

(wedge-shaped consolidation in the lung periphery adjacent to the pleura), Westermark sign (abrupt cutoff of pulmonary vascularity distal to a PE), or a pleural effusion may also be seen.

- **Blood laboratories:** A D-dimer level can provide evidence of thrombus formation. D-Dimer is a fibrin degradation product.
- **Arterial blood gas testing:** Decreased PaO_2, decreased $PaCO_2$, increased pH, and increased A-a gradient.

TREATMENT

Supplemental oxygen if hypoxemic. Anticoagulation therapy, usually with IV heparin or low-molecular-weight heparin followed by oral warfarin for 3–6 months. Thrombolytic therapy may be useful in a subset of patients with massive PE and hypotension. Placement of a filtering device in the IVC can be used in patients who cannot tolerate anticoagulation due to an elevated bleeding risk.

PROGNOSIS

Variable, ranging from sudden death to asymptomatic resolution.

Pulmonary Hypertension

Pulmonary hypertension is the elevation of intravascular pressure within the pulmonary circulation and includes pulmonary artery hypertension as well as pulmonary venous hypertension. Pulmonary artery hypertension is defined as an arterial pressure > 25 mm Hg at rest or > 35 mm Hg with exertion. Idiopathic (primary) pulmonary arterial hypertension has no known cause and carries a poor prognosis. It occurs in the absence of underlying heart or lung disease and is more common in women than in men. Primary pulmonary hypertension is associated with mutations in genes linked to transforming growth factor beta (TGF-β) signaling and is characterized by vascular hyperreactivity with proliferation of smooth muscle. Congenital idiopathic pulmonary hypertension is associated with abnormally thickened vasculature.

Secondary pulmonary hypertension is more common and is related to lung or heart disease, including:

- Chronic thromboembolic disease.
- Loss of vessels by scarring or destruction of alveolar walls.
- Chronic hypoxemia.
- Increased flow (left-to-right shunt).
- Elevated left atrial pressure, as in CHF or mitral stenosis.
- Chronic respiratory acidosis (eg, chronic bronchitis, obstructive sleep apnea).
- Meconium aspiration at birth, the most common cause of persistent pulmonary hypertension of the newborn.

PRESENTATION

Dyspnea and exertional fatigue. Substernal chest pain, similar to angina pectoris, is sometimes seen. Occasionally, chest pain is more right-sided. If cardiac output falls enough, syncope can result.

DIAGNOSIS

- **Physical exam:**
    - Lung examination often normal unless pulmonary hypertension is due to concomitant lung disease.
    - Loud P_2, right-sided S_3 and S_4.
    - JVD.
    - Right ventricular heave.
- **CT:** Increased prominence and size of hilar pulmonary arteries, which rapidly taper off. Enlarged cardiac silhouette (particularly RV and RA enlargement). Redistribution of blood flow to the upper lungs (Figure 10-42).
- **PFT:** Spirometry and lung volumes usually normal, with a decreased D$_{LCO}$.
- **Arterial blood gas testing:** Useful in determining whether hypoxemia or acidosis plays a role in the disease's cause.
- **Pathology:** Intimal hyperplasia and medial hypertrophy of small arteries and arterioles, leading to obliteration of the lumen. Plexogenic (web-like) lesions are typically seen in idiopathic disease. Thickening of the walls of larger arteries is also seen. Right ventricular hypertrophy is also a feature.

TREATMENT

Supplemental O_2 therapy, various vasodilators (eg, sildenafil, endothelin receptor antagonists, or prostacyclins), inhaled nitric oxide, and anticoagulation therapy.

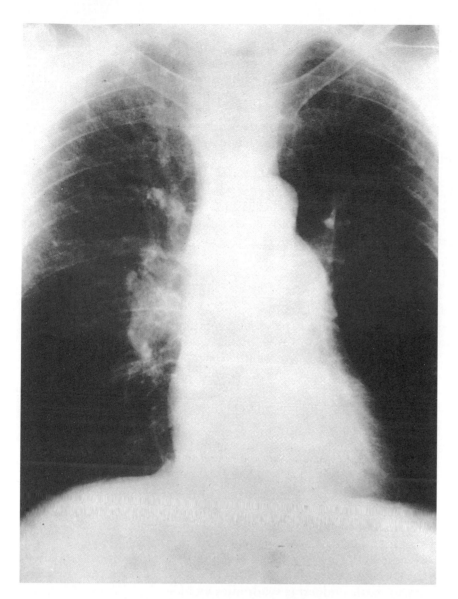

FIGURE 10-42. **Chest x-ray of a patient with pulmonary hypertension.** The pulmonary arteries are dilated with a lack of visible peripheral vasculature. (Reproduced with permission from Crawford MH. *Current Diagnosis & Treatment in Cardiology*, 2nd ed. New York: McGraw-Hill, 2003: 387.)

PROGNOSIS

- Right-sided heart failure can occur due to elevated right-sided pressures.
- Idiopathic (primary) pulmonary hypertension: Poor prognosis, often resulting in death within a few years of diagnosis if untreated.
- Secondary pulmonary hypertension: Treat the underlying disease.

RESPIRATORY TRACT CANCERS

Lung Cancer

Primary lung cancer is the leading cause of cancer-related death in both men and women, as well as the second most common cancer by incidence in both sexes. There are five major types of primary lung cancer: squamous cell carci-

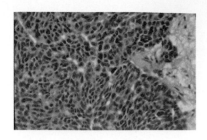

FIGURE 10-43. Photomicrograph of a patient with small-cell carcinoma. The cells are small, with little cytoplasm or other defining characteristics. (Courtesy of the Uniformed Services University of the Health Sciences.)

noma, adenocarcinoma (including the bronchioloalveolar subtype), small-cell carcinoma (Figure 10-43), large-cell carcinoma, and carcinoid tumors. Cigarette smoking is clearly related to certain subtypes of lung cancer, including squamous cell carcinoma, which is the most prevalent type of primary lung tumor, and small-cell carcinoma. Quitting reduces subsequent risk of developing lung cancer, but this risk likely never drops to that of a nonsmoker. Occupational exposures, including to asbestos (bronchogenic carcinoma > malignant mesothelioma), arsenic, haloethers, and polycyclic aromatic hydrocarbons, can predispose to lung cancer.

Areas of parenchymal scarring can serve as foci for the development of adenocarcinoma and, more specifically, bronchioloalveolar carcinoma. Most of the respiratory symptoms seen with lung cancer are due either to local tissue destruction by a growing tumor or airway obstruction.

PRESENTATION

The location of the tumor is a key determinant of presenting symptoms. For instance, an endobronchial tumor can manifest with cough and hemoptysis. Postobstructive pneumonia and dyspnea develop due to tumor obstructing an airway. If the pleura are involved, pleural effusion and chest pain can result. Secreted products may also contribute to symptoms (see following list of paraneoplastic endocrine syndromes). As with all malignancies, anorexia and weight loss are also seen. In certain cases, a recognizable syndrome may arise due to the specific circumstances of the tumor:

- **Superior vena cava syndrome:** Compression of the superior vena cava by tumor leads to facial swelling, cyanosis, and dilation of the veins of the head, neck, and upper extremities.
- **Pancoast tumor:** Eponym for lung cancer of any subtype that arises at the apex of the lung. Can manifest with **Horner syndrome** (ptosis, anhidrosis, miosis, enophthalmos, and loss of ciliospinal reflex) due to involvement of the cervical sympathetic plexus.
- Hoarseness due to paralysis of the **recurrent laryngeal nerve.**
- Distant metastases to the brain, bone, liver, or adrenals can manifest with organ-specific symptoms.
- **Paraneoplastic endocrine syndromes** include:
  - **Cushing syndrome** due to adrenocorticotropic hormone (ACTH) secreted by small-cell carcinoma.
  - **Syndrome of inappropriate secretion of diuretic hormone (SIADH)** with small-cell carcinoma.
  - **Hypercalcemia** due to parathyroid hormone-related protein (PTHrP) secreted by squamous cell carcinoma.

DIAGNOSIS

- **Chest film:** Nodule or mass within the lung.
  - **Centrally located:** Squamous and small cell.
  - **Peripherally located:** Adenocarcinoma and large cell. Involvement of the hilar lymph nodes or pleura can also be seen.
  - An exception to this is the bronchioloalveolar subtype of adenocarcinoma, which often has a more diffuse radiographic appearance, termed **ground-glass opacity,** similar to pneumonia.
- **CT or positron emission tomography (PET) scans:** To determine location, lymph node involvement, or metastasis for staging.
- **Cytologic examination** of sputum or washings from bronchoscopy, or tissue pathology from a **lung biopsy.**

- **PFT:** To assess whether a patient has the residual capacity to survive surgical resection of a tumor.
- **Pathology:** The major types of primary lung cancer and their key characteristics are listed in Table 10-13. Multiple tumors arising at once should raise suspicion for metastatic disease from a primary outside the lungs, as the lung's extensive vasculature makes it a nidus for hematogenous seeding.

TREATMENT

- **Small-cell carcinoma:** Metastases occur very early in the disease course, so surgery is not an option, only chemotherapy and/or radiation.
- **Non–small-cell carcinoma (NSCLC):** Surgical resection if there is no distant spread. If metastases are present, then chemotherapy and/or radiation.
- Conventional chemotherapeutics for lung cancer include the platinum cross-linkers (cisplatin), intercalating agents (doxorubicin), taxanes (pacli-

TABLE 10-13. Types of Lung Cancer

NAME	INCIDENCE AMONG PRIMARY LUNG CANCERS	ORIGIN	LOCATION	CHARACTERISTICS
Non–small-cell lung cancer (NSCLC)				
Squamous cell carcinoma	30%	Squamous epithelium of airways	Proximal large airways	Associated with smoking. Keratin pearls on histology. May cavitate. Associated with paraneoplastic syndrome—PTHrP (hypercalcemia).
Adenocarcinoma	50%	Mucus glands	Lung periphery, sites of scarring	**Bronchial** subtype is most common primary lung cancer seen in nonsmokers. **Bronchioloalveolar** subtype not clearly related to smoking; spreads along alveolar walls.
Large-cell carcinoma	< 5%	Epithelial cells, very poorly differentiated	Lung periphery	
Carcinoid	< 5%	Neuroendocrine cells in lungs or GI tract		Secretes serotonin; can cause carcinoid syndrome (flushing, diarrhea, wheezing, salivation).
Small-cell lung cancer (SCLC)				
Small cell ("oat cell," Figure 10-43)	20%	Kulchitsky neuroendocrine cells of primary and secondary bronchi	Central (bronchi)	Commonly associated with paraneoplastic syndromes such as ectopic ACTH and SIADH.
Other				
Mesothelioma		Pleural cells	Pleura	Associated with asbestos exposure; risk is greatly increased by cigarette smoking.

ACTH = adrenocorticotropic hormone; PTH = parathyroid hormone; SIADH = syndrome of inappropriate secretion of antidiuretic hormone.

taxel), vinca alkaloids (vincristine), and nucleoside analogs (gemcitabine). Targeted therapy is a more recent approach; agents (eg, gefitinib) which inhibit the epidermal growth factor receptor (EGFR) have been effective in patients with NSCLC harboring epidermal growth factor receptor (EGFR) mutations.

PROGNOSIS

Overall 5-year survival is about 14%. Squamous cell carcinoma has the best prognosis, and small-cell carcinoma has the worst. Early-stage disease, while rarely found, has a much better prognosis than late-stage disease.

Malignancies of the Upper Respiratory Tract

BENIGN LARYNGEAL TUMORS

The most common clinical presentation is hoarseness.

- **Vocal cord nodules:** Smooth hemispheric protrusions located on the true vocal cords. These occur chiefly in heavy smokers and singers.
- **Laryngeal papilloma:** A benign neoplasm on the true vocal cords that forms a soft, raspberry-like excrescence. Rarely more than 1 cm in diameter.
- **Juvenile laryngeal papillomas:** Usually singular in adults but multiple in children. Associated with human papillomavirus types 6 and 11.

LARYNGEAL CARCINOMA

Accounts for 2% of all cancers. Presents in patients aged > 40 years, more often in men than in women. Associated with smoking, alcohol consumption, and asbestos exposure. Manifests as persistent hoarseness.

- **Glottic tumors:** On the true vocal cords, usually keratinizing.
- **Supraglottic tumors:** Above the vocal cords; one-third metastasize.
- **Subglottic tumors:** Below the vocal cords.

NASOPHARYNGEAL CARCINOMA

Strong link to Epstein-Barr virus (EBV) infection. EBV infects the host by replicating in the nasopharyngeal epithelium and then infecting nearby tonsillar B lymphocytes. High frequency in the Chinese population.

PULMONARY INFECTIONS

Pneumonia

Infection of the lung parenchyma is a major cause of morbidity and mortality, accounting for nearly 10% of all hospital admissions and approximately 55,000 deaths in the United States each year, according to the Centers for Disease Control and Prevention. Pneumonia is often classified as either being community-acquired or nosocomial (ie, occurring in patients who have been in the hospital and therefore exposed to a different set of causative agents as well as medical conditions or interventions that may predispose to particular routes of infection). An additional subtype of pneumonia is aspiration pneumonia, in which oral flora (including anaerobes) are aspirated into the lung, often due to loss of consciousness, neuromuscular disease, and/or seizure. Infectious causes include bacterial, viral, and fungal pathogens, the most common being *Streptococcus pneumoniae* (Table 10-14). Some clinicians

KEY FACT

Sites for metastasis of primary lung cancers (ranked by frequency):
1. Hilar lymph nodes
2. Adrenal glands
3. Liver
4. Brain
5. Bone (osteolytic)

FLASH BACK

EBV produces several proteins that modulate growth signaling in B lymphocytes. This property explains why EBV infection can lead to Burkitt lymphoma, Hodgkin lymphoma, or nasopharyngeal carcinoma, in addition to many other lymphoproliferative disorders.

TABLE 10-14.   **Common Causes of Pneumonia**

Organism	Characteristics	Complications	Treatment
Gram-Positive Bacteria			
Streptococcus pneumoniae	Gram-positive diplococci; most frequent community-acquired cause; most common in elderly or debilitated persons; **rust-colored sputum; lobar pneumonia.**	Empyema.	Penicillins, cephalosporins, macrolides, some quinolones.
Staphylococcus aureus	Gram-positive cocci in clusters; often a complication of influenza, viral pneumonias, or blood-borne infection in IV drug users; seen in hospitalized patients, the elderly, and those with chronic lung disease; **bronchopneumonia.**	Abscess formation or empyema not uncommon; bacterial endocarditis and brain and kidney abscesses possible from hematogenous spread.	Oxacillin, nafcillin, vancomycin (for MRSA), linezolid.
Gram-Negative Bacteria			
Haemophilus influenzae	Gram-negative coccobacillus requiring hematin and NAD$^+$ for culture; usually seen in infants and children, but may occur in adults with COPD; **bronchopneumonia.**	Meningitis and epiglottitis in infants and children.	Second- or third-generation cephalosporins, TMP-SMX.
Klebsiella pneumoniae	Gram-negative rod; most frequent in diabetic or alcoholic patients; high mortality rate in the elderly; **red currant-jelly sputum; bronchopneumonia.**	Large amount of damage to the alveolar walls leading to necrosis and abscess formation.	Aminoglycosides, third-generation cephalosporins.
Pseudomonas aeruginosa	Gram-negative rod; appears blue-green when cultured; common cause of nosocomial pneumonia and pneumonia in immunocompromised and CF patients.	Focal hemorrhage and necrosis.	Combination therapy using ticarcillin, piperacillin, ciprofloxacin, cefepime, or gentamicin.
Legionella pneumophila	Gram-negative coccobacillus requiring charcoal yeast agar plus iron and cysteine for culture; stains poorly; infection spreads by inhalation of aerosol from contaminated water; affects both healthy and debilitated adults; **often lobar, but no characteristic pattern.**	Relatively high mortality rate if untreated.	Macrolides, quinolones.
Moraxella catarrhalis	Gram-negative diplococcus; seen in the elderly and patients with COPD. **Bronchopneumonia.**		Second- or third-generation cephalosporins, macrolides, quinolones.

(continues)

TABLE 10-14.   Common Causes of Pneumonia *(continued)*

ORGANISM	CHARACTERISTICS	COMPLICATIONS	TREATMENT
Other Bacteria (anaerobes and intracellulars)			
Anaerobes	**Aspiration pneumonia:** due to aspiration of secretions from the oropharynx into the tracheobronchial tree; patients with impaired consciousness or difficulty swallowing are at highest risk; often located in dependent segments of lung. Can be gram-negative or gram-positive; agents are often normal part of oral flora.	Abscess or empyema formation is common.	Penicillin, clindamycin.
Mycoplasma pneumoniae	Frequent cause of **interstitial pneumonia** in young adults; insidious onset with mild, limited course; associated with **nonspecific cold agglutinins.**		Macrolides, quinolones, tetracyclines such as doxycycline. Inherently β-lactam resistant because it has no cell wall.
Chlamydophila pneumoniae and *C psittaci*	Obligate intracellular bacteria that target columnar epithelium and cause **interstitial pneumonia.** *C psittaci* is found in parrot feces and causes **psittacosis.**		Macrolides (erythromycin), Tetracyclines (doxycycline).
Coxiella burnetii	Rickettsial organism—obligate intracellular; infects people working with cattle or sheep, or those who drink unpasteurized milk from infected animals; **interstitial pneumonia.**	Can cause hepatitis or myocarditis.	Doxycycline.
Viruses and Fungi			
Viral pneumonia	Most common pneumonia of childhood. Caused by influenza viruses, adenoviruses, rhinovirus, and RSV; measles virus produces giant-cell pneumonia.		■ Influenza A: Amantadine and rimantadine. ■ Influenza A and B: Zanamivir and oseltamivir. ■ RSV (prophylaxis): Palivizumab and ribavirin.
Pneumocystis jiroveci (formerly *Pneumocystis carinii*)	**PCP:** Unicellular fungus; identified as alveolar cysts on silver stain; most common opportunistic infection in AIDS patients—**AIDS-defining illness; ground-glass opacities** on CT.		TMP-SMX. Always give prophylactically if CD4+ count is < 200/mm^3.

COPD = chronic obstructive pulmonary disease; MRSA = methicillin-resistant *Staphylococcus aureus*; NAD$^+$ = nicotinamide adenine dinucleotide; PCP = pneumocystis pneumonia; RSV = respiratory syncytial virus; TMP-SMX = trimethoprim-sulfamethoxazole.

subdivide these organisms into those that cause typical versus atypical pneumonias, although this is not a rigid distinction. Generally speaking, typical pneumonias (caused by *S pneumoniae, Staphylococcus aureus, Haemophilus, Klebsiella,* and others) tend to manifest with more lobar consolidation, alveolar exudate, and sputum production than do atypical pneumonias (caused by *Mycoplasma, Chlamydophila, Coxiella, Legionella,* viruses, and others). The term *typical pneumonia* encompasses both lobar pneumonia and bronchopneumonia, whereas *atypical pneumonia* is roughly synonymous with interstitial pneumonia.

The most important causes of pneumonia vary with the patient's age, with neonates being particularly susceptible to *Streptococcus agalactiae* (group B) and *Escherichia coli,* children susceptible to viral pneumonia, and the elderly succumbing to gram-negative bacilli. *S pneumoniae, Mycoplasma,* and *Chlamydophila* are common causes of pneumonia and may be seen at any age from childhood onward.

Risk factors for developing pneumonia include viral upper respiratory infection, alcohol abuse, cigarette smoking, and COPD. Infection can spread to the lungs by inhalation, aspiration, and hematogenous spread from other sites. Inflammation and infection of the distal air spaces leads to a reduction in ventilation to those areas. If perfusion is maintained, then $\dot{V}/\dot{Q}$ mismatch results, with or without shunting.

PRESENTATION

Fever (with or without chills), cough (with or without sputum production), and dyspnea. A nonproductive cough suggests viral or mycoplasmal pneumonia. Blood-tinged or rusty sputum suggests bacterial pneumonia. Pleuritic chest pain due to inflammation adjacent to the pleura.

DIAGNOSIS

- **Physical exam:**
    - Tachycardia, tachypnea, and fever.
    - Crackles over the affected area on auscultation.
    - Bronchial breath sounds, increased tactile fremitus, and egophony.
    - Dullness to percussion if there is frank consolidation or associated effusion.
- **Laboratory tests:** Leukocytosis with left shift (increased polymorphonuclear neutrophil [PMN] fraction of WBCs) and increased bands (immature granulocytes) in bacterial pneumonia.
- **CT:** Allows classification as a lobar, patchy, or interstitial pattern of distribution. Pleural effusions may accompany a bacterial pneumonia.
    - **Lobar pneumonia (typical):** Infection tends to spread through the entire lobe, with intra-alveolar exudates. *Streptococcus pneumoniae* is the classic pathogen (Figure 10-44).
    - **Bronchopneumonia (typical):** Patchy distribution involving more than one lobe, with distal airway inflammation and alveolar disease. Caused by a wide variety of organisms.
    - **Interstitial pneumonia (atypical):** Diffuse, patchy inflammation of the interstitial walls, which is sometimes very subtle on radiograph (Figure 10-45).
- **Sputum Gram stain and culture:** *Mycoplasma, Chlamydia,* and *Legionella* require additional serology and antigen testing.
- **Nasal swab.**
- **Arterial blood gas testing:** Reduced PaO_2 with normal or reduced $PaCO_2$ due to hyperventilation.

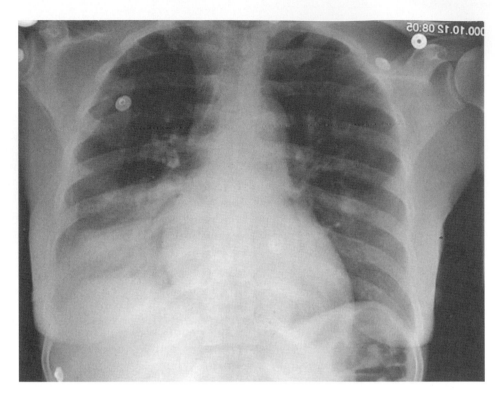

FIGURE 10-44. **Lobar pneumonia.** Radiographic appearance of a right lower lobe pneumonia. (Reproduced with permission from Stone CK, Humphries RL. *Current Diagnosis & Treatment: Emergency Medicine*, 6th ed. New York: McGraw-Hill, 2008: Figure 11-6.)

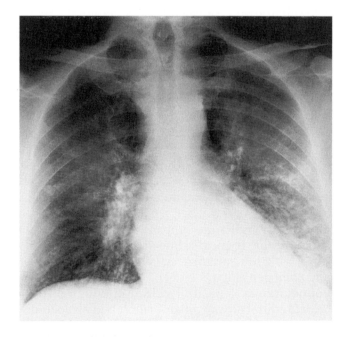

FIGURE 10-45. **Interstitial pneumonia.** Chest film of a patient with mycoplasmal pneumonia. Diffuse interstitial and alveolar infiltrates can be seen. (Reproduced with permission from Hall JB, Schmidt GA, Wood LDH. *Principles of Critical Care*, 3rd ed. New York: McGraw-Hill, 2005: 826.)

TREATMENT

Antibiotic therapy is the mainstay for bacterial and fungal pneumonia (Table 10-15). Supportive care for most viral pneumonias. Antivirals available for influenza infection.

TABLE 10-15. **Fungal Infections of the Lungs**

ORGANISM	PRESENTATION	CHARACTERISTICS	TREATMENT
Candida albicans (yeast)—candidiasis	Fever, tachypnea, patchy infiltrates on chest film.	Uncommon cause of pneumonia; hematogenous spread seen in immunocompromised patients.	Amphotericin B and fluconazole.
Cryptococcus neoformans (yeast)—cryptococcosis	Often asymptomatic, but can have productive cough, fever, weight loss.	Associated with pigeon droppings; can also produce **cryptococcal meningitis;** organism's encapsulated appearance can be seen with India ink stain but definitively diagnosed with latex agglutination test.	Cryptococcal meningitis: Amphotericin B plus flucytosine. Non-CNS cryptococcosis: Fluconazole.
Aspergillus (mold)—aspergillosis	Wheezing, dyspnea, and cough with **allergic bronchopulmonary aspergillosis;** fever, cough, dyspnea, pleuritic chest pain, and hemoptysis seen in invasive forms, usually in immunocompromised patients	Fungal balls (aspergillomas) can form in preexisting cavities; the invasive form of aspergillosis has a tendency to grow into vessels with widespread hematogenous dissemination; seen as narrow-angle (< 45 degrees) branching hyphae in tissue.	Amphotericin B or itraconazole.
Blastomyces dermatitidis (dimorphic)—blastomycosis	Fever, chills, productive cough. May also present with skin lesions, bone lesions, or genitourinary involvement.	Found in the midwestern and southeastern United States; broad-based budding yeast. Inhaled from soil. Causes pneumonia-like lung disease and may progress to disseminated disease.	Amphotericin B or itraconazole.
Histoplasma capsulatum (dimorphic)—histoplasmosis	Often asymptomatic; the young or immunocompromised may have disseminated or chronic disease with fever, fatigue, and weight loss.	Found in the river valleys of the central United States, and in soil contaminated by bird or bat droppings; elicits caseating granuloma formation in tissue; the disseminated form is marked by multisystem involvement with infiltrates of macrophages filled with intracellular fungi; round or oval yeast forms in tissue.	Amphotericin B +/− itraconazole.
Coccidioides immitis (dimorphic)—coccidioidomycosis	Fever, cough, headache, chest pain; disseminated or chronic disease produces systemic symptoms.	Found in the southwestern United States, Mexico, and South America; may have acute, disseminated, or chronic course. Fungal spherules containing endospores are found within granulomas.	Amphotericin B; surgery may also have a role.

In most cases, appropriate treatment results in complete recovery without long-term sequelae, but morbidity and mortality increase with age. Complications include:

- **Lung abscess:** Pus collection often caused by bacterial pneumonia, bronchial obstruction, or aspiration. Often due to *Staphylococcus, Pseudomonas, Klebsiella, Proteus,* or anaerobic organisms. Requires antibiotics and drainage.
- **Empyema:** Pus in the pleural space. Often caused by anaerobes and staphylococci. Requires drainage.

Tuberculosis

Approximately one-third of the world's population has been infected with TB, which results in 2–3 million deaths each year. The burden of disease is greatest in developing countries.

TB is primarily caused by *Mycobacterium tuberculosis*, an aerobic, rod-shaped, acid-fast bacterium (colloquially termed "red snappers" due to their appearance on Ziehl-Neelsen acid-fast stain), which is transmitted by airborne droplets from infected patients. The disease is so named because of the immune system's attempt to quarantine mycobacteria within dense granulomas ("tubercles") consisting of a core of macrophages surrounded by supporting T lymphocytes. There are three forms of TB: primary, secondary, and miliary.

- **Primary TB:** At initial infection, a **Ghon complex** develops, consisting of a peripheral parenchymal lesion called a **Ghon focus** and granulomas in involved hilar lymph nodes. The Ghon focus develops into a granuloma and eventually undergoes caseating necrosis at its core. Over time, the Ghon complex may calcify and heal into a Ranke complex.
- **Secondary (reactivation) TB:** Results from reactivation of a prior site of infection, where the bacteria became dormant but were never cleared. Lesions are localized to the lung apices (region of greatest aeration) with hilar lymph node involvement. Granulomatous lesions form and rupture, resulting in cavitary lesions. Scarring and calcification may be seen.
- **Miliary TB:** Disseminated disease caused by hematogenous spread of bacteria. It may follow from primary or secondary TB. The granuloma-filled lung takes the appearance of being filled with millet seeds, hence the name. Prognosis is very poor without treatment.

Pulmonary symptoms include chronic productive cough and hemoptysis. Respiratory function is generally well-preserved, perhaps because of localization of the destructive disease to the Ghon complex in primary TB and to the apices in secondary TB. Systemic symptoms include weight loss, fever, and night sweats.

- **Physical exam:**
  - **Primary TB:** Fever, chest pain. Often fairly normal physical exam.
  - **Secondary TB:** Cough (evolving into hemoptysis), weight loss, wasting, night sweats.
  - Crackles over the affected area on auscultation.
- **Tuberculin skin test (PPD or Mantoux test):** Acts through a type IV hypersensitivity reaction. A small amount of purified protein derivative

(PPD) from *M tuberculosis* is injected subcutaneously. Induration or swelling at the site after 48–72 hours indicates prior exposure to TB. This does not differentiate between active and prior infections, and false-positives occur in individuals with prior vaccination with the variably effective BCG (bacillus Calmette-Guérin) vaccine.

- **Chest film:**
    - **Primary TB:** Nonspecific, often lower lobe infiltrate, hilar lymph node enlargement, and pleural effusion.
    - **Secondary TB:** Lesions located in the apices or superior segment of a lower lobe. Infiltrates, cavities, nodules, scarring, and/or contraction may be seen (Figure 10-46).
    - Culture of the organism from sputum is needed for a definitive diagnosis. **Acid-fast staining** is useful for quicker results.

TREATMENT

Six months of treatment with isoniazid (INH), pyridoxine (vitamin B_6), and rifampin, supplemented during the first 2 months with pyrazinamide and ethambutol. A current global challenge is the rise of multidrug-resistant (MDR) and, more recently, extensively drug-resistant (XDR) tuberculosis. MDR-TB is resistant to at least rifampin and isoniazid; XDR-TB is additionally resistant to several second-line therapies. The treatment of drug-resistant TB depends heavily on culture sensitivities.

Latent tuberculosis infection (LTBI) treatment for individuals with a positive PPD but no active disease generally consists of 9 months of INH plus pyridoxine. Note that this is not an appropriate regimen for active TB.

PROGNOSIS

Most patients with primary TB are asymptomatic. Lifetime risk of reactivation is about 10% in immunocompetent patients. This is elevated in patients with AIDS or other immunosuppressive states. Reactivation TB can be com

MNEMONIC

The **4 R's** of Rifampin: **R**amps up cytochrome P450 metabolism; causes **R**ed or orange urine; leads to rapid **R**esistance when used alone; acts by inhibiting **R**NA polymerase.

MNEMONIC

The anti-TB drugs can be remembered with the acronym **RIPES:**
Rifampin
Isoniazid (INH)
Pyrazinamide
Ethambutol
Streptomycin
Even though streptomycin is no longer a first-line drug for TB, it has historical significance as the first drug to be discovered that could cure tuberculosis.

CLINICAL CORRELATION

The major side effects of **isoniazid** are hepatotoxicity, peripheral neuropathy, and CNS effects. The latter two are due to depletion of pyridoxine (vitamin B_6). Therefore, patients are given pyridoxine supplementation during isoniazid therapy.

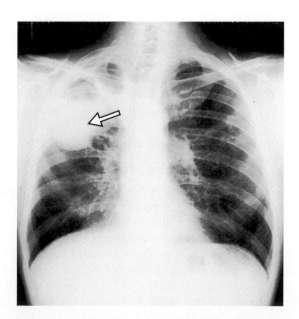

FIGURE 10-46. Tuberculosis. Chest x-ray of a patient with reactivation TB, hilar lymphadenopathy, and a cavitary lesion in the right upper lobe (*arrow*). (Reproduced with permission from Doherty GM, Way LW, *Current Surgical Diagnosis & Treatment*, 12th ed, New York: McGraw-Hill, 2006: 371.)

plicated by miliary TB, in which distal organs are seeded with innumerable small lesions. Extrapulmonary TB includes tuberculous meningitis, Potts disease of the spine, psoas abscesses, paravertebral abscesses, tuberculous cervical lymphadenitis (scrofula), pericarditis, and kidney and GI involvement.

Upper Respiratory Tract Infections

Fever, sore throat, drooling, and difficulty breathing may be presenting symptoms. The age of the patient is also helpful in diagnosis. Physical exam may show a reddened oropharynx.

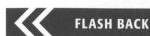

FLASH BACK

Acute rheumatic fever (see Pathology section in Chapter 1) may occur following group A streptococcal pharyngitis only, whereas poststreptococcal glomerulonephritis (see section on Nephritic Syndrome in Chapter 8) may occur following pharyngitis or skin infections (eg, impetigo).

- **Pharyngitis:** Inflammation of the pharynx; manifests as a sore throat. Viral etiology is more likely than bacterial, but individuals with pharyngitis should be tested for *Streptococcus pyogenes* ("strep throat") because timely treatment with penicillin V is important for the prevention of serious sequelae such as rheumatic fever, although treatment does not prevent poststreptococcal (acute proliferative) glomerulonephritis.
- **Epiglottitis:** Syndrome of young children with an infection of the epiglottis (most frequently caused by *H influenzae*) causing pain and airway obstruction, often manifesting with uncontrollable drooling. The incidence of epiglottitis has fallen dramatically with the introduction of the *H influenzae* type b (Hib) vaccine.
- **Croup (laryngotracheobronchitis):** Croup is a common illness in children caused most often by the parainfluenza virus, influenza viruses, or respiratory syncytial virus (RSV). The typical presentation is a febrile child with barking cough, stridor, and hoarseness.

Fungal Infections

A variety of fungal pathogens can cause pulmonary infection (see Table 10-15) including *jiroveci Pneumocystis jiroveci* (see Table 10-14).

OTHER RESPIRATORY DISEASES

Spontaneous Pneumothorax

- **Primary spontaneous pneumothorax:** Associated with specific body habitus or trauma. The classic patient is a tall, thin male adolescent or young adult with sudden onset of shortness of breath and chest pain, often without exertion. The usual cause of primary spontaneous pneumothorax is the rupture of an air-filled lung bleb, but a ruptured airway may also be a cause.
- **Secondary spontaneous pneumothorax:** Occurs due to rupture of blebs secondary to disease processes such as COPD, TB, pneumonia, asthma, or CF.
- A subset of pneumothoraces are termed **tension pneumothoraces** independent of cause. Generally, a pneumothorax falls under the tension subtype if the patient has an ipsilateral intrapleural pressure *greater than* atmospheric pressure during expiration (and possibly at other times during the respiratory cycle). This net positive pressure pushes the mediastinum *away* from the pneumothorax and may reduce venous return to the heart and cardiac output. Note, however, that intake of air into the intrapleural space (ie, development of the pneumothorax) only occurs while the intrapleural pressure is *less than* atmospheric pressure.

DIAGNOSIS

The deflated lung produces the following signs on examination of the ipsilateral chest:

- **Decreased breath sounds** on the affected side.
- Asymmetrical expansion.
- Absent fremitus.
- Hyperresonance on percussion.
- Tracheal deviation ("mediastinal shift") away from the lesion seen in tension pneumothorax.

In addition, the collapsed lung may be identified on a chest radiograph, as shown in Figure 10-47.

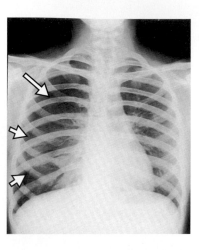

TREATMENT

- Supplemental oxygen to increase the rate of resorption of intrapleural air. In cases of a small asymptomatic pneumothorax, this may be sufficient for spontaneous recovery to occur.
- In larger and/or symptomatic pneumothoraces, air should be evacuated from the intrapleural space via **thoracentesis** (needle aspiration) or chest tube placement **(tube thoracostomy)** with a water seal, which acts as a one-way valve.
- In cases of recurrent pneumothorax, the pleurae may be sealed together through **pleurodesis,** in which chemical or mechanical irritation is employed in order to encourage fibrous scar tissue formation, sealing the visceral and parietal pleurae together. This effectively glues the lung to the chest wall.

FIGURE 10-47. Radiograph of spontaneous pneumothorax on the right side. The outline of the right lung is visible (*arrows*), abnormally separated from the parietal pleura. (Adapted with permission from Doherty GM, Way LW. *Current Surgical Diagnosis & Treatment*, 12th ed. New York: McGraw-Hill, 2006: 349.)

Allergy

PRESENTATION

The term *allergy* is typically used to refer to type I hypersensitivity, mediated by IgE cross-linking after exposure to an allergen, leading to mast cell degranulation and histamine-mediated vascular permeability. Allergies manifest in a myriad of ways, but many of the symptoms affect the respiratory system, in particular, allergic rhinitis ("hay fever" —congestion, sneezing, itching), extrinsic **asthma,** and **anaphylaxis.** Anaphylaxis is the most severe allergy syndrome, characterized by multiorgan involvement including urticaria, edema, airway obstruction, low blood pressure, GI symptoms, and anxiety. Any airway obstruction must be addressed immediately, as with the related *status asthmaticus,* usually through administration of epinephrine.

DIAGNOSIS

The symptoms of allergies are classic and generally sufficient to establish a diagnosis. However, specific testing for allergen sensitivities may be instructive in certain cases; this is accomplished through either a **radioallergosorbent test (RAST)** of the blood for ingestion/inhalation allergies or a skin test for contact allergies.

TREATMENT

In many cases, the main "treatment" of allergies is allergen avoidance, especially in the case of hypersensitivities to foods, animals, or materials. If this is not possible, several drug classes may be employed:

- **First-generation antihistamines** (diphenhydramine, chlorpheniramine, dimenhydrinate): Reversible inverse agonists at H_1 histamine receptors, thereby reversing the vascular permeability caused by mast cell degranulation. These drugs are used to relieve acute allergy symptoms such as rhinitis and urticaria. However, because they can cross the blood-brain barrier, they also induce somnolence; indeed, diphenhydramine is also indicated as a sleep aid. Other side-effects include low blood pressure, a "paradoxical reaction" (hyperactivity, palpitations, increased heart rate), anticholinergic effects (mAChR inhibition), and anti-β-adrenergic effects.

- **Second-generation antihistamines** (loratadine, fexofenadine, cetirizine, desloratadine): Similar mechanism of action as the first-generation drugs, but these do not cross the blood-brain barrier and therefore do not cause drowsiness, making them suitable for everyday use. Side-effects include headache, fatigue, dry mouth, thirst, dry nose, nervousness, rapid heartbeat, diarrhea.
- **Nasal decongestants** (pseudoephedrine, phenylephrine): Sometimes combined with second-generation antihistamines, these drugs act to reduce congestion and edema by increasing α_1-**adrenergic** signaling. Pseudoephedrine acts by stimulating release of norepinephrine and thus may cause side effects of agitation, palpitations, tachycardia. Phenylephrine is a direct α_1-agonist and may cause hypertension. Notably, phenylephrine as a nasal spray is effective but may lead to rebound congestion on discontinuation. Evidence is equivocal at best for its utility as a systemic drug.
- **Epinephrine:** In cases of anaphylactic shock, epinephrine should be administered intramuscularly immediately. Specialized injectors for this purpose should be carried by persons with a known anaphylactic reaction.

FLASH BACK

H_2 receptor blockers are used to prevent acid secretion in the stomach (see Chapter 3).

Another method occasionally employed to treat allergies is **immunotherapy,** in which successively escalating doses of allergen are injected with the goal of inducing tolerance. This is particularly useful for unpredictable and difficult-to-avoid allergens such as bee venom.

PROGNOSIS

Most cases of allergy are primarily a lifelong nuisance with seasonal or environmental variation. However, a severe allergic reaction may result in anaphylaxis, which has a poor prognosis unless immediately managed.

Hypersensitivity Pneumonitis

PRESENTATION

Results from inhalation of biological or chemical dust such as aerosolized mold or droppings, leading to a lymphocyte-mediated inflammatory response in the alveoli. Distinguished from asthma in that this is an alveolar disease rather than one of bronchi; additionally, unlike asthma and allergy, this is not type I hypersensitivity. Symptoms of acute disease include chest tightness, cough, wheezing, fever, and dyspnea, resolving hours after discontinuation of exposure. Symptoms of chronic disease include dyspnea, fatigue, cough, and weight loss.

DIAGNOSIS

- Probable diagnosis made with positive history of exposure, consistent CT scan (reticular, nodular, or ground glass opacities), bronchoalveolar lavage showing increased lymphocytes.
- Definitive diagnosis can be made with lung biopsy (findings include loosely organized granulomas) in conjunction with a consistent history.
- Differential diagnosis includes pneumoconiosis, IPF, COPD, and asthma.

TREATMENT

Avoid further exposure to offending dusts. Glucocorticoids may help resolve symptoms.

PROGNOSIS

Usually complete or near complete recovery of lung function following cessation of antigen exposure.

INDEX

About the Senior Editors

Tao Le, MD, MHS

Tao has been active in medical education for the past 19 years. As senior editor, he has led the expansion of *First Aid* into a global educational series. In addition, he is the founder of the *USMLERx* online test bank series as well as a cofounder of the *Underground Clinical Vignettes* series. As a medical student, he was editor-in-chief of the University of California, San Francisco, *Synapse*, a university newspaper with a weekly circulation of 9000. Tao earned his medical degree from the University of California, San Francisco, in 1996 and completed his residency training in internal medicine at Yale University and allergy and immunology fellowship training at Johns Hopkins University. At Yale, he was a regular guest lecturer on the USMLE review courses and an adviser to the Yale University School of Medicine curriculum committee. Tao subsequently went on to cofound Medsn and served as its chief medical officer. He is currently section chief of adult allergy and immunology at the University of Louisville.

Kendall Krause, MD

Kendall is currently a resident in preventive medicine/public health at the University of Colorado. This is Kendall's third tour of duty with *First Aid*—she cut her teeth as a junior editor for *First Aid Cases for the USMLE Step 1* and senior editor on the first edition of the *First Aid for the Basic Sciences*. Kendall attended the Yale School of Medicine before completing her internship in emergency medicine at Massachusetts General and Brigham and Women's Hospitals. Kendall has acted as an articles editor for the *Yale Journal of Health Policy, Law, and Ethics*, and a contributor for the ABC News Medical Unit. Her current work is focused on health equity, evidence-based practice, and health care delivery and systems in resource limited settings.

About the Editors

Elizabeth Eby Halvorson, MD

Elizabeth is currently a resident in pediatrics at Wake Forest Baptist Medical Center. She has completed two previous projects with First Aid while a medical student at Vanderbilt University School of Medicine, the first as junior editor of *First Aid for the Basic Sciences* and the second as senior editor of *First Aid Cases for the USMLE Step 2CK*. Elizabeth will complete a chief resident year at Wake Forest and then is planning to pursue a career as an academic pediatric hospitalist. Her research interests include infectious diseases and vaccines, pediatric obesity, and medical education. Outside of work, Elizabeth enjoys running, yoga, and spending time with her husband and two dogs.

William L. Hwang, MSc

William is currently an MD-PhD student and Soros Fellow in the Harvard-MIT Health Sciences and Technology and Biophysics programs. He earned an MSc in Chemistry at the University of Oxford on a Rhodes Scholarship. William's research interests include single-molecule biophysics, microfluidics, and imaging-based diagnostics. His scientific work has been featured in *Scientific American* and recognized by the *Lab on a Chip* Journal Prize, the Washington Academy of Science Outstanding Achievement in Research Award, and the Howard G. Clark Biomedical Engineering Research Award. William studied at Duke University on an Angier B. Duke full merit scholarship and graduated first in his class with degrees in biomedical engineering, physics, and electrical and computer engineering. He was named by *USA Today* to the 2006 All-USA College Academic First Team. In 2003, he founded United InnoWorks Academy (www.innoworks.org), a 501(c)(3) non-profit organization, to provide innovative science, engineering, and medicine programs for disadvantaged children at no cost. Serving as executive director for the past 8 years, William has led more than 600 volunteers at a dozen university-based chapters to mentor more than 1500 underprivileged grade-school students.

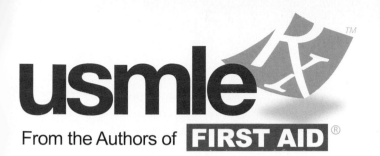

usmle Rx ™

From the Authors of **FIRST AID** ®

▷ **3000+** top rated Step 1 questions with detailed explanations

▷ Integrated with First Aid for the USMLE Step 1

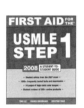

▷ Predictive of actual USMLE performance

▷ Pass guarantee – pass or we double your subscription*

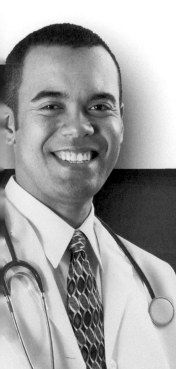

Students are raving

● *"I own Kaplan Qbank... but I heard so many good things about USMLERx that I just bought this and I love it! The explanations you provide are **awesome compared to Kaplan Qbank.**"*

● *"I used USMLERx and thought it was incredible... **I scored 99 on the exam.**"*

● *"Wow... USMLERx is badass... USMLERx was challenging... this is more representative of **what the real test is like.**"*

flash facts

● *World's largest online flash card deck for the USMLE Step 1!*

● ***10,000+** flash cards integrated with **First Aid for the USMLE Step 1**.*

● *Searchable by organ system, discipline, and topic.*

● *Discuss, annotate and mark your favorite First Aid topics.*

● *First Aid topics integrated with corrections and bonus content.*

www.**usmlerx**.com
Your Prescription for USMLE Success

*Subject to restrictions. See website for details.